The SAGE
Handbook *of*
Mental health
and Illness

The field of mental health is now an ideological and terminological battle ground. The diagnostic categories, and the terms used to refer to the people affected, are all strongly and validly contested. This important book helps policy makers, practitioners and researchers to pick their way across this minefield relatively unscathed, to appreciate in fine grain detail the social context within which mental illnesses unfurl, and how this context shapes (often in profoundly socially excluding ways) the lives of people with mental health problems. As a corrective to biological reductionism, this wise book actively expands our understanding of how social forces permeate all aspects of mental illness.
Professor Graham Thornicroft, Institute of Psychiatry, UK

Pilgrim, Rogers and Pescosolido's volume is a wide-ranging and cross-national examination of many core issues in the sociology of mental health. It presents a variety of perspectives on fundamental substantive and policy issues in mental health and illness. Its scope and range make it ideal for scholars and students in a variety of disciplines concerned with social aspects of psychological distress and disorder.
Professor Allan Horwitz, Rutgers University, USA

This book provides the reader with an updated, in-depth yet comprehensive, overview of key issues in our understanding of mental ill health and mental health. The text illustrates well changes in the way we conceptualise mental ill health and health over the last twenty years, referring us to past and present reasons for these changes, such as a greater emphasis on mental wellbeing, mental health promotion, recovery, and social inclusion. A number of countries, professions and disciplines are represented in the book by both well known authors in this field, and some newcomers to it. Together they have succeeded in offering the reader an impressive range of ideas, knowledge and evidence that challenge some of the cherished notions we have as a culture about mental ill health and mental health.
Professor Shula Ramon, Anglia Ruskin University, UK

The SAGE
Handbook *of*
Mental health
and Illness

Edited by

David Pilgrim,
Anne Rogers
and Bernice Pescosolido

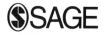

Los Angeles | London | New Delhi
Singapore | Washington DC

First published 2011

SAGE Publications Ltd
1 Oliver's Yard
55 City Road
London EC1Y 1SP

SAGE Publications Inc.
2455 Teller Road
Thousand Oaks, California 91320

SAGE Publications India Pvt Ltd
B 1/I 1 Mohan Cooperative Industrial Area
Mathura Road
New Delhi 110 044

SAGE Publications Asia-Pacific Pte Ltd
33 Pekin Street #02-01
Far East Square
Singapore 048763

Library of Congress Control Number: 2010927890

British Library Cataloguing in Publication data

A catalogue record for this book is available from the British Library

ISBN: 978-1-84787-382-8

Typeset by Glyph International, Bangalore, India
Printed by MPG Books Group, Bodmin, Cornwall
Printed on paper from sustainable resources

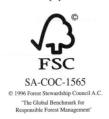

FSC
SA-COC-1565
© 1996 Forest Stewardship Council A.C.
'The Global Benchmark for
Responsible Forest Management'

Contents

Acknowledgement

The editors would like to offer their profound gratitude to Mary Elizabeth Hannah for her extensive support during the production of this Handbook.

List of Editors

David Pilgrim is Professor of Mental Health Policy in the School of Social Work at the University of Central Lancashire and Visiting Professor, University of Liverpool, UK. He has higher degrees in both psychology and sociology and his career has been divided between clinical work in the British National Health Service and research and teaching in academia, with a particular interest in professionalization, service innovations and service users' views. His *A Sociology of Mental Health and Illness* (Open University Press, 2005, with Anne Rogers), was winner of the 2006 British Medical Association's Medical Book of the Year Award. His other books include *Examining Trust in Health Care: A Multi-Disciplinary Perspective* (Palgrave, 2010, with Floris Tomasini and Ivalyo Vassilev), *Key Concepts in Mental Health* (SAGE, 2009), *A Straight Talking Introduction to Psychological Treatment* (PCCS Books, 2009) and *Mental Health and Inequality* (Palgrave, 2003, with Anne Rogers).

Anne Rogers is Professor of Sociology of Health Care at the University of Manchester. Her research interests lie broadly within the sociology of health care, mental health and most recently social networks, relationships and personal long term condition management. Her research has included exploring patients' experience of psychiatric services, the social patterning of mental health problems, lay epidemiology, professional knowledge and sociological analysis of old and new forms of treatment. She has published extensively in peer reviewed journal articles and has been an author or co-author of a number of books. These include *Experiencing Psychiatry: Users' Views of Services* (Macmillan, 1993, with David Pilgrim and Ron Lacey), *Demanding Patients? Analysing Primary Care Use* (Open University, 1998, with Karen Hassell and Gerry Nicolaas) and *Mental Health and Inequality* (Palgrave, 2003, with David Pilgrim). Her *A Sociology of Mental Health and Illness* (Open University Press, 2005, with David Pilgrim) was winner of the 2006 British Medical Association's Medical Book of the Year Award.

Bernice Pescosolido is Distinguished and Chancellor's Professor of Sociology and Director of the Indiana Consortium for Mental Health Services Research at Indiana University, USA. Pescosolido's research and teaching focus on how social networks connect individuals to their communities and institutional structures. Her Network Episode Model, developed in the early 1990s, focuses on how individuals recognize, respond to the onset of health problems and use health care services, providing new insights to understanding patterns and pathways to care, adherence to treatment and outcomes of health care. She initiated the first major national study of stigma of mental illness in the US in over 40 years, and with funding from the Fogarty International Center, led a team of researchers in the first international study of stigma.

List of Contributors

Gillian Bendelow is Professor of Sociology at the University of Sussex, UK, and worked as a community mental health nurse in East London before entering academia. She is an established medical sociologist who has made research contributions to the fields of chronic illness, pain and 'contested' conditions, lay concepts of health and illness and integrated models of mental and emotional health. She is regularly invited as a keynote/plenary speaker to international academic and policy-oriented events and is author of *Health, Emotion and the Body* (Polity, 2009), *Pain and Gender* (Pearson Education, 2000) and co-author of *Emotions in Social Life and The Lived Body* (Routledge,1998) as well as many edited books and journal articles.

Richard Bentall is Professor of Clinical Psychology at the University of Bangor, UK. He is interested in the problem of classification of mental illness and in the relationship between psychopathology and normal variations in human personality. This interest has led him to challenge traditional research strategies in psychopathology, which have focused on broadly defined syndromes such as 'schizophrenia', and to advocate research which focuses on particular classes of abnormal behaviour and experience ('symptoms'). In 1989, he was awarded the May Davidson Award from the British Psychological Society for contributions to the field of clinical psychology. He has edited and authored several books, most notably *Madness Explained* (Penguin, 2003), which was winner of the British Psychological Society Book Award 2004. The ideas in this were developed subsequently in his *Doctoring the Mind* (Allen Lane, 2009).

Michael Bloor is Professor of Sociology at the Universities of Cardiff and Glasgow, UK. His research interests include occupational health and safety, global governance, risk behaviour and health services research. His *Keywords in Qualitative Methods: a Vocabulary of Research Concepts* was published in 2006 (SAGE, with F. Wood).

Peter Campbell is a British mental health system survivor. He has been receiving services consistently for more than forty years and has been involved in action towards positive change since the mid-1980s. He works as a freelance teacher in the mental health field and has an Honorary Doctorate in Education at Anglia Ruskin University. He was a founder member of Survivors Speak Out

(1986) and Survivors' Poetry (1991). He is particularly interested in mental health nursing and in mental health legislation. Peter has provided chapters for a variety of mental health textbooks and contributes regularly to *OpenMind* and other magazines. He is co-editor (with Phil Barker and Ben Davidson) of *From the Ashes of Experience* (Whurr Publishers, 1999).

Carolyn Chew-Graham is Professor of Primary Care at the University of Manchester, UK and also works as a general practitioner in the city. She is a qualitative researcher and has published on general practitioners' attitudes to their work, particularly in the care of patients with distress, chronic illness and multiple symptoms, and care across the primary/secondary interface. Her externally funded work consists of developing and testing new interventions for patients with mental health problems in primary care. Carolyn has a particular interest in the mental health of older people. She is Royal College of General Practitioners' Clinical Champion, Mental Health, and co-Chair of the Forum for Primary Care Mental Health, a partnership between the RCGP and Royal College of Psychiatrists, aiming to influence policy, develop educational materials for GPs and improve care of people with mental health problems.

Angus Clarke is Professor and Consultant in Clinical Genetics in Cardiff University, UK. He studied medical sciences and genetics at Cambridge and qualified in medicine from Oxford University. After registration, he worked in general medicine and then paediatrics. He studied the clinical and molecular genetics of ectodermal dysplasia in Cardiff and then worked in clinical genetics and paediatric neurology in Newcastle upon Tyne, developing an interest in Rett syndrome and neuromuscular disorders. He returned to Cardiff in 1989 and has maintained these interests and developed further interests in genetic screening, the genetic counselling process and the social and ethical issues around human genetics. He represents the Chief Medical Officer for Wales on the UK Human Genetics Commission. He has (co)authored and edited six books, including *Genetics, Society and Clinical Practice* (Bios Scientific Publishers, 1997) and *Living with the Genome* (Palgrave, 2006). He established and directs the Cardiff MSc course in Genetic Counselling.

Jonathan Gabe is Professor of Sociology at Royal Holloway, University of London, UK. He has research interests in medical controversies, social relations of health care and patients' experience of chronic illness. Amongst his most reccent books are *The New Sociology of the Health Service* (Routledge, 2009, edited with Michael Calnan), *Pharmaceuticals and Society* (Wiley Blackwell, 2009, edited with Simon Williams and Peter Davis) and *Challenging Medicine* (Routledge, 2006, edited with Davide Kelleher and Gareth Williams). He is currently an editor of the international journal *Sociology of Health and Illness*.

Helen Herman is Professor of Psychiatry at the University of Melbourne and Director of the World Health Organization (WHO) Collaborating Centre for

Mental Health in Melbourne, Australia. She is a psychiatrist and public health practitioner with a particular interest in promoting mental health through population-based public health interventions as well as better health services for people living with mental illnesses. Her recent books include *Promoting Mental Health: Concepts, Evidence and Practice* (WHO, 2005, with Saxena and Moodie), *Depressive Disorders, Third Edition* (World Psychiatric Association (WPA) – Series Evidence and Experience in Psychiatry, Wiley-Blackwell, 2009 with Maj and Sartorius), *Contemporary Topics in Women's Mental Health* (WPA Series, Wiley-Blackwell, 2009 with first editor Chandra, Kastrup, Niaz, Rondon and Okasha), *Parenthood and Mental Health* (WPA Series, Wiley-Blackwell, 2010 with first editor Tyano, Keren and Cox) and *Substance Abuse* (WPA Series Evidence and Experience in Psychiatry, Wiley-Blackwell, 2010 with first editor Ghodse, Maj and Sartorius).

Karen Iley is Lecturer in Nursing in the School of Nursing Midwifery and Social Work at the University of Manchester, UK. She is a registered nurse having worked as a nurse manager in the British National Health Service before moving into an academic career. Her post-graduate degree is in the Sociology of Health and Healthcare. Her research interests include ethnic inequalities in mental healthcare, the organization and delivery of healthcare services and how patients access and use health care services.

Renata Kokanovic is Monash Fellow at the School of Political and Social Inquiry at the Monash University, Melbourne and Honorary Senior Research Fellow at the Department of General Practice at University of Melbourne, Australia. Her research is in the sociology of health and illness, focusing on medicalization of everyday life and cultural research on experiences of emotional distress. She has her work published in a number of academic journals, including *Sociology of Health and Illness Social Sciences Medicine and Qualitative Health Research.*

Ann McCranie is a PhD candidate in Sociology at Indiana University, Bloomington, USA. Her dissertation examines the scientific/intellectual movement of recovery, mental health services research and the impact that 'recovery-oriented' academic researchers in the United States have had on federal and state mental health policy. She is currently involved in a long-term NIMH-funded qualitative evaluation of a clinical and academic collaboration in community mental health. Her other research spans medical sociology, organizational research and social networks, but is focused on the treatment and lives of people with severe mental health problems.

Nick Manning is Professor of Social Policy and Sociology, and Director of the Institute of Mental Health at University of Nottingham/Nottinghamshire Healthcare NHS Trust, UK. He has higher degrees in sociology and social policy. His research interests are in the application of sociology to the field of mental health, social change in Eastern Europe and social theory. His recent books include *Health and Healthcare in the New Russia* (Ashgate, 2009), *Global Social Policy*, (SAGE, 2008), *Social Policy* (Oxford University Press, 2007), *International Encyclopaedia of Social Policy*, 3 volumes (Routledge, 2006), *A Culture of Enquiry: Research Evidence and the Therapeutic Community* (Jessica Kingsley, 2004) (translated into Italian in 2007), and *Poverty and Social Exclusion in the New Russia* (Ashgate, 2004).

Alison Munro is currently a Research Fellow in the Institute for Applied Social and Health Research at the University of the West of Scotland. She has a PhD in the area of attitudes of nurses and social workers to working with alcohol users and alcohol problems, and has a wide range of experience in alcohol, drugs and co-morbidity research.

James Nazroo is Professor of Sociology and Director of the Cathy Marsh Centre for Census and Survey Research, University of Manchester, UK. Much of his research has focussed on ethnic inequalities in health, with a concern to go beyond describing differences in health to assessing the contribution that social disadvantage might make to observed differences. Central to this has been developing an understanding of the links between ethnicity, racism, class and inequality. His research in this field has covered a variety of elements of social disadvantage, including socioeconomic position, racial discrimination and harassment, and ecological effects. It also covers a variety of health outcomes, including general health, mental health, cardiovascular disease and sexual health. He has taken an increasing focus on comparative analysis (across groups, time and place) to investigate underlying processes, research that has involved collaborations with colleagues in the US, Canada, Europe and New Zealand – as well as the UK.

Sigrun Olafsdottir is Assistant Professor of Sociology at Boston University, USA. She received her PhD from Indiana University in 2007. Her research focuses on medical sociology, sociology of mental health, political sociology and cultural sociology. Her dissertation, *Medicalizing Mental Health: A Comparative View of the Public, Private, and Professional Construction of Illness*, was selected the Best Dissertation in Mental Health by the Mental Health Section of the American Sociological Association and was awarded the Esther L. Kinsley PhD Dissertation Award for the Most Outstanding Dissertation by Indiana University. Her research articles have appeared in *The Journal of Health and Social Behavior, Social Science and Medicine, Sociological Perspectives, Sociological Forum* and *the Journal of the American Academy of Child and Adolescent Psychiatry*.

Brea Perry is Assistant Professor of Sociology and Faculty Associate in the Center for the Study of Violence Against Children at the University of Kentucky, USA. Her research focuses on the interrelated roles of social networks and interaction, social structure, culture and biological systems in disease etiology and the illness career. She has published research on dynamic social network processes, stigma and its consequences, youth in foster care, mental illness in children and adults, and gene–environment interactions in disease pathways. In 2009, she was honoured with two awards from the American Sociological Association for her dissertation. In addition, she is the recipient of the 2009 Eliot Freidson Outstanding Publication Award from the American Sociological Association Medical Sociology Section for 'Under the Influence of Genetics: How Transdisciplinarity Leads Us to Rethink Social Pathways to Illness' (*American Journal of Sociology*, 2008, with Bernice Pescosolido, J. Scott Long, Jack Martin, John Nurnberger and Victor Hesselbrock).

Benedikt Rogge is Research Associate in the Institute of Empirical and Applied Sociology at the University of Bremen, Germany. He has higher degrees in both psychology (University of Tuebingen) and sociology (University of Essex). He is particularly interested in the relationships between social inequalities and life events on the one hand and people's mental health and stress on the other. He is currently completing his PhD on a longitudinal interview study on how unemployment alters people's identity process and well-being. His forthcoming publications in English include 'Time structure or meaningfulness? Critically reviewing research on mental health and everyday life in unemployment' (in T. Kieselbach, T. and S. Mannila (eds), *Persistent Unemployment and Precarious Work: Research and Policy Issues*. Wiesbaden: VS) and 'Unemployment and its association with health-relevant actions: investigating the role of time perspective with German census data' (*International Journal of Public Health*, with Reinhard Schunck).

Diana Rose is an Academic Social Scientist and had a brief career from 1972 to 1984 in mainstream academia but lost that position because of her mental illness diagnosis. In 1996, she resumed an academic career, first in an NGO and then at the Institute of Psychiatry, King's College London where she is now Senior Lecturer in User-Led Research. Prior to this, she first became involved in the UK mental health services user movement in 1986 when she saw an advertisement for her local user group in a well-known London magazine. The meeting turned her view of services on its head – from a self-understanding of being manipulative and attention-seeking (the message from services) she came to understand that her human rights were being violated.

Susan Roxburgh is Associate Professor of Sociology at Kent State University, USA. She has published on topics such as gender differences in the work and well-being, relationship, race/gender differences in mental health, and parenthood and well-being have appeared in a number of journals including *Journal of Health and Social Behavior*, *Journal of Family and Economic Issues*, *Journal of Family Issues*, *Addictive Behaviors* and *Sociological Forum*. Her research on time pressure and health has been funded by the National Institutes of Health.

She has been a two-term member of the *Journal of Health and Social Behavior* editorial board and served on the American Sociological Association's distinguished book award committee between 2008 and 2010. Her current research projects include the relationship between childhood adversity and adult depression among the incarcerated and variations in the marriage–mental health relationship by race/ethnicity and gender.

Graham Scambler is Professor of Medical Sociology in the Research of Infection and Population Health, at University College London, UK. He is a member of the standing committee of the International Consortium for Research and Action Against Health-Related Stigma. His current research interests include comparative study of stigma as a barrier to health interventions with sex workers; sexual trafficking; the impact of biological, psychological and social mechanisms on epilepsy-related quality of life; class and health inequality; the differential prestige attaching to medical diagnoses; and patient education and empowerment. His books include *Coping with Chronic Illness and Disease* (London: Routledge) and *Sociology as Applied to Medicine* (London: Saunders).

Scott Schieman is Professor of Sociology at the University of Toronto, Canada. He is also the editor of *Sociology of Religion* and deputy editor at *Society and Mental Health*. His research interests focus on the personal and social conditions that influence stress processes and health. Recent projects deal with substantive areas in religion, work and the work–family interface. He recently received a grant award from the *Canadian Institutes of Health Research* to conduct a national survey of work, family, stress and well-being in Canada. He is also writing a book that investigates beliefs about God's involvement and causal influence in everyday life.

Mark Schmitz is Associate Professor in the School of Social Work in the College of Health Professions and Social Work at Temple University, USA. He has a PhD in sociology and primarily teaches research methods and statistics. His research interest has emphasized the evaluation of methods for diagnosing mental disorder, primarily through examining the validity of the diagnostic criteria for major depressive disorder used in the DSM. Studies of the bereavement exclusion for MDD and the clinical significance criterion have been recently published. His further work includes the examination of episode duration as a diagnostic criterion for MDD and a comparison of DSM-III-R and DSM-IV criteria for distinguishing depressive disorder from normal sadness episodes.

Andrew Scull is Distinguished Professor of Sociology and Science Studies at the University of California, San Diego, USA. Educated at Balliol College, Oxford and at Princeton, he has held faculty positions at the University of Pennsylvania, Princeton and UCSD. He has written extensively on the history of psychiatry in Britain and North America. His books include *Decarceration* (1977,

1984), *Museums of Madness* (1979), *Social Order/Mental Disorder* (1989), *The Asylum as Utopia* (1991), *The Most Solitary of Afflictions* (1993), *Masters of Bedlam* (1996), *Undertaker of the Mind* (2001), *Customers and Patrons of the Mad Trade* (2003), *Madhouse* (2005), *The Insanity of Place/The Place of Insanity* (2007) and *Hysteria* (2009). He has held fellowships from the American Council of Learned Societies and the Guggenheim Foundation, and is a past president of the Society for the Social History of Medicine.

Jenny Secker is Professor of Mental Health at Anglia Ruskin University, UK and the South Essex Partnership University NHS Foundation Trust, UK. She trained in Edinburgh, first as a mental health nurse and later as a social worker. After completing her PhD in the Department of Social Work and Social Policy at Edinburgh University, she worked as a researcher in a number of academic and practice organizations. Her main research interests are in the area of mental health and social inclusion. Her study of arts participation, *Mental Health, Social Inclusion and Arts: Developing the Evidence Base*, was awarded the Royal Society of Public Health 2009 Arts and Health Award for Arts and Mental Health Research. She has also published widely on employment and mental health, including *New Thinking about Mental Health and Employment* (Radcliffe, 2005, with Bob Grove and Patience Seebohm).

Philip Thomas is British psychiatrist and currently an Honorary Visiting Professor in the University of Bradford, UK and a Non Executive Director of Mersey Care NHS Trust. His interests include philosophy (post-structuralism and critical theory) and their application to psychiatry, psychology and medicine. He served as a Professor of Philosophy, Diversity and Mental Health in the University of Central Lancashire until May 2009, and is a founder member and co-chair of the Critical Psychiatry Network. He has published over 100 scholarly papers mostly in peer reviewed journals, and authored or co-authored three books including *The Dialectics of Schizophrenia* (Free Associations Books, 1997) and *Postpsychiatry: Mental Health in a Postmodern World* (with Pat Bracken, 2005, Oxford University Press, 2005).

Jane Ussher is Professor of Women's Health Psychology, and leader of the Gender Culture and Health Research Unit: PsyHealth, at the University of Western Sydney, Australia. She has published widely on the subject of the material-discursive construction and experience of health, in particular associated with women's mental health, the reproductive body and sexuality. She is editor of the Routledge *Women and Psychology* book series. She is author of a number of books, including *The Psychology of the Female Body* (Routledge, 1989), *Women's Madness: Misogyny or Mental Illness?* (Harvester Wheatsheaf, 1991), *Fantasies of Femininity: Reframing the Boundaries of Sex* (Penguin, 1997), *Managing the Monstrous Feminine: Regulating the Reproductive Body* (Routledge, 2006) and *The Madness of Women: Myths and Experience* (Routledge 2011).

Her current research focuses on sexual and reproductive health, with particular emphasis on premenstrual experiences, sexuality and cancer, and gendered issues in caring.

Jerome Wakefield is University Professor, Professor of Social Work and Professor of Psychiatry and Affiliate Faculty in Bioethics, in the Center for Ancient Studies, and in InSPIRES (Institute for Social and Psychiatric Initiatives – Research, Education and Services), at New York University, USA. He holds two doctorates, in Social Work and Philosophy, both from University of California at Berkeley, and has previously held faculty positions at University of Chicago, Columbia University, and Rutgers University. He writes primarily on the conceptual foundations of the mental health professions, especially the concept of mental disorder and the validity of psychiatric diagnostic criteria in distinguishing disorder from normal forms of suffering, with over 170 scholarly and public-intellectual publications. He is co-author with Allan Horwitz of *The Loss of Sadness: How Psychiatry Transformed Normal Sorrow into Depressive Disorder* (Oxford, 2007), named the best psychology book of 2007 by the Association of Professional and Scholarly Publishers.

Preface

We are grateful to all the contributors of this Handbook and hope that its readers find the chapters useful, informative and stimulating. Although not an exhaustive list of topics are covered (our field of interest is very broad and virtually unending), enough are available in the following pages to mirror much of the way in which mental health and mental disorder are currently explored in the Anglophone academy by and for social science. The book could be considered in its entirety as a fair sample of the work being done in the field indicated by its title or it could be used as a reference book by students of mental health and mental disorder with a particular interest.

Our choice of topics has been broadly divided into one section on mental health in its social context and another in which clinical and mental health policy matters are addressed more pointedly. This division is somewhat arbitrary and the allocation of a chapter in this or the other part of the book might be open to fair challenge. However, the partition is offered as a way of signalling the distinction between the general and the particular even if the two need to, or can, always be considered fruitfully in relation to one another. The two parts are merely the first of a few signposts for the reader picking up the book for the first time, which could have seemed a large picture to comprehend, if we had merely listed one chapter after another.

Each of the two parts will contain their own introduction to note the key points of each chapter and at times to offer our own commentary on points of contact or contrast between the contributions. As editors, we have made no demands on any of the contributors to write in this or that way about the topic they address. Our role has merely been one of feedback and trimming rather than academic guidance, as they are all experienced specialists in their field. In other words, when commissioning the chapters at the outset, our concern was to have a series of topics represented in the book and we turned to those we trusted to write well about the one allocated to them. We hope that the reader is rewarded by our policy of trust in the writers. Finally, we have taken the editors' privilege of supplying our own contributions at points in the book (with some help from friendly colleagues) and so that policy of trust also extends to ourselves.

DAVID PILGRIM
ANNE ROGERS
BERNICE PESCOSOLIDO

Mental Health and Mental Disorder in Social Context

Editors' Introduction

The first chapter is written by a medical geneticist, Angus Clarke. As will be clearer in later chapters (see Thomas and Bentall in Section 2) bio-reductionism remains a recurring point of contention and grievance for social scientists studying mental health. It is useful then to begin with this topic but written by a professional biologist with a critical eye about, and commitment to, 'the social'. Clarke explains in some detail how geneticists think about behaviour, dismissing at the outset strong claims from either side of the 'nature – nurture' debate. He provides a useful and informed discussion for readers with no background in genetics about how that broad field considers mental disorders. Not only does this field entail empirical complexity, it also implies some pre-empirical questions about conceptual coherence in relation to distinctions between the normal and the abnormal.

In line with these more fundamental pre-empirical questions, if the empirical link between genetics and behaviour in its social context is complicated it is not a simple matter either to 'measure' mental disorder as the next chapter indicates. Jerome Wakefield and Mark Schmitz address this vexed question, in particular relation to community samples, which contain people who have had no professional contact and do not (necessarily) view themselves as being mentally disordered. The problems of both reliability and construct validity for psychiatric epidemiology also remain for social scientists, especially those reliant on nosological systems, such as DSM (from the American Psychiatric Association) or ICD (from the World Health Organization). Funding agencies like the NIMH in turn demand their use (whatever doubts might be harboured by individual researchers). The detailed methodological challenges addressed in this chapter are particularly pertinent to consider in the light of the DSM now going into a fifth edition, due to appear in May 2013 (http://www.dsm5.org/pages/default.aspx). This further revision is being constructed at a time when hard and fast distinctions between particular disorders and between many disorders and normality are often still not easy to make.

In the next chapter, Benedikt Rogge offers a contribution from Germany (a special thanks to him, from us, for rising to the challenge, so admirably, of writing in a second language). He addresses the recent pre-occupation within social science and social policy about wellbeing and positive psychology and begins where the last chapter left off: mental health is a fuzzy concept. After the problems of defining mental health and mental disorder are addressed, Rogge then summarizes the shift towards 'positive psychology' and places it within a wider sociological context of debate about 'the self'. This draws our attention to the disciplinary separation (as well as potential common interest) between psychiatry, psychology and sociology. Positive psychology and the sociology of the self may now be complementary exercises to place alongside the clinical focus on defects, pathology and distress found in psychiatry and clinical psychology.

This prospect is also picked up in the next chapter by Gillian Bendelow, who begins as a sociologist with a focus on emotional health as a discourse to be considered separately from the concerns of clinical professionals. In particular she wants to start a discussion about mental health and the emotions with a reconsideration of the traditional psycho-somatic split, the legacy of Cartesian dualism. Her attention to medicalization and the limits of a focus on biomedical antecedents links to later chapters (particularly from Olafsdottir in this section and Thomas and Bentall in the next). However, Bendelow also cautions against the risks of new emphases on holism, which create the spectre of 'healthism' and invite new forms of surveillance and social control.

The next chapter returns us to social epidemiology, with a particular focus on ethnicity and race from a British viewpoint. James Nazroo and Karen Iley emphasize the role of social and economic inequalities in the production of both ethnic/racial differences in risk of severe mental illness. Those inequalities also construct the experience of ethnic/racial minorities, when their members experience mental health problems and have services contact. However, this chapter appears in this part of the book rather than the next because the process of service contact mirrors wider social processes about race and inequality. This and other chapters (see Chew-Graham, Hermann and Secker in the next section of the book) are a window into the established class gradient in mental health, which we simply take for granted now as social scientists (see our preface). The authors go on to examine methodological criticisms of studies in the field to date and round off their chapter with a consideration of the experience that ethnic/racial minorities have of their problems, which connect the experience of service contact with the shared wider racialised context which both patients and services are embedded in.

If race is one important dimension to the experience of mental health problems, so too is gender. This topic is discussed by Jane Ussher with a focus on the experience of depression. She looks at the extensive empirical evidence on gender differences in the diagnosed incidence of depression and prevalence but then goes on to explore competing explanations. The latter include hormonal, as well as psychological and sociological accounts, especially in relation to material and role inequalities. She also introduces other variables, which are important but contested; domestic violence and lesbian relationships (discussed as well later, in the chapter by Pilgrim and Rogers). Gender inequality is thus posited as an important source of mediation between social stressors and personal distress. Ussher also summarizes some evidence on cultural differences, which is extended in the next contribution, also written from Australia.

Renata Kokanovic discusses depression, but this time in relation to the cross-cultural challenges of formulating the meaning of experienced and expressed distress. Her examination of depression raises some important conceptual points suggested in earlier chapters; Ussher's just noted, but also those from Bendelow, Rogge and most fundamentally from Wakefield and Schmitz. Can we readily distinguish depression from normality and is misery experienced and expressed in the same way in all cultural contexts? Given that the World Health Organization has been concerned about a 'pandemic' of depression, the other question implied is 'a pandemic of what?' Kokanovic's exploration allows us to reflect on these questions and like Ussher raises some challenges for social scientists about the tensions between realist and constructivist accounts of common distress.

Questions of stress and experienced distress are then considered more extensively by Susan Roxburgh, who focuses on the stress process model. This consists of three primary elements: stressors, intervening explanatory variables and stress outcomes. Each of these elements is considered in turn by the author. The intervening variables include resources, such as social support, which are picked up for more consideration at the end of the book in the chapters by Secker and Pescosolido. Finally Roxburgh looks at the outcomes of stress, especially depression (sadness, demoralization and alienation) and anxiety (feelings of tension, restlessness and irritability). These are the main, often mixed, manifestations of 'common mental disorders' treated in primary care (see Chew-Graham in Section 2).

In the subsequent chapter by Scott Schieman, the stress process model is also used as a framework for understanding the relationship between faith and mental health. Despite a common assumption about secularization, belief in God as a causal agent remains important for many people (even if they have no agreed named religion or attend religious rituals regularly). For this reason, Schieman argues that it is important for students of mental health in society to look carefully at the interaction of faith, stressors and personal resources. This reminds us of the importance of 'intervening explanatory variables' in Roxburgh's earlier account. It is also an opportunity to rehearse competing arguments about whether religion is pathogenic or helpful in the lives of ordinary people.

In the next chapter, Brea Perry joins one of us (Pescosolido) to consider the emergence of stigma about mental disorder, especially in relation to that identified in early life. On the one hand, prevalence rates of recorded mental disorder are at their highest in the very young (and the very old), on the other we know little about public attitudes towards childhood problems. This chapter provides an empirical account from the USA of how the general public comprehends health conditions in childhood (ADHD, depression and asthma). This makes a start at producing an evidence base about ordinary understandings of childhood problems that might be the basis for public education and other policies.

Stigma is addressed in a more general way by Graham Scambler in the next chapter, which starts with Goffman and Wittgenstein as early authoritative discussants about the separation of normal from non-normal conduct in society. Stigma has to be considered in the same sociological breath as norms: it cannot be understood as a free-standing topic. Scambler places specific consideration about mental illness within a wider context of the sociology of stigma and in relation to labelling theory, biographical disruption and narratives of personal tragedy. He extends this to challenges from disability theory, moving on to a discussion about the possibility of stigma reduction programmes. Once more, this discussion brings in some ontological and epistemological aspects of social science, in relation to the tension between materialist and constructivist accounts.

If stigma is one outcome of norm transgression, then the re-framing of the latter, from sin and crime to illness, is the starting point of Sigrun Olafsdottir's exploration of medicalization, with attention being paid to the interests of the medical profession, the drug companies and managed healthcare. As she notes, this confluence of interests is at its most obvious in the USA and hence the stronger interest in the medicalization thesis there than in other parts of the world. The author provides a critique of this US-bias in theorizing medicalization and introduces a comparative approach as a corrective. This does not undermine the basic model of medicalization but it does imply a needed sensitivity to cross-national/cultural differences.

In the final chapter in this section of the book, two of us (Pilgrim and Rogers) start with a criticism of the taken-for-granted cultural assumption about mental disorder as the source of danger. We argue that a more valid account should understand it as a two way street. Danger is also a common source of mental disorder – in the home, on the streets, in the workplace and most dramatically in war zones. (The chapter by Roxburgh on stress is pertinent here, as is the part of Ussher's chapter that has already considered domestic violence.) The notion of danger is discussed in relation to both violence and risk and this permits us to note the tension, which exists in debates about mental health policy in relation to social control (serving the state and third party interests) and beneficent paternalism (the use of legal powers to ensure treatment of mental disorder). This policy emphasis starts to explore topics to appear in Section 2, especially in the chapters from Scull and Rose and Campbell.

1

The Limits to Psychiatric and Behavioural Genetics

Angus Clarke

INTRODUCTION

My starting assumption is that genes are 'involved in' behaviour; consequently, genetic variation contributes to variation in behaviour. To deny that would be not merely unreasonable but incoherent, although there is still some appetite for the old nature – nurture pseudo-controversy. The too-crude dismissal of the importance of genetic factors can still appeal to those who enjoy attacking the strawman genetic determinist, who is thought to argue for the 'primacy' of genetics over the environment (Sonuga-Barke, 2010). If there is any sense in talk of the 'primacy of genetics', it is that an individual's set of genes is given and fixed from conception and is from then on available for interaction with the (changing) environment. What does not make sense is to think of either an individual's genes or their environment as being the principal determinant of future behaviours in isolation from their environment or their genes (respectively).

A full repertoire of genes is required for all behaviour (whether the latter is designated as normal or abnormal). All but a few of the smallest chromosomal deletions, that result in some genes being present in one copy per cell instead of the usual two, are associated with cognitive impairment and therefore with difficulties for the individual in organizing their behaviour. Even chromosomal duplications – resulting in three copies of the relevant genes – usually affect cognition and behaviour as well as other aspects of growth and development.

Such chromosomal anomalies become interesting – and challenge our understanding – when we find that a particular deletion or duplication is associated not merely with a diffuse cognitive impairment but with some more specific and unusual behaviours. The idea that a disruption to the set of chromosomes leads to a 'spanner in the works' and thereby a disruption to thought and communication can be accommodated within a very primitive model of 'genes acting within the brain'; but how would a specific chromosomal anomaly lead to a specific behavioural anomaly?

The types of evidence we can draw upon to assess the effects of genetic variation on psychiatric disease and behaviour more generally include observations of people with disturbances of cognitive development and behaviour (including mental illness), where there is a good reason to accept a chromosomal or genetic basis for the disturbance. We might also observe the familial clustering of diagnosed mental illness or cognitive impairment, sometimes presented in terms of 'heritability'. In addition, we might have an apparent association of genetic variants from across the genome with diagnosed mental illness or a variation in behavioural traits.

In this chapter, I examine the types of evidence and argument that have been used to relate genetic factors to behaviour, primarily that deemed to be abnormal. We consider what types of conclusion such evidence is able, in principle, to support in the light of a realistic model of gene-environment interaction.

EVOLUTION AND ETHOLOGY

One context in which genes are related to behaviour is in discussions of our evolutionary past. It is clear that the behavioural patterns enabled by our genes have been compatible with our survival as a species. This has always entailed both cooperation and competition with our fellow humans; it is with whom one cooperates, with whom one competes that is important. Observations of primate behaviour can give insight into our remote past because our ancestors resembled contemporary primates (Cheney and Seyfarth, 2007). However, while such accounts may tell us something about the evolutionary success of different behavioural strategies, they do not allow us to draw inferences about how specific genes are related to particular behaviours. The genetic constitution of a species will impose constraints on the repertoire of behaviours available to an individual of that species but this gives us no access to understanding the way in which the genetic variation between individuals leads them to behave differently.

Armchair evolutionary reflection leads us to consider how the behaviour of an individual will let him or her contribute maximally to the next generation of the species. Such an approach focuses on competition within a species and forces us to acknowledge the importance of *sexual* selection, as well as the narrower type of natural selection for mere survival. While we must combat parasites and infectious diseases in order to survive, and be able to endure occasional injury and famine, such qualities will not be transmitted to the next generation if we leave no offspring, that is, if we cannot attract a mate and ensure that our children survive to maturity. A crude Darwinian approach starts from the position of 'selfishness' to identify the behavioural traits that will prove to be essential for individuals both to survive and to reproduce effectively. However, can we account through such reasoning for the range of human behaviours found in modern societies?

With such a question, as in science generally, one must search for the 'counter-examples' that could disprove a hypothesis. One obvious question has related to altruism. How can one make sense of apparently altruistic behaviour, such as issuing a warning cry about a predator or assisting members of the species in rearing their offspring, within a Darwinian framework? Risk-taking or burden-sharing by one individual on behalf of others can be accounted for through the conventional operation of natural selection, if those helped in this apparently 'altruistic' fashion are relatives. In such circumstances, the 'altruist' is promoting the survival of relatives and thereby the transmission of his/her own genes when they are passed on by a relative. Such considerations apply in particular to some of the social insects, as with sterile worker bees labouring to ensure the success of the hive, but also to birds and mammals with cooperative rearing of the young. More complex patterns of indirect reciprocity in human societies may have developed from such practices (Nowak and Sigmund, 2005) and looking for cooperation between non-kin does not provide clear counter-examples (Clutton-Brock, 2009).

Evolutionary psychology constitutes an attempt to account for a range of human behaviours and attributes – normal and abnormal – by postulating similarly 'natural' processes, explicable in terms of natural selection. Its weakness is that the processes it describes must have happened in the distant evolutionary past if they are to account for human behaviours, personality traits and psychopathology evident today. This field of enquiry is all too vulnerable to the criticism that it is essentially a series of Kiplingesque speculations in the tradition of the *Just So Stories*. The descriptions of human gender roles and personality types may ring true, or may at least be amusing, but the causal accounts are largely speculative, neither adding firm knowledge nor yielding useful (testable) hypotheses.

However, despite this criticism, there are of course good reasons for expecting different patterns of social behaviour in male and female humans, as in many other animals, not only primates. One especially important factor in recent human evolution may have been the appearance of spoken language, which may have led to the rapid development of 'wit' – in both senses – through female choice of mate and the processes of sexual selection. However, one can only speculate about the details and the naturalistic fallacy – arguing from 'is' to 'ought' – is all too common in this domain. From the possibility that our hunter-gatherer forebears may (at certain times, in certain places) have had a particular pattern of social organization, we can draw no conclusions about how we *should* organize our collective lives today.

Claims about 'intelligence' are related to the speculations of evolutionary psychology. Thus, the idea that the human X chromosome is especially involved in 'intelligence' receives a limited degree of support from some evidence. There does appear to be an excess of X chromosome genes among those in which mutation causes serious cognitive impairment (Turner, 1996), although that does not allow one to conclude that variation in genes on the X chromosome accounts for more than that chromosome's rightful share of the genetic contribution to variation in intelligence (however, this is measured). Such reasoning is entirely invalid. Furthermore, these claims ignore the greater chance of a gene on the X chromosome coming to attention through mutation and the greater chance of the mode of inheritance being apparent.

In summary, an evolutionary (Darwinian) approach to the study of animal (and human) behaviour is necessary – 'nothing in biology makes sense except in the light of evolution' – *but* such an approach is limited in what it can establish as fact about the past or as desirable about the present. There are altogether too many examples of popular science writing that seek for solutions to today's social and political problems through the application of crude ideas about our collective past.

'IT'S A KNOCK-OUT': STRUCTURE AND FUNCTION IN THE BRAIN

Other approaches in addition to genetics have been taken in the search for understanding of the central nervous system (CNS). These approaches all have in common a commitment to the reductionist project. This is not intended as a criticism because a reductionist approach has to be the starting point for any scientific study of the central nervous system. Only in this way can one recognize the limits of reductionist explanation – by coming up against them. Assigning functional roles to specific regions of the brain through the analysis of the effects of damage from tumour, infarction, haemorrhage or experimental lesions is a long-established approach that was essential in the early stages of neuroscience and remains so today. The central difficulty of this approach has been to understand the rules of inference from the observations made, which are remarkably similar between the different contexts of neuroscience and genetics. In neuroscience, what can one conclude about the function of part X of the brain if behaviour Y occurs when a lesion is produced there? In genetics, what can one conclude from the emergence of behaviour Q when gene P is inactivated or altered (mutated) in some other way?

In relation to neuroanatomy, there has been a progressive development of our ability to make such inferences as the working model of the brain has increased in sophistication through the accumulation of our knowledge of previous observations and experimental interventions. The *normal* function of one of the basal ganglia, for example, might not be most helpfully understood as the suppression of involuntary contra-lateral writhing movements, although that might be the most prominent feature of a lesion there, whether pathological or experimental.

There has been a similar process of sophistication in our understanding of the function of genes. The naming of genes is now more formalized but used to be based upon the phenotype that arose when a mutation occurred in the gene. The 'white-eye' gene of *Drosophila* usually produces eye pigment, which is not produced when the gene is mutated so that the eyes are then white. In one sense, this leads to a paradoxical naming of a normal gene or the corresponding protein by its opposite (as with the dystrophin protein, a lack of which results in Duchenne muscular dystrophy) or the naming of a gene by a disease-related feature irrelevant to the function of the normal gene (as with the archetypal example of the polyglutamine repeat disease, Huntington's disease and the huntingtin protein, whose normal function is related to the disease after which it has been named by coincidence only).

More recently, the role of particular neural circuits and pathways has been defined in animal models in increasing detail using these approaches of inferring function from the effects of the ablation of brain structures. Two recent illustrations, drawn almost at random from many, include the switching on or off of fear in mice (Herry et al., 2008) and the pursuit of rewards in rats (Burke et al., 2008).

Another productive, reductionist approach to structure-function relationships in the brain is that of imaging, including functional imaging, which is able to identify neural circuits active during specific tasks and sensory processing. As David Hume indicated long ago, the temporal association of two events does not establish causation. Such experiments may therefore not be able to distinguish the causal driver of a neural process from those associated circuits involved in its modulation, if indeed there is usually something corresponding to a 'causal driver' so that the distinction has a meaning (Logothetis, 2008).

With this approach, it may even be difficult to distinguish actual neural activity from anticipated but aborted activity, as blood flow in the cortex can be directed in anticipation of an imminent task that then fails to be carried through to performance (Sirotin and Das, 2009). Whether the findings of such studies are regarded as explanations or, more properly, as increasingly detailed descriptions of the phenomena to be explained, will depend upon the investigator's point of view.

This rather abstract argument is relevant to the topic of this chapter when considering the question of a behavioural phenotype and what shape an explanation of such a phenotype might take, if an explanation can be discerned at all. Let us look at the parallels in a closely related field. The recognition of an unusual pattern of physical features is the core activity in dysmorphology – the clinical study and delineation of patients with congenitally abnormal physical features, often also accompanied by abnormalities of the CNS and of cognitive development.

The early development of this discipline centred on the recognition of recurrent patterns of malformation or unusual physical features and whether these were usually sporadic events in a family or had a tendency to recur. Once cytogenetics had developed to the point of diagnostic applications, some conditions but not others were found to be associated with chromosomal anomalies, initially with an abnormal chromosome number (as in Down syndrome or Turner syndrome) and then with more subtle anomalies, such as chromosomal deletions or duplications. The extent to which trisomy 21 is not only associated with but can be said to 'explain' Down syndrome is an interesting question at many levels, with obvious parallels in the neurosciences. While trisomy 21 may explain why one child rather than another is affected by Down syndrome, it only permits a detailed mechanistic explanation of some of the physical and behavioural features of the condition. Even where it can account for the incidence of dementia at an early age in those with Down syndrome, *it is unable to account for why an individual has a specific lapse of memory on one occasion but not another.*

The interplay between clinical and laboratory genetics has been enormously productive in developing a taxonomy of dysmorphology. The recognition of an association between cases of a clinical disorder and particular cytogenetic or molecular genetic findings leads to the recognition of a subgroup of the clinical disorder where this association is not apparent. Such atypical cases will often have a different cause and may, in time, be recognized as an altogether different entity in their own right. One could mention the emergence of Noonan syndrome from Turner syndrome as an example, or the recognition of CDKL5-related disease from among the 'early onset of seizures' variant of Rett syndrome. To what extent can we expect similar progress in our understanding of the genetic basis of the disorders affecting behaviour?

SYNDROMES AND BEHAVIOUR

Many of the dysmorphic syndromes affecting embryogenesis and then physical and cognitive growth and development are associated with abnormal patterns of behaviour. These abnormal behaviours are most often the result of substantial cognitive impairments that restrict the assimilation of sensory input, its cognitive processing and then the behavioural responses. Some of these syndromes show very characteristic patterns of behaviour, such as the 'cocktail party' chatter of a child with Williams syndrome, the social awkwardness of some males with fragile X syndrome or the social interest but slow responses of someone with Rett syndrome. Such behaviours can sometimes be recognized as a part of the overall 'gestalt' of the condition or they may be more apparent when behaviour is studied with objective systems of description and measurement. In relation to the physical features of some dysmorphic syndromes, it is becoming possible to sketch out a plausible sequence of events from the underlying genetic cause of the condition through the consequences of that in the embryo and foetus to the physical features of the affected child or adult, as with the structural proteins disrupted in Williams syndrome (including a deletion of the elastin gene) or Marfan syndrome (a fibrillin gene mutation).

Are we then beginning to be able to give a coherent account of the pathway from the genetic alteration underlying a syndrome to the specific behavioural features found in that condition? The short answer – all we have space for here – is 'No!' Such explanatory pathways for these and other dysmorphic syndromes have not yet been constructed in a plausible fashion, except to state the obvious, that an abnormality in a gene required for normal brain development and function will have cognitive and behavioural consequences.

We must indeed be very cautious in attributing behaviours common in those with a specific condition directly to the primary genetic basis of the condition, rather than to some indirect habits of social interaction that develop because of the physical appearance of the young child, the pattern of their cognitive abilities or particular difficulties they have with the senses or with organizing motor activities. However, the observation of an association between a genetic anomaly, its particular physical features and a particular pattern of behaviour is not fundamentally in doubt, even if the mechanisms through which the genetic change leads to the pattern of behaviour often remain obscure.

SINGLE GENE EFFECTS

Are we any further forward with understanding the effects of single genes on behaviour in the absence of developmental problems and severe cognitive impairment? As with development of the brain, so with conditions which lead to its degeneration: single gene disorders that lead to the loss of neurons and neuronal connectivity lead to the loss of capacity and so to dementia – as in Huntington disease and the familial forms of early-onset Alzheimer disease. But what about the effects of single genes on more specific items or patterns of behaviour, other than simply causing severe cognitive impairment?

There are distinct single-gene (Mendelian) disorders and chromosomal deletion syndromes associated with patterns of behaviour more usually seen in the absence of a clear genetic anomaly. The behavioural pattern of autism, for example, is often found in children with tuberous sclerosis (TS) (caused by mutation in the TSC1 or TSC2 genes) and sometimes in children with constitutional PTEN gene mutations (Butler et al., 2005). The diagnosis of 'schizophrenia' occurs at a high frequency (more than 25 per cent) in adults with the 22q11 deletion typical of people affected by the DiGeorge and Shprintzen (velo-cardio-facial) syndromes. Children with TS usually develop benign intra-cerebral tumours (tubers) and those with mutations in PTEN – another tumour suppressor gene affecting growth in early life – often show macrocephaly and so the effect in both cases may be mediated by abnormal growth of the brain.

Other Mendelian loci in which mutation is associated with autism are those encoding the neuroligin proteins NLGN3 and NLGN4 (Jamain et al., 2003). These cell adhesion molecules are positioned on the postsynaptic side of synapses and are believed to interact specifically with neurexin 1 on the presynaptic side; it is of great interest – although perhaps tantalizing – that deletions and other disruptions of the neurexin 1 gene NRXN1 are implicated as contributing to 'schizophrenia' (Kirov et al., 2009). Such single gene effects, however, have been found in few cases of psychiatric disease and in no cases of behavioural variation 'within the normal range'. Given the high frequency of psychiatric disease, with 'schizophrenia' having a life-time incidence of ~1 per cent, and given the long history of investment in research into these conditions, what can we say about the contribution of genetic factors to these important disorders? Recent studies of genetic variation across the genome suggest an overlap between the factors contributing to 'autism' and to 'schizophrenia', raising the possibility that these conditions may not be distinct diagnostic entities.

PSYCHIATRIC DISORDERS AND MULTI-FACTORIAL INHERITANCE

Genetic research into psychotic disorders, such as 'schizophrenia' (SZ) and 'bipolar disease' (BPD) has long been justified by its proponents indicating studies of heritability, especially twin studies comparing identical twins with fraternal twins or siblings. These studies often show a high value of heritability (up to 80 per cent in many studies). As molecular genetic studies became feasible in the 1980s, researchers set out to identify familial cases of SZ and BPD in order to conduct linkage analyses and map the important loci.

Although there were a few positive results, it became clear that single genes of major effect segregating in families (i.e. Mendelian loci) are not contributing substantially to the incidence of these disorders. As molecular methods developed along with the statistical and bioinformatic methods required to interpret their findings, it became possible to search for loci of lower penetrance – less likely to cause disease – until with current methods it has become clear that even powerful genome-wide association studies (GWAS), with (cumulatively) many thousands of cases and controls, have been unable to identify genetic variation accounting for more than a small fraction of the supposed genetic contribution to the risk of these diseases.

However, it is important to note that a few loci, implicated through segregation of disease in those rare families where a gene of major effect does seem probable, have now also been implicated in these more recent GWAS studies as perhaps contributing weaker disease predispositions in a much greater number of cases (O'Donovan et al., 2009). Of particular interest is the finding that two of the loci at which variation is associated with SZ are also associated with the risk of BPD. This raises the possibility that the genetic predisposition to both disorders is at least partly shared, so that they may not be two distinct conditions but instead somewhat different manifestations of a single category of major psychosis. And these factors also overlap with those implicated in autism.

The research community now needs to learn from these findings what they can tell us about the mechanisms underlying these disorders: what cellular mechanisms and/or neural pathways become dysfunctional in the presence of the predisposing variants, and how does this increase the risk that an individual will become psychotic? Understanding these functional mechanisms – the basic neurophysiology – may give insight into new therapeutic possibilities for these common and immensely distressing and burdensome conditions. (For other accounts of psychosis see Bentall and Thomas, this handbook.)

LIMITATIONS OF THE COMPLEX DISEASE MODEL OF THE PSYCHOSES

Although the overview of current research into the genetic basis of SZ and BPD outlined above is fair, there are some complexities that need to be considered if we are to place the recent research findings in context. We need to question the evidence on which SZ has been considered so highly heritable and we need to think about what the term 'heritability' includes.

At this point, I should make explicit my 'ideological' position as both a paid-up realist (Bhaskar, 1975) and social constructionist (Berger and Luckmann, 1966). The world and our observations of it are real; the ideas we have about the world, however, are constructed and communicated in language and through processes of social interaction and negotiation. Diagnostic categories are social constructions that may correspond in more or less helpful and appropriate ways to observable reality; the construction of diagnoses in psychiatry has been and inevitably remains a more complex and contested area than in trauma surgery but the suffering associated with 'psychiatric disease' is real – incontestably – whatever labels we choose to employ.

First, it has become clear that some cases of diagnosed SZ are associated with the de novo occurrence (in the proband) of a small chromosomal deletion or, less often, a duplication. These are known collectively as copy number variants (CNVs) and are detected on DNA microarrrays (gene chips), which can compare the relative dosage of gene sequences from across the genome. The same technology is proving very useful in identifying the genetic basis of previously unexplained cases of dysmorphic syndromes and other disorders of physical and/or cognitive development.

What does this mean? Well, comparisons of identical and fraternal twins have been the mainstay of heritability studies in SZ, and if a condition has been caused by a new genetic change of major effect (such as a CNV) then it is likely to affect both of a pair of identical twins but only one of a pair of fraternal twins. A CNV arising as a new mutational event will therefore lead to a high estimate of heritability for the disorder simply because it is a new mutation of high penetrance affecting identical but not fraternal twins. This will lend unwarranted support to the ideas of the 'complex disease' origin of SZ, because the causal model underlying the estimate of heritability will have been misconceived. CNVs known to be associated with SZ are being recognized in 2–3 per cent of cases, and de novo CNVs in as many as 10 per cent of cases of SZ (Xu et al., 2008) although that figure is higher than other published figures (reviewed in O'Donovan et al., 2009).

What remains uncertain is whether the de novo CNVs found in SZ represent a small subgroup of SZ. In contrast, they could be the tip of the iceberg, with many other cases arising as de novo events undetected by microarray technology because they are much smaller, perhaps point mutations or other intragenic mutations within loci included in the CNV sites. It may take a few years for uncertainty to be clarified, especially if de novo events contribute to some classes of disease and not to others. If the CNVs constitute only the tip of an iceberg of new or recent mutations occurring in the last few generations, then this could account for both the high estimates of heritability and the lack of success of GWAS studies in accounting for more than a small fraction of the heritability. The new generation sequencing technologies will help to resolve the issue in the long term, as much greater volumes of sequence data become available from patients with different patterns of disease. In the short to medium term, however, such data will doubtless generate more information than can be interpreted with confidence, as more sequence variants of uncertain significance will be encountered.

The second complexity we need to address is the nature of the 'heritability' estimated in twin studies and other experimental designs. This is the proportion of the variance in a quantitative trait that can be attributed to variation in the relevant genetic factors as a fraction of the total phenotypic variance. So the term applies only to quantitative traits and not to categorical traits, and it includes all the relevant genetic factors and not only the straightforward (independent) components of these factors. If all the relevant genetic factors interacted by modifying the risk of disease in a simple, multiplicative fashion, as would be the case for combining independent risk factors, then there would be less reason to query the interpretation of heritability estimates (although the point made in the paragraphs above would still remain valid). From what we know of other (lower) organisms, however, it seems most unlikely that GxG and GxE effects can be ignored. The problem is that, for many reasons, humans are poor organisms for estimating interactions between (i.e. among) genes and between genes and the environment.

Specific gene-gene (GxG) interactions are difficult to identify unless one has access to information about the phenotypes associated with each genotype from among the range of those possible. Because of the vast range of genetic variation within the human species, the nonrandom pattern of mating among humans, the long time-course from birth to maturity and the quantity of phenotypic information required, it is doubtful if enough data could ever be captured to permit such analyses. Indeed, there may not be enough people alive for the range of relevant genotypes to be represented. And this puts to one side the question of analysis and of interactions with the environment.

Our environments, of course, are also highly complex and variable; we live for decades and early experience may well shape our later mental health; we do not often marry or mate 'at random' and our family sizes are small and becoming smaller. The possibility of gathering enough information about the mental health outcomes of a large enough set of individuals of known genotype to assess the risks of disease for a range of specific genotypes at numerous interacting loci and in the face of a range of different early and adult environments is therefore small unless one makes vastly simplifying assumptions as to what factors can be ignored. If the GWAS studies had shown (or come to show) that specified genetic factors do account for a large proportion of the (estimated) heritability, then that would have supported the simplifying assumptions underlying that work.

However, none of this has happened (yet). Given this complexity and uncertainty the methodological assumptions about psychosis and heritability in psychiatric genetics in the first part of the twentieth century were clearly flawed and driven by eugenic pre-suppositions. Indeed many of assumptions embedded in the legacy of that period in biological psychiatry remain highly speculative (Kingdon and Young, 2007). Put simply, the eugenic assumption of degeneracy pre-figured the desire to find confirmatory empirical evidence and weak methodologies of inquiry were deployed to find the latter (Marshall, 1990; Pilgrim, 2008).

GENE INTERACTIONS IN QUANTITATIVE TRAITS

In model organisms, where experimental designs are possible and mating can be controlled, such as with the fruitfly *Drosophila melanogaster* in particular, data can be collected that give us good insight into gene-gene (GxG) and gene-environment (GxE) interactions influencing a wide range of traits including important behaviours. Especially helpful has been a long series of studies by Trudy Mackay and her colleagues, often using recombinant inbred strains of flies kept in a small number of distinct environments and studied with the help of breeding programmes. Of course, none of these facilities exist in human populations but the difficulty of demonstrating or measuring in humans the effects that have been identified in fruit flies does not mean that they are absent from our species.

Trudy Mackay's work in *Drosophila* on both life-span (longevity) (Leips and Mackay, 2000; Vieira et al., 2000) and sensory bristle number (Dilda and Mackay, 2002) shows that there are strong interactions between genes, between genes and sex and between genes and the environment, especially temperature (as I have outlined in more detail elsewhere – Clarke, 2004). This work has been integrated with microarray studies of gene expression to identify genes likely to be important influences on lifespan (Geiger-Thornsberry and Mackay, 2004; Lai et al., 2007). The methods required for the quantitative genetic analysis of behavioural traits have been established some years ago (Anholt and Mackay, 2004) and have begun to yield important insights (Ayroles et al,. 2009), although it is interesting that research focused on mutagenic screens to identify single gene loci influencing such traits is still yielding the most important findings (Vosshall, 2007).

Such work demonstrates that the genetic architecture of complex traits involves many loci interacting in a truly complex fashion and suggests that the studies that could feasibly be conducted in humans will fail to identify many such effects, at least into the medium term. In addition, it seems that there are single genes of great importance for specific behaviours – and in which mutation will disrupt one or more such behaviours – but that many loci influence patterns of behaviour in a complex web of GxG and GxE interactions, even if they cannot all be identified in our own species. For this to be true, there must be a high level of genetic polymorphism that is of functional importance and that is maintained not merely by mutation and drift (the random consequences of breeding patterns) and not the effects of selection.

Is that likely? The answer has to be 'yes' in *Drosophila* and there is no reason why it would not also be true for our own species. Phenomena such as frequency-dependent selection, density-dependent selection, sexually antagonistic selection and other types of disruptive selection are well known (Rice et al., 1992; Sokolowski et al., 1997) so that there is no need to expect heterozygote advantage and drift as the only mechanisms to account for high levels of polymorphism. The evidence in favour of recent natural selection in humans is limited but this relates principally to shifts in allele frequency leaving evidence in the pattern of linkage disequilibrium; such findings tell us nothing about the maintenance of polymorphism as discussed here.

GENE-ENVIRONMENT INTERACTIONS IN MENTAL DISORDERS

Thoughtful reviews of the genetics of complex disorders in humans have indicated such difficulties as those identified above in looking at such traits and disorders in humans (Kendler and Greenspan, 2006; Lewis and Brunner, 2004; Weiss, 2008). It would clearly be immensely difficult to obtain data about GxG interactions across a range of standardized environments in our species, without assuming that other genes are not involved in the trait under investigation. Despite this, some information has been collected about the overall effect of specific single alleles in at least two different environments (i.e. the GxE interactions) for several psychiatric disorders.

Highly dramatic and largely unsupportable claims have been made about the contribution of genetic variation at the MAO locus to violent behaviour but more modest claims about the interaction of a functional polymorphism at this locus with a personal history of physical abuse as a child do have some supporting data, indicating that those subject to abuse in childhood and who have lower levels of MAOA activity are more likely to display antisocial behaviour as adults (Caspi et al., 2002).

Another example of GxE interactions evident in humans is of the association between a genetic variant in another enzyme influencing levels of amine neurotransmitters and antisocial behaviour. Among those given a label of ADHD, the frequency of antisocial behaviour differed with the alleles of a polymorphism at the COMT locus (Caspi et al., 2008) and similar findings have been made elsewhere (Fowler et al., 2009; Maestu et al., 2008). The interpretation of such findings, however, is not straightforward and needs great care to avoid erroneous over-generalizations (Thapar et al., 2007a). In particular, the intrauterine environment may modify the effects of genotype and postnatal environment as influences on subsequent psychopathology (Langley et al., 2007) and there are methods that could begin to disentangle such effects (Thapar et al., 2007b).

Turning to autism, the findings of an association with CNVs (deletions and duplications) as discussed above is of great interest, especially because of the implication of specific genomic regions containing plausibly 'relevant' gene loci (Glessner et al., 2009; Wang et al., 2009). While autism is clearly not a single disorder, and can be strongly associated with mutations at some specific genes (e.g. Butler et al., 2005), most cases are not associated with a clear Mendelian disease. Therefore, the extent to which the CNVs identified in these two 2009 studies have arisen de novo (or have been transmitted from an affected parent) is also of great interest because of the distorting (inflating) effects of such events on measures of heritability, as discussed above.

The degree to which common variants in the population modify the phenotype of autism while individually rare but cumulatively common major mutations (such as CNVs or the presence of rare Mendelian diseases) trigger the development of such problems remains to be determined; at least it is clear that these issues are now being addressed by the molecular researchers, who are not content to adopt a 'traditionally' deterministic stance (Happe et al., 2006; Stephan, 2008; Weiss et al., 2009).

In the area of 'depression', too, evidence is emerging that people of certain genetic constitutions are more liable than others to respond to stressful life events by becoming sad and distressed (Caspi et al., 2003; Risch et al., 2009). Such findings bring psychiatric genetics much closer to the lay perspective on causation of such illness as being in part triggered by circumstance, in part the result of personality.

In the case of SZ, some of the predisposing genetic factors appear to be the same as in autism and BPD (Lichtenstein et al., 2009 and references cited above). If these findings are upheld by further evidence, then these diagnostic categories will clearly require reassessment. The finding of post mortem epigenetic differences within specific regions of the brain between patients affected by SZ and controls lends some credibility to the idea that early life experience may contribute to disease through such a mechanism (Mill et al., 2008). While some familial mutations are known that can act as strong triggers of SZ (Blackwood et al., 2001), it is perhaps intrinsically unlikely that such inherited variants of major effect would be common as the fertility of those with disease is likely to have been impaired both by reduced survival (especially in the past, before effective treatments) and impaired social skills.

The frequent finding of novel CNVs affecting genes in neurodevelopmental pathways in cases of SZ (Walsh et al., 2008) suggests that many cases of such disorders arise de novo and that other such new mutation events undetectable by array CGH will account for further cases. The most plausible conclusion at present seems to be that major (and often new) events trigger disease and that common functional variants will modify the nature and course of disease and perhaps thereby influence the particular diagnosis made according to today's taxonomy; polymorphisms at the loci of major effect (e.g. Stefansson et al., 2003) may also act as such modifiers when the trigger is a major event elsewhere in the genome (Carroll and Owen, 2009).

GENETICS OF NORMAL TRAITS AND INTELLIGENCE

There is a long tradition of studies of 'intelligence', as measured by the Intelligence Quotient and its heritability. These have usually used twin and adoption studies and have indicated a high heritability (often of 0.6 – 0.8). These findings have then often been misused by those with a prior political commitment to support some particular social policy such as – typically – the uselessness of investing in the early education of those belonging to lower social classes or specific ethnic groups.

Such misapplications of research findings make the elementary error of treating heritability as if it were a fixed biological constant instead of being a variable that depends upon *the particular social environment* operating at the time. Moreover, this error is compounded when we consider that the environments to which different research groups were exposed were systematically different, as is the case in societies with wide socioeconomic differentials (Fischer et al., 1996; Lewontin, 1991). There is no need for us to recite these analyses here (Gould, 1981). Instead, let us simply recall that the prospect of misapplication of research findings in this area – looking at IQ differences between social and ethnic groups – is so great and the chance of 'useful' results contributing to the educational success of future generations so slim that the case for undertaking or supporting such research hardly exists (Clarke, 1997a; Harper, 1997). Some did believe in good faith that elucidating the genetic basis of variation in IQ within the normal range would help to understand the causes of severe cognitive impairment but these studies have failed to deliver that promise and were never likely to do so as the methodologies involved were intrinsically flawed.

It is clear that many measures of the heritability of IQ in contemporary society have been systematically inflated by the techniques employed (Devlin et al., 1997) and that IQ as measured is heavily dependent on socio-economic status (Turkheimer et al., 2003). Furthermore, the idea that there are 'genes for intelligence' seems implausible. *Rather, there will be specific patterns of alleles at multiple loci that interact with each other and the environment to modify a number of cognitive abilities.*

The suggestion that one particular allele at a locus will be consistently associated with superior 'wit' is most implausible. In that case, one would expect there to be strong selection – both conventional natural selection and, especially, sexual selection – in favour of that allele and it would then not remain polymorphic. Rather, it is much more likely that variation at loci important for cognition and communication is maintained by the advantages brought by each allele in different GxG and GxE circumstances – as discussed above for *Drosophila* longevity, for example. The whole sorry saga of the genetics of IQ appears to be a tale of misunderstandings by researchers who have either been politically motivated or who have simply placed too much value on a narrow, scholastic intellect that happens to have brought them a degree of academic success.

APPLICABILITY OF GENE-WIDE ASSOCIATION STUDIES (GWAS) TO CLINICAL RISK ASSESSMENT

The research into the association between common genetic variation and the risk of the common, complex diseases has been struggling to explain its lack of success in accounting for more than a small fraction of the heritability of disorders, from cancer and diabetes to 'schizophrenia' (Maniolo et al., 2009). The reader who has reached this point will be familiar with much of the explanation. We have seen inflated estimates of heritability, as well as the difficulty in assessing GxG and GxE interactions in our species. However, there are some additional factors to consider: epigenetic variation acquired in early life as a 'predictive adaptive response' (Moore and Williams, 2009); the often underestimated contribution of rare variants to common diseases (Bodmer and Bonilla, 2008); and the impossibility of pangenome panels of SNPs (Conrad et al., 2009; Estivill and Armengol, 2007) to capture CNVs that have relocated to other sites around the genome (Schrider et al., 2010).

Even in the case of disorders, where the nosology is relatively straightforward – and certainly much less contested than in psychiatric disease – the use of genetic association studies using the SNP-based GWAS approach is of little, if any, clinical utility. It is poor at assigning healthy individuals to clinically useful risk categories and so is generally of little, or no, value. If it could be justified as at least accurate, there would remain many reasons as to why it may not be helpful, such as the sometimes paradoxical (medically unhelpful) behavioural and psychological responses to high or low risk information (Clarke, 1995, 1997b). However, its power to account for the heritable fraction of disease risk is so limited, not even that inadequate justification is available to those who offer such 'services' on the open market (Edelman and Eng, 2009; Janssens et al., 2008). Such irresponsibility must surely be motivated by desire for a quick return on investment rather than any professional sense of good healthcare (Clarke, 1995, 1997b). The scientific value of the underlying research is not in doubt – it is only the *application* of the research findings to assign healthy individuals to risk categories that is unwarranted (Jakobsdottir et al., 2009).

The suggestion that such tests should be made available to assess the risk that an individual might suffer from psychiatric disease is still less justified for at least two important reasons (Braff and Freedman, 2008; Couzin, 2008). First, those likely to seek such testing will probably have a close family history of psychiatric disease. Accordingly, the SNP-based GWAS results will be irrelevant if the disease in the person's family is at least in part caused by an important de novo genetic event or at least one that has occurred within the last few generations. Second, such results could add to the stress known to precipitate at least some types of psychiatric morbidity.

CONCLUSION

Genetic variation contributes substantially to the occurrence of psychiatric disease and research into this is not only worthwhile but has recently begun to yield important results. However, from what we know of the genetic factors involved, the claims made about the genetic contribution to psychiatric disease in the past – especially some of the assessments of 'heritability' – appear to have been inflated and to have minimized the contribution to disease of the combined effects of many rare genetic variants and of Gene × Environment and Gene × Gene interactions. It is likely that our understanding of mental illness and its classification may well require a radical revision, when and if our understanding of the genetic factors involved has been consolidated; this reassessment may also prove to be very helpful in developing new therapeutic approaches.

REFERENCES

Anholt, R.R.H. and Mackay, T.F.C. (2004) Quantitative genetic analyses of complex behaviours in drosophilia. *Nature*, 5: 838–849.

Ayroles, J.F., Carbone, M.A., Stone, E.A. et al. (2009) Systems genetics of complex traits in *Drosophila melanogaster*. *Nature Genetics*, 41: 299–307.

Berger, P.L. and Luckmann, T. (1966) *The Social Construction of Reality*. Harmondsworth: Penguin Books.

Bhaskar, R. (1975) *A Realist Theory of Science*. London: Verso.

Blackwood, D.H.R., Fordyce, A., Walker, M.T. et al. (2001) Schizophrenia and affective disorders-cosegregation with a translocation at chromosome 1q42 that directly disrupts brain-expressed genes: clinical and P300 findings in a family. *American Journal of Human Genetics*, 69: 428–433.

Bodmer, W. and Bonilla, C. (2008) Common and rare variants in multifactorial susceptibility to common diseases. *Nature Genetics*, 40(6): 695–701.

Braff, D.L. and Freedman, R. (2008) Clinically responsible genetic testing in neuropsychiatric patients: a bridge too far and too soon? *American Journal of Psychiatry*, 165(8): 952–955.

Burke, K.A., Franz, T.M. Miller, D.N. and Schoenbaum, G. (2008) The role of the orbitofrontal cortex in the pursuit of happiness and more specific rewards. *Nature*, 454: 340–344.

Butler, M.G., Dasouki, M.J. and Zhou, X.-P. (2005) Subset of individuals with autism spectrum disorders and extreme macrocephaly associated with germline PTEN tumour suppressor gene mutations. *Journal of Medical Genetics*, 42: 318–321.

Carroll, L.S. and Owen, M.J. (2009) Genetic overlap between autism, schizophrenia and bipolar disorder. *Genome Medicine*, 1: 102.1–102.7.

Caspi, A., McClay, J., Moffitt, T.E. et al. (2002) Role of genotype in the cycle of violence in maltreated children. *Science,* 297: 851–854.

Caspi, A., Sugden, K., Moffitt, T.E. et al. (2003) Influence of life stress on depression: moderation by a polymorphism in the 5-HTT gene. *Science,* 310: 386–389.

Caspi, A., Langley, K., Milne, B. et al. (2008) A replicated molecular genetic basis for subtyping antisocial behaviour in children with attentional-deficit/hyperactivity disorder. *Archives of General Psychiatry,* 65(2): 203–210.

Cheney, D.L. and Seyfarth, R.M (2007) *Baboon Metaphysics. The Evolution of a Social Mind.* Chicago: Chicago University Press.

Clarke, A. (1995) Population screening for genetic susceptibility to disease. *British Medical Journal,* 311: 35–38.

Clarke, A. (1997a) Limits to Genetic Research: human diversity, intelligence and race. In P.S. Harpe and A. Clarke (eds) *Genetics, Society and Clinical Practice.* Oxford: Bios Scientific Publishers.

Clarke, A. (1997b) The genetic dissection of multifactorial disease: the implications of susceptibility screening. In P.S. Harpe and A. Clarke (eds) *Genetics, Society and Clinical Practice.* Oxford: Bios Scientific Publishers.

Clarke A. (2004) On dissecting the genetic basis of behaviour and intelligence. In D. Rees and S. Rose (eds) *The New Brain Sciences: Perils and Prospects.* Cambridge: Cambridge University Press.

Clutton-Brock, T. (2009) Cooperation between non-kin in animal societies. *Nature,* 462: 51–56.

Conrad, D.F., Pinto, D., Redon, R., Feuk, L., Gokcumen, O., Zhang, Y., Aerts, J., Andrews, T.D., Barnes, C., Campbell, P., Fitzgerald, T., Hu M, Ihm C.H., Kristiansson, K., Macarthur, D.G., Macdonald, J.R., Onyiah, I., Pang, A.W., Robson, S., Stirrups, K, Valsesia, A., Walter, K. and Wei, J., The Wellcome Trust Case Control Consortium, Tyler-Smith, C., Carter, N.P., Lee, C., Scherer, S.W. and Hurles, M.E. (2009) Origins and functional impact of copy number variation in the human genome. *Nature,* e-pub ahead of print. PMID: 19812545.

Couzin, J. (2008) Gene tests for psychiatric risk polarize researchers. *Science,* 319: 274–277.

Devlin, B., Daniels, M. and Roeder, K. (1997) The heritability of IQ. *Nature,* 388: 468–471.

Dilda, C.L. and Mackay, T.F.C. (2002) The genetic architecture of *Drosophila* sensory bristle number. *Genetics,* 162: 1655–1674.

Edelman, E. and Eng, C. (2009) A practical guide to interpretation and clinical application of personal genomic screening. *British Medical Journal,* 339:1136–1140.

Estivill, X. and Armengol, L. (2007) Copy number variants and common disorders: filling the gaps and exploring complexity in genome-wide association studies. *PLoS Genetics,* 3(10): 1787–1799.

Fischer, C.S., Hout, M., Jankowski, M.S., Lucas, S.R., Swidler, A. and Voss, K. (1996) *Inequality by Design: Cracking the Bell Curve Myth.* Princeton University Press: Princeton, New Jersey.

Fowler, T., Langley, K., Rice, F. et al. (2009) Psychopathy trait scores in adolescents with childhood ADHD: the contribution of genotypes affecting MAOA, 5HTT and COMT activity. *Psychiatric Genetics,* 19: 312–319.

Geiger-Thornsberry, G.L. and Mackay, T.F.C. (2004) Quantitative trait loci affecting natural variation in *Drosophila* longevity. *Mechanisms of Ageing and Development,* 125: 179–189.

Glessner, J.T., Wang, K., Cai, G. et al. (2009) Autism genome-wide copy number variation reveals ubiquitin and neuronal genes. *Nature,* 459: 569–573.

Gould, S.J. (1981) *The Mismeasure of Man.* Harmondsworth: Penguin.

Happé, F., Ronald, A. and Plomin, R. (2006) Time to give up on a single explanation for autism. *Nature Neuroscience,* 9(10): 1218–1220.

Harper, P.S. (1997) Genetic Research and IQ. In P.S. Harpe and A. Clarke (eds) *Genetics, Society and Clinical Practice.* Oxford: Bios Scientific Publishers.

Herry, C., Ciocchi, S., Senn, V., Demmou, L., Müller, C. and Lüthi A. (2008) Switching on and off fear by distinct neuronal circuits. *Nature,* 454: 600–606.

Jakobsdottir, J., Gorin, M.B., Conley, Y.P. et al. (2009) Interpretation of genetic association studies: markers with replicated highly significant odds ratios may be poor classifiers. *PLoS Genetics,* 5(2).

Jamain, S., Quach, H., Betancu, C., Råstam, M., Colineaux, C., Gillberg, I.C., Soderstrom, H., Giros, B., Leboyer, M., Gillberg, C., Bourgeron, T. and the Paris Autism Research International Sibpair Study (2003) Mutations of the X-linked genes encoding neuroligins NLGN3 and NLGN4 are associated with autism. *Nature Genetics,* 34: 27–29.

Janssens, C.A.J.W., Gwinn, M., Bradley, L.A. et al. (2008) A critical appraisal of the scientific basis of commercial genomic profiles used to assess health risks and personalize health interventions. *American Journal of Human Genetics,* 82: 593–599.

Kendler, K.S. and Greenspan, R.J. (2006) The nature of genetic influences on behaviour: Lessons from 'simpler' organisms. *American Journal of Psychiatry,* 163: 1683–1694.

Kingdon, D. and Young, A.H. (2007) Research into putative biological mechanisms of mental disorders has been of no value to clinical psychiatry. *British Journal of Psychiatry,* 191: 285–90.

Kirov, G., Rujescu, D., Ingason, A., Collier, D.A., O'Donovan, M.C. and Owen, M.J. (2009) Neurexin 1 (NRXN1) deletions in schizophrenia. *Schizophrenia Bulletin,* 35(5): 851–854.

Lai, C., Parnell, L.D, Lyman, R.F. et al. (2007) Candidate genes affecting *Drosophila* life span identified by integrating microarray gene expression analysis and QTL mapping. *Mechanisms of Ageing and Development,* 128: 237–249.

Langley, K., Holmans, P.A., van den Bree, M.B.M. et al. (2007) Effects of low birth weight, maternal smoking in pregnancy and social class on the phenotypic manifestation of attentional deficit hyperactivity disorder and associated antisocial behaviour: investigation in a clinical sample. *BioMed Central,* 7: 26.

Leips, J. and Mackay, T.F.C. (2000) Quantitative trait loci for life span in *Drosophila melanogaster.* interactions with genetic background and larval density. *Genetics,* 155: 1773–1788.

Lewis, S.J. and Brunner, E.J. (2004) Methodological problems in genetic association studies of longevity-the apolipoprotein E gene as an example. *International Journal Epidemiological,* 33: 962–970.

Lewontin R. (1991) *The Doctrine of DNA: Biology as Ideology.* Harmondsworth: Penguin.

Lichtenstein, P., Yi, B.H., Bjork, C., Pawitan, Y., Cannon, T.D., Sullivan, P.F. and Hultman, C.M. (2009) Common genetic determinants of schizophrenia and bipolar disorder in Swedish families: a population-based study. *Lancet,* 373: 234–239.

Logothetis, N.K. (2008) What we can do and what we cannot do with fMRI. *Nature,* 453: 869–878.

Mäestu, J., Allik, J., Merenäkk, L. et al. (2008) Associations between an alpha 2a adrenergic receptor gene polymorphism and adolescent personality. *American Journal of Medical Genetics,* 147B: 418–423.

Manolio, T.A., Collins, F.S., Cox, N.J. et al. (2009) Finding the missing heritability of complex diseases. *Nature,* 461: 747–753.

Marshall, J.R. (1990) The genetics of schizophrenia: axiom or hypothesis? In R.P. Bentall (ed.) *Reconstructing Schizophrenia.* London: Routledge.

Mill, J., Tang, M., Kaminsky. Z., Khare, T., Yazdanpanah, S., Bouchard, L., Jia, P., Assadzadeh, A., Flanagan, J., Schumacher, A., Wang, S-C. and Petronis, A. (2008) Epigenomic profiling reveals DNA-methylation changes associated with major psychosis. *American Journal of Human Genetics,* 82: 696–711.

Moore, J.H. and Williams, S.M. (2009) Epistasis and its implications for personal genetics. *American Journal of Human Genetics,* 85: 309–320.

Nowak, M.A. and Sigmund, K. (2005) Evolution of indirect reciprocity. *Nature,* 437: 1291–1298.

O'Donovan, M.C, Craddock, N.J. and Owen, M.J. (2009) Genetics of psychosis; insights from views across the genome. *Human Genetics,* 126: 3–12.

Pilgrim, D. (2008) The eugenic legacy in psychology and psychiatry. *International Journal of Social Psychiatry,* 54, (3) 272–284.

Rice, W.R. (1992) Sexually antagonistic genes: experimental evidence. *Science,* 256: 1436–1439.

Risch, N., Herrell, R., Lehner, T. et al. (2009) Interaction between the serotonin transporter gene (5-HTTLPR), stressful life events, and risk of depression. *Journal of American Medical Association,* 301(23): 2462–2471.

Schrider, D.R. and Hahn, M.W. (2010) Lower linkage disequilibrium at CNVs is due to both recurrent mutation and transposing duplications. *Molecular Biology and Evolution*, 27(1): 103–111.

Sirotin, Y.B. and Das, A. (2009) Anticipatory haemodynamic signals in sensory cortex not predicted by local neuronal activity. *Nature*, 475–479.

Sokolowski, M.B., Pereira, H.S. and Hughes, K. (1997) Evolution of foraging behaviour in *Drosophila* by density-dependent selection. *Proceedings of the National Academy of Science USA*, 94: 7373–7377.

Sonuga-Barke, E.J.S. (2010) Editorial: 'It's the environment stupid!' On epigenetics, programming and plasticity in child mental health. *Journal of Child Psychology and Psychiatry*, 51: 113–115.

Stefansson, H., Sarginson, J., Kong, A. et al. (2003) Association of neuregulin 1 with schizophrenia confirmed in a Scottish population. *American Journal of Human Genetics*, 72: 83–87.

Stephan, D.A. (2008) Unraveling autism. *American Journal of Human Genetics*, 82: 7–9.

Thapar, A., Langley, K., Asherson, P. et al. (2007a) Gene–environment interplay in attention-deficit hyperactivity disorder and the importance of a developmental perspective. *British Journal of Psychiatry*, 190: 1–3.

Thapar, A., Harold, G., Rice F. et al. (2007b) Do intrauterine or genetic influences explain the foetal origins of chronic disease? A novel experimental method for disentangling effects. *BMC Medical Research Methodology*, 7: 25.

Turkheimer, E., Haley, A., Waldron, M. et al. (2003) Socioeconomic status modifies heritability of IQ in young children. *Psychological Science*, 14(6): 623–628.

Turner, G. (1996) Intelligence and the X chromosome. *Lancet*, 347: 1814–1815.

Vieira, C., Pasyukova, E.G. Zeng, Z. et al. (2000) Genotype–environment interaction for quantitative trait loci affecting life span in *Drosophila melanogaster*. *Genetics*, 154: 213–227.

Vosshall, L.B. (2007) Into the mind of a fly. *Nature*, 450: 193–197.

Walsh, T., McClellan, J.M., McCarthy, S.E. et al. (2008) Rare structural variants disrupt multiple genes in neurodevelopmental pathways in schizophrenia. *Science*, 320: 539–543.

Wang, K., Zhang, H., Ma, D. et al. (2009) Common genetic variants on 5p14.1 associate with autism spectrum disorders. *Nature*, 459: 528–533.

Weiss, K.M. (2008) Tilting at quixotic trait loci (QTL): An evolutionary perspective on genetic causation. *Genetics,* 179: 1741–1756.

Weiss, L.A., Arking, D.A. et al. (2009) A genome-wide linkage and association scan reveals novel loci for autism. *Nature*, 461: 802–808.

Xu, B., Roos, J.L., Levy, S, van Rensburg, E.J., Gogos, J.A. and Karayiorgou, M. (2008) Strong association of de novo copy number mutations with sporadic schizophrenia. *Nature Genetics*, 40(7): 880–885.

2

The Challenge of Measurement of Mental Disorder in Community Surveys

Jerome C. Wakefield and
Mark F. Schmitz

INTRODUCTION

Community studies in psychiatric epidemiology attempt to determine the number of people suffering from mental disorder in general and from each specific type of mental disorder, and to identify the characteristics and risk factors correlated with each disorder and possible etiological factors in the disorder's occurrence. The information derived from such community studies influences mental health policy, guides prevention and screening efforts, impacts the planning for efficient distribution of mental health care, and forms the primary justification for decisions regarding the level of funding of mental health services and research. To accomplish the aims of such community studies, researchers must develop measures that can assess psychiatric symptoms among individuals who often neither consider themselves to be mentally ill nor seek mental health treatment and so have never been professionally diagnosed. Since the beginning of psychiatric epidemiology, formulating reliable and valid indicators of disorder to use in such surveys has represented a major challenge to the ingenuity of researchers.

Well-trained clinicians, with the help of an adequately detailed history and diagnostic interview, can generally identify a case of mental disorder when they see one. However, identifying people with a mental disorder in the general population, most of whom have never seen a clinician, is a very different matter. It is generally too expensive to use mental health professionals to survey large samples, so lay interviewers with a fixed set of questions are almost always used in such studies. Consequently, epidemiological surveys lack many of the safeguards and corrective mechanisms available in a clinical evaluation by a trained mental health professional who can flexibly explore the nature and sources of a patient's distress. Thus, even though they attempt to replicate clinical diagnoses in the community population, such studies can be more prone to diagnostic error.

In order to try to capture the judgment of a clinician, the main strategy that has been used in recent years in constructing epidemiologic instruments to measure mental disorder is simply to take the diagnostic criteria sets that clinicians use to diagnose patients, presented in the American Psychiatric Association's *Diagnostic and Statistical Manual of Mental Disorders* (2000), and to translate those criteria into questions in a research instrument. This chapter will explore the special problems that have arisen in epidemiologists' attempts to transfer diagnostic criteria from the domain of clinical evaluation to the much different epidemiological arena where disorder is measured in the general population by survey.

WHY CLINICAL SAMPLES ARE INADEQUATE MEASURES OF COMMUNITY PREVALENCE

Early attempts at obtaining prevalence estimates of mental disorder in the community used clinical samples and simply surveyed how many individuals had received treatment in hospitals, private practices, and other service venues. There are several fundamental problems with estimating community prevalence in this way. Not all disordered individuals have access to mental health services, and many either do not recognize that they have a disorder or prefer not to seek help even if they do. Moreover, it is common for individuals to consult professionals and even to receive treatment for normal conditions of intense grief or concern about life events. One can get a sense of how much of a difference clinical sampling versus direct community sampling of a population can make to prevalence estimates from Srole et al.'s (1978) classic study of mental disorders in midtown Manhattan. Srole's group studied both a clinical sample and a community sample within the same area. Based on the clinical sample, the prevalence of mental disorder was estimated to be 12.9 percent – in an area saturated with mental health services and professionals. Yet, based on the community survey, the prevalence according to a conservative criterion was estimated to be 23.4 percent and by a looser criterion 81.5 percent (Manis et al., 1964).

In addition to providing misleading estimates of prevalence, clinical samples may also provide more subtly biased answers to other questions that epidemiological studies are designed to answer, such as questions about the demographic breakdown of mental disorders. A good example of the sorts of problems to which clinical sampling is prone can be found in the seemingly contradictory socioeconomic-level prevalence data in two classic clinical-prevalence studies, Hollingshead and Redlich's (1958) study of New Haven and Srole et al.'s (1978) study of midtown Manhattan. Hollingshead and Redlich's clinical data, based on a census of New Haven mental treatment centers, including public and private hospitals and outpatient offices and facilities, indicated dramatically higher disorder prevalence rates in lower socioeconomic (SES) classes, whereas Srole et al.'s clinical data indicated higher rates of disorder in the upper classes. Hollingshead and Redlich's finding that the lower the class, the greater the proportion of psychiatric patients, was claimed by them to support the etiological hypothesis that social stress is a primary cause of mental illness. Hollingshead and Redlich found the following clinical prevalence rates per 100,000 population in various socioeconomic classes: I–II (highest), 556; III, 538; IV, 642; and V (lowest), 1,659.

These findings are in stark contrast to the results of the Midtown Manhattan study of clinical venues, which found the following total patient rate per 100,000 in three SES classes: Upper, 1,703; Middle, 1,178; Lower, 1,060. Aside from the fact that the rate is overall much higher, there is the striking fact that the direction of the relationship between SES and treatment rate is reversed; it seems that in New Haven, the poor get ill more frequently, whereas in Manhattan, the rich get ill more frequently. Do these data reflect an actual difference in the relationship between SES and mental disorder in the two locations?

Almost certainly they do not, because Srole et al. also did a community study and their population statistics (as opposed to their clinical prevalence rates) indicated that lower socioeconomic classes do have higher rates of disorder. How, then, did it come out that Srole et al.'s clinical prevalence rates indicated the opposite of both Hollingshead and Redlich's results and their own community study?

The answer seems to have more to do with treatment availability than with a correlation between SES and disorder. When the Midtown SES data are broken down by treatment site, they look as follows: Public Hospitals: 98 (upper); 383 (middle); 646 (lower), Private Hospitals: 104; 39; 18, Clinics: 61; 160; 218, Office Therapists: 1,440; 596; 178. These dramatic differences in direction of relationship between SES and patient population in different settings exist also in the New Haven data, as a reanalysis by Srole et al. revealed. In fact, the direction of the relationship between SES and patient population is the same for each category in both studies; in both cases, more poor people use public hospitals and more middle or upper SES people use office therapists. The difference in the overall prevalence rates is due to the fact that the mix of available services is different in the two locations. New Haven's services are more oriented toward public hospitals, which are used disproportionately by the poor, whereas Manhattan's services (at least at the time of Srole et al.'s study) contain a much greater proportion of private outpatient therapists, who are used by the better off. It appears that different services are used by different SES segments of the population, and the mix of services offered in a given locale may substantially affect the rates at which individuals from given SES categories use the services.

Even in community studies that directly interview samples of community members rather than patients, the service-based bias can still arise in an indirect and more subtle form. This can happen if the criteria used in identifying the community members who are disordered contain features that refer to service use as a way of trying to distinguish disorder from normal distress. This approach has been used in some recent psychiatric epidemiologic surveys as well as some prominent reanalyses of those data sets (Narrow et al., 2002). This approach can reintroduce the same biases based on service access or inclination to seek help that afflicted clinical surveys.

GENERAL SYMPTOM CHECKLISTS AND THE PROBLEM OF FALSE POSITIVES

Before the new wave of instruments used in most recent epidemiological studies (which we will shortly consider), most studies used instruments consisting of general symptom checklists, and simply defined some threshhold of number of symptoms as the point above which an individual is considered disordered. These instruments yielded an overall, unidimensional score of disordered status rather than specific diagnoses, although specific diagnoses could sometimes be derived from suggested subscales. For example, the Langner (1962) scale, used in the landmark "Midtown Manhattan Study," contained 22 questions.

LANGNER SCALE QUESTIONS

1 I feel weak all over much of the time.
2 I have had periods of days, weeks, or months when I couldn't take care of things because I couldn't "get going."
3 In general, would you say that most of the time you are in high (very good) spirits, good spirits, low spirits, or very low spirits?
4 Every so often I suddenly feel hot all over.
5 Have you ever been bothered by your heart beating hard? Would you say: often, sometimes, or never?
6 Would you say your appetite is poor, fair, good, or too good?
7 I have periods of such great restlessness that I cannot sit long in a chair (cannot sit still very long).
8 Are you the worrying type (a worrier)?
9 Have you ever been bothered by shortness of breath when you were *not* exercising or working hard? Would you say: often, sometimes, or never?
10 Are you ever bothered by nervousness (irritable, fidgety, tense)? Would you say: often, sometimes, or never?
11 Have you ever had any fainting spells (lost consciousness)? Would you say: never, a few times, or more than a few times?

12 Do you ever have any trouble in getting to sleep or staying asleep? Would you say: often, sometimes, or never?
13 I am bothered by acid (sour) stomach several times a week.
14 My memory seems to be all right (good).
15 Have you ever been bothered by "cold sweats"? Would you say: often, sometimes, or never?
16 Do your hands ever tremble enough to bother you? Would you say: often, sometimes, or never?
17 There seems to be a fullness (clogging) in my head or nose much of the time.
18 I have personal worries that get me down physically (make me physically ill).
19 Do you feel somewhat apart even among friends (apart, isolated, alone)?
20 Nothing ever turns out for me the way I want it to (turns out, happens, comes about, that is, my wishes aren't fulfilled).
21 Are you ever troubled with headaches or pains in the head? Would you say: often, sometimes, or never?
22 You sometimes can't help wondering if anything is worthwhile anymore.

In general, a score of four or more positive answers to questions on the Langner scale was considered to indicate disorder. Looking at the scale's questions, one immediately sees two weak points. First, one might easily answer four or more questions positively for reasons other than that one has a mental disorder. Many of the listed symptoms could be normal reactions to misfortunes in life, or even symptoms of physical disorder. It has been commonly observed that many of the listed symptoms in this and comparable instruments – from feeling alone or that one's wishes are not fulfilled to feelings of worry, nervousness, or low spirits – could easily indicate a normal response of *demoralization* to negative life events. If one is reacting normally to a difficult environment, one is not disordered, but the Langer scale and other symptom scales might classify one as disordered. A second important weak point is that general scales like Langner's scale do not distinguish among different disorders.

It turns out that the number of false positives with the Langner scale is considerable (Dohrenwend and Dohrenwend, 1982). Based on statistics provided by Langner (1962), one can calculate that, in a community sample diagnosed by mental health professionals (and using these professionals' diagnoses – which themselves may contain false positives – as the "gold standard" criterion against which Langner's scale is tested), the scale substantially over-reported the rate of mental disorder. The rate of disorder goes from a "true" rate of 23 percent (as measured by the professionals' diagnoses) to a measured rate of 31 percent. The challenge of the false positives problem is also brought out by the fact that, in Srole et al.'s (1978) study, fully 82 percent of the surveyed community population reported some psychiatric symptomatology. The 82 percent estimate of the prevalence of psychiatric symptoms has often been cited in critiques as a *reductio ad absurdam* of the validity of psychiatric epidemiological estimates based on symptom checklists. What it really shows, though, is that to have a useful epidemiological instrument, one must pay extremely careful attention to the false-positives problem and distinguish true disorders from normal distress. General symptom checklists of the Langner-scale type did not adequately make such distinctions.

TRANSITION TO THE USE OF DSM CRITERIA AS THE BASIS FOR MEASUREMENT OF MENTAL DISORDER IN EPIDEMIOLOGIC SURVEYS

The major approach taken in psychiatric epidemiology since the 1970s and the development of *DSM-III* (American Psychiatric Association, 1980, 1987) has been the use of operationalized symptom-based measures of specific mental disorders derived from *DSM* diagnostic criteria. Such measures base diagnosis on what essentially comes to a symptom checklist, in which a certain number of symptoms is necessary and sufficient for diagnosis of a specific disorder. These measures are "decontextualized" in the sense that they look only at symptoms and do not consider the subject's circumstances or what those circumstances might mean to the particular subject. Such criteria have the advantage that they provide standardized outcomes that do not vary from interviewer to interviewer. Because they do not require (or even permit) probes about the personal meaning of responses, interviewers do not need clinical training. This considerably lowers the cost of administering surveys, an especially important consideration in epidemiological research where large samples are necessary to adequately study a variety of disorders many of which occur rather rarely in the population.

As we saw, earlier studies also used de-contextualized symptoms, but in a generalized scale that confused distress with disorder. In more recently devised instruments, the problems of general symptom checklists are dealt with in several ways. First, separate sets of symptoms are presented for each disorder, so that disorders can be discriminated from each other. Second, a disorder may be indicated by a large number of possible symptoms, with diagnosis being triggered only when the individual has a certain number out of a list of typical symptoms. Third, exclusion clauses are used to eliminate the possibility that symptoms are caused by problems other than the target disorder, such as physical disease; for example, the criteria for depressive disorder might include an exclusion clause that attempts to reflect the *DSM* requirement that: "The symptoms are not due to the direct physiological effects of a substance (e.g., a drug of abuse, a medication) or a general medical condition (e.g., hypothyroidism)" (American Psychiatric Association, 2000: 356). Some of these features are illustrated in examples presented later. As we shall see, even using all these strategies, false positives remain a challenging problem because of the as yet unresolved problem of distinguishing intense normal distress from mental disorder.

Because *DSM* diagnoses are based on symptoms, epidemiologists could develop standardized interview structures simply by translating *DSM* criteria into questions for surveys of the general population, using a symptom checklist approach similar to that of earlier studies but with more complex algorithms for making a diagnosis. Lay interviewers could ask these questions in standardized, preprogrammed formats, and the answers could then be analyzed by computer to categorize respondents as disordered or not. Epidemiologists relied on the *DSM* as the authoritative guide to diagnostic criteria, but also adopted the *DSM* approach as practical and cost-effective. There was little in the way of independent examination of whether the *DSM* criteria are valid when translated from the clinical setting to the very different context of the community survey (Dohrenwend and Dohrenwend, 1982).

The categorical system of the *DSM-III* and subsequent editions of the *DSM* was thus the basis and indeed part of the inspiration of all large American community studies of psychiatric disorders that have been implemented since the late 1970s. Simultaneously with the development of the *DSM-III*, the National Institute of Mental Health decided to launch the Epidemiologic Catchment Area Study (ECA), the first study that would measure the prevalence of particular types of mental disorder in the community (Robins and Regier, 1991). "Catchment areas" was the term used to specify areas covered by community mental health services in the legislation that led to the community mental health system, and the ECA studied a sample of five such areas – Los Angeles, CA, New Haven, CT, Durham, NC, Baltimore, MD and St. Louis, MO. Based on the *DSM-III*, ECA researchers constructed the Diagnostic Interview Schedule (DIS) to be used by the study, which in turn formed the basic approach of the Composite International Diagnostic Interview (CIDI) that was used in subsequent studies in the United States (on which we focus here) and internationally (Kessler et al., 1994, 2005a). These instruments measure specific diagnostic conditions in community populations that were supposed to be comparable to the major clinical entities found in the *DSM*.

Because the *DSM-III* required that conditions satisfy an extended criteria set before being classified as a specific disorder, psychiatric epidemiologists expected *DSM* diagnoses to provide not only category-specific diagnoses but also more realistic estimates of the amount of mental disorder in the community. The core assumption was that a structured diagnostic interview would allow researchers "to obtain psychiatric diagnoses comparable to those a psychiatrist would obtain" (Robins et al., 1985: 952). It was hoped that the results would provide good estimates of how much untreated mental disorder existed. These estimates, in turn, would provide policy makers with knowledge of how much unmet need existed for psychiatric services.

The rigid standardization of structured interviews had the advantage of improving the consistency of symptom assessment across interviewers and research sites and the consequent reliability of diagnostic decisions (Wittchen, 1994). However, the standardized questions and scoring procedures in community studies preclude the possibility of using discretion and thus treat all symptoms, regardless of their context, as signs of pathology. For example, the sorts of experiences that produce normal sadness responses – breakups of romantic relationships and marriages, job losses, severe physical illness, disappointed career goals, and the like – are rampant in community populations and produce feelings and "symptoms" of blueness, fatigue, lack of appetite and so on that are much like those in depressive disorder (Horwitz and Wakefield, 2007; Wakefield et al., 2007), yet these experiences of normal sadness might end up being counted as symptoms of disorder using the symptom checklist approach (see next).

RELIABILITY AND RECALL PROBLEMS IN MEASUREMENT OF DISORDER IN RECENT PSYCHIATRIC EPIDEMIOLOGY

Three large-scale, heavily funded projects have been the primary sources of information about the occurrence of mental disorders in the US population: the Epidemiologic Catchment Area study (ECA: Robins and Regier, 1991), the National Comorbidity Survey (NCS: Kessler et al., 1994), and the National Comorbidity Survey Replication (NCS-R: Kessler et al., 2005a). Each of these projects used structured interviews, administered by lay interviewers. In the ECA, the measurement tool for assessing mental disorders was the Diagnostic Interview Schedule (DIS), which was based on *DSM-III* diagnostic criteria. In the NCS, the measurement tool was the University of Michigan version of the Composite International Diagnostic Interview (UM-CIDI), which was based on *DSM-III-R* diagnostic criteria. The NCS-R served as a replication and extension of the NCS, and used the World Mental Health Initiative revision of the CIDI (WMH-CIDI), which was mainly an update of the CIDI to *DSM-IV* criteria.

The changes from the ECA to the NCS not only incorporated the changes in diagnostic criteria from *DSM-III* to *DSM-III-R*, but also involved several key modifications in the implementation of the lay interviews, in order to improve the recall process of the respondents (Kessler et al., 1998). A main reason for these modifications was that serious problems emerged in the test–retest reliability of the ECA instrument. These problems were revealed when the data from the one-year ECA follow-up were compared to the data for the same sample from the original ECA data collection and yielded some serious discrepancies in symptom reports. It turned out that many respondents to the second wave provided reports about what symptoms they had ever had that were inconsistent with the reports they provided on the first ECA wave (Simon and VonKorff, 1995). For example, a respondent might report in the second wave never having experienced a symptom that he or she had reported in the first wave as having been experienced; or an individual might report never having experienced a symptom in the first wave and then in the second wave report having had the symptom prior to the time of the first wave.

Based on the assumption that the ECA inconsistencies were due in part to a memory retrieval problem, the NCS made several changes to address such issues. For example, important stem questions for each diagnosis were placed at the beginning of the entire interview so that fatigue would not be a factor; the inter-viewer emphasized to the respondent the importance of carefully examining her/his memory; and the questions were asked at a slower pace to stress active recall during the interview. The NCS did produce generally higher levels of symptom reports, but because there was no one-year follow-up of the NCS sample, it remains unknown whether the methods it used actually increased reliability and validity of recall or merely increased reports of symptoms of questionable relation to disorder.

Thus, the question of reliability remains a serious and unresolved concern for psychiatric epidemiology. The degree of potential urgency of this concern has not become generally appreciated because, perhaps unsurprisingly, very little published research resulted from the second wave of the ECA (Kessler et al., 1998). However, other studies in which respondents were interviewed multiple times suggest the problem of reliability of symptom reports is a serious one that extends beyond the ECA (Wells and Horwood, 2004).

Of particular importance for understanding the test–retest reliability problems in the ECA is that instruments like the DIS and CIDI may be based on faulty assump-tions about human memory, especially when using questions beginning with the phrase "Have you ever…" (Rogler et al., 1992). The key issue is that these struc-tured interviews entail problems associated with episodic memory, which requires the respondent to accurately recall whether and when an episode happened (Barsky, 2002; Belli, 1998; Rogler et al., 1992). Of the three main problems in episodic memory, encoding, storage, and retrieval, the last may be the most malleable to variations in interview methodologies (Rogler et al., 1992). This is the target of the main changes in memory aid processes implemented in the NCS: place the main stem questions at the beginning of the questionnaire, emphasize the importance of the respondent to carefully examine her/his memory, and provide a slower pace of the questions to stress active recall during the interview (Kessler et al., 1998).

Many studies have examined the test–retest reliability of epidemiologic instruments in the past 20 years, including extensive studies of the DIS and the CIDI. Unfortunately many of these studies use clinical samples and very short time intervals between the interviews, some as short as one day (Andrews and Peters, 1998; Hasin et al., 2006; Ross et al., 1995; Rubio-Stipec et al., 1999; Wacker et al., 1990; Wittchen, 1994; Wittchen et al., 1998). It has been noted that although reliability can be quite good in samples having high disorder prevalence, such as clinically based samples, the reliability in community samples can be considerably worse (Wells et al., 1988).

Results from prospective studies further indicate the problems in retrospective studies such as the ECA and NCS/NCS-R, by finding dramatically higher life-time prevalence estimates when disorders are assessed longitudinally (Mattison et al., 2007; Moffitt et al., 2007; Wells and Horwood, 2004). For example, in considering respondents aged 32 and younger, the NCS-R found lifetime preva-lence estimates of 25 percent for Major Depressive Disorder and 6 percent for Generalized Anxiety Disorder (Kessler et al., 2005a), whereas results from the

Dunedin Study, using repeated assessments in which the assessment instrument was administered several times over a period of years, showed estimates of 44 percent and 15 percent for those two disorders by age 32 (Moffitt et al., 2007).

Note that the higher Dunedin prevalence rates are achieved by diagnosing a lifetime disorder for all respondents who qualify for an episode of the disorder in any one or more of the assessments. One finding that suggests that this approach may have some validity is that similar values for one-year prevalence estimates are obtained from the Dunedin Study and from the NCS-R. However, this cumulative approach does not recognize that false positive diagnoses may greatly inflate the resulting lifetime prevalence estimates.

DSM AND THE PROBLEM OF FALSE POSITIVES

Although the goal of diagnosis in *DSM* and epidemiological instruments is primarily the same, namely, obtaining valid diagnoses using operationalized criteria for specific mental disorders, the distinct features of clinical and epidemiological contexts can result in potentially serious problems of false positive diagnoses in epidemiological instruments. For a variety of reasons, persons who in a clinical setting might readily be identified as nondisordered are more likely to be wrongly identified as disordered in an epidemiological study using the same *DSM* criteria.

For one thing, clinical interviewing and treatment extend over time and allow the clinician the luxury of correcting a mistaken initial diagnosis based on later findings. As new information emerges, the clinician might even conclude that there were extenuating circumstances and that the individual does not genuinely suffer from a disorder after all.

The clinician can even "disagree" with the official *DSM* criteria when the context of symptoms warrants such an exception. For these and other reasons, the cost of an initial false positive diagnosis in a clinical setting is not as great as the cost of a false negative, where an individual may not get treatment that is needed. And, even if there is a false positive, some purpose may be served because treatment may still be useful with subclinical conditions. In contrast, epidemiological diagnoses are almost always based on one contact and there are no feedback loops or corrective mechanisms by which diagnostic evaluations can be reconsidered in light of emerging information. Nor is there second-guessing the criteria; epidemiological surveys rely exclusively on the diagnostic criteria in the epidemiological instrument in an algorithmic all-or-none fashion. Thus, false positives remain false positives. And, false positives defeat the essential point of an epidemiological study, which is to count disorders.

Moreover, clinical populations are highly self-selected and contain individuals who have been willing to undergo considerable inconvenience to obtain help with their problems. The psychological and institutional obstacles that help-seekers must overcome mean that members of the clinical population are likely to be suffering from very high levels of distress, disability, or other harm, which may be indicative of a genuine disorder. This tends to make the issue of conceptual specificity superfluous. Diagnosis becomes a matter of choosing the category of disorder that best applies to the patient. This is a very different kind of problem than the one that faces epidemiologists. Epidemiological surveys encompass many people who report problems similar to those of clinical populations but who have never sought out a mental health professional. In such cases, the seriousness of the condition, and thus its disorder status, may be questionable. These divergent features of clinical and epidemiological contexts should make one wary about uncritically transposing clinically derived criteria into the epidemiological domain.

But the problem also lies with the *DSM* criteria themselves. It turns out (Wakefield, 1993, 1996) that many *DSM* criteria are inconsistent even with *DSM*'s own definition of disorder and consequently are prone to give rise to false positives. In particular, two of *DSM*'s definitional requirements for disorder are frequently violated by its own criteria. The first is that the condition must be due to a psychological or biological dysfunction; many of the criteria describe human harms (e.g., intense anxiety, excessive use of alcohol) that need not originate in dysfunctions. The second requirement that is often violated is the stipulation that the harm cannot be the result of social conflict or the attempt by society to control disapproved behavior; many of the criteria involve "symptoms" that are clearly manifestations of social conflict (e.g., arrest for use of illegal drugs, disapproval of one's alcohol use by one's family) and are not harms directly caused by dysfunctions. Here are just a few examples of how *DSM*'s rules for diagnosis diverge from the concept of disorder and encompass nondisordered problems of living (we thank the American Psychological Association for permission to use here some material previously published in Wakefield [1996]).

Major depressive disorder

Diagnosis of major depressive disorder is based on having several out of a set of symptoms typical of an extreme sadness response, for example, sadness, emptiness, lack of enjoyment in one's usual activities, loss of appetite, lack of concentration, trouble sleeping, and so on. The criteria correctly contain an exclusion for uncomplicated bereavement (i.e., one is not diagnosed as disordered if the symptoms are due to a normal-range response to having recently lost a loved one, with up to two months of symptoms allowed as normal), but they contain no exclusions for equally normal reactions to other losses, such as a terminal medical diagnosis in oneself or a loved one, separation from one's spouse, or losing one's job. If in grappling with such a loss, one's reaction includes just two weeks of depressed mood, diminished pleasure in usual activities, insomnia, fatigue, and diminished ability to concentrate on work tasks, then one satisfies *DSM* criteria for major depressive disorder, even though such a reaction need not imply pathology any more than it does in bereavement.

Separation anxiety disorder

Separation anxiety disorder is diagnosed in children on the basis of symptoms indicating age-inappropriate, excessive anxiety concerning separation from home or from those to whom the individual is attached, lasting at least four weeks. The symptoms (e.g., excessive distress when separation occurs, worry that some event will lead to separation, refusal to go to school because of fear of separation, reluctance to be alone or without major attachment figure) are just the sorts of things children experience when they have a normal, intense separation anxiety response. The criteria do not distinguish between a true disorder, in which separation responses are triggered inappropriately, and normal responses to perceived threats to the child's primary bond due to an unreliable caregiver or other serious disruptions. For example, in a study of children of military personnel at three bases that happened to occur at the time of Desert Storm, when many parents of the children were in fact leaving for the Middle East and where children knew other children whose parent had been killed or injured, the level of separation anxiety was high enough among many of the children for them to qualify as having separation anxiety disorder according to *DSM* standards, but in fact they were responding with a normal-range separation response to an unusual environment in which they had realistic concerns that the parent would not come back (A.M. Brannan, personal communication).

Disorder of written expression

An op-ed piece on *DSM-IV* in the *New York Times* by Stuart Kirk and Herb Kutchins (1994), which the *Times* titled "Is Bad Writing a Mental Disorder?" used disorder of written expression from the category of learning disorders as an example of the "nonsense" that is in the Manual. Because *DSM-IV* criteria for this and other learning disorders require only that the child's achievement level be substantially below average, it is true that the criteria do not distinguish very bad penmanship from disorder. Clearly, a distinction is needed here: bad penmanship is not a disorder in itself, but bad penmanship caused by a dysfunction in one of the mechanisms that enable children to learn to write is a disorder (Kirk and Kutchins acknowledged that this distinction could be made). This sort of distinction has been common in the learning disorders community for decades, and it requires that before diagnosing a child with a learning disorder, one must attempt to eliminate possible "normal" causes of the lack of achievement, such as family distractions, lack of motivation, or inability to understand the language of instruction. Because *DSM-IV* criteria fail to make this distinction, there is no adequate answer to the op-ed piece's embarrassing question. In actuality, the problem is not with the category of disorder of written expression but with the invalid *DSM-IV* criteria. The danger is that when *DSM-IV* puts forward criteria that are open to such ridicule, the legitimate distinction can easily get lost. In the case of the learning disorders, this distinction is critical not only for diagnosis but for the integrity and public support of special education programs.

Antisocial personality disorder

Sheer criminal behavior must be distinguished from antisocial disorders of personality. Traditionally, this distinction was made by requiring that an antisocial mental disorder must involve a dysfunction in one of the mechanisms that usually inhibit such behavior, such as those that provide the capacity for guilt, anxiety, remorse, learning from mistakes, or capacity for loyalty. *DSM-III* and *DSM-III-R* criteria failed to make this distinction adequately. The *DSM-IV* criteria for antisocial personality disorder are the following: In addition to having been conduct disordered before age 15, the adult must meet three or more of the following criteria: either inconsistent work history or failure to honor financial obligations, breaking the law, irritability and aggressiveness, impulsivity, deceitfulness, recklessness, and lack of remorse. These criteria do not adequately distinguish between career criminals and the mentally disordered (see Pilgrim and Rogers, this handbook). The criminal certainly meets the illegal activity criterion and may well meet the work/finance criterion (criminal activity is not "work" as intended in this criterion), the deceit criterion (criminal careers often involve substantial deceit), and one or more of the impulsivity, irritability/aggressiveness, or recklessness criteria (by the very nature of criminal activity). The "remorse" criterion was added as a concession to the traditional approach to validity, but because only three criteria are necessary for diagnosis, the inclusion of a seventh "remorse" criterion does nothing to prevent false positives on the basis of three out of the other six criteria.

EXTENDED EXAMPLE: GENERALIZED ANXIETY DISORDER

In this section, we present an extended example of a recent attempt to use *DSM*-derived criteria in an epidemiological study to measure the prevalence of a particular mental disorder, namely, generalized anxiety disorder. We selected this example because it is among the disorders with the highest prevalence rates, it concerns an affect – anxiety – that occurs in normal individuals and thus potentially poses a false-positive problem, and in a quest for validity of measurement has undergone considerable changes in criteria in the different versions of the *DSM* (Ruscio et al., 2007).

Generalized anxiety disorder (GAD) is a disorder of chronic anxiety arousal. Lifetime prevalence in the general population is estimated by the NCS-R to be 5.7 percent (Kessler et al., 2005a). The commonness of GAD, combined with other features of the data to be explored below, led Blazer et al. (1991), in considering results from the ECA (in which the GAD prevalence rate was even higher), to question whether the conditions diagnosed as GAD are really disorders: "Generalized anxiety disorder is a common condition, even among people not suffering from any other disorder. Its association with a number of social risk factors makes us wonder whether it is a disorder in the ordinary sense of the word. Could it be a residual of symptoms reflecting poor life satisfaction or generalized stress?" (p. 199). In other words, given all the stresses in our environment, there is a question whether the diagnostic criteria used in epidemiologic studies correctly distinguish disordered anxiety reactions from normal reactions to stressful environments.

The NCS-R diagnoses of GAD are made on the basis of the *DSM-IV* criteria operationalized by the CIDI as below.

WMH-CIDI OPERATIONALIZATION OF DSM-IV GAD

A. Excessive anxiety and worry, occurring more days than not for at least 6 months, about a number of events or activities: Assessed by having Part 1, Part 2, and Part 3.

Part 1: "Yes" answer to one of the following three "gate" questions:

"Did you ever have a time in your life when you were a worrier – that is, when you worried a lot more about things than other people with the same problems as you?"

"Did you ever have a time in your life when you were much more nervous or anxious than most people with the same problems as you?"

"Did you ever have a period lasting one month or longer when you were anxious and worried most days?"

Part 2: The duration of worry lasts longer than 6 months, assessed by:

"What is the longest period of months or years in a row you ever had when you were worried or anxious most days?"

Part 3: Anxiety about a number of events or activities, assessed by:

"Earlier you mentioned having a time in your life when you were "a worrier." The next questions are about that time. Looking at pages 18–19 in your booklet, what sort of things were you worried or nervous or anxious about during that time?" This criterion is satisfied if two or more activities are identified out of 32 listed activities, such as finances, success at school, relationships with family, health or welfare of loved ones.

B. The person finds it difficult to control the worry: Assessed by:

"How often do you find it difficult to control your anxiety or worry – often, sometimes, rarely, or never?" If respondent says "often" or "sometimes," then this criterion is satisfied.

C. The anxiety and worry are associated with three (or more) of the following six symptoms (with at least some of the symptoms present for more days than not for the past six months): (1) restlessness or feeling keyed up or on edge, (2) being easily fatigued, (3) difficulty concentrating or keeping mind on activity, (4) irritability, (5) tense, sore, or aching muscles, and (6) trouble falling or staying asleep. This criterion is assessed by "Yes" responses to six questions directly phrased as above, with the following preamble:

Think of your worst period lasting (one month/six months) or longer when you were worried or anxious: During that episode, did you often have any of the following associated problems.

D. The focus of the anxiety and worry is not confined to features of an Axis I disorder, such as Panic Disorder, Social Phobia, Obsessive-Compulsive Disorder, Separation Anxiety Disorder, Anorexia Nervosa, Somatization Disorder, or Hypochandriasis, and the anxiety and worry do not occur exclusively during Posttraumatic Stress Disorder. The PTSD portion of this criterion is not operationalized in the WMH-CIDI. The other portion of the criterion is assessed by at least one "Yes" response to a subset of the events and activities used in Part 3 of Criterion A.

E. The anxiety, worry, or physical symptoms cause clinically significant distress or impairment in social, occupational, or other important areas of functioning. This is criterion is satisfied by having either Part 1 or Part 2.

Part 1: An answer of "often" or "sometimes" to "How often were you so nervous or worried that you could not think about anything else, no matter how hard you tried – often, sometimes, rarely, or never?" Or an answer of "moderate," "severe," or "very severe" to "How much emotional distress did you ever experience because of your worry or anxiety – no distress, mild distress, moderate distress, severe distress, or very severe distress?"

Part 2: An answer of "some", "a lot", or "extremely" to "How much did your worry or anxiety ever interfere with either your work, your social life, or your personal relationships – not at all, a little, some, a lot, or extremely?" Or an answer of "often", "sometimes", or "rarely" to "How much were you unable to carry out your daily activities because of your worry or anxiety – often, sometimes, rarely, or never?" Or at least one answer out of four activities indicating moderate, severe, or very severe interference to "How much did your worry or anxiety interfere with (a) home management, (b) ability to work, (c) ability to form and maintain close relationships with other people, (d) your social life?" Or an answer of at least 5 days to "About how many days out of 365 in the past 12 months were you totally unable to work or carry out your normal activities because of your worry or anxiety?" Or an answer of "Yes" to "Did you ever in your life talk to a medical doctor or other professional about your worry or anxiety?"

F. The disturbance is not due to the direct physiological effects of a substance or due to a general medical condition, and does not occur exclusively during a mood disorder, a psychotic disorder or a pervasive developmental disorder. The psychotic disorder and pervasive developmental disorder hierarchies were not operationalized in the WMH-CIDI. The substance/medical condition hierarchy was assessed by not having a "Yes" response to "Do you think your worry and anxiety were always the result of physical causes?" The mood disorder hierarchy was assessed using the WMH-CIDI Major depressive disorder, minor depression, dysthymia disorder, and mania algorithms. If none of these mood disorders were present, then the criterion was satisfied. If at least one of the mood disorders was present, then if the GAD onset preceded the onset of the mood disorder, or the GAD was more recent or more persistent (assessed by number and length of episodes) than the mood disorders, then this criterion was satisfied.

The central problem in inferring an anxiety dysfunction is that anxiety reactions are a natural part of life. Human beings are designed to experience anxious arousal when experiencing various kinds of threats and stressors, from momentary dangers to chronically overwhelming demands. Thus, the sheer occurrence of anxiety, even intense anxiety, is not enough of a basis on which to infer internal dysfunction. Moreover, there is no natural limit to the length of time during which people can appropriately respond with anxiety to an ongoing environmental stressor, so the persistence of anxiety in itself is not a good indicator of dysfunction. Because chronic anxiety is a normal response to some situations, more than just chronic anxiety is needed to warrant diagnosis of an anxiety disorder. Perhaps the best circumstantial evidence for the existence of an anxiety dysfunction is intense, persistent anxiety that is not in any coherent or proportional way related to environmental stressors.

Unfortunately, the WMH-CIDI criteria for GAD simply assess anxiety and do not address the problem of distinguishing normal anxiety from pathological anxiety; such a distinction may be practically challenging but is crucial to validity. The excessive worry criterion only partially deals with proportionality of the anxiety to situational stressors, by having the respondents consider what they think other people might feel in similar circumstances. The comparative feature does establish that either the respondent is more intensely reactive than the average person, or that there are special circumstances that made the situation more anxiety provoking than it would normally be, but that does not really establish that the anxiety was "excessive" in the sense of pathological versus just the upper part of the distribution of normal responsiveness. Moreover, the third possible way to satisfy criterion A, that the respondent simply was anxious or worried most days over some period of a month or longer, abandons the comparative requirement altogether.

The list of activities used in the excessive worry criterion do not help matters much; for example, one can be legitimately worried for periods of six months or longer regarding finances or the health of a family member – indeed, one might easily be worried about both of these simultaneously because health problems often entail financial worries – and nothing in the wording of the list of activities suggests that the respondent is being asked to identify only excessive or unreasonable instances of worry. Thus, the excessive worry criterion provides no basis whatever for sorting dysfunction from normal anxiety responses, nor does the question about whether the respondent can control the worry (criterion B above) in that humans are not designed necessarily to control feelings and worry, except up to a degree. A person could easily experience intense anxiety over a period of several months due to stressful life circumstances, such as the ups and downs of a life-threatening illness in a loved one; the ongoing threat of losing one's job; the process of preparing for doctoral examinations, bar exams, or some other school or occupational challenge; or watching one's savings evaporate in a stock market plunge. The critical issue is to distinguish chronic anxiety that is a normal response to chronic stressors from chronic anxiety that results from a malfunction of anxiety-regulating mechanisms. To do that, the feelings would presumably have to be related to their context.

To assess the C criterion above, the respondent is asked a series of questions about specific symptoms. To meet diagnostic criteria, at least three symptoms must be reported as having occurred during the worst period of anxiety. But, the symptoms are just the components of any intense anxiety response, and such responses can be normal or pathological. So, the symptom questions add nothing to the conceptual validity of the criteria because they fail to distinguish anxiety caused by a dysfunction from normal anxiety. The D criterion is designed to provide some consideration of the distinction of GAD symptoms from potentially similar symptoms caused by other disorders. Unfortunately, this criterion is essentially ignored in the WMH-CIDI, by basically replicating a portion of the operationalization of the A criterion, with no consideration of distinguishing GAD symptoms from the symptoms of other disorders.

The E criterion functions as the clinical significance criterion, which formed a key component of the changes in criteria sets provided by *DSM-IV*. The problem is that anxiety is an emotion that by its very nature is distressing and to some extent impairing of usual role functioning. It is hard to imagine many individuals who satisfy the other criteria, including intense worry and various anxiety symptoms, reporting that they experienced no distress or lessening of routine role functioning. The clinical significance criterion thus seems more or less redundant in this set of criteria, and unlikely to help in distinguishing false positives from true disorders. The problem is that intense normal anxiety is itself generally "clinically significant" in the sense specified. The clinical significance criterion offered in *DSM-IV* has been broadly criticized across disorders for numerous reasons, including redundancy with symptoms, lack of empirical support, and the fundamentally tautological nature of the criterion in recognizing disorder – because for the criterion to work, "clinically significant" must mean "indicative of disorder," but whether the condition is indicative of disorder is exactly what the criterion is supposed to help one decide (Beals et al., 2004; Coyne and Marcus, 2006; Wakefield and Spitzer, 2002). A particularly problematic aspect of the clinical significance criterion is that it reflects a basic misunderstanding of the main problem underlying false positives. The underlying assumption in the criterion is that a condition is pathological if it causes sufficient distress or impairment in social or role functioning. However, *DSM* false positives are most often due not to a failure of symptoms to reach a threshold of harmfulness but to a failure of symptomatic criteria to indicate the presence of an underlying dysfunction. For example, the most obvious potential false positive in the Manual, uncomplicated bereavement as distinguished from major depressive disorder, must be dealt with in an additional special exclusion clause and is not eliminated by the clinical significance criterion that is added to the criteria set, because normal grief can be just as distressful and role impairing as pathological depression, even though it is not caused by a dysfunction. The operationalization of the clinical significance criterion for GAD in the WMH-CIDI (criterion E above) is particularly weak due to the large number of vague questions that allow a respondent to be identified as having "clinically significant" GAD.

The overall inadequacy of the DSM-style criteria for GAD is illustrated in a classic study by Breslau and Davis (1985). When Breslau and Davis evaluated 357 mothers of chronically ill children using *DSM-III* criteria in the DIS, they found an astonishingly high lifetime GAD rate of 45 percent. It seems plausible to suggest that, rather than all of the diagnosed women being disordered, most of these women were reacting normally to an extremely stressful situation. Breslau and Davis themselves interpreted their findings to mean that the criteria lacked specificity. The results of Breslau and Davis's study suggest that normal people facing a chronic stressor easily meet *DSM-III* GAD criteria. These results triggered the investigation of changes in the GAD criteria in *DSM-III-R*, with further revisions occurring in the GAD criteria in *DSM-IV* (Kessler et al., 2004), upon which the WMH-CIDI algorithm described above are based.

The NCS-R results, which used the WMH-CIDI, are in certain respects reminiscent of Breslau and Davis's findings. For example, Ruscio et al. (2005) found that lifetime GAD is significantly more prevalent among the unemployed than the employed, and unemployed respondents are more likely to be in a financially precarious position and thus respond positively to most of the above questions. Despite these results suggesting false positives, Ruscio et al. (2005) attempt to extend the criteria for GAD to be more inclusive by eliminating the excessive worry criterion. Kessler et al. (2005b) similarly explored the reduction of the GAD duration criterion from six months to various shorter periods.

The efforts in both of these studies have been towards broadening diagnosis of GAD to include subthreshold cases, by examining similarities between subthreshold cases and so-called disordered cases of GAD. We believe the results from these studies simply show the inadequacy of the GAD criteria to distinguish dysfunction from normal reactions to stressful environmental circumstances. Also, while it is always possible that those with anxiety disorders have fared worse in life due to the disorder, the most plausible interpretation of these findings is that the stress of financial and related problems causes anxiety symptoms. However, such people are not necessarily disordered, any more than are the mothers of chronically ill children in Breslau and Davis's study. The upshot of this analysis is that it appears that the NCS-R data provide no grounds for making even a rough guess of the true prevalence of GAD, as a genuine disorder of anxiety arousal.

RECENT ISSUES: DIMENSIONALITY AND "SUB-THRESHOLD DISORDER"

In preparations for the fifth edition of the *DSM*, a vigorous debate has arisen regarding the basic categorical approach used in the manual. Because epidemiologic studies, such as the NCS and NCS-R, find very high comorbidity among disorders as well as extensive variability within disorders regarding types of symptoms exhibited and disorder prognosis, and a lack of discrete cutoffs in symptom distribution (Krueger et al., 2005), several authors have proposed adopting a dimensional typology in assessing disorder in the *DSM* (Clark, 2005; Krueger et al., 2005; Watson, 2005; Widiger and Samuel, 2005).

It has been argued that dimensional approaches, when linked to research-derived measures, can give higher levels of diagnostic reliability and validity (Widiger and Samuel, 2005), although the problem of false positives and whether what is being validly measured is a genuine disorder has not been much addressed. However, other authors argue that the most important issue is the clinical utility of diagnosis, and that a dimensional approach to diagnosis, while perhaps more effective for researchers, may not be so helpful for clinicians (First, 2005). Proposals for including dimensional components in clinical diagnosis are being explored, with the possible addition of indicators of symptom severity and patient functioning (First and Westen, 2007).

In a related issue, numerous authors have advocated the inclusion as disorders of cases that do not meet the minimum symptom count for a given diagnosis (Angst et al., 2003; Kendler and Gardner, 1998; Kessler et al., 2003). Rather, such "subthreshold" conditions, it is argued, should be conceived as milder disorders on a continuum. For example, cases of depression exhibiting four symptoms or fewer would be identified as mild depression (Judd et al., 1997; Kramer, 2005; Sullivan et al., 1998). Subthreshold cases of depression have been found to exhibit similar correlates as major depression, as well as significant levels of impairment (Kessler et al., 1997). These authors conclude that minor depression cannot be dismissed as nondisorder, and that prevalence estimates of depressive disorder, based on the five-symptom cutoff, are actually much too low.

Similar conclusions have been reached regarding the prevalence and comorbidity of subthreshold cases of GAD, where "subthreshold" is defined by reducing the requirement of six-month symptom duration to one-month (Kessler et al., 2005b) and eliminating the excessive worry criterion (Ruscio et al., 2005). Making such changes greatly increases the prevalence estimates of GAD, while slightly reducing the comorbidity of GAD with other disorders (Ruscio et al., 2007). Importantly, these changes greatly increase the likelihood of misdiagnosing normal anxiety responses to environmental circumstances as disordered. Little attention has been paid to this potential problem by those putting forward such proposals.

Granted, the symptom cutoffs in diagnoses are rather arbitrary. And there are people exhibiting only a few symptoms who are experiencing conditions that should be diagnosed as disordered. However, the key is to distinguish normal responses to circumstances from dysfunctional responses to those circumstances, and emphasizing the counting of symptoms simply misses this fundamental point regarding the assessment of dysfunction and disorder. Any number of symptoms may or may not indicate disorder, depending on the environmental context of those symptoms. Likewise, the duration of the symptoms only gives an indication of disorder when the environmental context would indicate that symptoms should no longer be present. Dimensionalization of diagnosis, in which less symptoms or less duration are allowed for diagnosis, would make most sense if combined with an effort to address the problem of the upsurge in false positives that might occur due to such a change.

CONCLUSION

The field of psychiatric epidemiology may be said to have a logical structure like that of an upside-down pyramid; the integrity and meaningfulness of an enormous, expensive research enterprise rests on the validity of a few definitions of mental disorders incorporated into its measuring instruments, generally taken from DSM. Yet, if the argument above is correct, there is reason to believe that these definitions do not give a clear and valid picture of the domain of disorder. Instead, they seem to fuzzily encompass a broad range of abnormal and normal situations in which human beings feel distress or are impaired in their usual functioning. For all their innovation and sophistication, DSM-derived criteria do not overcome some of the problems in distinguishing disorder from nondisorder that beset the earlier symptom checklists. If subthreshold conditions are included as disorders as is now being discussed, the problem would become acutely worse. Dimensionalization of diagnostic criteria would also serve to leave the distinction between disorder and nondisorder even more unclear than it is now.

Yet these problems seem resolvable through such means as methodological innovations and revisions in criteria. Regarding methodological innovations, for example, future epidemiological studies might use a two-stage process in which subjects are first screened using DSM or comparable criteria and then those meeting DSM criteria for disorder are interviewed by a professional to distinguish genuine cases from false positives. As to changes in criteria, such revisions might take account of situational context in judging whether distress is pathological.

Current studies, though flawed, do provide large amounts of valuable data on the prevalence of disorder, distress, and impairment. However, for now, the question remains open as to whether or when psychiatric epidemiology will reach its ultimate goal of accurately measuring the true prevalence of mental disorder in community populations.

REFERENCES

American Psychiatric Association (1980) *Diagnostic and Statistical Manual of Mental Disorders* (third edition). Washington, D.C.: Author. (*DSM-III*).

American Psychiatric Association (1987) *Diagnostic and Statistical Manual of Mental Disorders* (third edition, revised). Washington, D.C.: Author. (*DSM-III-R*).

American Psychiatric Association (2000) *Diagnostic and Statistical Manual of Mental Disorders* (fourth edition – text revision). Washington, D.C.: Author. (*DSM-IV*).

Andrews, G. and Peters, L. (1998) The psychometric properties of the Composite International Diagnostic Interview. *Social Psychiatry and Psychiatric Epidemiology,* 33: 80–88.

Angst, J., Gamma, A., Benazzi, F., Vladeta, A., Eich, D., and Rossler, W. (2003) Toward a definition of subthreshold bipolarity: Epidemiology and proposed criteria for Bipolar-II, Minor Bipolar Disorders and Hypomania. *Journal of Affective Disorders,* 73: 133–146.

Barsky, A.J. (2002) Forgetting, fabricating, and telescoping: The instability of the medical history. *Archives of Internal Medicine,* 162: 981–984.

Beals, J., Novins, D.K., Spicer, P., Orton, H.D., Mitchell, C.M., Baron, A.E., Manson, S.M., and the AI-SUPERPFP Team (2004) Challenges in operationalizing the *DSM-IV* clinical significance criterion. *Archives of General Psychiatry,* 61: 1197–1207.

Belli, R.F. (1998) The structure of autobiographical memory and the event history calendar: Potential improvements in the quality of retrospective reports in surveys *Memory,* 6: 383–406.

Blazer, D.G., Hughes, D., George, L.K., Swartz, M., and Boyer, R. (1991) Generalized Anxiety Disorder, in L.N. Robins and D.A. Regier (eds), *Psychiatric Disorders in America: The Epidemiologic Catchment Area Study.* New York: Free Press. pp. 180–203.

Breslau, N. and Davis, G.C. (1985) *DSM-III* Generalized Anxiety Disorder: An empirical investigation of more stringent criteria. *Psychiatry Research,* 15: 231.

Clark, L.A. (2005) Temperament as a unifying basis for personality and psychopathology. *Journal of Abnormal Psychology,* 114: 505–521.

Coyne, J.C. and Marcus, S.C. (2006) Health disparities in care for depression possibly obscured by the clinical significance criterion. *American Journal of Psychiatry,* 163: 1577–1579.

Dohrenwend, B.P. and Dohrenwend, B.S. (1982) Perspectives on the past and future of psychiatric epidemiology. *American Journal of Public Health,* 72: 1271–1279.

First, M.B. (2005) Clinical utility: A prerequisite for the adoption of a dimensional approach in *DSM. Journal of Abnormal Psychology,* 114: 560–654.

First, M.B. and Westen, D. (2007) Classification for clinical practice: How to make *ICD* and *DSM* better able to serve clinicians. *International Review of Psychiatry,* 19: 473–481.

Hasin, D.S., Samet, S., Nunes, E., Meydan, J., Matseoane, K., and Waxman, R. (2006) Diagnosis of comorbid psychiatric disorders in substance users assessed with the Psychiatric Research Interview for Substance and Mental Disorders for *DSM-IV. American Journal of Psychiatry,* 163: 689–696.

Hollingshead, A.B. and Redlich, F.C. (1958) *Social Class and Mental Illness.* New York: John Wiley.

Horwitz, A.V. and Wakefield, J.C. (2007) *The Loss of Sadness: How Psychiatry Transformed Normal Sorrow into Depressive Disorder.* New York: Oxford University Press.

Judd, L.L., Akiskal, H.S., and Paulus, M.P. (1997) The role and clinical significance of subsyndromal depressive symptoms (SSD) in Unipolar Major Depressive Disorder. *Journal of Affective Disorders,* 45: 5–18.

Kendler, K.S. and Gardner, C.O. (1998) Boundaries of major depression: An evaluation of *DSM-IV* criteria. *American Journal of Psychiatry,* 155: 172–177.

Kessler, R.C. McGonagle, K.A., Zhao, S., Nelson, C.B., Hughes, M., Eshleman, S., Wittchen, H.-U., and Kendler, K.S. (1994) Lifetime and 12-month prevalence of *DSM-III-R* psychiatric disorders in the United States: Results from the National Comorbidity Survey. *Archives of General Psychiatry,* 51: 8–19.

Kessler, R.C., Berglund, P., Demler, O., Jin, R., and Walters, E.E. (2005a) Lifetime prevalence and age-of-onset distributions of *DSM-IV* Disorders in the National Comorbidity Survey Replication. *Archives of General Psychiatry,* 62: 593–602.

Kessler, R.C., Brandenburg, N., Lane, M., Roy-Byrne, P., Stang, P.D., Stein, D.J., and Wittchen, H.-U. (2005b) Rethinking the duration requirement for Generalized Anxiety Disorder: Evidence from the National Comorbidity Survey Replication. *Psychological Medicine,* 35: 1073–1082.

Kessler, R.C., Merikangas, K.R., Berglund, P., Eaton, W.W., Koretz, D.S., and Walters, Ellen E. (2003) Mild disorders should not be eliminated from the *DSM-V. Archives of General Psychiatry,* 60: 1117–1122.

Kessler, R.C., Walters, E.E., and Wittchen, H.-U. (2004) Epidemiology, in R.G. Heimberg, C.L. Turk, and D.S. Mennin (eds), *Generalized Anxiety Disorder: Advances in Research and Practice.* New York: Guilford Press. pp. 29–50.

Kessler, R.C., Wittchen, H.-U., Abelson, J.M., McGonagle, K.A. et al. (1998) Methodological studies of the Composite International Diagnostic Interview (CIDI) in the US National Comorbidity Survey (NCS). *International Journal of Methods in Psychiatric Research,* 7: 33–55.

Kessler, R.C., Zhao, S., Blazer, D.G., and Swartz, M. (1997) Prevalence, correlates, and course of minor depression and major depression in the National Comorbidity Survey. *Journal of Affective Disorders,* 45:19–30.

Kirk, S.A. and Kutchins, H. (1994) Is bad writing a mental disorder? *New York Times*, 6/20/94, p. A17.

Kramer, P.D. (2005) *Against Depression*. New York: Viking.

Krueger, R.F., Watson, D., and Barlow, D.H. (2005) Introduction to the special section: Toward a dimensionally based taxonomy of psychopathology. *Journal of Abnormal Psychology*, 114: 491–493.

Langner, T.S. (1962) A twenty-two item screening score of psychiatric symptoms indicating impairment. *Journal of Health and Human Behavior*, 3: 269–276.

Manis, J.G., Brawer, M.J., Hunt, C.L., and Kercher, L.C. (1964) Estimating the prevalence of mental illness. *American Sociological Review*, 29: 84–89.

Mattisson, C., Bogren, M., Horstmann, V., Munk-Jorgensen, P., and Nettelbladt, P. (2007) The long-term course of depression in the Lundby Study. *Psychological Medicine*, 37: 883–891.

Moffitt, T.E., Harrington, H.L., Caspi, A., Kim-Cohen, J., Goldberg, D., Gregory, A.M., and Poulton, R. (2007) Depression and Generalized Anxiety Disorder: Cumulative and sequential comorbidity in a birth cohort followed prospectively to age 32 years. *Archives of General Psychiatry*, 64: 651–660.

Narrow, W.E., Rae, D.S., Robbins, L.N., and Regier, D.A. (2002) Revised prevalence estimates of mental disorders in the United States. *Archives of General Psychiatry*, 59: 115–123.

Robins, L.N., Helzer, J.E., Orvaschel, H., Anthony, J.C., Blazer, D.G., Burnam, A., and Burke, J.D., Jr. (1985) The diagnostic interview schedule, in W.W. Eaton and L.G. Kessler (eds), *Epidemiologic Field Methods in Psychiatry: The NIMH Epidemiologic Catchment Area Program*. New York: Academic Press. pp. 143–170.

Robins, L.N. and Regier, D.A. (eds) (1991) *Psychiatric Disorders in America: The Epidemiologic Catchment Area Study*. New York: Free Press.

Rogler, L.H., Malgady, R.G., and Tryon, W.W. (1992) Issues of memory in the Diagnostic Interview Schedule. *Journal of Nervous and Mental Disease*, 180: 215–222.

Ross, H.E., Swinson, R., Doumani, S., and Larkin, E.J. (1995) Diagnosing comorbidity in substance-abusers: A comparison of the test–retest reliability of two interviews. *American Journal of Drug and Alcohol Abuse*, 21: 167–185.

Rubio-Stipec, M., Peters, L., and Andrews, G. (1999) Test–retest reliability of the computerized CIDI (CIDI-Auto): Substance abuse modules. *Substance Abuse*, 20: 263–272.

Ruscio, A.M., Chiu, W.T., Roy-Byrne, P., Stang, P.E., Steing, D.J., Wittchen, H.-U., and Kessler, R.C. (2007) Broadening the definition of Generalized Anxiety Disorder: Effects on prevalence and associations with other disorders in the National Comorbidity Survey Replication. *Journal of Anxiety Disorders*, 21: 662–676.

Ruscio, A.M., Lane, M., Roy-Byrne, P., Stang, P.E., Stein, D.J., Wittchen, H.-U., and Kessler, R.C. (2005) Should excessive worry be required for a diagnosis of Generalized Anxiety Disorder? Results from the US National Comorbidity Survey Replication. *Psychological Medicine*, 35: 1761–1772.

Simon, G.E. and VonKorff, M. (1995) Recall of psychiatric history in cross-sectional surveys: Implications for epidemiologic research. *Epidemiologic Reviews*, 17: 221–227.

Srole, L., Langner, T.S., Michael, S.T., Kirkpatrick, P., Opler, M.K., and Rennie, T.A.C. (1978) *Mental Health in the Metropolis: The Midtown Manhattan Study* (Revised edition, with five new chapters, edited by L. Srole and A.K. Fischer). New York: New York University Press.

Sullivan, P.F., Kessler, R.C., and Kendler, K.S. (1998) Latent class analysis of lifetime depressive symptoms in the National Comorbidity Survey. *American Journal of Psychiatry*, 155: 1398–1406.

Wacker, H.R., Battegay, R., Muellejans, R., and Schloesser, C. (1990) Using the CIDI-C in the general population, in C.N. Stefanis, A.D. Rabavilas and C.R. Soldatos (eds), *Psychiatry: A World Perspective*. Amsterdam: Elsevier Science. pp. 138–143.

Wakefield, J.C. (1993) Limits of operationalization: A critique of Spitzer and Endicotts (1978) proposed operational criteria for mental disorder. *Journal of Abnormal Psychology*, 102: 160–172.

Wakefield, J.C. (1996) *DSM-IV*: Are We Making Diagnostic Progress? *Contemporary Psychology*, 41: 646–652.

Wakefield, J.C., Schmitz, M.F., First, M.B., and Horwitz, A.V. (2007) Extending the bereavement exclusion for major depression to other losses: Evidence from the National Comorbidity Survey. *Archives of General Psychiatry*, 64: 433–440.

Wakefield, J.C. and Spitzer, R.L. (2002) Why requiring clinical significance does not solve epidemiology's and *DSM*'s validity problem, in J.E. Helzer and J.J. Hudziak (eds), *Defining Psychopathology in the 21st Century: DSM-V and Beyond*. Washington, DC: American Psychiatric Publishing, Inc. pp. 31–40.

Watson, D. (2005) Rethinking the mood and anxiety disorders: A quantitative hierarchical model for *DSM-V*. *Journal of Abnormal Psychology*, 114: 522–536.

Wells, J.E. and Horwood, L.J. (2004) How accurate is recall of key symptoms of depression? A comparison of recall and longitudinal reports. *Psychological Medicine*, 34: 1001–1011.

Wells, K.B., Burnham, M. A., Leake, B., and Robins, L.N. (1988) Agreement between face-to-face and telephone-administered versions of the depression section of the NIMH Diagnostic Interview Schedule. *Journal of Psychiatric Research*, 22: 207–220.

Widiger, T.A., and Samuel, D.B. (2005) Diagnostic categories or dimensions? A question for the *Diagnostic and Statistical Manual of Mental Disorders – Fifth Edition*. *Journal of Abnormal Psychology*, 114: 494–504.

Wittchen, H.-U. (1994) Reliability and validity studies of the WHO-Composite International Diagnostic Interview (CIDI): A critical review. *Journal of Psychiatric Research*, 28: 57–84.

Wittchen, H.-U., Lachner, G., Wunderlich, U., and Pfister, H. (1998) Test–retest reliability of the computerized *DSM-IV* version of the Munich-Composite International Diagnostic Interview (M-CIDI). *Social Psychiatry and Psychiatric Epidemiology*, 33: 568–578.

3

Mental Health, Positive Psychology and the Sociology of the Self

Benedikt Rogge

INTRODUCTION

Mental health is a fuzzy concept. It is intertwined with social and cultural values, which are characteristically and legitimately diverse (Fulford, 2001). Hence, there is no bird's eye view of it but a variety of different perspectives (Pilgrim, 2005: 438). Established approaches to mental health focus on psychiatric disorder or psychological distress. That is they see mental health as the absence of symptoms of psychopathology. In this chapter, two different perspectives are described from positive psychology and the sociology of the self. Both have developed distinct theoretical concepts and delivered empirical evidence that complement the psychopathological view and are of high relevance to researchers and practitioners in the field of mental health.

The present contribution is structured as follows. First, as a background the psychiatric disorder and the psychological distress concept are briefly recapitulated. Then, I highlight the approach and contributions of positive psychology. Subsequently, I deal with the sociology of the self. For both perspectives, emergence, main theoretical assumptions, central empirical findings and merits and criticisms are described. The contribution ends with a short conclusion.

BACKGROUND: THE DISORDER AND THE DISTRESS APPROACH

Both the psychiatric disorder and the psychological distress approach (see for example Payton, 2009) conceive mental health indirectly as the absence of symptoms. Mental health is thus defined negatively by the absence of pathology, operationalized by cognitive, emotional, behavioural and (occasional) physical symptoms, defined in psychiatric classifications, such as DSM and ICD (Rogers and Pilgrim, 2005). However, there are major differences between these deficit approaches. First, proponents of the disorder concept assume a dichotomous illness entity (Kessler, 2002) whereas those championing the distress concept regard mental health as a continuum (Mirowsky and Ross, 2002). Thus, in the disorder concept, which is notably but not only advocated by psychiatrists, there is either a total absence or a total presence of psychiatric disorder (Horwitz, 2002: 145). Proponents of the distress concept have criticized this rationale as pathologizing. Instead, they focus on the relative absence of psychological burden (Mirowsky and Ross, 2003). Many of them see no qualitative difference between the depressive symptoms of a person with and a person without a diagnosis.

Second, the disciplinary affinities and aetiological assumptions differ. Rooted in the medical model of illness, the disorder concept traditionally pays special attention to the genetic, neurological and physiological determinants of mental health (Pilgrim, 2005). Disorders are seen as objective dysfunctions and assessed by a medically trained clinician. By contrast and emerging mainly from the social sciences, the distress approach considers nonpsychotic problems, for example, symptoms of anxiety and depression, as appearances of unusual stress (Mirowsky and Ross, 2003). Emphasis is put on the social causes of psychological problems, that is negative life events, chronic stressors or daily hassles.

Third, as a consequence, the involvement of subjects in the assessment of mental health differs. While the disorder approach does acknowledge subjective distress as a potential criterion for many disorders, ultimately the clinician's assessment is independent from it. The clinical diagnosis of an ego-syntonic disorder that is a disorder with an individual feeling no distress, for example the diagnosis of histrionic personality disorder, illustrates this reasoning. The distress approach, however, rejects the idea of an objective assessment of mental health and lets the subject assess her own psychological state. Methodically, instead of diagnostic inventories it draws on self-report scales consisting of standardized symptom checklists, for example the CES-D, BSI, GHQ (Mirowsky and Ross, 2002).

Finally, the two approaches use different reference norms. The clinical judgement in the disorder concept is based on the duration rules and cut-off points determined in the psychiatric classifications and manuals (Kessler, 2002). The distress concept, by contrast, refers to social reference norms, as provided by large scale survey data (a statistic or actuarial approach).

THE APPROACH OF POSITIVE PSYCHOLOGY

The emergence of positive psychology

Positive psychology represents one variant of a positive view of mental health to which, for example, the salutogenetic model of Antonovsky, Sen's capability approach and sociological quality of life research can all be subsumed. Positive psychology seeks to balance the emphasis on psychopathology that prevailed for so long in mental health research. It focuses on why people are and stay healthy and well; on their flourishing and functioning rather than on their dysfunctions and disorders. It centres around notions such as 'well-being', 'happiness', 'flourishing', 'positive affect', 'life satisfaction' and 'domain satisfaction'. As a historical point of reference, scholars often cite Aristotle, who suggested that all things aimed at 'the good', which he called 'eudaimonia'. Aristotle saw eudaimonia as the most perfect and worthwhile of all things, as, so to speak, the 'most final' of all goals (Ackrill, 2006: 46–47).

The more recent roots of positive psychology lie in the humanistic psychology movement of the 1950s and 1960s (Ryan and Deci, 2001). It claimed that humans strived for self-actualization and the realization of their potential. Scholars such as Abraham Maslow and Carl Rogers created the vision of a fully-functioning, healthy and happy individual. They criticized the widespread focus on psychopathology and sought to deliver a positive view of mental health. In an oft-quoted sentence, Maslow (1968) put it like this: 'It is as if Freud supplied us the sick half of psychology and we must now fill it out with the healthy half'.

From the 1980s on, what Diener and colleagues (2009: 16) call an 'affective revolution' put positive feelings as a major topic onto the agenda of academic psychology. Ever since, research on well-being and happiness has increased. In 1998, the US psychologist Martin Seligman adopted Maslow's term 'positive psychology' to group previous studies and initiate a further boost of research (Seligman and Csikszentmihalyi, 2000). In the meantime, positive psychology has greatly expanded. Research centres, academic conferences, awards, a dedicated section of the America Psychological Association, an Oxford University Press Series, Master's study schemes and a significant number of book publications all contain the label 'positive psychology'. Moreover, the amount of journal publications devoted to the study of happiness and human flourishing has seen a tremendous upsurge. In addition, positive psychologists have published self-help books, as well as specific practical applications and interventions for counsellors and therapists (e.g. Magyar-Moe, 2009). So far, positive psychology has predominantly been rooted in and promoted by the work of North American researchers. It is yet becoming increasingly international.

Central assumptions of positive psychology

Positive psychology studies 'the processes and conditions that contribute to optimal functioning and flourishing in human beings' (Lucas, 2007b: 686).

Its starting assumption is that people all over the world seek happiness and well-being (Diener et al., 2003a: 420). Individual happiness is seen as a source of health, prosocial behaviour, work productivity and other markers of success and functioning (Lyubomirsky et al., 2005). It helps individuals to broaden and build resources for the future, for example to acquire new skills (Fredrickson, 2001). Thus, it is considered as beneficial for both the individual and society.

The notions of well-being and happiness are often used interchangeably. In the narrow sense, happiness is a specific emotion referring to feelings of pleasure or comfort. Well-being refers to 'being well in general', an individual's global evaluation of her life as a whole (Lucas, 2007a). Here, I concentrate on the latter. As to the problem of objectivity and subjectivity in the conception of well-being, two different theoretical variants have developed, the 'hedonic approach' and the 'eudaimonic approach' (Ryan and Deci, 2001).

The hedonic approach uses the notion of 'subjective well-being' (SWB) as its core research construct (Huppert and Baylis, 2004). 'A person is said to have high [SWB] if she or he experiences life satisfaction and frequent joy' (Diener et al., 1997: 25). SWB is viewed as residing within the individual who is seen as the only knowledgeable informant on it (Diener, 1993). SWB researchers thus claim to fully adopt the respondent's perspective. The SWB concept is not grounded in clinical symptoms as the disorder and the distress concept. Specifically, it focuses on emotional and cognitive processes rather than behavioural criteria.

According to Ed Diener, one of the leading psychological researchers in the field, SWB is an umbrella term encompassing four more specific concepts (Diener et al., 2003b). These are: (a) pleasant affect, for example joy, elation, happiness, mental health; (b) unpleasant affect, for example guilt, shame, sadness, anxiety, worry, anger, stress, depression; (c) global satisfaction with one's life; (d) domain satisfaction, for example work, family, leisure, health, finances. Having deep roots in survey research, the SWB approach uses mostly quantitative self-report measures that operationalize people's everyday feelings. Life satisfaction scales, for instance, include items such as, 'Taking all things together, how would you say things are these days – would you say you are very happy, pretty happy, or not too happy?' (Schwarz and Strack, 1999). In sum, the SWB concept delivers a positive, nonsymptom-based, continuous, bottom-up oriented and subjective approach to mental health. In a reversal of deficit approaches, note that the second grouping about negative affect conceives SWB in terms of the relative absence of these feelings.

The eudaimonic approach, by contrast, centres around the notion of 'psychological well-being' (PWB). It postulates a human need for self-actualization using various criteria that are specified by the researcher. Ryff and colleagues (e.g. Ryff, 1989) suggested six dimensions of PWB that are autonomy, environmental mastery, personal growth, positive relations with others, purpose in life and self-acceptance. These are operationalized by items such as 'I like most parts of my personality' (self-acceptance) and 'I sometimes feel as if I've done all there is to do in life' (purpose in life). The concept of 'flourishing' (Ryff and Singer, 1998) additionally incorporates 'social well-being'. Others have conceptualised PWB as 'happiness plus meaning' (Seligman, 2002). For these authors, meaning stands, for example for the feeling to lead a purposeful life and to be part of something larger.

Compared to the SWB approach, the PWB concept is characterized by a relativization of subjectivity. In this regard, it resembles the disorder concept. Both approaches draw on the concept of functioning, in terms of a 'dysfunction' and a 'fully functioning individual' respectively. Critics have argued against the culture-specificity and Western normativity of such approaches (Rogers and Pilgrim, 2005). Still others have noted the deficit of construct validity in PWB, as determinants and outcomes are mixed up (Veenhoven, 2008). In the following, I restrict myself to psychological research on SWB.

Empirical research in positive psychology

A leitmotif and central finding of empirical research in positive psychology is that SWB is weakly related to external circumstances and strongly related to personality (e.g. Sheldon and Lyubomirsky, 2009).[1] External circumstances, here, are meant to include an individual's financial situation, work situation, living situation, sex, age, ethnicity, health and also major life events. The only exceptions are social relationships and marital status that are positively related to SWB (Ryan and Deci, 2001). As a consequence, positive psychologists see SWB as a fairly stable phenomenon with much inter-individual but little intra-individual variance.

What does positive psychology base its observation on? To begin with, empirical studies found there was no strong, linear association between income and well-being. Cross-sectional data demonstrated that wealthier people were happier, particularly within poorer groups and nations (Diener and Biswas-Diener, 2002). Yet the picture changed with longitudinal evidence. The economist Easterlin (Easterlin, 1974) famously made the point that economic circumstances only had a small effect on SWB. One oft-quoted, illustrative study found that lottery winners did not report higher well-being levels than the investigated control group (Brickman et al., 1978). Subsequent research confirmed the finding that income increases were not accompanied by proportional increases in SWB, particularly past a threshold where an individual's basic needs are satisfied (Easterlin, 2003).

To explain this, positive psychologists suggested an adaptation effect. Humans are assumed to find themselves in a 'hedonic treadmill' (Frederick, 2007). This metaphor suggests that throughout their lives, individuals pursue greater happiness but their happiness remains constant because they adjust to the changed circumstances. This idea was then related to the one of a genetically determined set-point for SWB (Headey and Wearing, 1989). According to the set-point model, each person enjoys an individual, stable SWB set-point to which he or she inevitably returns after any change. This included major positive and negative life events such as marriage, job loss, divorce or widowhood. Consequently, an individual's SWB level remains in a constant, dynamic equilibrium. Empirical research delivered some support for the adaptation hypothesis. Besides, the set-point argument was backed up by heritability studies. The twin study by Tellegen and colleagues (Tellegen et al., 1988) showed that monozygotic twins were much more similar in SWB than dizygotic twins even when growing up in different environments. The conclusion drawn from these studies was that genes account for 80 percent of the stable variance in long-term reports of SWB and of 50 percent of immediate SWB (Lykken and Tellegen, 1996).

So it was concluded that SWB was largely independent of external circumstances. Yet, considerable differences were found between individuals. Positive psychologists assume that a large part of this variance is accounted for by personality traits. Extraversion and neuroticism were reported to be primary links between personality and SWB (Diener and Lucas, 1999; Diener et al., 2003a). Extroverts were found to have better SWB whereas people with high levels of neuroticism have lower SWB scores. Optimism was also reported to positively relate to SWB, agreeableness and conscientiousness only slightly. The assumed stability of personality traits over time explained the relative stability of SWB. Three different explanations for the association of personality and SWB have been advanced (Diener et al., 2003a: 408): (a) differential set-points of SWB, as seen above; (b) differential emotional reactivities; (c) differential cognitive processing of emotional information. Particularly the latter explanation stimulated vast research. Overly positive self-evaluations, (exaggerated) perceptions of mastery, external attributions of failure and internal attributions of success and downward comparisons were found to be correlated with SWB (Ryan and Deci, 2001). Taylor and Brown (1999) explicitly speak of the 'illusion of mental health' as distorting information in a positive direction. Finally, also behavioural and motivational parameters, for example the pursuit of personally meaningful goals, were found to relate to SWB (Diener et al., 1999).[2]

The devaluation of external circumstances in positive psychology differs markedly from the traditional focus in mental health research in the social sciences and in sociology in particular. In the meantime, however, growing empirical evidence, including from within positive psychology, indicates this devaluation as well as the assumption of SWB stability were too hasty. Economic circumstances have turned out to be more important than previously suggested. Headey and colleagues (Headey et al., 2004), for instance, show that the combined effects of wealth, income and consumption affect SWB more than assumed so far. In particular, life events matter considerably more to SWB than thought. This point is elaborated below. Numerous national panel studies have yielded four major findings that contradict some core tenets of set-point theory:

- First, there are life events after which complete adaptation does not occur. One of the most researched examples is unemployment (Clark, 2006; Clark and Oswald, 1994; Lucas, 2007a; Lucas et al., 2004). In fact, in Western societies people who experience unemployment do not return to baseline levels of SWB, even years after becoming re-employed. Besides, long-term unemployment does not entail SWB habituation. Similar applies to disability.
- Second, SWB effects differ across life events (Diener et al., 2006). Whilst adaptation to marriage seems to be fairly quick on average, adaptation to widowhood can take several years (Lucas, 2007a).
- Third and very importantly, there are substantial differences among individuals in their reactions to life events. After marriage, for instance, people who primordially react strongly are still far from baseline levels several years later (Lucas et al., 2003). This includes long-lasting positive changes in SWB for some and significant declines for others.
- Fourth, SWB is not independent from external circumstances. One example is the 'social norm effect of unemployment'. Clark and colleagues (Clark, 2003; Clark et al., 2008) found that the more people are unemployed within an unemployed person's context (partnership, household, reference group), the better off he or she is in terms of SWB. This association has been replicated by many other studies. Other circumstantial factors are likely to be of greater relevance to SWB than assumed in positive psychology, too. Sociological SWB research has provided supporting evidence for this (Veenhoven, 2008). Recently, Diener and colleagues acknowledged the role of circumstances and the immense inter-individual variability in reaction to life events and developed an updated version of adaptation theory (Diener et al., 2006).

Merits and criticisms of positive psychology

A clear merit of the positive psychology movement is its promotion of a positive view of mental health. Not the absence of pathological symptoms but the presence of emotional well-being is key: this is a corrective to a defect-only approach from psychiatry and clinical psychology. It fruitfully complements and might even challenge the negative approach to mental health. Also, psychological SWB research looks at people's subjective perceptions. By this, it has greatly contributed to establishing an understanding of well-being beyond pecuniary and economic factors, as it was long prevalent not only within economics. By investigating the association of cognitive, motivational and behavioural factors with SWB, it illuminates in what ways individuals make a difference. For example, sociologists might learn from this to take the individual's role more seriously. Incorporating individual parameters to a greater extent in their research will help to overcome their often one-sided focus on structural and contextual determinants of mental health outcomes (Thoits, 2006).

As for the critique of positive psychology, the uncritical devaluation of external circumstances has been mentioned. Some psychologists still continue it despite the empirical evidence. Besides, inter-individual variance needs to be borne in mind. The strict assumption of SWB set-points was falsified. Future research needs to scrutinize closely how people vary in SWB and in what affects it. Actually, this point has already been made in the path-breaking studies by George Brown and colleagues about 20 years ago (Brown, 2005; Brown and Harris, 1989). They had found that critical life events spawn differential mental health impacts depending on the meaning individuals ascribe to them and contextual conditions.

A further weakness of positive psychology is that it largely de-contextualises SWB. Yet, cognitive, motivational and behavioural processes need to be related to social background characteristics. They are not equally distributed within society. For example, mastery is less prevalent in lower social status groups (Pearlin et al., 2007). Investigating the interface of personal, social and structural processes will prove rewarding in the future (see also Schnittker and McLeod, 2005).

Some clinicians have criticized SWB methodology arguing that survey data cannot distinguish between the façade and the reality of well-being (e.g. Shedler et al., 1993). Empirical evidence shows that the façade of well-being, for example defence mechanisms such as a repressive coping style, is linked to negative psychophysiological outcomes and mental disease (Weinberger, 1990).

SWB research has also been criticized on methodological grounds with regard to difficulties of interpreting scores from SWB self-report scales. Beyond an individual's contexts and situational moods (Schwarz and Strack, 1999), differential response patterns are likely to distort SWB scores as people exhibit internalized habits of displaying emotions that, again, vary with social characteristics (Bendelow, in this handbook). In addition, it is unclear how individuals interpret SWB scales and in particular the scale end points (Frederick, 2007). With time, a subject's interpretation of the scale points might change rather than the SWB level itself.[3]

Finally, positive psychology has been criticized at a normative level. One reproach is that the construct of well-being is a specific corollary of Western individualistic culture (Carlisle et al., 2009). Then, a Foucauldian argument would be that SWB research constructs new normalities by placing on the individual the onus of well-being (ibid.). Conceptions such as the Sustainable Happiness model by Lyubomirski and Sheldon (Lyubomirsky et al., 2005) seem to suggest that greater happiness can be achieved by anyone who is only willing to steadily work on his or her daily activities, for example by gratitude visits, strength dates, thought control and the performance of selfless acts. SWB research is thus criticized for following the ideological rationale of individualization and permanent optimization. In this, it differs from the discrepancy-oriented focus of the disorder and the distress approach. It is therefore said to establish and spread happiness as a social norm echoing the growing medicalization and pathologization of negative feelings by psychiatry (Horwitz and Wakefield, 2007).

THE APPROACH OF THE SOCIOLOGY OF THE SELF

The emergence of the sociology of the self

The sociology of the self conceives mental health as intricately interwoven with an individual's identity process. It neither adopts a negative, nor a positive view of mental health but follows an ipsative[4] rationale concentrating, in the first place, on how the individual sees their social reality. Other theoretical approaches sharing the emphasis on the self are, *inter alia*, psychological self-discrepancy theory (Higgins, 1987), psychological self-concept theory (Rosenberg, 1979) and psychotherapeutical consistency theory (Grawe, 2004). The sociology of the self centres around the notions of 'self' and 'identity' combining them with concepts such as 'congruence', 'consistency', 'coherence' or 'discrepancy'. Its relevance for mental health research is grounded in the assumption that self-consistency and self-congruence are to be considered as basic human needs (Grawe, 2004). The emergence of well-being, distress and disorder are thus closely related to whether an individual lives in agreement with herself or not. Besides, the sociology of the self addresses some of the problems we have encountered in the approach of positive psychology.

Historically, the sociology of the self[5] goes back to Northern American pragmatism of the early twentieth century and symbolic interactionism (Callero, 2003). The work of George H. Mead (1934) is still a crucial point of reference. In the second part of the twentieth century, the sociology of the self was refined (e.g. McCall and Simmons, 1966) and a structural variant emerged (Stryker, 1980: 2008). Towards the end of the century, it was further backed up by the renaissance of interactionist thinking in the social sciences (Plummer, 2000). Since then, the sociology of the self has been used in mental health research (e.g. Thoits, 1992). In general, it seems to be increasingly acknowledged in the sociology of health (Schnittker and McLeod, 2005).

Central assumptions of the sociology of the self

To outline the theoretical contours of the sociology of the self, we need to go back a little. Mead (1934) suggested understanding the self as a dialogic structure between a plurality of 'me's on the one hand, and the 'I' on the other hand. The 'me's stand for the expectations that others have towards an individual, as assumed and internalized by the individual herself. They structure, albeit never fully determine, the 'I' which represents spontaneity, creativity and a 'constitutional surplus of impulse's (Joas, 1997: 118). Most importantly, the 'me's become part of the individual's self-identity that is how she sees and reflexively thinks about herself. There are at least three different types of 'me's (Stets, 2006). First, there are social identities, that is the social categories an individual thinks she belongs to, for instance, 'female', 'elderly' or 'white'. Second, there are role identities bundling the social expectations an individual sees herself exposed to, for example 'mother', 'friend' or 'boss'. Whilst social identities are based on the supposed, general uniformity of the group members, role identities refer to a specific complementary relationship between interacting individuals. Role identities differ in their psychological centrality for an individual forming what some have called a prominence hierarchy (McCall and Simmons, 1966). Third, there are 'person identities' spanning across all roles and situations and standing for a person's view of her individual characteristics, for example dominance or submissiveness.[6]

Along with a focus on the notion of self goes a focus on the notion of meaning that is the ways people make sense of the social reality they live in. The individual attribution of meaning goes hand in hand with the above-described structures of the self and vice versa. However, self and meaning are to be located within context. In a very broad sense, the notion of context encompasses historical, structural, cultural, social and situational conditions (Callero, 2003). These conditions restrict and enable the attribution of meaning that, in turn, structures an individual's action.

The identity process as a whole is conceived as a permanent dynamic. Characteristically, it is guided by the basic need for self-consistency. That is an individual's view of herself strives towards matching with her perceptions of herself in social reality and vice versa. This process can be called self-verification (Stets, 2006). The need for self-consistency includes at least two separate concepts. Self-concordance that is the degree to which an individual's goals or role identities are compatible and do not conflict with each other. And self-congruence that is, as described, the degree to which an individual perceives the self as verified.[7] Enduring feelings of self-incongruence make it likely that perceptions of reality are changed, for example through change of her own action, or that her self-identity is modified, for example through a reordering of her prominence hierarchy (Burke, 2006). The process of self-verification is affected by both social context factors, such as major life events and personal agency, for example the purposeful acquirement of new social roles (Thoits, 2003, 2006).

Importantly, an individual's feelings of self-incongruence are assumed to relate to lower self-esteem, lower well-being and increased subjective distress. Burke (1991, 1996) and colleagues even hypothesized that situational identity verification produced positive emotion and situational nonverification negative emotion. Theoretically, it is assumed that enduring feelings of self-incongruence relate to the experience of subjective distress. Besides, they are considered to operate as triggers or accelerators in the development of psychiatric disorders (Grawe, 2004).

The sociology of the self is not rooted in a homogeneous methodical tradition. Many researchers use qualitative methods in order not to bypass individual's accounts of meaning (Simon, 1997: 260). Semi-structured and in-depth interviews are seen as particularly pertinent for a fine-grained analysis of an individual's self (Kvale, 1996). Positive psychologists such as Ed Diener also recommended the use of qualitative methods to gather information that 'can be customized to a specific respondent's life' (Diener, 1993: 143). Specifically, qualitative methods help to address the neglect of inter-individual variability as seen in the criticisms of positive psychology. However, quantitative methods are also applied by sociologists of the self. Characteristically, they explore individuals' prominence hierarchies and levels of identity congruence. Interesting methodical instruments have been delivered by the psychologists Grawe and colleagues (Holtforth and Grawe, 2000, 2003). With the help of their congruence scales, they explore people's motivational goals and their perceptions to what extent these are achieved.

Empirical research in the sociology of the self

Theory and empiricism in the sociology of the self are less uniform than, for example, the paradigm of positive psychology. It delivers a broad framework encompassing many empirical studies not dealing with the concepts of self-congruence and self-consistency. In the following, I restrict myself to depicting research that is relevant in the context of mental health.

A specific characteristic of empirical research within the framework of the sociology of the self is its focus on self-congruence as emerging within an individual's proximal contexts of interaction. Within these interactional contexts, 'reflected appraisals' are of high relevance. Reflected appraisals are an individual's 'perceptions of self-relevant meanings' (Burke, 1991: 837). For example, in a study on the identity process of homosexuals, Kaufman and Johnson (2004) showed that negative reactions, particularly from friends and family, impaired the respondents' feelings of self-congruence. Other studies confirmed that negative reflected appraisals reduce self-congruence. These appraisals are, in turn, associated with more general social categories. For instance, Sheeran and Abraham (1994) found that unemployed people think significant others evaluate them considerably worse than employed people. In addition, social structure comes into play. The higher the social rank of the person to which the reflected appraisal is attributed, the more important an individual deems it (Cast et al., 1999). Reflected appraisals can also increase feelings of self-congruence. Social approval of particular activities increases their relevance for an individual's identity process (Ball and Orford, 2002).

Other studies have dealt with the relations of an individual's identity process and the attribution of meaning. Life events such as marriage, unemployment and divorce have different meanings for individuals (Reynolds and Turner, 2008). Unemployment, for instance, is interpreted as an existential tragedy by some but others might experience it as a release from a burden (Ezzy, 2001). This depends on the social context. In a study of chronically ill people, Charmaz (1983) showed that many of their respondents displayed discrediting definitions of self. These perceptions of self were related to the respondents' feeling of not meeting the expectations of significant others. The perception of supportive and alleviating others, by contrast, bolstered the identity process of the participants and increased their feelings of self-congruence. Similarly, Francis (1997) set out how the meaning individuals give to their divorce and widowhood can be positively reconstructed within support groups. The redefinition of the respondents' life situation within the context of the support groups improved their self-congruence and emotional well-being.

The likelihood of feelings of self-congruence is not equally distributed in society. It depends on individual's material, social and cultural resources.

Williams (1998) suggested the concept of 'emotional capital' to better understand social inequalities in this process. He stresses that individuals' capability to protect the boundaries of the self is linked to the material and psychosocial conditions they live in. But also socio-cultural norms and institutional mechanisms affect levels of self-congruence. Stigma research illustrates this. On the one hand, there is no direct relation between stigma and self-evaluation as modified labelling theory has made clear. Camp and colleagues (Camp et al., 2002), for instance, show how women with the diagnosis of a psychiatric disorder manage to distance themselves from the stigma of being mentally ill and to maintain levels of self-congruence. On the other hand, labelled persons are confronted with disapproval, rejection and exclusion in numerous interactional contexts due to the gravity of their stigmatization. This makes the challenge of conserving self-congruence generally more difficult for them (Rogers and Pilgrim, 2005: 27).

This of course applies to other stigmatized social categories, too, as the disabled, the unemployed, etc. Equally, it is valid for an individual's subjective social rank. The lower a person locates herself on the ladder of social stratification, the less likely is she to experience self-congruence which, in turn, is associated with increased depressive symptoms (Gilbert, 2000). In this context, some authors have criticized the general neglect of culture in mental health research (McLeod and Lively, 2007; Simon, 2000, 2007). They argue social norms, collective values and shared beliefs affect self-congruence and mental health outcomes and deserve further scrutiny.

A number of studies has explicitly scrutinized the association of self-congruence and other mental health outcomes. Paul and Moser (2006), for instance, investigated people's work identities. They operationalized identity incongruence as levels of employment commitment that are incompatible with a person's employment situation, that is having high employment commitment while being unemployed and vice versa. Incongruence in the work role was found to be associated with well-being, distress, depression and anxiety. Burke and Stets even assumed that situational self-verification registered positive emotion and incongruence and lack of self-verification registered negative emotion (Stets, 2006). They found some empirical support for these hypotheses. For instance, self-verification was found to be associated with self-esteem and mastery (Stets and Harrod, 2002). Incongruence in a positive direction that is, for example, social reactions that are more positive than expected, does yet not entail negative but positive emotion. Stets and Asencio (2008) thus stress the necessity to also include the need for self-enhancement in theorizing on the relationship between the identity process and emotions.

Finally, narrative and biographical researchers have explored how individuals give meaning to their past as a whole. They have placed special emphasis on the construct of narrative coherence, that is the temporal, autobiographical, causal and thematic coherence of an individual's self-narrative (McAdams, 2006). Narrative coherence also follows the principle of consistency and is directly related to an individual's view of herself. People vary considerably in narrative coherence. Sufferers from chronic illness, for instance, use different frameworks to tell their life story. Specifically, they vary in to what extent they describe their illness as biographically disruptive (Richardson et al., 2006). Similar applies to the narratives of job loss that can be heroic or tragic (Ezzy, 2001). Importantly, narrative coherence has been found to be positively related with happiness and life satisfaction (Baerger and McAdams, 1999). Besides, therapists and counsellors have recognized the potentially healing effects of storytelling (Rosenthal, 2003).

Merits and criticisms of the sociology of the self

The most obvious merit of the sociology of the self is its focus on concepts such as self-congruence, self-consistency and self-coherence. By this, it delivers a perspective with a pronounced idiosyncratic ('idiographic') appreciation of the individual. The individual's perceptions and attributions of meaning are placed centre stage. Particularly if linked to the use of qualitative research methods, it is capable of providing a detailed account of an individual's concerns, meanings and life worlds. The neglect of inter-individual variance, for example as seen in life event research in positive psychology, can be countered by this approach.

However, as a consequence of this there is a tendency of some researchers to overemphasize the power of the subject and neglect the role of structural and contextual conditions. We have already seen this criticism in relation to the positive psychology movement. Other sociologists of the self, by contrast, conceive the identity process as a social automatism. Actually, neither seems to be inherent to the wider theoretical framework. The sociology of the self, as depicted here, seeks to avoid any sort of reductionism and attempts to deal with both structure and agency (Thoits, 2006). It addresses the complexity of the identity process and mental health dynamics. Specifically, it concentrates on the complex mediating mechanisms that explain mental health. In doing so, it looks at dynamic processes rather than states (McLeod and Lively, 2007: 290). Then, it focuses on an individual's proximal contexts of social interaction that is usually neglected by other approaches while yet being of crucial relevance to mental health. Besides, being interested in the inter-linkage of macro- and micro-levels, it helps researchers to bridge two perspectives that are often seen in opposition to each other. By this, the sociology of the self contributes to integrating the psychological focus on personality and the sociological focus on structure. The variance within both individuals and groups can thereby be further illuminated (Schnittker and McLeod, 2005).

Finally, the sociology of the self delivers perhaps the least heteronomous and ideological approach to mental health as it focuses on the individual's view of herself and reality. Yet, as with subjective well-being research, the lack of an objective assessment of the individual's state can be criticized from a clinical perspective.

CONCLUSION

Positive psychology and the sociology of the self complement extant research on psychiatric disorder and psychological distress. They deliver perspectives in their own right and contribute to an improved understanding of mental health processes. A very interesting avenue for further study is to explore the relations between the different constructs dealt with here. Self-incongruence and low well-being are conceptually distinct from psychological distress and psychiatric disorder (Payton, 2009). However, they are likely to operate as precursors of psychiatric disorder. As Grawe (2004) suggests, enduring feelings of self-incongruence may lead to the onset of psychiatric disorder. Investigating the dynamic transformation of self-incongruence into psychiatric disorder and how this is linked to structural, interactional and individual factors will be a highly interesting topic for future research.

NOTES

1 Note, however, that economic and sociological SWB research differs in this regard (Veenhoven, 2008). The so-called, 'livability paradigm' has defended and evidenced the influence of external circumstances on SWB.

2 Note that, for reasons of scope, I do not deal with the dynamics of SWB over the life course nor its variance across nations and cultures but see, for example Easterlin (2006) and Diener et al. (1995).

3 For instance, at a specific point of time, the scale point 'very happy' might stand for a family home with a kid whilst five years later, 'very happy' might represent a family home with two kids plus two cars. I think this is not only a methodological problem. An underlying question is if human SWB is conceived as a homeostatic or a heterostatic entity. Much of SWB research seems to follow a homeostatic rationale (e.g. Diener et al., 2009: S. 16). Yet, other scholars such as Antonovsky and Frankl have proposed a heterostatic view of life satisfaction emphasizing the human need to permanently create new goals – and thus never ever reach the scale end point.

4 In psychological methods, an 'ipsative assessment' indicates an assessment of an individual's state with regard to prior assessments rather than social norms or external criteria (Broverman, 1962). However, here I use the term in a conceptual sense rather than a methodological one.

5 The theoretical conception of the self depicted in the following is rooted in the tradition of sociological social psychology (McLeod and Lively, 2007). The Foucauldian approach to the self is not dealt with here despite its potential usefulness for mental health research (but see Callero, 2003).

6 However, there is a difference to the concept of personality traits as conceived by psychologists. Person identities are subject to individuals' reflexive view of themselves and no fixed, stable entities as personality traits.

7 Other authors such as Burke (1991) speak of 'identity congruence' which relates to the congruence within one particular role rather than the self as a whole.

REFERENCES

Ackrill, J.L. (2006) Aristotle on eudaimonia. In O. Höffe, (ed.) *Aristoteles. Nikomachische Ethik.* Berlin: Akademie Verlag. pp. 39–62.

Baerger, D.R. and McAdams, D.P. (1999) Life story coherence and its relation to psychological well-being. *Narrative Inquiry,* 9: 69–96.

Ball, M. and Orford, J. (2002) Meaningful patterns of activity amongst the long-term inner city unemployed: A qualitative study. *Journal of Community and Applied Social Psychology,* 12: 377–396.

Brickman, P., Coates, D. and Janoff-Bulman, R. (1978) Lottery winners and accident victims: Is happiness relative? *Journal of Personality and Social Psychology,* 36: 917–927.

Broverman, D.M. (1962) Normative and ipsative measurement in psychology. *Psychological Review,* 69: 295–305.

Brown, G.W. (2005) The social origins of depression and the role of meaning. In A., Heath, J. Ermisch and D. Gallie, (eds) *Understanding Social Change.* Oxford: Oxford University Press. pp. 255–290.

Brown, G.W. and Harris, T.O. (1989) *Life Events and Illness.* London: Unwin Hyman.

Burke, P.J. (1991) Identity processes and social stress. *American Sociological Review*, 56: 836–849.

Burke, P.J. (1996) Social identities and psychosocial stress. In H.B. Kaplan, (ed.) *Psychosocial Stress. Perspectives on Structure, Theory, Life-course, and Methods.* San Diego: Academic Press. pp. 141–174.

Burke, P.J. (2006) Identity change. *Social Psychology Quarterly*, 69: 81–96.

Callero, P.L. (2003) The sociology of the self. *Annual Review of Sociology*, 29: 115–133.

Camp, D.L., Finlay, W.M.L. and Lyons, E. (2002) Is low self-esteem an inevitable consequence of stigma? An example from women with chronic mental health problems. *Social Science and Medicine*, 55: 823–834.

Carlisle, S., Henderson, G. and Hanlon, P.W. (2009) 'Wellbeing': a collateral casualty of modernity. *Social Science and Medicine*, 69: 1556–1560.

Cast, A.D., Stets, J.E. and Burke, P.J. (1999) Does the self conform to the view of others? *Social Psychology Quarterly*, 62: 68–82.

Charmaz, K. (1983) Loss of self: a fundamental form of suffering in the chronically ill. *Sociology of Health and Illness*, 5: 168–195.

Clark, A.E. (2003) Unemployment as a social norm: psychological evidence from panel data. *Journal of Labor Economics*, 21: 323–351.

Clark, A.E. (2006) A note on unhappiness and unemployment duration. *IZA Discussion Papers*, 2406:

Clark, A.E. and Oswald, A.J. (1994) Unhappiness and unemployment. *Economic Journal*, 104: 648–659.

Clark, A.E. Knabe, A. and Rätzel, S. (2008) Unemployment as a social norm in Germany. *SOE Papers on Multidisciplinary Panel Data Research*, 132.

Diener, E. (1993) Assessing subjective well-being: progress and opportunities. *Social Indicators Research*, 31: 103–157.

Diener, E. and Biswas-Diener, R. (2002) Will money increase subjective well-being? A literature review and guide to needed research. *Social Indicators Research*, 57: 119–169.

Diener, E. and Lucas, R.E. (1999) Personality and subjective well-being. In D., Kahnemann, E., Diener, and N. Schwarz, (eds) *Well-being: the Foundations of Hedonic Psychology.* New York: Russell Sage Foundation. pp. 213–229.

Diener, E., Diener, M. and Diener, C. (1995) Factors predicting the subjective well-being of nations. *Journal of Personality and Social Psychology*, 69: 851–864.

Diener, E., Suh, E. and Oishi, S. (1997) Recent findings on subjective well-being. *Indian Journal of Clinical Psychology*, 24: 25–41.

Diener, E., Suh, E.M., Lucas, R.E. and Smith, H.L. (1999) Subjective well-being. Three decades of progress. *Psychological Bulletin*, 125: 276–302.

Diener, E., Oishi, S. and Lucas, R.E. (2003a) Personality, culture, and subjective well-being: Emotional and cognitive evaluations of life. *Annual Review of Psychology*, 54: 403–425.

Diener, E., Scollon, C.N. and Lucas, R.E. (2003b) The evolving concept of subjective well-being: the multifaceted nature of happiness. *Advances in Cell Agina and Gerontology*, 15: 187–219.

Diener, E., Lucas, R.E. and Scollon, C.N. (2006) Beyond the hedonic treadmill: revising the adaptation theory of well-being. *American Psychologist*, 61: 305–314.

Diener, E., Lucas, R.E., Schimmack, U. and Helliwell, J.F. (2009) *Well-being for Public Policy.* Oxford: Oxford University Press.

Easterlin, R.A. (1974) Does economic growth improve the human lot? Some empirical evidence. In P.A. David, and M.W. Reder, (eds) *Nations and Households in Economic Growth: Essays in Honour of Moses Abramowitz.* New York: Academy Press. pp. 89–125.

Easterlin, R.A. (2003) Building a better theory of well-being. *IZA Discussion Papers*, 742.

Easterlin, R.A. (2006) Life cycle happiness and its sources – Intersections of psychology, economics, and demography. *Journal of Economic Psychology*, 27: 463–482.

Ezzy, D. (2001) *Narrating Unemployment.* Burlington: Ashgate.

Francis, L.E. (1997) Ideology and interpersonal emotion management: Redefining identity in two support groups. *Social Psychology Quarterly*, 60: 153–171.

Frederick, S. (2007) Hedonic treadmill. In R. Baumeister, and Vohs (eds) *Encyclopedia of Social Psychology*. London: SAGE. pp. 419–420.

Fredrickson, B.L. (2001) The role of positive emotions in positive psychology: the broaden-and-build theory of positive emotions. *American Psychologist*, 56: 218–226.

Fulford, K.W.M. (2001) 'What is (mental) disease?': an open letter to Christopher Boorse. *Journal of Medical Ethics*, 27: 80–85.

Gilbert, P. (2000) The relationship of shame, social anxiety and depression: the role of the evaluation of social rank. *Clinical Psychology and Psychotherapy*, 7: 174–189.

Grawe, K. (2004) *Psychological Therapy*. Seattle: Hogrefe & Huber.

Headey, B. and Wearing, A. (1989) Personality, life events, and subjective well-being: toward a dynamic equilibrium model. *Journal of Personality and Social Psychology*, 57: 731–739.

Headey, B., Muffels, R. and Mark, W. (2004) Money doesn't buy happiness ... Or does it? A reconsideration based on the combined effects of wealth, income and consumption. *IZA Discussion Papers*, 1218.

Higgins, E.T. (1987) Self-discrepancy – a theory relating self and affect. *Psychological Review*, 94: 319–340.

Holtforth, M.G. and Grawe, K. (2000) Questionnaire for the analysis of motivational schemas. *Zeitschrift fur Klinische Psychologie-Forschung und Praxis*, 29: 170–179.

Holtforth, M.G. and Grawe, K. (2003) The incongruence questionnaire (INK). An instrument for the analysis of motivational incongruence. *Zeitschrift fur Klinische Psychologie und Psychotherapie*, 32: 315–323.

Horwitz, A.V. (2002) Outcomes in the sociology of mental health and illness: Where have we been and where are we going? *Journal of Health and Social Behavior*, 43: 143–151.

Horwitz, A.V. and Wakefield, J.C. (2007) *The Loss of Sadness. How Psychiatry Transformed Normal Sorrow into Depressive Disorder*. Oxford: Oxford University Press.

Huppert, F.A. and Baylis, N. (2004) Well-being: toward an integration of psychology, neurobiology, and social science. *Philosophical Transactions of the Royal Society London B*, 359: 1447–1451.

Joas, H. (1997) *G.H. Mead. A Contemporary Re-examination of his Thought*. Cambridge, MA: MIT Press.

Kaufman, J.M. and Johnson, C. (2004) Stigmatized individuals and the process of identity. *The Sociological Quarterly*, 45: 807–833.

Kessler, R.C. (2002) The categorical versus dimensionsal assessment controversy in the sociology of mental illness. *Journal of Health and Social Behavior*, 43: 171–188.

Kvale, S. (1996) *Interviews: an Introduction to Qualitative Research Interviewing*. London: SAGE.

Lucas, R.E. (2007a) Adaptation and the set-point model of subjective well-being. Does happiness change after major life events? *Current Directions in Psychological Science*, 16: 75–79.

Lucas, R.E. (2007b) Happiness. In Baumeister, R. and Vohs (eds) *Encyclopedia of Social Psychology*. London: SAGE. pp. 411–414.

Lucas, R.E., Clark, A.E., Georgellis, Y. and Diener, E. (2003) Reexamining adaptation and the set point model of happiness: Reactions to changes in marital status. *Journal of Personality and Social Psychology*, 84: 527–539.

Lucas, R.E., Clark, A.E., Georgellis, Y. and Diener, E. (2004) Unemployment alters the set point for life satisfaction. *Psychological Science*, 15: 8–13.

Lykken, D. and Tellegen, A. (1996) Happiness is a stochastic phenomenon. *Psychological Science*, 7: 186–189.

Lyubomirsky, S., Sheldon, K.M. and Schkade, D. (2005) Pursuing happiness: The architecture of sustainable change. *Review of General Psychology*, 9: 111–131.

Magyar-Moe, J.L. (2009) *Therapist's Guide to Positive Psychology Interventions (Practical Resources for the Mental Health Professional)*. Oxford: Elsevier.

Maslow, A. (1968) *Toward a Psycholog of Being*. New York: D. Van Nostrand Co.

McAdams, D.P. (2006) The problem of narrative coherence. *Journal of Constructivist Psychology*, 19: 109–125.

McCall, G.J. and Simmons, J.L. (1966) *Identities and Interactions*. New York: The Free Press.

McLeod, J.D. and Lively, K.J. (2007) Social psychology and stress research. In W.R. Avison, J.D. McLeod, and B.A. Pescosolido, (eds) *Mental Health, Social Mirror*. New York: Springer. pp. 275–303.

Mead, G.H. (1934) *Mind, Self, and Society. From the Standpoint of a Social Behaviorist*. Chicago: University of Chicago Press.

Mirowsky, J. and Ross, C.E. (2002) Measurement for a human science. *Journal of Health and Social Behavior*, 43: 152–170.

Mirowsky, J. and Ross, C.E. (2003) *Social Causes of Psychological Distress*. New York: Aldine de Gruyter.

Paul, K.I. and Moser, K. (2006) Incongruence as an explanation for the negative mental health effects of unemployment: Meta-analytic evidence. *Journal of Occupational and Organizational Psychology*, 79: 595–621.

Payton, A.R. (2009) Mental health, mental illness, and psychological distress: same continuum or distinct phenomena? *Journal of Health and Social Behavior*, 50: 213–227.

Pearlin, L.I., Nguyen, K.B., Schieman, S. and Milkie, M.A. (2007) The life-course origins of mastery among older people. *Journal of Health and Social Behavior*, 48: 164–179.

Pilgrim, D. (2005) Defining mental disorder: tautology in the service of sanity in British mental health legislation. *Journal of Mental Health*, 14: 435–443.

Plummer, K. (2000) Symbolic interactionism in the twentieth century. In B. Turner, (ed.) *The Blackwell Companion to Social Theory*. Oxford: Blackwell. pp. 193–222.

Reynolds, J.R. and Turner, R.J. (2008) Major life events: Their personal meaning, resolution, and mental health significance. *Journal of Health and Social Behavior*, 49: 223–237.

Richardson, J.C., Ong, B.N., and Sim, J. (2006) Is chronic widespread pain biographically disruptive? *Social Science and Medicine*, 63: 1573–1585.

Rogers, A. and Pilgrim, D. (2005) *A Sociology of Mental Health and Illness*. Maidenhead: Open University Press.

Rosenberg, M. (1979) *Conceiving the Self*. New York: Basic Books.

Rosenthal, G. (2003) The healing effects of storytelling. On the conditions of curative story-telling in the context of research and counseling. *Qualitative Inquiry*, 9: 915–933.

Ryan, R.M. and Deci, E.L. (2001) On happiness and human potentials: A review of research on hedonic and eudaimonic well-being. *Annual Review of Psychology*, 52: 141–166.

Ryff, C.D. (1989) Happiness is everything, or is it? Explorations on the meaning of psychological well-being. *Journal of Personality and Social Psychology*, 57: 1069–1081.

Ryff, C.D. and Singer, B. (1998) The contours of positive human health. *Psychological Inquiry*, 9: 1–28.

Schnittker, J. and McLeod, J.D. (2005) The social psychology of health disparities. *Annual Review of Sociology*, 31: 75–103.

Schwarz, N. and Strack, F. (1999) Reports of subjective well-being: judgmental processes and their methodological implications. In D. Kahnemann, E. Diener, and N. Schwarz, (eds) *Well-being: the Foundations of Hedonic Psychology*. New York: Russell Sage Foundation. pp. 60–84.

Seligman, M.E.P. (2002) *Authentic Happiness: Using the New Positive Psychology to Realize Your Potential for Lasting Fulfillment*. New York: Simon and Schuster.

Seligman, M.E.P. and Csikszentmihalyi, M. (2000) Positive psychology: an introduction. *American Psychologist*, 55: 5–14.

Shedler, J., Mayman, M. and Manis, M. (1993) The illusion of mental health. *American Psychologist*, 48: 1117–1131.

Sheeran, P. and Abraham, C. (1994) Unemployment and self-conception – a symbolic interactionist analysis. *Journal of Community and Applied Social Psychology*, 4: 115–129.

Sheldon, K.M. and Lyubomirsky, S. (2009) Change your actions, not your circumstances: an experimental text of the Sustainable Happiness model. In A.K. Dutt, and B. Radcliff, (eds) *Happiness, Economics, and Politics: Towards a Multi-Disciplinary Approach.* Cheltenham, UK: Edward Elgar. pp. 324–342.

Simon, R.W. (1997) The meanings individuals attach to role identities and their implications for mental health. *Journal of Health and Social Behavior,* 38: 256–274.

Simon, R.W. (2000) The importance of culture in sociological theory and research on stress and mental health. A missing link? In C.F. Bird, P. Conrad, and A.M. Fremont (eds) *Handbook of Medical Sociology.* New Jersey: Prentice Hall. pp. 68–78.

Simon, R.W. (2007) Contributions of the sociology of mental health for understanding the social antecnts, social regulation, and social distribution of emotion. In W.R. Avison, J.D. McLeod, and B.A. Pescosolido, (eds) *Mental Health, Social Mirror.* New York: Springer. pp. 239–274.

Stets, J.E. (2006) Identity theory and emotions. In J.E. Stets, and J.H. Turner (eds) *Handbook of the Sociology of Emotions.* New York: Springer. pp. 203–223.

Stets, J.E. and Asencio, E.K. (2008) Consistency and enhancement processes in understanding emotions. *Social Forces,* 86: 1055–1078.

Stets, J.E. and Harrod, M.M. (2002) Verification across multiple identities: The role of status. *Social Psychology Quarterly,* 67: 155–171.

Stryker, S. (1980) *Symbolic Interactionism: a Social Structural Version.* Reading, MA: Benjamin-Cummings Pub. Co.

Stryker, S. (2008) From Mead to a structural symbolic interactionism and beyond. *Annual Review of Sociology,* 34: 15–31.

Taylor, S.E. and Brown, J.D. (1999) Illusion and well-being: a social psychologicl perspective on mental health. In R. Baumeister, (ed.) *The Self in Social Psychology.* Philadelphia: Taylor and Francis. pp. 43–66.

Tellegen, A., Lykken, D., Bouchard, T.J., Wilcox, K.J., Segal, N.L. and Rich, S. (1988) Personality similarity in twins reared apart and together. *Journal of Personality and Social Psychology,* 54: 1031–1039.

Thoits, P.A. (1992) Identity structures and psychological well-being: Gender and marital status comparisons. *Social Psychology Quarterly,* 55: 236–256.

Thoits, P.A. (2003) Personal agency in the accumulation of multiple role-identities. In P.J. Burke, T.J. Owens, R.T. Serpe, and P.A. Thoits, (eds) *Advances in Identity Theory and Research.* New York: Kluwer Academic/Plenum Publishers. pp. 179–194.

Thoits, P.A. (2006) Personal agency in the stress process. *Journal of Health and Social Behavior,* 47: 309–323.

Veenhoven, R. (2008) Sociological theories of subjective well-being. In M. Eid, and R. Larsen, (eds) *The Science of Subjective Well-being: a Tribute to Ed Diener.* New York: Guilford Publications. pp. 44–61.

Weinberger, D.A. (1990) The construct validity of repressive coping style. In J.L. Singer, (ed.) *Repression and Dissociation.* Chicago: The University of Chicago Press. pp. 337–386.

Williams, S.J. (1998) 'Capitalising' on emotions? Rethinking the inequalities in health debate. *Sociology,* 32: 121–139.

4

Sociological Aspects of the Emotions

Gillian Bendelow

INTRODUCTION

As Rogers and Pilgrim (1998, 2005) have consistently emphasized, the manifestation of emotional distress is endemic across all cultures, although interpretation and responses may vary widely. Across most of so-called 'western' society, madness and emotional instability have always aroused public response and intervention. Since the nineteenth century, these interventions in the form of scientific medicine in general, and psychiatry in particular, has meant that medicalization has been the most dominant means of response (Foucault, 1965; Porter, 2002). Although psychoanalysis enjoyed a particularly significant influence in 'western' psychiatric practice until the 1940s (which still resonates to some extent with the popularity of talking cures and counselling), the development of biological and neuropsychiatry has largely dominated therapeutic responses to emotional distress from severe psychotic mental illnesses at one end of the spectrum to the ever-widening range of neurotic, anxiety and minor depressive disorders at the other. It is no small irony that most of what is termed *mental illness* has largely been treated with physical or biological interventions, including psychosurgery and electroconvulsive therapy. Although medicalized responses to emotional distress have acknowledged pluralistic approaches such as talking cures and psychosocial interventions, biological treatments, particularly in the form of pharmaceuticals have dominated the field of psychiatry and emotional health, and continue to do so with the renewed emphasis on seeking biological and genetic causes.

However, the limitations of this biomedical response are subject to enormous controversy in the form of *pharmaskepticism*, namely the dominant tendency to rely on pharmaceutical or technical interventions for simplistic solutions to highly complex illness syndromes.

In this chapter, I hope to explore the implications of contemplating emotional distress or mental disorder in terms of emotional health rather than mental illness. First, the role of emotion and stress in contemporary patterns of health and illness demands considerable rethinking across the mind/body divide and the traditional divisions between mental and physical conditions. In turn, this entails a re-examination of critique of the medicalization of emotional distress/disorder, with a particular emphasis on the limitations of the biomedical approach to aetiological factors, with subsequent consequences for diagnosis and treatment. Finally, the benefits of the more holistic and seemingly enlightened rubric of emotional health need to be considered against the backdrop of the potential for surveillance and social manipulation that the spectre of *healthism* raises.

LIMITATIONS OF THE BIOMEDICAL APPROACH TO MENTAL/EMOTIONAL DISTRESS

The limitations and inadequacies of scientific medicine in separating mind and body, reducing individuals to 'body machines' as discussed earlier, have long been a source of controversy highlighted by social scientists working within health and illness, particularly through the second wave feminists accounts of women's experiences of medicalization, and more recently through the burgeoning body of work on illness narratives. These critiques have influenced the turn to more holistic integrative models of health and illness, which are now permeating medical education and practice (Wade and Halligan, 2004) and serve to highlight further the outmoded relevance of mental/physical labels. Interest in how far physical or psychiatric disorder may be a result of living in a particular form of economic and political organization or domestic environment can be traced back to Marx's and Engels' concern with the social relations of capitalism, and with the links between these and individual health and well-being. Whilst recognizing the potential in terms of progress and civilization of the (then embryonic) new economic system, Marx predicted the detriment of health and well-being which alienation, the result of inevitable class exploitation, would result in the worker being:

> mutilate(d) ... into a fragment of a man, degrade him to the level of an appendage to a machine, destroy every remnant of charm in his work, and turn it into hated toil; they estrange him from the intellectual potentialities of the labour process in the same proportion as science is incorporated in it as an independent power; they distort the conditions under which he works, subject him during the labour process to a despotism more hateful for its meanness, they drag his wife and child beneath the wheels of the juggernaut of capital. (Marx 1906–1909, 1: 708)

Despite fundamental differences in the two conceptions of society, similar concerns can be found in the works of Durkheim (1897), most famously in *Suicide*, where the concept of anomie was used to identify the social causes of suicide by relating their rates in different social groups to social characteristics of those groups.

Wilkinson (2004) advocates the necessity to take on board how emotional qualities of empathy, compassion and pity must constitute part of our understanding of risk perception and to subsequently frame social responses to 'risk' more as a reaction to human pain and suffering:

> While suffering has always comprised the experience of humanity, we cannot impassively accept this as a normal and inevitable part of our human condition. This is because suffering hurts too much. The problem with suffering is that it involves us in far *too much* pain. The pain of suffering so dominates its senses that it cannot be simply ignored or blithely returned to its proper place. It is all at once excruciating and overwhelming, and as such it is entirely unacceptable. It must be fought against. (Wilkinson 2004: 2)

Medicalized responses to pain are ambivalent about the role of suffering in measuring and evaluating pain (Bendelow, 2006), and there is a tendency for suffering to be subsumed under the psychiatric rubric as *trauma,* a term traditionally ascribed to the after-effects of experience of very extreme events such as natural disaster and war. Experiences of trauma began to be medicalized during the twentieth century, influenced by Freudian concepts of hysteria. Traditional psychiatric diagnoses and treatment were challenged by middle class officers displaying symptoms of shellshock after their horrendous experiences in the First World War in the UK, but post traumatic stress disorder (PTSD) is thought to have become a credible psychiatric diagnosis after the Vietnam war (Summerfield, 2001). Summerfield points out that the disorder is constructed from socio-political concepts, rather than psychiatric observations and his critique of the development of PTSD as an illness challenges the twin assumptions that a psychiatric diagnosis constitutes a disease and that distress or suffering automatically implies a psychpathology:

> Post-traumatic stress disorder is the diagnosis for an age of disenchantment. Today there is often more social utility attached to expressions of victimhood than to 'survivorhood'; this is perhaps the reverse of 50 years ago. (Summerfield 2001: 322)

He claims that since the condition was given medical legitimation, trauma is conflated with any form of distress, rather than a reaction to extreme events and rewards 'medicalized victims rather than feisty survivors'.

The clinical criteria involves mood anxiety and sleep patterns, common to many other psychiatric disorders, but given the hierarchies of stigma across the range of contested conditions, PTSD has higher prestige than many and is subsequently a more desirable diagnosis.

For example, the meaning of trauma in the conventional western context was resisted in Leibling's extraordinary study of Bagandan women who had experienced civil war in Uganda through sexual violations, multiple rapes, impregnation and destruction of foetuses. These extreme acts of sexual transgression have been attributed to causing a crisis of identity in Bagandan women and men, but in this context war trauma was understood as a breakdown in cultural identity, manifested in psychological, social, cultural and physical effects, which are integrated and inseparable, not split between mind/body and society (Leibling, 2004; Leibling et al., 2007). However, this study reveals how women war survivors reconstructed their identities by taking on male roles as well as engaging in collective activities. Their ability to voice their experiences as a political act of resistance, resulted in a shared identity and a decrease in reported levels of depression. For instance, at the end of one heart rending interview in which a woman shared experiences of horrendous sexual savagery, she was asked what could happen to make her life improve. Her poignant but starkly simple reply to request '*a goat*' does not belittle the severity of her dreadful experience, but perhaps supports Summerfield's thesis that she is not 'ill' as a result of her experience, she is indeed 'a feisty survivor'.

EMOTION, STRESS AND HEALTH

Crucial to our understanding of the link between mind and body, the study of emotion has been theorized across a variety of perspectives ranging from a deterministically biological position at one end of the spectrum to being entirely socially constructed at the other. However, the *interactionist* approach, seemingly premised upon a non-dualistic ontology which seeks to unite both the biological and social realms of emotional being, offers the most relevant insights in the context of health and illness. Hochschild (1979, 1983, 2003) has played a key role in developing this highly influential approach to understanding emotion, drawing on a number of interactionist theorists including John Dewey, C.Wright Mills (1959) and Erving Goffman (1971).

   In her social theory of emotion, Hochschild (1983, 2003) stresses that although emotions have biological substrates, they are socially shaped and managed and therefore subject to hierarchical manipulation. *Feeling rules* are the ideological strategies we develop to deal with uncomfortable, distressing or inappropriate emotions and feelings, and may involve *deep acting,* as per Goffman's notion of unconsciously making oneself believe the socially desirable adaptation. Thus, *emotion management* is the type of work it takes to cope with these feeling rules and Hochschild applies this mainly in the realm of gender, class and work. For instance, she argues that 'meaning-making' jobs, which tend to be more common in the middle-class, put more of a premium on the individual's capacity to *do* emotion work. In this way, she maintains each class psychologically reproduces the class structure (Hochschild, 1983; 2003). The concept of *emotion work* involves the management of emotions of the individual in order to conform with the demands of the particular social situation and include subjective states, as well as more public bodily displays. Hochschild (1983) also coined the phrase *status shields* to describe the socially distributed resources that people have for protecting their sense of self in differing social situations.

The interactionist approach sees emotion through the notion of the 'mindful body', as the mediatrix of phenomenological experience, social and the body politic (Scheper-Hughes and Lock, 1987). Grief, for instance, is an example of emotional pain which is inseparable from its 'gut churning, nauseating experience', whilst physical pain bears within it a 'component of displeasure, and often of anxiety, sadness and anger that are fully emotional' (Leder 1990: 261). On the other hand, pain may also signal something positive. In this respect pain may bring us to an authentic recognition of our own limitations and possibilities. It may also be creative, not only in the sense of childbirth but also in terms of physical, emotional, artistic and spiritual achievements, or it may serve as a catalyst for much needed changes in our lives (Leder, 1990–5).

As Scheper-Hughes and Lock (1987) argue, emotions affect the way in which the body, illness and pain are experienced and are projected in images of the well and poorly functioning social and body politic: 'Insofar as emotions entail both feelings and cognitive orientations, public morality and cultural ideology, we suggest that they provide an important "missing link" capable of bridging mind and body, individual, society and body politic' (1987: 28–29). In this respect, explorations of sickness, madness, pain, disability and death are human events which are literally 'seething with emotion' (Scheper-Hughes and Lock, 1987).

The ability to bridge mind, body and society is an exciting proposition for understanding of the role of emotion in health and illness, and the work of Peter Freund has taken the notion of dramaturgical stress forward in this area.

However contested, there does seem to be some consensus that disorders of emotion result in difficulties of coping with a perceived, real or imagined threat to one's physical, mental, spiritual or emotional wellbeing, which in turn results in a series of physiological responses and adaptations. The psycho-social causes of disease and the role of factors such as life events and difficulties, and social support in the onset of physical and mental illness have been well established in the scientific as well as the social scientific literature, but the development of Hochschild's work by Freund has consistently held up the 'expressive body' as a common ground for the sociology of emotions and health and illness (1990, 1998, 2003) and maintains that the embodied self is so intimately meshed with social life, thus offering endless potential for socially constructing emotions and psychological responses. and suggests that human bodies should be seen as 'acting mind-body unities' (Freund, 1990: 457). Thus emotions as a form of communication can be physically expressed in motor activity (e.g. facial expression) or neuro-hormonally in different configurations of biological information – in other words the highly developed subjectivity of humans – mediates material-physical reality (Freund, 1990: 457). It is from this important set of propositions, that Freund is able to develop an existential-phenomenological perspective, one which emphasizes subjectivity and the active, expressive body, in order to bridge the mind–body–society split so necessary in understanding processes of health and illness. Inevitably, in this model external social structural factors such as one's position in different systems of hierarchy or various forms of social control can influence the conditions of our existence, how we respond and apprehend these conditions and our sense of embodied self. These conditions can also affect our physical functioning (Freund, 1990: 461).In order to elaborate this position further, Freund draws on the writings of Hochschild on emotion work and status shields in the context of status and social control. As he notes, one's position in the social hierarchy and the activities involved in insuring social control are two features of social structure that influence feelings, which in turn influence our physiology:

> since the body is a means of expressing meaning, including socio-cultural meaning, it is not unrealistic to suppose that people might express somatically the conditions of their existence. ... cultural factors can shape the language of the body. (Freund, 1990: 463)

In other words, one's position in any system of social hierarchy and the manner in which social relationships are managed both affect and are affected by bio-chemical states and other aspects of 'bodyliness' (Freund, 1990: 465). Therefore, a person's social position and status will determine the resources they have at their disposal in order to define and protect the boundaries of the self and counter the potential for invalidation by powerful and significant others. In other words, those who occupy less powerful positions in the social hierarchy are at greater risk of being invalidated, of feeling instrumentally powerless, insecure, unable to speak their mind and of experiencing 'unpleasant emotionality or emotional modes of being' (Freund, 1990: 466). Less powerful people, therefore, face a structurally in-built 'handicap' in the management of their own and others emotion. As Goffman (1959) and later Hochschild (1979, 2003) suggest, the emotion work involved in self presentation and role playing is stressful and if, as in the widely accepted adaptation model, this stress becomes chronic it may, for instance, affect neurohormonal regulation in the body. It is these forms of stress which Freund refers to as *dramaturgical stress,* and which are linked to the health capital model as social status provides *status shields* available to protect the boundaries and integrity of the self (Hochschild, 1979, 1983).

THE MEDICALIZATION OF EMOTIONAL DISTRESS

Although the concept of emotional health can be employed to address the mind/body divide and has enabled some destigmatization of 'mental disorders' (at least those which are not associated with psychosis or 'dangerousness') to some extent, it still tends to be the case that illnesses without clear and demonstrable scientific physiopathology remain at the bottom of the hierarchy. Across the whole range of medical care and practice, psychiatry and psychiatric treatments have always been, and still are, subject to huge controversy, less prestige and receive less funding for research.

Throughout history, the mentally 'disordered' have always been socially and legally marginalized as citizens. For instance, in the UK, since the eighteenth century, under English common law, land could be confiscated from those deemed either lunatics (*non compos mentis*) or idiots (*purus idiota*) by a jury of twelve (Scull, 1993). In the first half of the twentieth century, there was an administrative and geographical separation of those termed mentally ill and mentally defective. The term 'mentally defective/deficient' included congenital imbecility and feeble-mindedness and were cared for chronic institutions whose main function was training. In contemporary UK society, under the more generic but still contested term of disability, care and treatment is completely separate from those designated as mentally ill who were cared for in mental hospitals, the reformed Victorian asylum. Reaching their peak between the 1950s and 1970s, the criteria for hospital beds for the mentally ill included the 'morally deficient', but the aim was cure through medical treatment, often administered involuntarily with the aid of the 1953 and 1983 Mental Health Acts. Distinctions have always been made between psychotic and neurotic manifestations of mental disorder, with the former signifying a rupture with reality, however reality may be defined, which of course is much debated. Psychotic illness and its association with dangerousness defined by the Mental Health Act (1983) as the propensity to harm self or others tends to be categorized as serious mental illness (SMI) and despite the closure of many of the old asylums and mental hospitals throughout the 1980s and 1990s, are largely treated through psychiatric units and mental health teams.

Busfield (2002) has provided us with a helpful distinction between disorders of thought, emotion and behaviour and contemporary mental health care practice which can be translated into patterns of diagnosis and health care in contemporary Britain (see Table 4.1). As Table 4.1 indicates, the dwindling mental health services are increasingly directed towards chronic psychotic illness (SMI). Neurotic disorders are largely subsumed under the disorders of emotion rubric, and are treated predominantly through primary care, mainly GP prescriptions for pharmaceuticals. The controversial behavioural conditions such as substance misuse and personality disorders (including parasuicide and self-harm) are increasingly treated outside the NHS, if they are indeed treated at all.

In other words, there is distinction between psychoses (i.e. 'real' mental illness which abdicates individual responsibility and requires treatment, which may be coercive) and the disorders of emotion and behaviour health. Paradoxically, although there is more apparent openness, as well as access to knowledge and information about conditions such as reactive (not psychotic) depression, anxiety disorders and even of the range of addictive behaviours, emotional health has the propensity to place the onus of responsibility very squarely on the individual. Many of the conditions included under the category of emotion and behaviour, such as ADHD, anorexia and substance abuse, are highly contested as to whether they constitute 'real' illnesses, and are subject to great controversy within the

Table 4.1   Diagnosis and treatment of 'emotional disorder' in contemporary Britain

Disorder category (after Busfield, 2002)	Diagnosis	Treatment provider	Nature of treatment
Thought	Serious mental illness, e.g. schizophrenia, biopolar disorder, psychotic depression	Referral mainly through GP or primary care to Mental Health Services (hospital and community care) or private clinics	Psychotropic drugs and depot injections. Physical treatments, e.g. ECT, brain surgery. Behavioural and psychodynamic therapies
Emotion	Anxiety and depressive disorders Behavioural (e.g. ADHD) Eating (e.g. anorexia) and sleep disorders	80–90 percent of treatment primary care (GPs) Some specialist referral on NHS or private consultations	Pharmaceuticals: mainly SSRI's, Ritalin, etc. Behavioural and psychodynamic therapies
Behaviour	Substance misuse and addictions, e.g. drugs, alcohol, sexual offenders, personality disorders	Outside mainstream NHS health care, specialist services Some self referral and private 'rehab' clinics	Detoxification regimes, behavioural and psychodynamic therapies

Source: Bendelow (2009: 67)

medical press and the media. In turn, treatments and therapies for these conditions, unless privately funded by the individual, compete alongside other constrained resources, including the mental health services. To an even greater degree, the Substance Misuse Services remain low priority, much as they always have been and addictive or self-harming behaviour may be portrayed almost a lifestyle 'choice'. Thus, in terms of treatment, there are enormous socio-economic differences, as illustrated by the highly publicized celebrity rehab culture in contrast to the grim reality of the addict living on the streets.

HEALTHISM AND THE THERAPEUTIC CRITIQUE

Over the last decade or so, a movement often termed the 'therapeutic critique' has combined critiques of healthism with those of *disease mongering* and *pharmaskepticism*. It takes as its starting point Beck's (1992) notion of an overanxious insecure 'risk' society as characterized by the fragmentation of social networks and communities and the atomisation of individual (i.e. the isolation of individuals within homogenous social groups), Within this context, health now becomes a goal to be endlessly pursued if rarely achieved, and it has become inextricably linked with individual attitudes, commitment and personal responsibility. Perfect health involves self-transformation, 'not just of our bodies and our minds but even of our emotions' (Coward, 1989: 46). In his insightful book *The Importance of Disappointment*, Craib described a process of:

cultural pressures, often normal pressures which have to do with wanting to help people, to ease suffering, to be effective, to be good at our jobs, make us vulnerable to the denial of necessity and inevitability of certain forms of human suffering. We set out to cure and we construct blueprints of what people ought to be feeling, ought to be like, and we can too easily set about trying to manipulate or even force people into these blueprints. (Craib, 1994: 8)

Before his own untimely death, his warnings chime with the explosion of *quick fix culture*, the idiomatic term for the tendency to rely on medical interventions, especially in the form of pharmaceuticals, to banish discomfort and distress, or indeed any negative experience. Lyon (1996) aptly terms this rapidly growing propensity in modern society as *cosmetic psychopharmamcology*. She expresses concern about the vagueness of diagnostic criteria, resulting in the seemingly endless expansion of the boundaries of clinical depression through the diagnostic classification of conditions like *dysthymia*. Inevitably, she claims, the solution to this dysfunctionality is medicinal, further resulting in 'chemically assisted selves' (Lyon, 1996). Despite increased life expectancy and relative material wellbeing the so-called 'happiness gap' can thus be characterized as a chemical reaction to the difference between the dreams we are sold and the daily reality of life in advanced capitalism, as epitomized in Wurtzel's *Prozac Nation* (1997). What was previously seen in lay terms as common-sense social support is now the professionalisation of emotionality:

the counsel of parents, grandparents, aunts and uncles, ministers, priests and rabbis holds relatively less weight than it would a century ago, that of professional therapists, television talk show hosts, radio commentators, ... agony aunts assume relatively more weight. (Hochschild, 1994: 2)

There is certainly a popular argument that the socio-economic improvements of life in the western world have meant that whereas most of us in the 'west' never experience severe hunger or poverty, droughts and extreme climate conditions or infectious diseases that kill, we are in the midst of epidemics of depression, anxiety, substance misuse and eating disorders. These have been interpreted as a socially constructed luxury of a spoiled narcissistic society obsessed by material envy, body image, celebrity and reality TV. The concept of *affluenza* has been enthusiastically adopted by broadsheet media to describe this paradox of 'luxury fever' in quasi-medicinal terms – a middle class 'virus' brought on by the social and material envy of a society obsessed by:

flash holidays, luxury furniture, big salaries and expensive cars ... individualism replaced by consumerism as the aspirational middle classes shackle themselves to unfulfilling jobs, working excessively long hours and cutting themselves off from proper relationships. (James, 2007)

Critics of individualism and consumerism such as Furedi (2004) have indicated a growing tendency for social problems to be interpreted as emotional, and for the highly individualized idiom of therapeutic discourse to be used to make sense of social isolation, through discourses of being 'stressed out', 'burnt out' or having 'mid-life crisis'. In this model, personal inadequacies, guilt feelings, conflicts and neuroses which are being used to replace abstract, almost invisible social influences such as globalization, market forces, cultural and political institutions is a source of great concern to some contemporary writers reflecting on 'modern life'. Furedi (2004) has railed against the tendency for 'social and cultural influence to be discounted in favour of narrow psychological contemplation'. He contends that the emphasis on achievement of personal happiness and fulfilment through self-discovery, self assessment and self-actualization has resulted in self esteem becoming *the* important explanatory variable. In turn, low self esteem becomes an over-arching explanation for socially perceived 'problem' groups such as teenagers, unemployed, elderly, mentally ill, lone parents or the disabled. Furthermore, the avoidance of negative emotion, where it is seen as 'unhealthy' or 'pathological' to feel dissatisfied, disillusioned or miserable is all too readily absorbed into post Thatcher/Reaganite culture of 1980s individualism and, he argues, is *not* an enlightened shift (Furedi, 2004: 23). Thus, psychosocial overdeterminism in understanding health and illness is, for some critics, potentially as dangerous and as reductionist as biological supremacy. Bearing the therapeutic critique in mind, in particular as regards the warning that 'society is much more comfortable dealing with poverty as a mental health problem rather than a social issue' (Furedi, 2004: 27), it is essential not to overplay this factoring of the equation to the exclusion of all others, and to achieve conceptual, political and practical balance.

EMOTIONAL HEALTH: INTEGRATED MODELS OF HEALTH AND ILLNESS

Integrated models of health and illness are increasingly permeating contemporary healthcare, and are gaining popularity and credibility within the mainstream medical literature and research, as the limits of biomedicine become increasingly evident in contemporary times (Wade and Halligan 2004). Integrated models also challenge traditional sociological assumptions that doctors are only concerned with biological (disease) and that the social (illness) is of concern outside medicine as 'in everyday clinical practice doctors constantly faced with issues relating to social causes of ill-health and the social contexts of ill-health and lifestyle provide doctors with a framework to talk about the social' (Hansen and Easthope, 2006).

In the mental health arena, post-psychiatry has been heralded as a major challenge to the biomedical model providing a pragmatic and viable new direction for intervention into emotional distress (Bracken and Thomas, 2006). Beginning with the proposition that modernist psychiatry relies upon three elements, namely technical reasoning and a belief in science, exploration of the individual self and coercion and control of madness. The advocates of this movement assert that this agenda is no longer tenable because of various post-modern challenges to its basis, which question over-simplified notions of progress and scientific expertise, with the rise of the user movement being seen as of particular importance in challenging the biomedical model of mental illness (Bracken and Thomas, 2001, 2006).

Although the movement builds upon the conceptual frameworks of anti-psychiatry, practitioners of post psychiatry accept that emotional or mental distress is 'real' in the sense that clinical intervention is needed to alleviate the often severe problems experienced by individuals. They also accept that psychiatry is the dominant mode of dealing with distress, however limited diagnoses and treatments may be, but engage with the principles of value based medicine (VBM) which begin with the premise that values affect every stage of the clinical encounter, and by accepting and working with the diversity of values, opportunities arise for discussion, consultation and negotiation. In other words, the medical model is used as the basis of providing intervention, but diagnosis and treatment are negotiated with the client/user/sufferer (terminology may vary but 'patient' is less likely to be used).

Built on the principle of *ethical reasoning*, this approach emphasizes the significance of social, political and cultural contexts for the understanding of mental illness and draws attention to the importance of values, rather than causes, in research and practice, giving rise to a so-called 'new philosophy of psychiatry' (Fulford et al., 2002). Whilst recognizing the importance of empirical knowledge, it gives priority to interpretation and to meaningful experiences. User movements have long argued the need for open, genuine and democratic debate across the lay/professional divide and in this model, mental health practice does not need to be based on an individualistic framework centred on medical diagnosis and treatment. In addition, recent government policy emphases on social exclusion and partnership in health are viewed as an opportunity for a new deal between professionals and service users. Post-psychiatry proposes a new relationship between society and the emotionally distressed, challenging doctors to rethink their role and responsibilities, by building on critiques of anti-psychiatry and the failures of community care.

Recent socio-political (the rise of the risk society), epidemiological (the return of infectious disease epidemics) and ecological (the visible material impacts of global climate change) shifts are precipitating a conceptual and practical reorganization of medical ideologies and practices. Samson (1999) points out that residues of Hippocratic concepts of health and disease exist within medical practice specifically and within society more generally 'a medical system that is both environmental and psychosomatic. It is open to the possibility that the state of the body is influenced by natural phenomena, external and internal to the person … [and] also suggests that frames of mind and psychological states profoundly affect the body' (1999: 64). Certainly, the concept of *balance,* which is intrinsically holistic and based on the Hippocratic view of the body as a microcosm of Nature is crucial to the process of intellectual and conceptual thinking, as it is in understanding and constructing models of health care. The dissolution of the artificial divides between mental and physical health is an essential part of this rapprochement, and understanding the role of emotions with their propensity to link 'private troubles and public issues' (Wright Mills, 1959) is crucial to developing a mind/body/society perspective, as well as enlightened mental/emotional healthcare.

REFERENCES

Beck, U. (1992) *Risk Society; Towards a New Modernity.* London: SAGE.

Bendelow, G. (2006) Pain, suffering and risk. *Health Risk and Society,* 8(1): 1–12.

Bendelow G. (2009) *Health, emotion and the body.* Cambridge: Polity Press.

Bracken, P. and Thomas, P. (2001) Postpsychiatry: a new direction for mental health? *British Medical Journal,* 322: 724–727.

Bracken, P. and Thomas, P. (2006) *Postpsychiatry: Mental Health in a Postmodern World.* Oxford: Oxford University Press.

Busfield, J. (2002) The archaeology of psychiatric disorder: thought, emotion and behaviour. In G. Bendelow, M. Carpenter, C. Vautier and S. Williams (eds) *Gender, Health and Healing: the Public/Private Divide.* London: Routledge.

Coward, R. (1989) *The Whole Truth.* London: Faber and Faber.

Craib, I. (1994) *The Importance of Disappointment.* London: Routledge.

Durkheim, E. (1897) *Suicide: a Study in Sociology.* London: Routledge and Kegan Paul.

Foucault, M. (1965) *Madness and Civilisation: a History of Insanity in the Age of Reason.* New York: Random House Inc.

Freund, P. (1990) The expressive body: a common ground for the sociology of emotions and health and illness. *Sociology of Health and Illness,* 12(4): 452–477.

Freund, P. (1998) Social performances and their discontents. In G. Bendelow and S. Williams (eds) *Emotions in Social Life.* London : Routledge.

Freund, P., McGuire, M. and Podhurst, L. (2003) *Health Illness and the Social Body,* 4th edition. Prentice Hall.

Fulford, K.W.M., Dickenson, D. and Murray, T. (2002) *Healthcare Ethics and Human Values.* Oxford: Blackwell.

Furedi, F. (2004) *Therapy Culture: Cultivating Vulnerability in the Modern Age.* London: Routledge.

Goffman, E. (1971) *The Presentation of Self in Everyday Life.* Harmondsworth: Penguin.

Hanson, E. and Easthope, G. (2006) *Lifestyle in Medicine.* Critical Studies in Health and Medicine Series. London: Routledge.

Hochschild, A. (1979) Emotion work, feeling rules and social structure. *American Journal of Sociology,* 85: 551–575.

Hochschild, A. (1983, 2003) *The Managed Heart: the Commercialisation of Human Feeling.* Berkeley: University of California Press.

James, O. (2007) *Affluenza.* London: Vermillion.

Leder, D. (1990) *The Absent Body.* Chicago: Chicago University Press.

Leibling H. (2004) Ugandan women's experiences of sexual violence and torture during civil war years in Luwero District: Implications for health policy, welfare and human rights. *Psychology of Women Section Review,* 6(2): 29–37, autumn edition, BPS.

Liebling-Kalifani, H., Marshall, A., Ojiambo-Ochieng, R. and Nassozi, M. (2007) Experiences of women war-torture survivors in Uganda: implications for health and human rights. *Journal of International Women's Studies,* 8(4): 1–17.

Lyon, M. (1996) C. Wright Mills meets Prozac: the relevance of 'social emotion' to the sociology of health and illness. In V. James and J. Gabe (1996) *Health and the Sociology of Emotions.* Oxford: Blackwell.

Marx, K. (1906) *Capital: A Critique of Political Economy,* Vol. Chicago: Charles Kerr and Co 1: 708.

Rogers, A. and Pilgrim, D. (1998)[2005] *A Sociology of Mental Health and Illness* (3rd edition). Milton Keynes: Open University Press.

Pilgrim, D. (2005) *Key Concepts in Mental Health.* London: SAGE.

Porter, R. (ed) (2002) *The Faber Book of Madness.* London: Faber and Faber.

Sansom, C. (ed.) (1999) *Critical Health Studies.* Oxford: Blackwell.

Scheper-Hughes, N. and Lock, M. (1987) The mindful body: a prolegemonon to future work in medical anthropology. *Medical Anthropology Quarterly,* 1(1): 6–41.

Summerfield, D. (2001) The invention of post-traumatic stress disorder and the social usefulness of a psychiatric category. *British Medical Journal*, 322: 95–98.

Wade, D. and Halligan, P. (2004) Do biomedical models of illness make for good healthcare systems? *British Medical Journal*, 329(7479): 1398.

Wilkinson, I. (2004) *Suffering: a Sociological Introduction.* Oxford: Polity Press.

Wright Mills, C. (1959*) The Sociological Imagination.* London: Penguin.

Wurtzel, E. (1997) *Prozac Nation: Young and Depressed in America.* New York: Riverhead Tradition.

5

Ethnicity, Race and Mental Disorder in the UK

James Nazroo and Karen Iley

INTRODUCTION

One of the most striking findings in the literature on inequalities in health in the UK – perhaps the most striking finding – is that Black Caribbean people are three to five times more likely to be admitted to a psychiatric hospital with a diagnosis of first episode of psychosis than white people (Cochrane and Bal, 1989; Harrison et al., 1988; McGovern and Cope, 1987; Van Os et al., 1996), and some have reported even higher rates (Fearon et al., 2006). This difference is larger than that for any other condition or ethnic group in the UK except diabetes, where differences between white and most ethnic minority groups are of a similar order of magnitude (Erens et al., 2001; Nazroo, 2001; Sproston and Mindell, 2006). And this greater risk of psychotic illness is apparent for Black populations in other developed countries (e.g. Breshnahan et al., 2007; Cantor-Graae et al., 2005; Cantor-Graae and Selten, 2005; Robins and Reiger, 1991; Selten et al., 1997, 2001; Veling et al., 2006).

Although there is universal agreement that such findings are a matter of great concern, variations in how they are interpreted and therefore the object of such concern, have led to great disagreement and controversy. This is, perhaps, not surprising, given that the topic has the potential to align mental disorder with ethnic/racial identity (Sashidharan, 1993), whereby the increased risk of such illnesses is considered to be driven by essential characteristics of the ethnic/racial group.

The variations in how such findings are interpreted range from the view that they reflect the character and circumstances of people in different ethnic/race groups, to the claim that they reflect racism and racist research agendas. So, if the research evidence is accepted at face value, it can be seen as an opportunity for a further exploration of risk factors for mental illness, through an exploration of the characteristics of those ethnic minority groups with higher rates. Insofar as such differences might be considered to be a consequence of the social and economic inequalities ethnic minority groups face, such evidence can be used to press for policy development to address these inequalities. However, those who have regarded the data more critically have identified a range of methodological flaws in existing research, leading them to question the uncritical acceptance of the findings by the majority of the research and policy community, how this aligns with existing stereotypes about the lives and experiences of ethnic minority people, and how this leads to a reinforcing of racial stereotypes and the failure to identify racism as a key component of ethnic/racial minority people's interactions with both psychiatric services and the research community. These contrasting positions are reflected in the comments of Singh and Burns (2006) and Fernando (2003). Singh and Burns state:

> The excess of psychosis in the African-Caribbean community in the UK is real and well accepted by epidemiologists and researchers. (2006: 649)

and:

> Construing racism as the main explanation for the excess of detentions under the Mental Health Act among ethnic minorities adds little to the debate and prevents the search for the real causes of these differences. (2006: 649–50)

Their targets in making these comments are those who claim that psychiatric practice is institutionally racist. Fernando is an example of this. He writes:

> there is now an extensive body of theory and research documenting the ways in which race, ethnicity, gender and class … are causally linked to mental health problems, The problem is that none of this research seems to touch medical psychiatric research. (2003: 203)

and:

> the main and perhaps most serious problem is institutional racism that pervades all major systems affecting British people, including mental health services and the main disciplines that inform such services, namely psychology and psychiatry. (2003: 25)

In this chapter we adopt a position that emphasizes the role of social and economic inequalities in the production of both ethnic/racial differences in risk of severe mental illness, and in constructing the experience of ethnic/racial minorities in psychiatric care. We take this approach because of the growing evidence on the significance of social and economic inequalities in determining the ethnic/racial patterning of health (Nazroo and Williams, 2005), evidence that is often neglected in detailed discussion of policy development, but also because there is little focus within the inequalities field on how the provision and operation of services is influenced by and may reinforce such inequalities.

We will begin by outlining the key findings that have emerged on ethnic differences in psychotic illnesses, with a particular focus on the UK. Following this we review potential explanations for the sometimes contradictory findings that have been reported. We will then critically review the sources of data that have produced these findings, particularly focusing on the validity of statistics based on treatment rates, with the intention of allowing the reader to more carefully judge the validity of the conclusions that have been drawn. This will be followed by a discussion of ethnic minority people's experiences of mental health services and the implications this has for health care provision and practice.

We will finish with a discussion of the conclusions we can draw on ethnic inequalities in mental health, placing emphasis on how these are embedded in the experiences of ethnic minority people in developed countries and how psychiatric institutions and practices are also embedded in these wider inequalities. Throughout this we make most use of the example of Black people's high risk of treatment for psychotic illnesses, because it is here that the alignment of mental disorder with ethnicity is most apparent, although in places we draw on other examples to illustrate our points.

ETHNICITY/RACE AND PSYCHOTIC ILLNESS: A SUMMARY OF KEY FINDINGS

Most research on ethnic differences in psychotic illnesses has been based on studies of treatment rates. This is not surprising, the low prevalence of these conditions (about one in one hundred people, but see Bentall, this handbook), the difficulty of their measurement and the relatively small proportion of the population made up of ethnic minorities in most developed countries (in the UK only 7.9 per cent of the population described themselves as non-white at the 2001 Census) makes the conduct of such studies in the community extremely difficult. Over the past three decades, studies of treatment rates in the UK have consistently shown elevated rates of diagnosed schizophrenia among Black Caribbean people compared with the white population. Black Caribbean people are typically reported to be three to five times more likely than whites to be admitted to hospital with a first diagnosis of schizophrenia (Bagley, 1971; Cochrane and Bal, 1989; Harrison et al., 1988; Littlewood and Lipsedge, 1988; McGovern and Cope, 1987; Van Os et al., 1996).

These findings have been repeated in studies that have looked at first contact with all forms of treatment, rather than just hospital services (Fearon et al., 2006; King et al., 1994), although the rates in one such study were 'only' twice those of the white population (Bhugra et al., 1997). Some of the more recent of these studies have also looked at those of African ethnicity and have reported similarly raised rates of psychotic illness in this group (Fearon et al., 2006; King et al., 1994; Van Os et al., 1996). And such findings are reflected in research on the less extensively studied minority populations of the US and the Netherlands, where

Black populations are also shown to have rates of psychotic illness that are around three times greater than those for the white population (Breshnahan et al., 2007; Cantor-Graae and Selten, 2005; Robins and Reiger, 1991; Selten et al., 1997, 2001; Veling et al., 2006).

Explorations of the demographic characteristics of Black people admitted to hospital with a psychotic illness suggest that these illnesses are particularly common among young men (Cochrane and Bal, 1989), and some studies have suggested that the rates of diagnosed schizophrenia for Black Caribbean people born in Britain are even higher than for those who migrated – one widely cited study reported that young British-born Black Caribbean men were 18 times more likely than average to experience an admission for a first episode of psychosis (Harrison et al., 1988; see also McGovern and Cope, 1987).

Given the consistency of the evidence based on treatment statistics, it is somewhat surprising that they are not repeated in the two national community based surveys of mental illness among ethnic minority groups in the UK, the Fourth National Survey of Ethnic Minorities (FNS) (Nazroo, 1997) and the EMPIRIC study (Sproston and Nazroo, 2002). Overall, these studies found that Caribbean people had rates of psychotic illness that were atmost twice as high as those in the general population. For example, in the FNS (Nazroo, 1997) the annual prevalence of psychotic illness for Black Caribbean people was 14 per thousand, in comparison with the rate of 8 per thousand for the white group (i.e. 75 per cent higher in the Caribbean group).

And when differences were considered across gender, age and migrant/ non-migrant groups it was found that the prevalence of psychotic illness among: men; young men; and non-migrant men; was no greater than that for equivalent white people. For example, the annual prevalence of psychotic disorder among Caribbean men was estimated as 10 per thousand while among white British men it was estimated as 8 per thousand (Nazroo, 1997). This contrast with treatment data, where the largest differences have been reported for young men; indeed the higher rate found for Caribbean people in the community surveys was entirely driven by the higher rate found for Caribbean women.

Findings on rates of psychotic illness among other ethnic minority groups in the UK are more mixed. Studies of hospital based treatment suggest that rates of admission for psychotic illness among South Asian people are similar to those among white people (Cochrane and Bal, 1989). A more comprehensive prospective study of first contact for schizophrenia with *all* treatment services in one area of London (whose South Asian population is predominantly of Indian origin) confirmed this (Bhugra et al., 1997), but an earlier study using the same methods in another London district suggested that rates of psychotic illness among South Asian people (of Indian and Pakistani origin) were raised to similar levels to those found among Black Caribbean people (King et al., 1994). Indeed, King et al.'s study suggested that rates of psychotic illness among all ethnic minority groups studied were similarly raised in comparison with a white group, and that among the white people identified as having a first onset of psychotic illness the majority were not of British origin (King et al., 1994). Elsewhere the authors state that: 'Most [patients] were from an ethnic minority background, including those people defined as White' (Cole et al., 1995: 771). This, of course, suggests that it is misleading to maintain an exclusive focus on those of Black Caribbean origin when examining ethnic differences in psychotic illness in the UK.

In contrast to some of the findings for contact with treatment services, the community based FNS and EMPIRIC prevalence studies suggested that rates of psychotic illness might not be raised for South Asian people generally, and may be lower for Bangladeshi people than those for white British people (Nazroo, 1997; Sproston and Nazroo, 2002). In support of the conclusions drawn by King et al. (1994) and Cole et al. (1995), the FNS data also showed a high rate of psychosis among white people who were not of British origin, who had a 75 per cent higher rate than the white British group (Nazroo, 1997), although this finding was not replicated in the oversample of Irish people in the EMPIRIC study (Sproston and Nazroo, 2004).

Returning to the situation of Black Caribbean people, it is worth noting that treatment statistics suggest very low rates of *depression* compared with white people (Cochrane and Bal, 1989; Lloyd, 1993). This marked contrast with psychotic illness is a puzzle, because most (non-genetic) factors that might be implicated in the higher rates of psychotic disorders should also lead to a higher rate of other mental illnesses. Such statistics become more puzzling when considered alongside evidence from the FNS suggesting that the prevalence of depression among Black Caribbean people in the community is, in fact, more than 50 per cent higher than that among white people (Nazroo, 1997). Moreover, that study also suggested that despite this higher prevalence, rates of treatment for depression among Black Caribbean people were much lower than those for any other group (Nazroo, 1997).

As this review of evidence from the UK shows, the interpretation of statistics on the high rates of psychotic illness among Black populations in developed countries is problematic. Nevertheless, they have formed the basis for the discussion and research of possible underlying causes for the higher risk. So, before we go on to examine the methodological underpinnings of these statistics more critically, we next discuss possible explanations for a 'real' higher risk, contrasting those that focus on the characteristics of ethnic/race groups and those that focus on the inequalities faced by minority groups.

EXPLAINING ETHNIC INEQUALITIES IN RISK OF PSYCHOTIC ILLNESS

The kind of explanations considered for the observed greater risk of Black people for psychotic illnesses are similar to those considered more generally in the epidemiological literature on ethnic inequalities in health (Nazroo, 2001, 2003), which in turn reflect those discussed as long ago as the 'Black Report' on inequalities in health in the UK (Townsend and Davidson, 1982). Here we discuss non-health service related factors (which are discussed fully in the next two sections of this chapter), under four broad headings. The first three, migration, genetics and culture, reflect identification of the characteristics of those under greater risk that are assumed to be relevant (the assumption being that ethnicity equates to genetic and cultural difference, and migration), while the final heading, social and economic inequalities, reflects the contexts of their lives.

Migration

Within the European context ethnic differences in health are often considered in relation to processes of migration, because the presence of significant non-white populations in Europe is a result of the relatively recent post-Second World War migration. So, in this context different rates of psychotic illness across Black Caribbean and white groups in the UK (and more generally in Europe) could be a consequence of factors related to the process of migration and post-migration life in Europe. Here most emphasis has been placed on two possibilities: that social selection into a migrant group could have favoured those with a higher (or, theoretically in this case, lower) risk of developing illness; and that the stresses associated with migration might have increased risks. There is evidence to both support and counter these suggestions. Investigations of the rates of diagnosed schizophrenia in Jamaica and Trinidad suggest that they are much lower than those for Black Caribbean people in the UK and, in fact, that they are similar to those of the white population of the UK (Bhugra et al., 1996; Hickling, 1991; Hickling and Rodgers-Johnson, 1995). This would suggest that the higher rates for Black Caribbean people in the UK are either a consequence of factors related to the migration process, and/or the greater stresses surrounding the lives of ethnic minority people in the UK.

However, if the higher rates were a consequence of stress around migration, we would expect other migrant groups also to have higher rates of mental illness. As described earlier, evidence here is contradictory. On the whole studies have suggested that other migrants to Britain, in particular South Asian people, do not have similarly raised rates (Cochrane and Bal, 1989), although King et al. (1994) strongly came to the conclusion that the risk of schizophrenia was markedly higher in all migrant groups (including white migrant groups). In addition, if the higher rates of psychotic illness among Black Caribbean people were a consequence of selection into a migrant group, or the stresses associated with migration, one would expect the rates for those born in Britain to begin to approximate those of the white population. However, also as described earlier, studies have suggested that rates of diagnosed schizophrenia for second generation Black Caribbean people are markedly higher than for the first generation (Harrison et al., 1988; see also McGovern and Cope, 1987). This indicates that factors relating directly to the process of migration may not be involved, although these data (like most work in this area) are dependent on a very small number of identified cases.

Genetic differences

In much of the research on ethnicity and health, ethnicity is equated with geneti-cally defined races, and genetic difference is mobilized as a potential explanation for observed differences in health. Not surprisingly, then, there has been some discussion of the possibility that differences in risk of psychotic illness between Black and white people may be a consequence of genetic factors that correlate with ethnic/racial background, but little supporting evidence has been marshalled. In fact, what evidence there is suggests large differences in risk *within* ethnic/racial categories, implying that any genetic basis for such mental illness does not correlate closely with ethnic/racial background *per se*. For example, the evidence on 'schizophrenia' cited in the previous section, which shows that there are important differences between Black Caribbean people who stayed in Jamaica or Trinidad (who do not have raised rates), those who migrated to Britain (who appear to have raised rates) and those who were born in Britain (who appear to have markedly raised rates) suggests that the higher rates cannot be a straight-forward consequence of ethnic differences in genetic risk.

Culture

As for claims to genetic differences, explanations based on claims of the signifi-cance of cultural difference are often mobilized by those attempting to interpret research showing ethnic difference in health. And, perhaps not surprisingly, such an approach to explanation typically bases the cultural argument on speculative and stereotyped characterisations of the cultures of ethnic minority groups, which do not acknowledge the dynamic nature of culture (Ahmad, 1996). In the case of the higher risk of psychotic illness among Black Caribbean people in the UK explanations have often focussed on the higher rates of lone parenthood among Black Caribbean families, or the supposed higher consumption of risky forms of cannabis. But an examination of discussions in the UK around the higher risk of death from suicide among young female migrants from South Asia is more illustrative of the main points relating to the inadequacy of explanations that resort to crude cultural stereotypes.

Research evidence has shown that South Asian people in general have a low or average risk of depression (Cochrane and Stopes-Roe, 1981; Cochrane and Bal, 1989; Gillian et al., 1989; Nazroo, 1997; Sproston and Nazroo, 2002), but that migrant women from South Asia in the 15 to 24 age group have a two to three times greater risk of death from suicide than the national average – a greater risk that is not found for older women or men (Soni Raleigh et al., 1990; Soni Raleigh and Balarajan, 1992; Karmi et al., 1994).

To explain both these low and high rates, the same stereotype is used in mark-edly different ways. So, in language that is reminiscent of the concept of social capital (though it predates its relatively recent popularity in the health inequali-ties field), it has been suggested that the overall lower rates of mental illness among South Asian people could be a consequence of an Asian culture that provides extended and strong communities with protective social support networks (Cochrane and Bal, 1989). In contrast, in the attempt to explain the high mortality rates from suicide among young women born in South Asia, close and extended South Asian communities are portrayed as demanding of young people, constraining and conflictual, leading to the oppression of young women and contributing to the higher suicide rates (e.g. Soni Raleigh and Balarajan, 1992), rather than as supportive and cohesive.

Of course, a closer examination shows that such stereotypes may not hold. For example, despite the focus on patriarchal 'South Asian' families, there are in fact, great similarities between the motives of white and South Asian patients for their suicidal actions. In one study of attempted suicide Handy et al. (1991) report that arguments with parents were a common factor for both white and Asian children, and in another study of attempted suicide Merrill and Owens' (1986) examples of 'restrictive Asian customs (e.g. not allowing them to go out at night, mix with boys, or take further education)' (p. 709) are not greatly different from what one might find in a dispute between a young white woman and her parents. Indeed, a study of coroners' reports on actual suicides in London found that only one third of the twelve South Asian women who had committed suicide had 'family conflict' cited among the reasons for the suicide, and only by stretching the imagination could these be considered as specific to South Asian cultures (Karmi et al., 1994).

It is also worth noting that the literature attempting to explain these high rates of death from suicide was largely generated in the early 1990s. In contemporary times it seems strange to be talking in the UK of 'South Asian' women in this way, rather the stereotype offered is one that is now typically, and routinely, applied to Muslim communities and Muslim women. It is, then, perhaps surprising to find that these high death rates do not apply to women born in the predominantly Muslim countries of Pakistan and Bangladesh. A more recent paper showed that rates for those women are, in fact, very low, with the high rates exclusively present for those born in India and East Africa (Soni Raleigh, 1996). This example illustrates both how the significance of a particular ethnic identity can change dramatically over a short period of time, with a shift from a discussion of 'South Asians' to one of 'Muslims' and also how this shift in significance has the potential to shape how we respond to research evidence.

Socioeconomic inequalities and the impact of racism

A focus on social causation is rare in the literature examining the aetiology of psychotic illness (Jarvis, 2007), in part because in much of this literature social inequalities are hypothesized to result from illness rather than the other way around. However, the broader literature on ethnic/racial inequalities in health clearly demonstrates the significance of socioeconomic inequalities, both within and across ethnic groups (Nazroo, 1998, 2001, 2003). So, within an ethnic/racial group greater socioeconomic resources correlate with better health, and differences between ethnic/racial groups in the level of health are largely accounted for by socioeconomic inequalities. This is the case for a wide range of health outcomes and in a range of national contexts (Nazroo and Williams, 2005).

It would not be surprising, of course, if the poor, run down, inner city environments and poor housing that many ethnic minority people live in, and their poorer employment prospects and standards of living, led to greater mental distress and increased risk of psychotic illness (King et al., 1994). Although many have speculated that this may be the case, socioeconomic inequalities have not been a primary area of empirical investigation in this field, perhaps because of data limitations (studies of contact with treatment services do not, on the whole, collect information on socioeconomic position). And where socioeconomic inequalities have been studied, the methods have often been inappropriate (Nazroo, 1998). There has been considerable criticism of this failure, with commentators suggesting that ignoring the possibility that the relationship between ethnicity and mental health is a consequence of social disadvantage allows the theoretical alignment of psychiatric disorder with an essentialized ethnic difference and encourages a focus on genetic or cultural explanations (Sashidharan, 1993; Sashidharan and Francis, 1993).

Perhaps not surprisingly, where the connection with socioeconomic inequalities has been investigated small numbers of cases have given limited statistical power, but suggested that socioeconomic inequalities might be important for risk of psychotic illness in the Black Caribbean group (Nazroo, 1997; Sproston and Nazroo, 2002). And if a broader spectrum of mental illnesses is considered, findings from the FNS show a marked socioeconomic patterning within all of the ethnic groups it covered, and that this patterning contributes to differences across groups (Nazroo, 1997).

Different rates in mental health across different ethnic groups might also be a consequence of the experiences of discrimination and racism that ethnic minority people face in developed countries. The empirical investigation of the relationship between experiences of racial harassment and discrimination and mental health is far from straightforward (Karlsen and Nazroo, 2006). Most important is the difficulty in measuring exposure to racism and discrimination accurately, given that these are a central, but often subtly expressed, feature of the lives of ethnic minority people and one that may be more likely to be reported by those experiencing mental distress. Nevertheless, experiences of racial harassment and discrimination appear to be related to mental health in the few but growing number of studies that have been conducted. Studies in the US and New Zealand have shown a relationship between self-reported experiences of racial harassment and a range of health outcomes, including psychological distress (Harris et al., 2006; Williams et al., 2003). In the UK, findings from the Fourth National Survey of Ethnic Minorities suggested a relationship between experiences of racial harassment, perceptions of racial discrimination and a range of health outcomes across ethnic groups, including psychotic illness (Karlsen and Nazroo, 2002). This analysis showed that for ethnic minority people as a whole, reporting experiences of racial harassment and perceiving employers to discriminate were related to an increased likelihood of having a psychotic illness independently of each other, and that this relationship was also independent of socioeconomic effects as indexed by occupational class. More recent analysis of the EMPIRIC study confirmed this, and was able to show that risk of psychotic illness for Black Caribbean people was greatly increased by experiencing any of racial harassment/ attack, discrimination in employment, or believing that British employers discriminate (Karlsen et al., 2005).

Perhaps the most important conclusion to be drawn from these findings is that there is nothing inevitable, or inherent, in being a member of a particular ethnic/ race category and risk of psychotic illness. It is misleading to consider Black Caribbean people in the UK to be uniformly at higher risk, those who are in a higher class, for example, have a lower risk (Sproston and Nazroo, 2002). This points to the need to move beyond explanations that appeal to essentialized, or fixed, ethnic/race effects, and to consider context and socioeconomic inequalities. It could be argued that the measures of socioeconomic inequality that have been considered in empirical work represent three dimensions operating simultaneously, economic disadvantage (as measured by occupational class), a sense of being a member of a devalued, low status, group (e.g. reporting the belief that British employers discriminate), and the personal insult and stress of being a victim of racial harassment or discrimination. Broadly these inequalities can be considered to be a consequence of the ways in which ethnic minority groups are racialized in contemporary societies, which in turn reflects a historical legacy of racism. This relates to claims that both psychiatric practice and psychiatric research reflect a racist agenda, as demonstrated by the uncritical acceptance of findings based on evidence drawn from treatment settings. We now turn to a discussion of the use of treatment data.

USING TREATMENT DATA TO IDENTIFY DIFFERENCES IN RISK OF MENTAL ILLNESS: WHAT CONCLUSIONS CAN WE DRAW?

One of the central problems with work on ethnicity and mental illness arises from the reliance of most work on data based on contact with treatment services. Contact with treatment services, even when access is universal as in the UK, reflects illness behaviour (i.e. the way that symptoms are perceived, evaluated and acted upon), rather than illness *per se* (Blane et al., 1996). This raises a number of linked problems when interpreting differences in treatment rates across ethnic groups, particularly as illness behaviour is likely to be affected by a number of factors that vary by ethnicity, such as socioeconomic position, health beliefs, expectations of the sick role and lay referral systems. And these problems become particularly important for work on rates of psychosis, where contact with services might be against the patient's wishes. So, despite the consistency of research findings showing that Black Caribbean people have higher rates of treatment for psychosis in the UK, some commentators have not accepted the validity of the interpretation of these data and continue to suggest that a higher incidence (rather than a higher treatment rate) remains unproven, because of the serious methodological flaws with the research that has been carried out. (See Sashidharan (1993) and Sashidharan and Francis (1993) for comprehensive reviews of this, and Adebimpe (1994) for a comment on the similar situation in the US.)

There are, as with all research, a number of technical problems facing studies using treatment data. For example, although these data can identify the number of patients, alternative data sources need to be used to identify the size of the population from which they are drawn. Typically this would be estimated from a population census, but the use of census data to provide a denominator requires: collection of appropriate data in the census; treatment data that are collected at the same time as the census and using census categories to classify patients; and accurate estimations of the geographical limit of the population that is covered by the treatment service. Here it is worth noting that a census typically underestimates the numbers of certain groups in the population, including ethnic/racial minority groups (OPCS, 1994), that the 'catchment' areas covered by treatment centres are rarely tightly defined, and that both of these make it difficult to estimate the size of the population from which cases are drawn (although not to the extent that could explain the many times higher rates of admission that are reported for Black Caribbean people and psychotic illnesses).

It is also possible that there are problems with the count of cases, with an overestimation of first onsets of psychosis, because of a variation across ethnic/race groups in the degree of under-identification of previous episodes. In the UK context it has been argued that this overestimation may occur for Black Caribbean people, because of high geographical mobility leading to records of previous admissions being missed and a reluctance to disclose previous diagnoses, because of a concern about the impact of these on how they might be managed (Lipsedge, 1993). The count of those receiving treatment might also be biased by variations in the route of admission to treatment by ethnicity, with Black people overrepresented among patients compulsorily detained in psychiatric hospital, more likely to have been in contact with the police or forensic services prior to admission, and more likely to have been referred to these services by a stranger rather than by a relative or neighbour. And this is despite studies in the UK showing the Black Caribbean patients are both less likely than whites to display evidence of self-harm and no more likely to be aggressive to others prior to admission (Davies et al., 1996; Harrison et al., 1989; McKenzie et al., 1995; Rogers, 1990). Of course this might not be significant if all cases appeared in the treatment settings used for studies, but this is unlikely to be the case – a recent US study indicates that 39 of 183 (21 per cent) people with possible psychosis had not received hospital treatment over a sixteen year follow-up (Bresnahan et al., 2007), and within the UK those who are treated in the private healthcare sector (estimated to be 14 per cent of patients) are not included in either treatment statistics or research studies (Raleigh and Deery, 2008).

It is also possible that differences in the attitudes of health care workers to different ethnic groups coupled with difficulties in the diagnosis of schizophrenia may be involved. For example, McKenzie et al. (1995) showed that Black Caribbean people with psychosis were less likely than equivalent whites to have received psychotherapy or antidepressants; Harrison et al. (1989) showed that although Black Caribbean people were no more likely to have been aggressive at the time of admission, once admitted staff were more likely to perceive them as potentially dangerous both to themselves and to others; and Rogers (1990) showed that psychiatrists were *more* likely than police to consider Black Caribbean patients detained in an emergency as dangerous to others. Coupled with difficulties in diagnosis, these pieces of evidence suggest that the stereo-types that inform the behaviour of health care workers may make them more likely to diagnose Black Caribbean people as psychotic. And although studies based on case notes show that the validity of diagnosis does not relate to the ethnicity of the patient, such studies cannot account for the ways in which race is written into such case notes. In contrast, studies examining diagnostic practice (Neighbors et al., 1989, 2003; Strakowski et al., 1993) and robust studies using vignettes (Loring and Powell, 1988) suggest that Black people are more likely than white people to be diagnosed as schizophrenic and more likely to be seen as dangerous.

Taken together, the comments above suggest that there are a variety of potential problems with studies based on treatment rates and, consequently, that their find-ings should not be taken at face value. There must remain some doubt about the claims of studies based on treatment rates regarding the higher rates of psychosis among African Caribbean people.

In addition to these difficulties, there is a large literature that queries the cross-cultural validity of psychiatric diagnostic practices. The concern is that members of different ethnic groups will have different symptomatic experiences when mentally ill, because of cultural differences in the idioms used to express mental distress. For example, it has been suggested that South Asian people in the UK may experience particular 'culture-bound' syndromes, that is a cluster of symp-toms which is restricted to a particular culture, such as sinking heart (Krause, 1989; see also Fenton and Sadiq-Sangster, 1996), and consequently not be identi-fied as mentally ill by standard diagnostic practices and research instruments. Kleinman (1987) argues that the different idioms for expressing mental distress in different cultures allows for a 'category fallacy', where the use of a category of illness that was developed in one cultural group for research or treatment in another culture group may fail to identify many to whom it can apply, because it lacks coherence in that culture. The idioms of mental distress in the researched group are simply different from those used in the research tool. So, Kleinman (1987) points out the obvious fallacy in attempting to identify the prevalence of 'semen loss' or 'soul loss' in white western groups. This may, of course, equally be the case for instruments designed to detect western expressions of mental distress when applied to other cultures. Indeed, Jadhav (1996) has been able to describe the historical and regional development of 'western depression', leading him to suggest that this apparently universal disorder is culturally specific. However, the findings of Nazroo and O'Connor (2002) suggest that the problem may not be in the broader construct, but in the detail of the idioms used to express distress.

This problem applies not just to treatment data, but also to survey data, such as those provided by the FNS and EMPIRIC studies. The interpretation of survey data, presents a number of additional problems. First, many surveys of ethnic minority people are carried out in particular locations and consequently have restricted generalizability beyond that geographical context (e.g. Bhugra et al., 1997). Second, many studies that claim to be nationally representative often only cover areas with large ethnic minority populations, so ethnic minority people living in predominantly white areas are not included. Third, even survey data that address these sampling biases, such as the FNS and EMPIRIC studies, inevitably suffer from a non-response problem, where some of those who are identified for inclusion in the survey refuse to co-operate, and such non-response may be related to the condition under study. Fourth, the condition under study might be sufficiently rare in the community and be sufficiently hard to detect (as, e.g. in the case of psychotic disorders) as to require both large samples and complicated procedures for estimating prevalence, making the estimate imprecise (so leaving large standard errors).

MENTAL HEALTH SERVICES

In addition to considering the impact of racism on health, either direct or through consequent adverse socioeconomic circumstances, it is also important to explore and address how such social disadvantage influences ethnic minority patients' experiences of and uptake of mental health services, and the implications of this for practice. Here we concentrate on evidence from the UK.

Generally, regardless of their ethnic background, people with mental health problems are critical of the services they receive (Keating et al., 2003; Sainsbury Centre for Mental Health (SCMH), 1998a, b). Common criticisms revolve around the fact that the mainstay of services are acute hospital units that are poorly staffed, leading to a lack of therapeutic intervention and a lack of information giving from staff. Complaints that are echoed in recent comments from the President of the UK Royal College of Psychiatrists (Bhugra, 2008; Observer, 2008), Not surprisingly, this has lead to suggestions that services could be improved by providing more support in the community and by engaging with service-user groups.

A number of more specific issues have been raised when the mental health care needs of ethnic minority people in the UK have been considered (King's Fund, 1998; SCMH, 1998a). Common criticisms have included a feeling that the contact they have with mental health services show staff to be culturally insensitive and that treatment is based on standard assessment tools that do not reflect their or their families' needs, of not being listened to, and families and carers feeling that they are not respected (Bowl, 2007a, b; SCMH, 2002). Such cultural insensitivity is likely to be reflected in the stereotypes used by health care workers when dealing with ethnic minority people (Audini and Lelliott, 2002; Keating et al., 2003). Stereotypes such as African Caribbean people being considered as 'Big, Black and dangerous' (Keating, 2007; Webbe, 1998), or 'loud and difficult to manage' (Kings Fund, 2003) continue to exist and it has been suggested that they contribute to the higher rates of detention experienced by such paptients (SCMH, 2002). There is a clear possibility that such cultural stereotypes extend to other elements of psychiatric practice. For example, one study has shown that when South Asian patients consult with their GPs about mental health problems, their symptoms often go undiagnosed (Commander et al., 1997). And the FNS found that Caribbean people who had scored on a depression inventory were far less likely than white people with equivalent scores to be receiving treatment, despite being as likely to have contacted their GP (Nazroo, 1997). This is further borne out by studies that show that Black Caribbean people are less likely than white or South Asian people to be referred to specialist services (Bhui and Bhugra, 2002; Burnett et al., 1999; Commander et al., 1997).

Ethnic minority carers and users of mental health services have also indicated that they are suspicious of statutory mental health services, a suspicion that appears to be based on previous negative experiences. Some users have reported that they are fearful of dying in hospital as a result of the over use of medication and the aggressive restraining techniques employed by staff (SCMH, 2002, 2006). This view fits with evidence that Black patients are more likely to be compulsorily treated, despite not being more likely to be a danger to themselves or others (Audini and Lelliot, 2002; Davies et al., 1996; Harrison et al., 1989; McKenzie et al., 1995; Morgan et al., 2005a; Rogers, 1990; SCMH, 2006). So they are more likely to be in psychiatric intensive care units and medium secure units, and more likely to be secluded or physically restrained (SCMH, 2006). They are also more likely to have contact with assertive outreach teams in the community, suggesting a lack of engagement with communities until crisis levels are reached (SCMH, 2006). Similarly, Black Caribbean patients with a diagnosis of psychosis remain in acute hospital care longer than white patients and have more frequent outpatient follow-up contacts, despite having fewer negative symptoms (Commander et al., 2003; Takei et al., 1998). Yet, despite this over-representation in the acute sector, when discharged into the community it seems that Black Caribbean patients receive variable and often inadequate support from community mental health teams and primary care services (Bhui and Bhugra, 2002; Bhui et al., 2003).

Concern about these findings has led to several policy initiatives in the UK. The backdrop to these has been a broader shift in the legislative framework as a result of The Human Rights Act 1998 and the Race Relations (Amendment) Act 2000, which followed the Macpherson Inquiry into the police investigation of the racist murder of a teenager (Steven Lawrence) in London (Macpherson, 1999). One focus of the Macpherson Inquiry was 'institutional racism', defined as:

> The collective failure of an organisation to provide an appropriate and professional service to people because of their colour, culture or ethnic origin. It can be seen or detected in processes, attitudes and behaviour which amount to discrimination through unwitting prejudice, ignorance, thoughtlessness and racist stereotyping which disadvantages ethnic minority people. (Macpherson, 1999: 28)

Following the Macpherson Inquiry, there has been a widespread acknowledgement that institutional racism operates in mental health services in the UK, and that this has contributed to failures in the care and treatment of ethnic minority people (Blofeld, 2003; DH, 2005). Not surprisingly, however, such an acknowledgment has not sat easily with some psychiatrists, who are concerned that they and their services are being labelled as racist and that this will have a negative impact on patient care (Murray and Fearon, 2007; Patel and Heginbotham, 2007; Singh, 2007). Nevertheless, the Race Relations (Amendment) Act, which followed the Macpherson Inquiry, specifically requires providers of public services to be pro-active in ensuring the elimination of practices and procedures that discriminate against particular ethnic groups. This legislation has been followed by a number of policy documents that aim to tackle ethnic inequalities in the health field. For example, the National Service Framework for Mental Health (DH, 1999) explicitly acknowledges the over-representation of Black groups in secure services and their greater likelihood to receive physical rather than psychological treatments and states that discrimination should be combated. More recently the Delivering Race Equality in Mental Health Care document (DH, 2005) provided a five year action plan to develop mental health services and improve the training of healthcare professionals. It has also led to the appointment of a National Director for mental health and ethnicity, who is supported by nine regional 'race equality leads' concerned with eliminating discrimination, with the intention of strengthening leadership for mental health services for ethnic minority patients. This programme is also trying to improve engagement with communities by establishing 'community development workers' (DH, 2005) and improving liaison between General Practitioners (or primary care teams) and community mental health teams (Bhui and Bhugra, 2002). There have also been calls for a related set of initiatives to improve liaison with the criminal justice system (Challal and Iqbal, 2004), given the involvement of the police in many admissions (Morgan et al., 2005b), something that appears to be more likely if the patient does not have a GP to support them (Bhui and Bhugra, 2002; Keating, 2007). Such initiatives are clearly intended to tackle a range of connected problems, however, it remains uncertain whether they can be successful. For example, Fernando (2005) has pointed out that the 'race equality leads' have only an advisory role, so may have limited effectiveness; an evaluation of such initiatives is sorely needed.

A related and recurring theme in discussions of how to improve services is the need for healthcare professionals to receive training and education about cultural diversity. This need is seen across UK health services (DH, 2005), where it is suggested that stereotypical images of ethnic minority people continue to persist in part because of the lack of cultural diversity and cultural competence training during, for example, nurse education (Gerrish et al., 1996; Webbe, 1998), so such stereotypes are rarely challenged and can become deeply rooted in clinical practice. In the mental health field, where such issues might be very visible, it has been noted that many healthcare professionals are uncomfortable about discussing race, culture and racism (Keating, 2007; SCMH, 2002). To address such concerns, cultural competency training and the promotion of anti-discriminatory practice has now been incorporated into healthcare education. For example, it features on pre-registration nursing programmes in the UK (NMC, 2004), and more recently there has been a stronger focus on this both in the pre-registration education programmes for mental health nurses and as a component of their continuing education post-qualification (DH, 2006). Indeed, a recent review of mental health nursing in the UK has included in its recommendations a requirement to attend cultural competency training every three years, along with specifying standards to address ethnic service inequalities and non-discriminatory practice (DH, 2006).

However, effective cultural competency training is neither easy, nor straight-forward, to achieve. Certainly, many attempts to address cultural diversity in educational materials have failed or, worse still, been based on stereotypical images of ethnic minority groups. Indeed, in this new culturally aware climate it has been suggested that service users experience a new form of stereotyping, where practitioners make assumptions about their culture and identity as a result of simple generalizations (Challal and Iqbal, 2004; SCMH, 2002). So, such reforms to services may simply produce a set of assumptions and generalisations about ethnicity and culture that can, at worst, just translate into a narrow focus on assumed dietary and spiritual needs (Keating, 2007). Fernando (2003) argues that this is exactly why an approach that focuses on cultural difference can reinforce a racist environment. So, although these recent policy shifts have produced some optimism, tackling the institutional racism that lies at the route of these problems will not be straightforward to address (Burr and Chapman, 1998). It is possible that legislation and policies to overcome discrimination will not have a great impact on practice.

CONCLUDING COMMENTS

Our account suggests that many basic questions concerning the relationship between ethnicity/race and mental health remain unanswered. There remains a question of whether the use of western psychiatric instruments for the cross-cultural measurement of psychiatric disorder is valid and produces a genuine assessment of the differences between different ethnic groups (Jadhav, 1996; Kleinman, 1987; Littlewood, 1992). In the UK this has been raised particularly in relation to the low detection and treatment rates for depressive disorders among South Asians, but it may apply to other disorders and other ethnic/racial minority groups. It is also likely that treatment-based statistics reflect more than the health experiences of the populations from which those in treatment are drawn, that they also reflect the operation of public institutions in an environment where social identities remain racialized. The investigation of these issues is far from straightforward, not least because such phenomena are deeply embedded in specific contexts. Complex social phenomena are not easily reduced to gross empirical observations.

This is very apparent when we reflect on how ethnicity/race becomes reduced to simple observed categories, including within our own research. Within the wider theoretical literature many writers emphasize a notion of ethnicity as a social identity that reflects self-identification with cultural traditions that provide meaning, but also boundaries (fluid) between groups. Although such a conceptualization of ethnicity reflects identification with sets of shared values, beliefs, customs and lifestyles, it has to be understood dynamically, as an active social process (Smaje, 1996). In particular, the influence of a cultural affiliation on individuals and groups, and on their health, has to be properly contextualized to take account of different periods and different elements of an identity, such as class, gender and caste (Ahmad, 1996). What it means, for example, to be Black Caribbean might vary greatly in the different contexts of the US and the UK (Nazroo et al., 2007). So, ethnicity is also a hybrid identity (Modood, 1998; Hall, 1992) that is not just given, but which is also the target of social action, changing across contexts and over time, fused with elements from other cultures, and which exists alongside other competing and complementary identities (such as gender and class).

Nevertheless, and as any discussion of racism or socioeconomic inequality implies, it is important to consider the structural determinants of ethnicity/race. Here Miles' (1989) portrayal of racism as central to an understanding of ethnic/ race relations is of great use. When discussing the emergence of ethnic or 'race' categories within a society (the 'ethnic moment') Miles emphasizes how ethnic difference can be essentialized as a product of 'nature' and how this becomes a justification for exclusionary and discriminatory treatment (Miles, 1996). In addition to the implicit critique of health research that adopts essentialist notions of ethnicity as culture or biology, this also reminds us that a core component of ethnic relations involves the categorization of the Other and the exclusion of the Other. Central to Miles' argument is the suggestion that the construction of ethnic boundaries are economically determined, they occur within a wider set of class relations (Miles, 1996). This is a reminder both that ethnic identity – and the meaning of particular ethnic identities – are assigned as well as adopted (and assigned on the basis of power relations) and that ethnic minority status is closely associated with particular class positions.

Such complexity indicates that explaining ethnic/race differences in mental illness, or the role of psychiatric institutions, is not a straightforward task.

Perhaps, as others have pointed out (Sashidharan and Francis, 1993), the most important conclusion to draw is that it is vital to avoid essentializing ethnic differences in mental health (i.e. reducing them to stereotyped notions of cultural or biological difference), there is a need to explore the factors associated with ethnicity that may explain any relationship between ethnicity and mental health, such as the various forms of social disadvantage that ethnic minority people face. And it remains important to explore how racism and the social disadvantages that this leads to structure the experiences of ethnic minority people when they come into contact with mental health services. Despite this, the focus on biological explanations for mental illness, and neglect of social explanations continues in both the USA and the UK (Jarvis, 2007; Munro, 1999), and media fuelled public concerns about the dangers associated with mental illness appear to continue to influence policy (Munro, 1999). This has implications for the success of attempts to reform mental health services, which we described earlier, with a risk of a return to more coercive services that will present major difficulties for those working in an environment that is also attempting to be Delivering Race Equality in Mental Health Care (DH, 2005) in a context where young men are racialized as 'Big, Black and dangerous' (Webbe, 1998; Keating, 2007).

REFERENCES

Adebimpe, V.R. (1994) Race, racism, and epidemiological surveys, *Hospital and Community Psychiatry*, 45(1): 27–31.

Ahmad, W.I.U. (1996) The trouble with culture. In D. Kelleher and S. Hillier (eds), *Researching Cultural Differences in Health*. London: Routledge.

Audini, B. and Lelliott, P. (2002) Age, gender and ethnicity of those detained under Part ll of the Mental Health Act 1983, *British Journal of Psychiatry*, 280: 222–226.

Bagley, C. (1971) The social aetiology of schizophrenia in immigrant groups, *International Journal of Social Psychiatry*, 17: 292–304.

Bhugra, D. (2008) Renewing psychiatry's contract with society, *Psychiatric Bulletin*, 32, 281–283.

Bhugra, D., Hilwig, M., Hossein, B., Marceau, H., Neehall, J., Leff, J., Mallett, R. and Der, G. (1996) First-contact incidence rates of schizophrenia in Trinidad and one-year follow-up, *British Journal of Psychiatry*, 169: 587–592.

Bhugra, D., Leff, J., Mallett, R., Der, G., Corridan, B. and Rudge, S. (1997) Incidence and outcome of schizophrenia in whites, African-Caribbeans and Asians in London, *Psychological Medicine*, 27: 791–798.

Bhui, K. and Bhugra, D. (2002) Mental illness in Black and Asian ethnic minorities: pathways to care and outcomes, *Advances in Psychiatric Treatment*, 8: 26–33.

Bhui, K., Stansfield, S., Hull, S., Priebe, S., Mole, F. and Feder, G. (2003) Ethnic variations in pathways to and use of specialist mental health services, *British Journal of Psychiatry*, 182: 105–116.

Blane, D., Power, C. and Bartley, M. (1996) Illness behaviour and the measurement of class differentials in morbidity, *Journal of the Royal Statistical Society*, 156(1): 77–92.

Blofeld, J. (2003) *Independent Inquiry into the Death of David Bennett*. Norfolk, Suffolk and Cambridgeshire Strategic Health Authority, Norwich.

Bowl, R. (2007a) The need for Change in UK Mental Health Services: South Asian Service User's Views, *Ethnicity and Health*, 12: 1–19.

Bowl, R. (2007b) Responding to ethnic diversity: black service users' views of mental health services in the UK, *Diversity in Health and Social Care*, 4: 201–210.

Bresnahan, M., Begg. M.D., Brown, A., Schaefer, C., Sohler, N., Insel, B., Vella, L. and Susser, E. (2007) Race and risk of schizophrenia in a US birth cohort: another example of health disparity?, *International Journal of Epidemiology*, 36: 751–758.

Burnett, R., Mallet, R., Bugra, D., Hutchinson, G., Der, G. and Leff, J. (1999) The first contact of patients with schizophrenia with psychiatric services: social factors and pathways to care in a multi-ethnic population, *Psychological Medicine*, 29: 475–483.

Burr, J.A. and Chapman, T. (1998) Some reflections on cultural and social considerations in mental health nursing, *Journal of Psychiatric and Mental Health Nursing*, 5: 431–437.

Cantor-Graae, E. and Selten, J.P. (2005) Schizophrenia and migration: a meta-analysis and review, *American Journal of Psychiatry*, 162: 12–24.

Cantor-Graae, E., Zolkowska, K. and McNeil, T.F. (2005) Increased risk of psychotic disorder among immigrants in Malmo: a 3-year first-contact study, *Psychological Medicine*, 35: 1155–1163.

Challal, K. and Iqbal, A. (2004) *Foundations Experiencing Ethnicity: Discrimination and Service Provision.* York: Joseph Rowntree Foundation.

Cochrane, R. and Bal, S.S. (1989) Mental hospital admission rates of immigrants to England: a comparison of 1971 and 1981, *Social Psychiatry and Psychiatric Epidemiology*, 24: 2–11.

Cochrane, R. and Stopes-Roe, M. (1981) Psychological symptom levels in Indian immigrants to England – a comparison with native English, *Psychological Medicine*, 11: 319–327.

Cole, E., Leavey, G., King, M., Johnson-Sabine, E. and Hoar, A. (1995) Pathways to care for patients with a first episode of psychosis: a comparison of ethnic groups, *British Journal of Psychiatry*, 167: 770–776.

Commander, M.J., Dharan, S.P., Odell, S.M. and Surtees, P.G. (1997) Access to mental health care in an inner city health district. II: Association with demographic factors, *British Journal of Psychiatry*, 170: 317–320.

Commander, M., Odell, S., Surlees, P. and Sashidharan, S. (2003) Characteristics of patients and patterns of psychiatric service user in ethnic minorities, *International Journal of Social Psychiatry*, 49: 216–224.

Davies, S., Thornicroft, G., Leese, M., Higgingbotham, A. and Phelan, M. (1996) Ethnic differences in risk of compulsory psychiatric admission among representative cases of psychosis in London, *British Medical Journal*, 312: 533–537.

Dein, S. (1997) ABC of mental health in a multiethnic society, *British Medical Journal*, 315: 473–476.

Department of Health (1999) *The National Health Framework for Mental Health*. London: Department of Health.

Department of Health (2005) *Delivering Race Equality in Mental Health Care: an Action Plan for Reform Inside and Outside Services: and the Governments Response to the Independent Inquiry into the Death of David Bennett*. London: Department of Health.

Department of Health (2006) *From Values to Action: The Chief Nursing Officer's Review of Mental Health Nursing*. London: Department of Health.

Erens B., Primatesta P. and Prior G. (2001) Health Survey for England 1999: *The Health of Minority Ethnic Groups*. London: The Stationery Office.

Fearon, P., Kirkbiride, J.B., Morgan, C., Dazzan, P., Morgan, K., Lloyd, T., Hutchinson, G., Tarrant, J., Fung, W.L., Holloway, J., Mallett, R., Harrison, G., Leff, J., Jones, P.B. and Murray, R.M. (2006) Incidence of schizophrenia and other psychoses in ethnic minority groups: results from the MRC AESOP Study, *Psychological Medicine*, 36: 1541–1550.

Fenton, S. and Sadiq-Sangster, A. (1996) Culture, relativism and the expression of mental distress: South Asian women in Britain, *Sociology of Health and Illness*, 18(1): 66–85.

Fernando, S. (2003) *Cultural Diversity, Mental Health and Psychiatry. The Struggle Against Racism*. Hove and New York: Brunner–Routledge.

Fernando, S. (2005) Multicultural mental health services: projects for ethnic minority communities in England, *Transcultural Psychiatry*, 42: 420–436.

Gerrish., K., Husband, C. and Mackenzie, J. (1996) Ethnicity, the Minority Ethnic Community and Health Care Delivery. In W.I.U. Ahmad and C. Husband (eds) *'Race', Health and Social Care*. Birmingham: Open University Press.

Gilliam, S.J., Jarman, B., White, P. and Law, R. (1989) Ethnic differences in consultation rates in urban general practice, *British Medical Journal*, 299: 953–957.

Hall, S. (1992) The question of cultural identity. In S. Hall, D. Held and T. McGrew (eds) *Modernity and its Futures*. Cambridge: Polity.

Handy, S., Chithiramohan, R.N., Ballard, C.G. and Silveira, W.R. (1991) Ethnic differences in adolescent self–poisoning: a comparison of Asian and Caucasian groups, *Journal of Adolescence*, 14: 157–162.

Harris, R., Tobias, M., Jeffreys, M., Waldegrave, K., Karlsen, S. and Nazroo, J. (2006) Racism and health: The relationship between experience of racial discrimination and health in New Zealand, *Social Science and Medicine*, 63(6): 1428–1441.

Harrison, G., Owens, D., Holton, A., Neilson, D. and Boot, D. (1988) A prospective study of severe mental disorder in Afro-Caribbean patients, *Psychological Medicine*, 18: 643–657.

Harrison, G., Holton, A., Neilson, D., Owens, D., Boot, D. and Cooper, J. (1989) Severe mental disorder in Afro-Caribbean patients: some social, demographic and service factors, *Psychological Medicine*, 19: 683–696.

Hickling, F.W. (1991) Psychiatric hospital admission rates in Jamaica, *British Journal of Psychiatry*, 159: 817–821.

Hickling, F.W. and Rodgers-Johnson, P. (1995) The Incidence of First Contact Schizophrenia in Jamaica, *British Journal of Psychiatry*, 167: 193–196.

Jadhav, S. (1996) The cultural origins of Western depression, *International Journal of Social Psychiatry*, 42(4): 269–286.

Jarvis, G.E. (2007) The social causes of psychosis in North American psychiatry: a review of a disappearing literature, *The Canadian Journal of Psychiatry*, 52: 287–294.

Karlsen, S. and Nazroo, J.Y. (2002) The relationship between racial discrimination, social class and health among ethnic minority groups, *American Journal of Public Health*, 92(4): 624–631.

Karlsen, S. and Nazroo, J. (2006) Measuring and analyzing 'race', racism and racial discrimination. In J. Oakes and J. Kaufman (eds) *Methods in Social Epidemiology*, San Francisco: Jossey-Bass. 86–111.

Karlsen, S., Nazroo, J.Y., McKenzie, K., Bhui, K. and Weich, S. (2005) Racism, psychosis and common mental disorder among ethnic minority groups in England, *Psychological Medicine*, 35(12): 1795–1803.

Karmi, G., Abdulrahim, D., Pierpoint, T. and McKeigue, P. (1994) *Suicide among Ethnic Minorities and Refugees in the UK*. London: NE and NW Thames RHA.

Keating, F. (2007) *African and Caribbean Men and Mental Health*, Better Health Briefing 5. London: Race Equality Foundation.

Keating, F., Robertson, D. and Kotecha, N. (2003) *Ethnic Diversity and Mental Health in London:Recent Developments*, Working Paper, Kings Fund.

King, M., Coker, E., Leavey, G., Hoare, A. and Johnson-Sabine, E. (1994) Incidence of psychotic illness in London: comparison of ethnic groups, *British Medical Journal*, 309: 1115–1119.

King's Fund (1998) *London's Mental Health. The Report to the King's Fund London Commission*. London: King's Fund Publishing.

Kleinman, A. (1987) Anthropology and psychiatry: the role of culture in cross-cultural research on illness, *British Journal of Psychiatry*, 151: 447–454.

Krause, I. (1989) Sinking heart: a Punjabi communication of distress, *Social Science and Medicine*, 29(4): 563–575.

Lipsedge, M. (1993) Mental health: access to care for black and ethnic minority people. In A. Hopkins and V. Bahl (eds) *Access to Health Care for People from Black and Ethnic Minorities*, London: Royal College of Physicians.

Littlewood, R. (1992) Psychiatric diagnosis and racial bias: empirical and interpretative approaches, *Social Science and Medicine*, 34(2): 141–149.

Littlewood, R. and Lipsedge, M. (1988) Psychiatric illness among British Afro-Caribbeans, *British Medical Journal*, 296: 950–951.

Lloyd, K. (1993) Depression and anxiety among Afro-Caribbean general practice attenders in Britain, *International Journal of Social Psychiatry*, 39: 1–9.

Loring, M. and Powell, B. (1988) Gender, race and DSM-III: a study of the objectivity of psychiatric diagnostic behavior, *Journal of Health and Social Behavior*, 29: 1–22.

McGovern, D. and Cope, R. (1987) First psychiatric admission rates of first and second generation Afro–Caribbeans, *Social Psychiatry*, 22:139–149.

McKenzie, K., van Os, J., Fahy, T., Jones, P., Harvey, I., Toone, B. and Murray, R. (1995) Psychosis with good prognosis in Afro-Caribbean people now living in the United Kingdom, *British Medical Journal*, 311: 1325–1328.

Macpherson, W. (1999) *The Stephen Lawrence Inquiry: Report of an Inquiry by Sir William Macpherson of Cluny,* Cm 4261–1. London: The Stationary Office.

Merrill, J. and Owens, J. (1986) Ethnic differences in self-poisoning: a comparison of Asian and White groups, *British Journal of Psychiatry*, 148: 708–712.

Miles, R. (1989) *Racism.* London: Routledge.

Miles, R. (1996) Racism and Nationalism in the United Kingdom: a view from the periphery. In R. Barot (ed.) *The Racism Problematic: Contemporary Sociological Debates on Race and Ethnicity.* Lewiston: The Edwin Mellen Press.

Modood, T. (1998) Anti-essentialism, multiculturalism and the 'recognition' of religious groups, *The Journal of Political Philosophy*, 6(4): 378–399.

Morgan, C., Mallet, R., Hutchinson, G., Bagalkote, K., Morgan, K., Fearon, P., Dazzon, J., Boydell, K., McKenzie, K., Harrison, G., Murray, R., Jones, P., Craig, T. and Ieff, J. (2005a) Pathways to care and ethnicity. 1: Sample characteristics and compulsory admission, *British Journal of Psychiatry*, *186*: 281–289.

Morgan, C., Mallet, R., Hutchinson, G., Bagalkote, K., Morgan, K., Fearon, P., Dazzon, J., Boydell, K., McKenzie, K., Harrison, G., Murray, R., Jones, P., Craig, T. and Ieff, J. (2005b) Pathways to care and ethnicity 2: Source of referral and help-seeking, *British Journal of Psychiatry*, 186: 290–296.

Munro, R. (1999) There's sin in them there genes, *Nursing Times*, 95(33): 28–29.

Murray, R. and Fearon, P. (2007) Searching for racists under the psychiatric bed: commentary on … institutional racism in psychiatry, *Psychiatric Bulletin*, 31: 365–366.

Nazroo, J.Y. (1997) *Ethnicity and Mental Health: Findings from a National Community Survey.* London: Policy Studies Institute.

Nazroo J.Y. (1998) Genetic, cultural or socio-economic vulnerability? Explaining ethnic inequalities in health, *Sociology of Health and Illness*, 20(5): 710–730.

Nazroo, J.Y. (2001) *Ethnicity, Class and Health.* London: Policy Studies Institute.

Nazroo, J. Y. (2003) The structuring of ethnic inequalities in health: economic position, racial discrimination and racism, *American Journal of Public Health*, 93(2):277–284.

Nazroo, J.Y. and O'Connor, W. (2002) Idioms of mental distress. In O'Connor, W. and Nazroo, J. (eds) *Ethnic Differences in the Context and Experience of Psychiatric Illness: A Qualitative Study.* London: The Stationery Office.

Nazroo, J.Y. and Williams, D.R. (2005) The social determination of ethnic/racial inequalities in health. In M. Marmot and R.G. Wilkinson (eds) *Social Determinants of Health* (Second Edition). Oxford: Oxford University Press, pp. 238–266.

Nazroo, J.Y., Jackson, J., Karlsen, S. and Torres, M. (2007) The black diaspora and health inequalities in the US and England: does where you go and how you get there make a difference?, *Sociology of Health and Illness*, 26: 811–830.

Neighbors, H.W., Jackson, J.S., Campbell. L. and Williams, D. (1989) The influence of racial factors on psychiatric diagnosis, *Community Mental Health*, 44: 237–256.

Neighbors, H.W., Trierweiler, S.J., Ford, B.C. and Murof, J.R. (2003) Racial differences in DSM diagnosis using a semi-structured instrument: the importance of clinical judgement in the diagnosis of Blacks, *Journal of Health and Social Behaviour*, 44: 237–256.

Nursing Midwifery Council (2004) *Standards of Proficiency for Pre-registration Nurse Education.* London: Nursing Midwifery Council.

Observer (2008) Psychiatric patients 'feel lost and unsafe', June 29, http://www.guardian.co.uk/society/2008/jun/29/mentalhealth.health3 (accessed 24 October, 2008).

Office of Population Censuses and Surveys (1994) *Undercoverage in Great Britain (Census User Guide no. 58).* London: HMSO.

Patel, K. and Heginbotham, C. (2007) Institutional racism in mental health services does not imply racism in individual psychiatrists: Commentary on Institutional racism in psychiatry, *Psychiatric Bulletin*, 31: 367–368.

Raleigh, V. and Deery, A. (2008) Care quality data on mental health is too hard to pin down. *Health Service Journal.*

Robins, L.N. and Reiger, D.A. (1991) *Psychiatric Disorders in America: The Epidemiologic Catchment Area Study.* New York: Free Press.

Rogers, A. (1990) Policing mental disorder: controversies, myths and realities, *Social Policy and Administration*, 24(3): 226–236.

Sainsburys Centre for Mental Health (1998a) *Keys to Engagement: Review of Care for People with Severe Mental Illness Who Are Hard to Engage With Services.* London: Sainsburys Centre for Mental Health.

Sainsburys Centre for Mental Health (1998b) *Acute Problems: A Survey of the Quality of Care in Acute Psychiatric Wards.* London: Sainsburys Centre for Mental Health.

Sainsbury Centre for Mental Health (2002) *Breaking the Circles of Fear.* London: Sainsbury Centre for Mental Health.

Sainsbury Centre for Mental Health (2006) *Policy Paper 6 The Costs of Race Inequality.* London: Sainsbury Centre for Mental Health.

Sashidharan, S.P. (1993) Afro-Caribbeans and schizophrenia: the ethnic vulnerability hypothesis re-examined, *International Review of Psychiatry*, 5: 129–144.

Sashidharan, S. and Francis, E. (1993) Epidemiology, ethnicity and schizophrenia. In Ahmad, W.I.U. (ed.) *'Race' and Health in Contemporary Britain.* Buckingham: Open University Press.

Selten, J.P., Slaets, J.P.J. and Kahn, R.S. (1997) Schizophrenia in Surinamese and Dutch Antillean immigrants to The Netherlands: evidence of an increased incidence, *Psychological Medicine*, 27: 807–811.

Selten, J.P., Veen, N.N., Feller, W., Blom, J.D., Schols, D., Camoenië, W., Oolders, J., Van der Velden, M., Hoek, H.W., Vladár Rivero, V.M., Van der Graaf, Y. and Kahn, R. (2001) Incidence of psychotic disorders in immigrant groups to The Netherlands, *British Journal of Psychiatry*, 178: 367–372.

Singh, S. (2007) Institutional racism in psychiatry, *Psychiatric Bulletin*, 31: 363–365.

Singh, S.P. and Burns, T. (2006) Race and mental health: there is more to race than racism, *British Medical Journal*, 333: 648–651.

Smaje, C. (1996) The ethnic patterning of health: new directions for theory and research, *Sociology of Health and Illness*, 18(2): 139–171.

Soni Raleigh, V. (1996) Suicide patterns and trends in people of Indian subcontinent and Caribbean origin in England and Wales, *Ethnicity and Health*, 1(1): 55–63.

Soni Raleigh, V. and Balarajan, R. (1992) Suicide and self-burning among Indians and West Indians in England and Wales, *British Journal of Psychiatry*, 161: 365–368.

Soni Raleigh, V., Bulusu, L. and Balarajan, R. (1990) Suicides among immigrants from the Indian subcontinent, *British Journal of Psychiatry*, 156: 46–50.

Sproston, K. and Mindell, J. (2006) *Health Survey for England 2004: The Health of Minority Ethnic Groups.* London: National Centre for Social Research.

Sproston, K. and Nazroo, J. (eds) (2002) *Ethnic Minority Psychiatric Illness Rates in the Community (EMPIRIC).* London: The Stationery Office.

Strakowski, S.M., Shelton, R.C. and Kolbrener, M.L. (1993) The effects of race and comorbidity on clinical diagnosis in patients with psychosis, *Journal of Clinical Psychiatry*, 54: 96–102.

Takei, N., Persaud, R., Woodruff, P., Brockington, I. and Murray, R.M. (1998) First episodes of psychosis in Afro-Caribbean and white people, *British Journal of Psychiatry*, 172: 147–153.

Townsend, P. and Davidson, N. (1982) *Inequalities in Health (the Black Report).* Middlesex: Penguin.

Van Os, J., Castle, D.J., Takei, N., Der, G. and Murray, R.M. (1996) Psychotic illness in ethnic minorities: clarification from the 1991 Census, *Psychological Medicine*, 26: 203–208.

Veling, W., Selten, J.P., Veen, N., Laan, W., Blom, J.D. and Hoek, H.W. (2006) Incidence of schizophrenia among ethnic minorities in the Netherlands: a four-year first-contact study, *Schizophrenia Research*, 86: 189–193.

Webbe, A. (1998) Ethnicity and mental health, *Psychiatric Care*, 5(1): 12–16.

Williams, D.R., Neighbors, H.W. and Jackson, J.S. (2003) Racial/ethnic discrimination and health: findings from community studies, *American Journal of Public Health*, 93: 200–208.

6

Gender Matters:
Differences in Depression
between Women and Men

Jane M. Ussher

INTRODUCTION

Mental health is not gender neutral. There is incontrovertible evidence that gender differences exist in diagnosis of a range of mental health problems, with women more likely than men to be diagnosed with mood and anxiety disorders; somatoform or factitious disorder; dissociative identity or depersonalization disorder; eating disorders; sleep and adjustment disorder; and borderline, histrionic or dependent personality disorder (Cosgrove and Riddle, 2004). Men are more likely to be diagnosed with drug or alcohol abuse, and antisocial personality disorder, than women (Bebbington, 1996; Kuehner, 2003). Whether this is a sex difference tied to biology, or a gender difference located in social conditions and roles, or indeed a combination of the two, is a matter of considerable debate – as is the very legitimacy of psychiatric diagnosis. This is a debate not simply of interest to those with an interest in gendered experience. Understanding the aetiology and course of differences in mental health between women and men can have significant implications for all programmes of prevention and amelioration. It is thus a matter which all researchers and clinicians working in the field of mental health should consider.

This chapter will focus on the issue of depression, the most prevalent mental health condition affecting individuals worldwide, estimated to become the second most significant cause of disease and disability by 2020 (Murray and Lopez, 1996). Depression is also the central focus of analyses of gender differences in mental health, accounting for 41.9 per cent of the burden of disability related to neurological and psychiatric disorders for women, compared to 29.3 per cent in men (Blehar, 2006: 143), and standing as the fifth greatest burden for women and the seventh greatest burden for men across all physical and mental illnesses (Desjarlais et al., 1996). I will begin by examining epidemiological research which demonstrates the existence of gender differences in unipolar depression.[1] This will be followed by an exploration of the explanations put forward to explain this difference – biological, socio-cultural and psychological – ending with a critical examination of the epistemological underpinnings of research in this field and of the concept of depression as a diagnostic category.

Throughout, I will use the term 'gender' rather than 'sex' when referring to differences observed between men and women, in order to indicate the socially located nature of what it means to be woman or man. This does not imply that there is no biological or corporeal aspect to differences in depression between men and women. It simply means that biology does not have a direct causal influence which is not mediated by the social and cultural construction of masculinity and femininity, and the social roles of women and men.

GENDER DIFFERENCES IN DEPRESSION – EXAMINING THE EVIDENCE

The evidence that women experience prolonged misery, categorized as depression within current psychiatric taxonomies,[2] at significantly higher rates than men appears to be indisputable. Epidemiological research examining life time occurrence of depression in community samples reports that women outnumber men at a ratio of 2:1 (Bebbington, 1996; Kessler et al., 1994; Maier et al., 1999; Weissman et al., 1996); however, disparities as high as 4:1 have been reported (Perugi et al., 1990). Studies examining prevalence in the previous 1–12 months report that women are between 1.2 and 2.7 times more likely to have experienced depression than men, and women significantly out-number men in first admission rates for hospital treatment for depression, and on register studies where incidence is calculated by contact with services (see Bebbington, 1996). Women are also estimated to be twice as likely as men to be prescribed psychotropic medication for depression (Hamilton et al., 1996), in particular Serotonin Re-uptake Inhibitors (SSRIs) (Currie, 2005).

Gender differences in depression are not uniform across the lifespan. There is consistent evidence that prior to adolescence, boys outnumber girls over the whole gamut of mental health problems (Angold et al., 1998; Nolen-Hoeksema et al., 1991). Post adolescence, the gender balance is reversed. For example, in the National Comorbidity Survey of a nationally representative sample of 8098 US citizens, the increased rate of female depression occurred at age 10–14 (Kessler et al., 1993). Other studies are more precise, specifying age 13 (Peterson et al., 1991), or achievement of pubertal status, rather than simple chronological age (Angold et al., 1998). Whilst girls' depression increases at puberty, boys experience a significant reduction, leading to the conclusion that 'the transition to mid-puberty appeared transiently to protect boys from depression' (Angold et al., 1998: 59).

There is inconsistent evidence as to the continuity of this gender difference across the adult life span. It has been reported that higher rates of depression in women are maintained in later life (Beekman et al., 1999). However, two large scale population studies conducted in the US (Kessler et al., 1993) and the UK (Bebbington et al., 1998) reported that gender differences in depression do not persist after the mid-50s, 'due an absolute fall in female prevalences' (Bebbington et al., 1998: 16). The size and representativeness of the sample in the latter two studies has led to the conclusion that 'considerable weight' should be placed on the findings (Bebbington, 1998: 2) .

This epidemiological research appears to undermine earlier suggestions that gender differences in depression are an artefact – the result of women being more likely than men to report either mild symptoms of depression (Newman, 1984), or symptoms that last a few days (Craig and Nightingale, 1979), or conversely, men being more likely to forget their depressive symptoms than women (Kessler et al., 1993), or to underplay the severity of past episodes (Wilhelm and Parker, 1994). Whilst there are a number of studies which report no evidence of under-reporting of depression on the part of women (Fennig et al., 1994; Nazroo et al., 1998), Bebbington (1996) has also argued that any gender differences in reporting that did exist would be unlikely to be of a magnitude to explain the substantial differences in rates between women and men. Equally, whilst it has been argued that rates of women's depression are equivalent to rates of alcohol and drug use in men (Meltzer et al., 1995), the demographics of each group are very different (alcohol and drug use is highest in young single men, and depression highest in married women, or those with children, as outlined below), suggesting that depression and substance use 'are not alternative outcomes for men and women in the same situation' (Nazroo et al., 1998: 323).

Explaining the cause of gender differences in depression has consumed the attention of researchers from a range of academic disciplines. Within competing models from medicine, psychology and sociology, this pathological condition is located within the woman, in her faulty biology, her irrational (or dysfunctional) cognitions or her reactions to stressful life circumstances. Many feminist critics have argued that this acts to decontextualize what is often a social problem, legitimize expert intervention and negate the political, economic and discursive aspects of women's experience (LaFrance, 2009; Stoppard, 2000a; Ussher, 1991). However, as this chapter will demonstrate, the most widely accepted theories of gender differences in depression still ignore the gendered construction of women's prolonged misery. This has implications for the prevention and amelioration of women's distress, for the ways in which researchers and health professionals interact with women as 'experts' in this field, and for the ways in which women experience and position their own unhappiness.

BIOLOGY AS DESTINY: RAGING HORMONES AND REPRODUCTIVE DEBILITATION

Since the emergence of psychiatry as a profession in the mid-nineteenth century, depression has been positioned as a bio-medical condition, caused by biological dysfunction and ameliorated by pharmacological treatment (Pilgrim and Bentall, 1999; Pilgrim et al., forthcoming). It is thus not surprising to find that biological reductionism has been adopted by many in their attempts to explain gender differences in depression, in this instance the female reproductive body being positioned as to blame – the myth of the monstrous feminine (Ussher, 2006). Thus the emergence of gender differences in depression at puberty, with a reduction post-menopause, has led to the argument that 'the female prevalence in depression is linked to women's reproductive years' (Cyranowski et al., 2000: 25). Indeed, fecundity is positioned as so detrimental to women's mental health, that the 'sex hormone', oestrogen, is positioned as the cause. As John Studd argues:

> The excess of depression in women compared with men occurs at times of great hormonal fluctuations – at the time of puberty, in the postnatal period, and premenstrually – and it is worst in the few years before menstrual cycles end. At this time the worsening symptoms of premenstrual tension with age blend with the worst years of the climacteric. These wretchedly depressed women in their 40s usually respond well to oestrogen treatment rather than to the psychoactive drugs that remain the first line treatment of psychiatrists. (Studd, 1997: 977)

Or as Angold et al. (1999: 1044) argue, 'in later life (after age 55), the female excess of depressions diminishes; mostly because of falling rates in women at a time when their oestrogen levels are again low'.

There has been a substantial amount of research examining the relationship between hormones and depression, and the results are more equivocal than the confident statements cited above would suggest. For many researchers, the key to understanding gender differences in depression lies in understanding adolescent onset. For example, Kessler et al. (1993) have argued that the higher prevalence of 12 month depression for women which they observed in the National Comorbidity Survey is 'largely due to women having a higher risk for first onset' (p. 85). In one study it was argued that the 'turning on' of the endocrine system in girls as they emerge from pre to post-puberty might explain increases in depression at this stage in the life-cycle. However, only 4 per cent of the variance was accounted for by oestrogen levels, with life events and the interaction of oestrogen levels and life events, accounted for 17 per cent (Brooks-Gunn and Warren, 1989). One study which reported consistent evidence of an association between testosterone and oestrogen in the increasing prevalence adolescent girls' depression (Angold et al., 1999) is oft cited as evidence of a biological causal root to women's depression (e.g. Kuehner, 2003: 167). However, the authors themselves are more equivocal, concluding that:

> This is not to say that depression is simply caused by increased levels of androgens and oestrogen – that could scarcely be the case … Other exogenous (such as life events or daily hassles)

or endogenous (such as cognitive style) factors are required to explain the development of individual episodes of the disorder. (p. 1050)

Equally, Buchanan et al. (1992), in a thorough review of the role of hormones in adolescent mood and behaviour, which concludes that hormones 'do exert some influence over moods and behaviour' (p. 68), comments that 'environmental, social and cultural factors certainly play a role on the behaviours linked with estrogen – depression, anxiety, irritability, general feelings of wellbeing – and perhaps themselves influence hormone concentrations' (p. 68). Thus a solely hormonal explanation for differences between adolescent girls and boys appears to be unsupportable, even amongst those who adopt a bio-medical standpoint in their research.

The evidence for an association between hormones and depression during adulthood is also unequivocal. It has been suggested that sex hormones and genetics may combine to produce depression in adult women (Blehar, 2006: 152). However, a meta-analysis of four community and two twin studies, containing 20,000 participants, did not find any consistent gender difference in heritability (Sullivan et al., 2000), leading to the conclusion that 'the relative importance of genetic effects in major depression is the same in women and men' (Kuehner, 2003: 166). In looking to women's 'times of great hormonal fluctuation', there is strong evidence that premenstrual depression is more strongly associated with women's social and relationship context than with her hormonal status (Ussher, 2006), with over-responsibility, relationship dissatisfaction and communication problems leading to distress (Ussher, 2003a, 2004), whilst social support and positive communication within relationships leads to tolerance of premenstrual change outside of a pathological framework (Ussher and Perz, 2008, 2010). Equally, it is widely accepted that depression in the post-natal period is not hormonally related (Whiffen, 1992), with prolonged misery being deemed an understandable reaction to the strains of early motherhood (Nicolson, 1998), activating a pre-existing risk for depression (Williamson, 1993). As is the case with PMS, the social context of women's lives, and cultural constructions of motherhood, are also important, with high and unrealistic expectations of motherhood (Mauthner, 2000), combined with low social support (Bifulco et al., 1998), being major risk factors for post-natal depression. The final major hormonal transition in women's lives, menopause, is also not a time of 'psychological turmoil'. Community studies report that the majority of peri-menopausal and menopausal women are not depressed (e.g. Avis et al., 1994; Dennerstein, 1996), with social context and women's negotiation of midlife change, being the factors which lead to (or protect against), depression – not the menopausal body (McQuaide, 1998; Perz and Ussher, 2008).

These negative findings do not mean that hopes of a bio-medical explanation for gender differences in depression have been expunged. In a review of women's health as a 'biomedical field', Blehar (2006) concluded that 'with the exception of post-partum onset affective psychosis and bipolar disorder, there is relatively little evidence for a causal role of sex steroids in clinical disorders' (p. 151). However, she goes on to say: 'A limiting factor in studies of hormones may be methodological. In the near future, sensitive technologies to image in vivo brain function may allow researchers to test hormonal hypotheses more directly'. Indeed, Blehar confirms that 'the role of sex steroid in the etiology, manifestation, and course of mental illness remains a important emphasis area' (p. 40) for the National Institute of Health (NIH), the primary funding agency for bio-medical research in the US. It seems that researchers will continue looking until they find what they are searching for – an embodied cause of women's depression, tied to the reproductive body.

Yet the majority of researchers working in this field have shifted their attention away from the body, simply acknowledging the interaction of biological and psycho-social factors in the genesis of gender differences in depression, within a broadly bio psycho-social model. As two recent reviewers conclude:

> There seems no doubt that biological factors are involved in the emergence of depressive disorder, it is just difficult to argue that they are responsible for the sex difference. This pushes towards a consideration of physical and social environment. (Bebbington, 1998: 5)

> The key to understanding the higher rates of depression among women than men lies in an investigation of the joint effects of biological vulnerabilities and environmental provoking experiences. (Kessler, 2003: 5)

These multi-factorial models may appear to be a step forward from reductionist and body blaming biological standpoints. However, as will be outlined below, depression is still reified as a pathological condition, and the location of the problem is positioned within the woman, even when the social environment is acknowledged to be a diathesis factor in her distress.

SOCIO-CULTURAL FACTORS IMPLICATED IN GENDER DIFFERENCES IN DEPRESSION

Inequality, discrimination and violence

Gendered inequalities in society, leading to the discriminatory treatment of women, have been positioned as a significant factor in the development of depression. In the World Mental Health Report (Desjarlais et al., 1996), the social roots of women's mental health problems in low income countries were identified as under-nourishment, low paid work and domestic violence, leading to a plea for co-ordinated efforts to economically empower women and reduce violence in all of its forms. In European countries, women's life satisfaction increased after the introduction of abortion rights and birth control (Pezzini, 2005), and in the US, women who live in States which are high on the economic autonomy index, and where they have reproductive rights, experience significantly less depression (Chen et al., 2005). This has lead to the conclusion that depression can be reduced by increasing women's access to economic resources and employment, as well as facilitating autonomy over reproductive decisions.

Discrimination operating at an individual level is also an influential factor. Research has demonstrated that women who experience frequent sexism (Klonoff et al., 2000), or who perceive themselves to be subjected to personal discrimination (Dambrun, 2007), report higher levels of distress than those who report little sexism or low levels of discrimination. More specifically, the experience of physical and sexual violence has been linked to a range of mental health problems, including depression, anxiety, substance abuse and post traumatic stress syndrome (Cabral and Astbury, 2000; Cortina and Kubiak, 2006; Kendler et al., 2000; Molnar et al., 2001), as well as to physical health problems (Kendall-Tackett, 2007). Violence against women is so prevalent across cultures that it is now recognized as a primary health and human right issue by the World Health Organization (2000). More specifically, women's higher risk of having experienced child sexual abuse (Molnar et al., 2001) or adult sexual violence (Koss et al., 2003) has been described as going 'a considerable way to explaining the adult sex difference in depressive disorders' (Bebbington, 1998: 4). Indeed, in one study, it was estimated that 35 per cent of the differences in rates of depression between women and men could be accounted for by sexual abuse occurring before the age of 18 (Cutler and Nolen-Hoeksema, 1991).

Gender roles

The construction and experience of gendered roles has also been positioned as a significant factor in the development of depression. It has been posited that gender intensification occurs at puberty, leading to the parental and peer expectation of girls' conformity to 'restrictive social roles' (Nolen-Hoeksema and Girgus, 1994: 436). Girls who resist feminine gender typed activities, assert their intelligence, or pursue 'masculine type activities' risk rejection by boys, acting to 'contribute to their propensity to depression' (Nolen-Hoeksema and Girgus, 1994: 436). Conversely, masculinity as a trait has been deemed to protect against depression, operating through perceived competence (Wilson and Cairns, 1988). However, Bebbington (1996) has argued that as masculinity remains fairly stable throughout adolescence for girls, it cannot explain the gender difference in depression which emerges at this time.

Masculinity is not a necessarily positive trait for men: research has demonstrated an association between traditional characteristics of masculinity and risk taking or self destructive behaviour, stress, increased anxiety and anger, emotional expressiveness and poor health related behaviours (Batty, 2006). Male gender role conflict, the strain resulting from attempting to adhere to ideals of masculinity, such as success, power and restricted emotionality, accompanied by fear of qualities deemed feminine (O'Neil et al., 1986), has been reported to be associated with 'personal restriction, devaluation, or violation of others or self' (O'Neil, 1990: 25). Men who report high levels of gender role conflict also report higher levels of depression (Cormoyer and Mahalik, 1995), and are also more reluctant to seek help for psychological problems (Good et al., 1989), than men with low gender role conflict. At the same time, the higher rates of youth suicide recorded in men have been found to be associated with individualism, in particular indices of personal freedom and control, reflecting a failure of Western societies to provide appropriate sites or sources of male social identity and attachment, combined with the tendency to promote unrealistic or inappropriate expectations of individual freedom and autonomy (Eckersley and Dear, 2002).

Gender roles have also been linked to the negotiation and experience of life events. There is consistent evidence that depression is associated with both severe life events (Bifulco et al., 1998; Brown and Harris, 1989b), and cumulative adversity (Turner and Lloyd, 1995), for women and men. Indeed, one explanation for higher rates of depression in adolescent girls, when compared to boys, is the higher levels of challenges (Nolen-Hoeksema and Girgus, 1994) and life events (Gore et al., 1992) girls experience at this time. Certain groups of women, particularly those caring for young children (Brown and Harris, 1978), those experiencing poverty (Belle, 1990) and those with negative close relationships (Bifulco et al., 1998), have also been reported to have a greater susceptibility to life events, and to experience depression as a result. There is also evidence that women and men respond differentially to certain life events than men, those involving children, housing and reproduction, because of the greater salience of these events to women's role identity (Nazroo et al., 1998). Described as 'network events' this is interpreted as being the result of women's greater involvement in the lives of those around them (Kessler McLeod, 1984: 620), with women's responsiveness representing a 'cost of caring' (Kessler et al., 1985) that leads to elevated levels of depression. Indeed, men and women have been found to be equally likely to remember their own life events, but men are less likely than women to remember life events affecting significant others, leading to the suggestion that men may avoid depression through 'blocking out', or not attending to, network events (Turner and Avison, 1989).

Cultural differences in women's depression

Another factor which can act as a moderating variable in the relationship between gender and depression is cultural background. For example, there is evidence that African American women have lower rates of depression than White women living in the US, whereas Latino women have higher rates (Kessler et al., 1994). Indeed, in one study where White adolescent girls reported higher rates of depression post-menarche than pre-menarche, this difference was not found for African-American girls and Hispanics, leading the researchers to conclude that 'the association between puberty and depression in girls may be context-dependent' (Hayward et al., 1999: 148).

Post-adolescence, life stresses, physical health problems, perceived discrimination and internalized racism have been put forward as explanations for higher rates of depression in particular cultural groups (Brown et al., 2003). Socio-economic factors are also a key contributor: two recent studies found no difference between levels of depression in Asian-American, African-American (Jackson-Triche et al., 2000) or Latino women (Alegria et al., 2008), when compared to White US women, when socio-economic differences were controlled for. Acculturation is also an important factor: in one study of Chinese women living in the US, those who were acculturated were twice as likely to experience depression as those who were not acculturated, a difference that was not found for men (Takeuchi et al., 1998). A similar pattern has been reported with Latino women, who report higher rates of depression if they were born in the US than if they are migrants (Alegria et al., 2008). Culture can also impact upon depression through the different meanings of illness across cultural groupings, which can lead to culturally specific constructions and interpretations of symptoms, and as a consequence, different expressions of distress or patterns of help seeking (Brown et al., 2003; Hwang et al., 2008). For example, in a study which compared depression at midlife in North American and Japanese women, Avis et al. (1993) reported that there were much lower rates in the Japanese group, reflecting the different cultural meaning of menopause and aging in Japan. The relationship between gender, culture and depression is thus clearly complex and multifaceted (for a model which explores this complexity see Hwang et al., 2008). This suggests that researchers and health professionals should not be either gender or culture blind when designing research studies or interventions, as has often been the case in the past and is unfortunately still the case with many psychological approaches to depression, to which we will now turn.

IT'S ALL IN THE MIND: PSYCHOLOGICAL EXPLANATIONS FOR GENDER DIFFERENCES IN DEPRESSION

A number of psychological explanations have been put forward for gender differences in depression, with researchers and theorists positing that psychological factors mediate between biological vulnerability or life stress, to exacerbate or reduce the risk of depression (see Bebbington, 1996). For example, drawing on meta-analytic research which demonstrates that women are more concerned with affiliation, whilst men are concerned with personal autonomy, instrumentality and agency (Fengold, 1994), Cyrnanowski and colleagues (2000) put forward a model to explain adolescent onset of depression in terms of girls' heightened affiliative needs, interacting with adolescent transition difficulties and negative life events, particularly those with interpersonal consequences. These heightened affiliative needs are deemed to have an evolutionary base, located in 'women's historically greater investment in offspring care and their relatively greater use of long term sexual mate selection strategies' (p. 22), linked to the 'mammalian neuropeptide oxytocin' (Cyranowski et al., 2000: 23). Oxytocin, in combination with female reproductive hormones and endogenous opioid peptide mechanisms, has also been positioned as at the 'core' of the 'tend and befriend' response to stress found in women, in contrast to the 'fight or flight' response of men (Taylor et al., 2000: 411), with the 'tend and befriend' tendency deemed a risk factor in relation to women's responses to life events. Absence of a secure parental base, leading to an insecure attachment style has also been posited as a potential contributory factor in Cyranowski et al.'s (2000) model, as insecure attachments are linked to lower self-esteem, lower social support, and greater symptoms of psychological distress (Cooper et al., 1998). Similarly, in her work on self-silencing, a pattern of behaviour involving a focus on others at the expense of the self, accompanied by repression of one's own needs and concerns, Jack (1991) has associated insecure attachment style with high levels of self-silencing, and as a consequence, with depression (Duarte and Thompson, 1999).

Gender differences in cognitive appraisal and coping style have been put forward as a further explanation of women's greater propensity to depression. Meta-analytic research has demonstrated that in the face of stress, women are more likely to use coping strategies that involve verbal expression to others or the self – seeking emotional support, rumination and positive self-talk – whereas men engage in avoidance in the face of stressors that involve relationships or other people (Tamres et al., 2002). There is consistent evidence that rumination, rather than taking distracting action or changing the situation, is associated with depression in both men and women, with adolescent girls and adult women being more likely to show ruminative tendencies than adolescent boys or men (Nolen-Hoeksema and Girgus, 1994; Nolen-Hoeksema et al., 1999).

In a similar vein, Hankin and Abramson (2001) position adolescent girls' greater tendency for rumination as a key aspect of their 'depressogenic attributional style' (p. 785). Drawing on a general cognitive-vulnerability theory of depression (Abramson et al., 1989; Beck, 1987), the emergence of gender differences in depression post puberty is deemed to result from an interaction of pre-existing vulnerabilities, negative life events, and cognitive vulnerabilities. Thus genetic risk for depression, girls' greater tendency to report neuroticism, and maltreatment (primarily sexual abuse), interact with negative body image and 'depressiogenic inferential style' (Hankin and Abramson, 2001: 785), manifested by rumination, in the context of girls' greater likelihood of experiencing negative life events, which they have a tendency to encode in greater detail than boys (Davis, 1999). The risk of depression is increased by parental socialization, involving high levels of control, which lead to girls' negative self-evaluations and greater tendency to take responsibility for failure, compared to boys (Pomerantz and Ruble, 1998).

THE NEGATION OF THE POLITICAL CONTEXT OF WOMEN'S MISERY

Whilst these environmental and psychological models of misery may appear to be a step forward in locating aetiology outside of the woman's body, and in suggesting that attention should be paid to cognitions or social environment, from a feminist perspective these are at best partial, and at worst, deeply flawed accounts, as they act to de-politicize the roots of women's distress, neutralizing the causal pathways under scrutiny as objective entities that can be simply measured or monitored. As Pilgrim and Bentall (1999) argue, whilst 'it is possible to talk about the "diagnosis of child sexual abuse" and the "diagnosis of depression" in its survivors, it is less mystifying to think about the enduring misery created by the sexual oppression of children by adults' (p. 270). Equally, gender-blind constructs such as 'stressful life events' or 'depressogenic attributional style' are stripped of their gendered context (Stoppard, 2000b: 81). And whilst we may correlate social inequalities, gender roles or adult sexual violence with women's prolonged misery, there is no analysis of the political context which maintains deeply entrenched gender divisions which disadvantage women. We need to question 'who benefits from the restriction of women's reproductive rights?' 'Why is it that domestic and sexual violence is so endemic, and that so few cases are prosecuted?' (see Gavey, 2005). 'Why are women still taking on the greater burden of childcare, resulting in their greater vulnerability to adverse life events?' To take just one example, whilst women may suffer on an individual basis from the 'cost of caring', if they eschew this traditional feminine role, the expenditure placed on the State would blow national budgets, as well as making demands on individual men, who currently do far less unpaid caring, or housework, than women (Sirianni and Negrey, 2000). Stripping accounts of women's misery of any acknowledgement of the historical or political context of women's lives, whilst paying lip service to environmental or psycho-social influences, thus serves to shore up the very structural factors that lead to distress in the first place, through making gender inequality an invisible issue.

There *are* examples of attempts by psychological researchers to demystify, and position the blame for misery outside of the women, even when psychological mechanisms, such as rumination, are the focus of attention. For example, in Nolen-Hoeksema et al.'s research, women's propensity to rumination is deemed to be tied to the chronic strain they experience, 'the grinding annoyances and burdens that come with women's social power (including) … a greater load of the housework and child care and more of the strain of parenting than men' as well as absence of affirmation by their partners (Nolen-Hoeksema et al., 1999: 1068). This is combined with women's lower social status, and their unequal power and status in relationships, leading to feelings of chronic lack of control, low self-mastery and learned helplessness, and as a consequence, depression. The solution put forward by Nolen-Hoeksema and colleagues is to help women to gain more mastery over their lives, but also to change their social circumstances so they 'don't have so much to ruminate about' (1999: 1068).

Laudable as these conclusions are, they still negate the hetero-patriarchal context which produces gender inequalities in the first place. A case in point is analysis of the relationship of marriage and depression. For many years marriage has been put forward as a risk factor for women's depression (Bebbington et al., 1991; Gove, 1972; Gove et al., 1973), with young married women with small children deemed to be at particularly high risk (Brown and Harris, 1978). Conversely, marriage has been said to act as a protective factor for men (Weissman et al., 1984), with one study reporting that wives experience over five times the rate of depression as husbands (Bebbington et al., 1981). However, a number of studies report that marriage is a protective factor for both men and women, as it acts to buffer psychological distress (e.g., Sachs-Ericsson et al., 2000), with divorced or separated individuals at high risk of depression (Bebbington et al., 1988). There is also consensus that single mothers are at higher high risk for depression than married mothers, due to the difficulties of child care and multiple role responsibilities in what are often disadvantaged circumstances (Bifulco et al., 1998; Meltzer et al., 1995; Sachs-Ericsson and Ciarlo, 2000), whilst women who have no children at home have a lower risk for depression (with the presence of children having no impact on depression in men) (Bebbington et al., 1998).

It is interesting to note that in countries where a high value is placed on the home making role, married women report low levels of depression (Bebbington, 1998). This suggests an interaction between socio-cultural norms and interpersonal relationships, and their effects. Indeed, the cultural norms of a nation have been linked to national depression levels. Nations high on masculinity, where traditional gender role stereotypes are valued, have been found to have higher rates of depression than 'feminine' nations (Arrindell et al., 2003). What characterizes the feminine nations is that 'men and women are offered equal opportunities for the fulfilment of multiple social roles' (Arrindell et al., 2003: 809), something which is good for the mental health of both genders (Sachs-Ericsson and Ciarlo, 2000).

In reporting research on 'marriage' and depression, I am not taking a naïve hetero-normative position, for it is 'marriage' between a man and a woman which has been the focus of research in this area. And whilst the importance of gender roles within marriage is often implicitly acknowledged by researchers (e.g. Brown et al., 1989a: 381), there is rarely, if ever, any critique of the underlying tenets of hetero-patriarchy which may be instrumental creating the particular conditions within 'marriage' which precipitate women's distress. Specific factors in heterosexual relationships which have been linked to women's depression include relationship distress and dissatisfaction (Whisman and Bruce, 1999), self-silencing (Whiffen et al., 2007), humiliation (Brown et al., 1995), partner violence towards the woman (Koss et al., 2003), dissatisfaction with decision making, financial issues and child-care (Byrne et al., 2004), inequality in relation to domestic responsibilities (Doyle, 1995), absence of partner support (Brown et al., 1986), the presence of demand–withdraw interactions (Byrne and Carr, 2000), communication problems (Byrne et al., 2004) and feelings of disempowerment (Price, 1991). Whilst Brown and colleagues (1995) describe these relational patterns as creating 'depressogenic effects', as Pilgrim and Bentall argue, 'this could be reframed by simply stating that miserable women live with oppressive men' (1999: 270).

If we look outside of a heterosexual matrix, where roles within relationships are not taken for granted and divided on gendered terms, these oppressive patterns of relating are less common, suggesting that it is not 'marriage' *per-se* which is a risk factor for women's depression, but particular aspects relationships which are more common in a hetero-patriarchal context. For researchers have reported that in comparison to heterosexual relationships, lesbian relationships are experienced as more satisfying (Green et al., 1996; Kurdek, 2003; Metz et al., 1994); communication is more likely to include open exploration of feelings, empathic attunement to non-verbals, negotiation and the absence of contempt (Connolly et al., 2006); conflict is resolved more effectively (Kurdek, 2004b; Metz et al., 1994), with less likelihood of a demand-withdrawal style of conflict resolution (Kurdek, 2004a); there is greater egalitarianism, in dealing with house-hold responsibilities (Green et al., 1996: 197), accompanied by adaptability in dealing with relational needs and domestic tasks (Connolly, 2005: 270); and higher levels of cohesion or connectedness (Green et al., 1996), linked to mutual empathy, empowerment and relational authenticity (Mencher, 1990). This has implications for mental health. For example, in a recent study on women's pre-menstrual distress, women in lesbian relationships reported less depression and anxiety and higher levels of premenstrual coping than women in heterosexual relationships. This was associated with empathy, support and positive communi-cation with their woman partner, compared to rejection, absence of communica-tion and lack of empathy on the part of many male partners (Perz and Ussher, 2009; Ussher and Perz, 2008). This suggests that it should be hetero-patriarchy which is the focus of critical attention, not decontextualized 'marital' factors, as is so often the case in analyses of the relational context of women's depression.

However, this is not to say that heterosexual relationships are inevitably bad for mental health – or that lesbians (or gay men) necessarily report lower rates of depression. In a recent meta-analysis, it was argued that there is substantial evi-dence to suggest that higher rates of mental health problems are experienced by gay men and lesbians, due to 'minority stress', the experience of stigma, preju-dice and discrimination which creates a hostile and stressful social environment (Meyer, 2003). However, in reviewing the evidence on sexual orientation and mental health, Herek and Garnets (2007) conclude that whilst the minority stress model is a useful way of understanding heightened risks for depression in non-heterosexual women and men, a number of studies have 'not found statistically significant differences among sexual orientation groups when relevant demo-graphic factors were statistically controlled for' (p. 359). Thus, gender, life-style, social support and the presence of other risk factors will interact with the potential of minority stress to produce (or protect against) depression.

DECONSTRUCTING 'DEPRESSION' AND EXAMINING EPISTEMOLOGY

A further problem with both bio-medical and psycho-social accounts of gender differences in depression is that both camps reify the construction of prolonged misery as a pathological disorder, 'depression', which negates the discursive context within which psychiatric diagnoses are constructed. Within a realist framework, depression is deemed to be a discrete clinical entity that occurs in a consistent and homogeneous way, with identifiable aetiology factors which are perceived to have *caused* the symptoms women report. In contrast, as many critics have argued, depression can be conceptualized as a social category created by a process of expert definition (Kirk and Kutchins, 1992; Littlewood and Lipsedge, 1982; Stoppard, 2000a; Ussher, 1991), with self-diagnosis or self-referral the result of active negotiation of symptomatology, current life events and lifestyle and cultural, medical or psychological discourse about depression.

The existence of human misery is not in dispute. However, its description as a unitary psychiatric disorder 'depression' which can be objectively measured, is assumed to be uniform across sufferers, and is deemed to *cause* the distress which individuals experience, has been the object of much criticism (Fee, 2000; Pilgrim et al., forthcoming; Ussher, 2000). The establishment of depression as a real entity which exists independent of perception, language or culture was first promoted by Kraeplin in the late nineteenth century, and has been embraced wholeheartedly by modern psychiatry, as well as the rest of the 'psy' professions, as is exemplified by the adoption of the DSM (Diagnostic and Statistical Manual of the American Psychiatric Association) diagnostic category of depression as unquestioned truth in both research and clinical practice (Kirk and Kutchins, 1992). However, rather than reflecting 'real' disorders, it has been argued that the DSM diagnostic categories are social constructions which function as tools for the defense of the establishment at the expense of the weak and powerless (Kutchins and Kirk, 1997). At the same time, the pharmaceutical industry, and its allies, have been accused of 'disease mongering' in their active encouragement of the medicalization of 'ordinary ailments' (Moynihan et al., 2002: 324), acting in conjunction with psychiatry to legitimate medical intervention for 'common personal and social problems' (Double, 2002: 900).

The problematic nature of the diagnostic category of depression as a gendered construction is an issue which merits particular scrutiny. It has long been argued by feminist critics that depression is a gendered illness (Chesler, 1998; Ussher, 1991, 2011), with medical practitioners more likely to identify and diagnose depression in women than in men (Potts et al., 1991), particularly if women present with 'masculine' symptoms (Waisberg and Page, 1988). Women are also at risk of distress and self-diagnosis if they deviate from traditional expectations of femininity, through eschewing a self-sacrificing caring role (O'Grady, 2005), which can lead to feelings of 'failure' in living up to the script of a perfect wife and mother (Jack, 1991; Ussher, 2006). It has also been argued that psychometric instruments used to measure depression are gender-biased, pathologizing behaviours such as crying or loss of interest in sex which are more common in women than men (Salokangas et al., 2002).

There is evidence that many women only label their unhappiness or despair as 'depression', and as a result take up a bio-medical model to explain their 'symptoms', after receiving medical diagnosis and treatment (Gammell and Stoppard, 2000;

LaFrance, 2007), suggesting that medicalization plays a significant role in constructing 'depression' at an individual level. However, the discursive construction of women's distress as depression in health policy (Gattuso et al., 2005), medical journals (Ussher, 2003b), self-help books (Rittenhouse, 1991), drug company literature (Metzl and Angel, 2004; Munce et al., 2004), women's magazines (Gattuso et al., 2005) and other mass circulated literature (Blum and Stracuzzi, 2004), also plays a significant role in women positioning their distress as an illness, 'depression'. Governments are also active in promoting depression literacy in everyday life (Gattuso et al., 2005), resulting in a widening of the boundaries of mental illness categories (Busfield, 2002). However, the gendered nature of medicalization results in an insidious creeping of pathologization into women's lives. For example, in a study which examined advertisements for SSRI antidepressants over the period 1985–2000, Metzl and Angel (2004) reported that there was a clear shift towards positioning normative reactions to life events associated with marriage, motherhood, menstruation or menopause as psychiatric illnesses which warrant SSRI medication, resulting in emotional experiences such as 'being overwhelmed with sadness', or 'never feeling happy' being positioned as depression. This stands in contrast to the biomedical positioning of men's depression as 'an illness with bio-chemical roots' (Metzl and Angel, 2004: 580), suggesting that normal reactions to life's vicissitudes are less likely to be pathologized in men. This overrepresentation of women in pharmaceutical advertising has been implicated in the greater likelihood of physicians providing a formal diagnosis of depression for women's problems (Munce et al., 2004). It may also provide an explanation for the finding that women are twice as likely as men to be prescribed psychotropic medication for depression (Hamilton et al., 1996). As SSRIs have been linked with increased risk of suicidality (Gunnell et al., 2005), this has worrying implications for women's health and well-being.

On an individual level, the diagnosis of depression can serve to validate to women that there is a 'real' problem, isolating prolonged misery from 'the character of the sufferer' (LaFrance, 2007: 130), in the same way that many women embrace a diagnosis of PMS (Ussher, 2003a) or post-natal depression (Mauthner, 2000) in order to assure themselves (and others) that they are not 'going crazy'. However, within this medicalized framework, the solution to depression is always positioned as being within the individual, with women entreated to either take medication (Metzl and Angel, 2004), or to engage in self-management strategies (Gattuso et al., 2005). This serves to maintain the *status quo* and produce more productive citizens (LaFrance, 2007) and ensures that social and political inequalities which lead to distress in the first place remain unchallenged. At the same time, with a few notable exceptions (e.g. Gammell and Stoppard, 2000; LaFrance, 2007; Mauthner, 2000), the complexity of women's experience of prolonged misery remains unexamined, as researchers and clinicians are wedded to causal models of a uni-dimensional or multi-factorial level, the majority of which negate women's subjective negotiation of misery as 'depression', and the meaning this has in their individual lives.

There is beginning to be a movement away from narrow realist models of gendered experiences of depression, with researchers adopting a constructivist epistemological standpoint (Stoppard, 2000b), and using qualitative methods to examine the complexity of experience (e.g. Gammell and Stoppard, 2000; LaFrance, 2007; Mauthner, 2000). Social-constructionist approaches take a critical stance towards taken-for-granted knowledge, recognizing cultural and historical specificity, the fact that knowledge is sustained by social practices, and that knowledge and social action go together (Burr, 1995). However, social constructionism has been criticized for negating the influence of embodiment (Cromby and Nightingale, 1999), or for relegating the body to a passive subsidiary role, which has meaning or interpretation imposed upon it (Yardley, 1996), as well as negating other aspects of materiality which may influence depression, such as social class, ethnicity, sexual identity, personal relationships, or a prior history of sexual abuse, as well as the intra-psychic (Ussher, 2005).

We need to acknowledge that depression is both a constructed and lived experience – with material, discursive and intrapsychic concomitants (Ussher, 2005). An epistemological shift to a critical realist framework allows us to incorporate these different aspects of experience, and the different types of expert knowledge about depression and gender, into one framework. Critical realism recognizes the materiality of the body, and other aspects of social or relational experience, but conceptualizes this materiality as mediated by culture, language and politics (Bhaskar, 1989); accepts the legitimacy of subjective experience, yet rejects the anti-empiricism of many strands of constructivism (Pilgrim and Rogers, 1997); and accepts the utilization of a variety of methodologies, both qualitative and quantitative, without one being privileged above the other (Sayer, 2000). Critical realism has been adopted as a way forward for health research, in order to address the limitations of both positivism and constructivism (Pilgrim and Rogers, 1997; Ussher, 1996; Williams, 2003), allowing us to incorporate the findings of both qualitative and quantitative research, conducted from a range of theoretical perspectives (bio-medical, psychological, socio-cultural, discursive) into one framework. Thus what may appear to be contradictions or irrevocable disagreements within a positivist/realist frame, are then transformed into different parts of the complex picture that is 'gender and depression'; a picture which only makes sense when all the different parts are considered together. This allows us to acknowledge the 'real' of women's prolonged misery, yet to conceptualize it as a complex phenomenon which has multiple concomitants, material, discursive and intrapsychic, which are located in the specific historical and cultural context in which a woman lives – in contrast to the narrow medicalized view of depression as simply an individual pathology (see Pilgrim and Bentall, 1999).

CONCLUSION

Thus, in summary, there is consistent evidence of a gender difference in reporting of prolonged misery between the ages of puberty and late middle age.

Whilst biological theories have been offered to explain this gender difference, in particular hormonal changes associated with the female reproductive cycle, there is general consensus that hormones simply act as a vulnerability factor, if they have any influence at all, with socio-cultural, psychological and discursive factors being more closely associated with women's increased propensity to report misery and despair.

The negation of the personal and political implications of the positioning of women's prolonged misery as an internal pathology 'depression', to be treated on an individual level, can be justified no longer, as there is a wealth of evidence to demonstrate the gendered nature of both this diagnostic category, and the causes of women's despair (Ussher, 2010, 2011). Researchers may adopt the traditional positivist stance of objectivity and apolitical neutrality when they expound their various theories of gender differences in depression, but regardless of whether they are taking a bio-medical, environmental or psychological stand-point, they are acting in a biased and political manner through negating the gendered construction and experience of this so-called disorder. As with all forms of medicalization, this decontextualizes what is essentially a social problem, puts it under medical (or psychological) control, and denies both the discursive construction of misery as internal pathology, and the difficult conditions of many women's lives. Therefore, in order to prevent and ameliorate women's despair, change needs to happen at a relational, social, political and discursive level, in order to impact on individual women at an intra-psychic level. This is not simply an issue for those concerned with mental health, it is about addressing gendered (in)equality in society, and in that sphere we still have a long way to go.

ACKNOWLEDGEMENTS

Thanks are offered to Dave Pilgrim, Nicola Gavey and Janette Perz for comments on an earlier version of this chapter. A further development of the arguments will appear in the book *The Madness of Women: Myth and Experience*, (Ussher, JM) published by Routledge in 2011.

NOTES

1 The findings on bi-polar depression are more equivocal, with some reviews reporting higher rates in women (Arnold, 2003) and others reporting no gender differences (Kuehner, 2003). Gender differences in the course and nature of manic depression have been reported however, with women reporting later age of onset, more depressive symptoms, a more rapidly cycling disorder, and greater co-morbidity with medical disorders, in comparison to men (Arnold, 2003).

2 For an analysis of the historical context within which misery came to be positioned as depression, a biomedical disease, see Pilgrim et al., forthcoming.

REFERENCES

Abramson, L.Y., Metalsky, G.I. and Alloy, L.B. (1989) Hopelessness depression: A theory based sub-type of depression. *Psychological Review,* 96: 358–372.

Alegria, M., Casino, G., Shrout, P.E., Woo, M., Duan, N., Vila, D. et al. (2008) Prevalence of mental illness in immigrant and non-immigrant U.S. *The American Journal of Psychiatry*, 165(3): 359–369.

Angold, A., Costello, E.J. and Worthman, C.M. (1998) Puberty and depression: the roles of age, pubertal status and pubertal timing. *Psychological Medicine*, 28: 51–61.

Angold, A., Costello, E.J., Erkanli, A. and Worthman, C.M. (1999) Pubertal changes in hormones levels and depression in girls. *Psychological Medicine*, 29: 1043–1053.

Arnold, L.M. (2003) Gender differences in bi-polar disorder. *Psychiatric Clinics of North America*, 26: 595–620.

Arrindell, W.A., Steptoe, A. and Wardle, J. (2003) Higher levels of state depression in masculine than in feminine nations. *Behaviour Research and Therapy*, 41: 809–817.

Avis, N., Brambilla, D., McKinlay, S.M. and Vass, K. (1994) A longitudinal analysis of the association between menopause and depression. Results from the Massachusetts women's health study. *Annals of Epidemiology*, 4(3): 214–220.

Avis, N., Kaufert, P.A., Lock, M., McKinlay, S.M. and Vass, K. (1993) The evolution of menopause symptoms. *International Practice and Research*, 7(1): 17–32.

Batty, Z. (2006) Masculinity and depression: Men's subjective experience of depression, coping and preferences for therapy and gender role conflict. Unpublished PhD Thesis, University of Western Sydney. School of Psychology: University of Western Sydney.

Bebbington, P.E. (1996) The origins of sex differences in depressive disorder: Bridging the gap. *International Review of Psychiatry*, 8(4): 295–332.

Bebbington, P.E. (1998) Sex and depression. *Psychological Medicine*, 28(1): 1–8.

Bebbington, P.E., Brugha, T., Maccarthy, B., Potter, J., Sturt, E. and Wykes, T. (1988) The Camberwell collaborative depression study. I. Depressed probands: Adversity and the form of depression. *British Journal of Psychiatry*, 152: 754–765.

Bebbington, P.E., Dean, C., Der, G., Hurry, J. and Tennant, C. (1991) Gender, parity and the prevalence of minor affective disorder. *British Journal of Psychiatry*, 158: 33–40.

Bebbington, P.E., Dunn, G., Jenkins, R., Lewis, G., Brugha, T., Farrell, M. et al. (1998) The influence of age and sex on the prevalence of depression conditions: Report from the National Survey of Psychiatric Morbidity. *Psychological Medicine*, 28(1): 9–19.

Bebbington, P.E., Hurry, J., Tennant, C., Sturt, E. and Wing, J.K. (1981) The epidemology of mental disorders in Camberwell. *Psychological Medicine*, 11: 561–566.

Beck, A.T. (1987) Cognitive models of depression. *Journal of Cognitive Psychotherapy: An International Quarterly*, 1: 5–37.

Beekman, A.T., Copeland, J.R. and Prince, M.J. (1999) Review of community prevalence of depression in later life. *British Journal of Psychiatry*, 174: 307–311.

Belle, D. (1990) Poverty and women's mental health. *American Psychologist*, 45: 385–389.

Bhaskar, R. (1989) *Reclaiming Reality: A Critical Introduction to Contemporary Philosophy*. London: Verso.

Bifulco, A., Brown, G.W., Moran, P., Ball, C. and Campbell, C. (1998) Predicting depression in women: the role of past and present vulnerability. *Psychological Medicine*, 28: 39–50.

Blehar, M.C. (2006) Women's mental health research: The emergence of a biomedical field. *Annual Review of Clinical Psychology*, 2: 135–160.

Blum, L. M. and Stracuzzi, N.F. (2004) Gender in the prozac nation: Popular discourse and productive femininity. *Gender and Society*, 18(3): 269–286.

Brooks-Gunn, J. and Warren, M. P. (1989) Biological and social contributions to negative affect in young adolescent girls. *Child Development*, 60: 40–55.

Brown, C., Abe-Kim, J. and Barrio, C. (2003) Depression in ethnically diverse women: Implications for treatment in primary care settings. *Professional Psychology: Research and Practice*, 34(1): 10–19.

Brown, G.W., Andrews, B., Harris, T.O. and Adler, Z. (1986) Social support, self-esteem and depression. *Psychological Medicine*, 16(4): 813–831.

Brown, G.W. and Harris, T. (1978) *Social Origins of Depression: A Study of Psychiatric Disorders in Women*. London: Tavistock.

Brown, G.W. and Harris, T.O. (1989a) Depression. In G.W. Brown and T.O. Harris (eds) *Life Events and Illness*, pp. 49–93. New York: Guilford Press.

Brown, G.W. and Harris, T.O. (eds) (1989b) *Life Events and Illness*. New York: The Guilford Press.

Brown, G.W., Harris, T.O. and Hepworth, C. (1995) Loss, humiliation and entrapment among women developing depression: a patient and non-patient comparison. *Psychological Medicine,* 25: 7–21.

Buchanan, C.M., Eccles, J.S. and Becker, J.B. (1992) Are adolescents victims of raging hormones: Evidence for activational effects of hormones on moods and behaviour at adolescence. *Psychological Bulletin,* 111: 62–107.

Burr, V. (1995) *An Introduction to Social Constructionism*. London: Routledge.

Busfield, J. (2002) *Rethinking the Sociology of Mental Illness*. London: Blackwell.

Byrne, M. and Carr, A. (2000) Depression and power in marriage. *Journal of Family Therapy,* 22: 408–427.

Byrne, M., Carr, A. and Clark, M. (2004) Power in relationships of women with depression. *Journal of Family Therapy,* 26: 407–429.

Cabral, M. and Astbury, J. (2000) *Women's Mental Health: An Evidence Based Review*. Geneva: World Health Organisation.

Chen, Y., Subramanian, S.V., Acevedo-Garcia, D. and Kawachi, I. (2005) Women's status and depressive symptoms: A mulitlevel analysis. *Social Science and Medicine,* 60: 49–60.

Chesler, P. (1998) *Women and Madness*. New York: Doubleday.

Connolly, C.M. (2005) A qualitative exploration of resilience in long-term lesbian couples. *The Family Journal: Counseling and Therapy for Couples and Families,* 13(3): 266–280.

Connolly, C.M. and Sicola, M.K. (2006) Listening to lesbian couples: communication competence in long term relationships. In J.J. Bigner (ed.) *An Introduction to GLBT Family Studies*. pp. 271–296. New York: Howarth Press.

Cooper, M.L., Shaver, P.R. and Collins, N.L. (1998) Attachment styles, emotion regulation and adjustment in adolescence. *Journal of Personality and Social Psychology,* 74: 1380–1397.

Cormoyer, R.J. and Mahalik, J.R. (1995) Cross sectional study of gender role conflict examining college-aged and middle aged men. *Journal of Counselling Psychology,* 42: 11–19.

Cortina, L.M. and Kubiak, S.P. (2006) Gender and post-traumatic stress: Sexual violence as an explanation for women's increased risk. *Journal of Abnormal Psychology,* 115(4): 753–759.

Cosgrove, L. and Riddle, B. (2004) Gender bias in sex distribution of mental disorders in the DSM-IV-TR. In P.J. Caplan and L. Cosgrove (eds) *Bias in Psychiatric Diagnosis*, pp. 127–140. New York: Jason Aronson.

Craig, T.J. and Van Notta, P.A. (1979) Influence of two demographic characteristics on two measures of depressive symptoms. *Archives of General Psychiatry,* 36: 149–154.

Cromby, J. and Nightingale, D.J. (1999) What's wrong with social constructionism? In D.J. Nightingale and J. Cromby (eds) *Social Constructionist Psychology: a Critical Analysis of Theory and Practice*, pp. 1–21. Buckingham: Open University Press.

Currie, J. (2005) The marketization of depression: The prescribing of SSRI antidepressants to women. *Women and Health Protection*, http://www.whp-apsf.ca/pdf/SSRIs.pdf. (accessed 15 July, 2009).

Cutler, S.E. and Nolen-Hoeksema, S. (1991) Accounting for sex differences in depression through female victimisation: Childhood sexual abuse. *Sex Roles,* 24: 425–438.

Cyranowski, J.M., Frank, E., Young, E. and Shear, M. K. (2000) Adolescent onset of the gender difference in lifetime rates of major depression. *Archives of General Psychiatry,* 57: 21–27.

Dambrun, M. (2007) Gender differences in mental health: The mediating role of perceived personal discrimination. *Journal of Applied Social Psychology,* 37(5): 1118–1129.

Davis, P.J. (1999) Gender differences in autobiographical memory for childhood emotional experiences. *Journal of Personality and Social Psychology,* 76: 498–510.

Dennerstein, L. (1996) Well-being, symptoms and the menopausal transition. *Maturitas,* 23: 147–157.

Desjarlais, R., Eisenberg, L., Good, B. and Kleinman, A. (1996) *World Mental Health: Problems and Priorities in Low Income Countries*. Oxford: Oxford University Press.

Double, D. (2002) The limits of psychiatry. *British Medical Journal,* 324: 900–904.

Doyle, L. (1995) *What Makes Women Sick? Gender and the Political Economy of Health*. New Brunswick: Rutgers University Press.

Duarte, L. M. and Thompson, J. M. (1999) Sex-differences in self-silencing. *Psychological Reports*, 85, 145–161.

Eckersley, R. and Dear, K. (2002) Cultural correlates of youth suicide. *Social Science and Medicine*, 55(11): 1891–1904.

Fee, D. (2000) *Pathology and the Postmodern: Mental Illness as Discourse and Experience*. London: SAGE.

Fengold, A. (1994) Gender differences in personality: A meta-analysis. *Psychological Bulletin*, 116: 429–456.

Fennig, S., Schwartz, J.E. and Bromet, E.J. (1994) Are diagnostic criteria, time of episode and occupational impairment important determinants of the female:male ratio for major depression? *Journal of Affective Disorders*, 30: 147–154.

Gammell, D.J. and Stoppard, J.M. (2000) Women's experience of treatment of depression: Medicalization or empowerment? *Canadian Psychology*, 40(2): 112–128.

Gattuso, S., Fullagar, S. and Young, I. (2005) Speaking of women's 'nameless misery': The everyday construction of depression in Australian women's magazines. *Social Science and Medicine*, 61: 1640–1648.

Gavey, N. (2005) Just sex? *The Cultural Scaffolding of Rape*. London: Routledge.

Good, G.E., Dell, D.M. and Mintz, L.B. (1989) Male role and male gender role conflict: Relations to help seeking in men. *Journal of Counselling Psychology*, 36: 295–300.

Gore, S., Aseltine, R.H. and Colton, M.E. (1992) Social structure, life stress and depressive symptoms in a high school aged population. *Journal of Health and Social Behaviour*, 33: 97–113.

Gove, W. (1972) Sex, marital status, and mental illness. *Social Forces*, 51: 34–55.

Gove, W. and Tudor, J. (1973) Adult sex roles and mental illness. *American Journal of Sociology*, 78: 812–835.

Green, R.J., Bettinger, M. and Zacks, E. (1996) Are lesbian couples fused and gay male couples disengaged? Questioning gender straightjackets. In J. Laird and R.-J. Green (eds) *Lesbians and Gays in Couples and Families: A Handbook for Therapists*, pp. 185–230. San Francisco: Jossey Bass.

Gunnell, D., Saperia, J. and Ashby, D. (2005) Selective serotonin reuptake inhibitors (SSRIs) and suicide in adults: Meta-analysis of drug company data from placebo controlled randomized controlled tirals submitted to MHRA's safety review. *British Medical Journal*, 330: 385.

Hamilton, J.A., Grant, M. and Jensvold, M.F. (1996) Sex and treatment of depressions: When does it matter? In J.A. Hamilton, M. Jensvold, E. Rothblum and E. Cole (eds) *Psychopharmacology of Women: Sex, Gender and Hormonal Considerations*, pp. 241–260. Washington, DC: American Psychiatric Press.

Hankin, B.J. and Abramson, L.Y. (2001) Development of gender differences in depression: An elaborated cognitive vulnerability-transactional stress theory. *Psychological Bulletin*, 127(6): 773–796.

Hayward, C., Gotlib, I.H., Schraedley, M.A. and Litt, I.F. (1999) Ethnic differences in the association between pubertal status and symptoms of depression in adolescent girls. *Journal of Adolescent Health*, 25: 143–149.

Herek, G.M. and Garnets, L.D. (2007) Sexual orientation and mental health. *Annual Review of Clinical Psychology*, 3: 353–375.

Hwang, W.C., Myers, H.F., Abe-Kim, J. and Ting, J. Y. (2008) A conceptual paradigm for understanding culture's influence on mental health: the cultural influences on mental health (CIMH) model. *Clinical Psychology Review*, 28: 211–227.

Jack, D.C. (1991) *Silencing the Self: Women and Depression*. Cambridge MΛ: Harvard University Press.

Jackson-Triche, M.E., Sullivan, J.G., Wells, K.B., Rogers, W., Camp, P. and Mazel, R. (2000) Depression and health-related quality of life in ethnic minorities seeking care in general medical settings. *Journal of Affective Disorders*, 58: 89–97.

Kendall-Tackett, K.A. (2007) Inflammation, cardiovascular disease, and metabolic syndrome as sequelae of violence against women. The role of depression, hostility and sleep disturbance. *Trauma, Violence and Abuse*, 8(2): 117–126.

Kendler, K.S., Bulik, C.M., Silberg, J., Hettema, J.M., Myers, J. K. and Prescott, C.A. (2000) Childhood sexual abuse and adult psychiatric and substance use disorders in women. *Archives of General Psychiatry,* 57: 953–959.

Kessler, R.C. (2003) Epidemiology of women and depression. *Journal of Affective Disorders,* 74: 5–13.

Kessler, R.C. and McLeod, J.D. (1984) Sex differences in vulnerability to undesirable life events. *American Sociological Review,* 49: 620–631.

Kessler, R.C., McLeod, J.D. and Wethington, E. (1985) The costs of caring: A perspective on the relationship between sex and psychological distress. In I.G. Sarason and B. Sarason (eds) *Social Support: Theory, Research and Applications*, pp. 491–506. Boston: Martinus Nijhoff.

Kessler, R.C., McGonagle, K.A., Swartz, M., Blazer, D.G. and Nelson, C.B. (1993) Sex and depression in the National Comorbidity Survey I: Lifetime prevalence, chronicity and recurrence. *Journal of Affective Disorders,* 29: 85–96.

Kessler, R.C., McGonagle, K.A., Zhao, S., Nelson, C.B., Hughes, M. and Eshleman, S. (1994) Lifetime and 12-month prevalence of DSM-II-R psychiatric disorders in the United States: Results from the National Co-morbidity Survey. *Archives of General Psychiatry,* 5(1): 8–19.

Kirk, S. and Kutchins, H. (1992) *The Selling of DSM : the Rhetoric of Science in Psychiatry*. New York: A. de Gruyter.

Klonoff, E. A., Landrine, H. and Campbell, R. (2000) Sexist discrimination may account for well-known gender differences in psychiatric symptoms. *Psychology of Women Quarterly,* 24: 93–99.

Koss, M.P., Bailey, J.A., Yuan, N.P., Herrera, V.M. and Lichter, E.L. (2003) Depression and PTSD in survivors of male violence: research and training initiatives to facilitate recovery. *Psychology of Women Quarterly,* 27: 130–142.

Kuehner, C. (2003) Gender differences in unipolar depression: an update of epidemiological findings and possible explanations. *Acta Psychiatr. Scand.,* 108: 163–174.

Kurdek, L.A. (2003) Differences between gay and lesbian cohabiting couples. *Journal of Social and Personal Relationships,* 20: 411–436.

Kurdek, L.A. (2004a) Are gay and lesbian cohabiting couples really different from heterosexual married couples? *Journal of Marriage and Family,* 66: 880–900.

Kurdek, L.A. (2004b) Gay men and lesbians: The family context. In M. Coleman and L.H. Ganong (eds) *Handbook of Contemporary Families: Considering the Past, Contemplating the Future*. pp. 96–105. Thousand Oaks, CA: SAGE.

Kutchins, H. and Kirk, S. (1997) *Making us Crazy: DSM: the Psychiatric Bible and the Creation of Mental Disorders*. New York: Free Press.

LaFrance, M.N. (2007) A bitter pill. A discursive analysis of women's medicalized accounts of depression. *Journal of Health Psychology,* 12(1): 127–140.

LaFrance, M.N. (2009) *Women and Depression: Recovery and Resistance*. London/New York: Routledge.

Littlewood, R. and Lipsedge, M. (1982) *Aliens and Alienists: Ethnic Minorities and Psychiatry*. Harmondsworth: Penguin.

Maier, W., Gansicke, M., Gater, R., Rezaki, M., Tiemens, B. and Urzula, R.F. (1999) Gender differences in the prevalence of depression: a survey in primary care. *Journal of Affective Disorders,* 53: 241–252.

Mauthner, N. (2000) Feeling low and feeling really bad about feeling low. Women's experience of motherhood and post-partum depression. *Canadian Psychology,* 40(2): 143–161.

McQuaide, S. (1998) Women at midlife. *Social Work,* 43(1): 21–31.

Meltzer, H., Gill, B., Petticrew, M. and Hinds, K. (1995) The prevalence of psychiatric morbidity among adults living in private households. *OPCS Survey of Psychiatric Morbidity in Great Britain. Report 1.* London: HMSO.

Mencher, J. (1990) Intimacy in lesbian relationships: A critical re-examination of fusion. Work in Progress No 42. Wellesley, MA: Wellesley College, Stone Center for Women's Development. Document Type: Book.Citation.

Metz, M.E., Rosser, B.R.R. and Strapko, N. (1994) Differences in conflict-resolution styles among hetero-sexual, gay, and lesbian couples. *The Journal of Sex Research*, 31(4): 293–308.

Metzl, J.M. and Angel, J. (2004) Assessing the impact of SSRI antidepressants on popular notions of women's depressive illness. *Social Science and Medicine*, 58: 577–584.

Meyer, I.H. (2003) Prejudice, social stress, and mental health in lesbian, gay, and bisexual populations: Conceptual issues and research evidence. *Psychological Bulletin*, 129: 674–697.

Molnar, B.E., Buka, S.L. and Kessler, R.C. (2001) Child sexual abuse and subsequent pathology: results from the national comorbidity survey. *American Journal of Public Health*, 91(5): 753–760.

Moynihan, R., Heath, I. and Henry, D. (2002) Selling sickness: the pharmaceutical indistry and disease mongering. *British Medical Journal*, 324: 886–890.

Munce, S., Robertson, E.P., Sansom, E.K. and Stewart, D.E. (2004) Who is portrayed in psychotropic drug advertisements? *Journal of Nervous and Mental Disease*, 192(4): 284–288.

Murray, J.L. and Lopez, A.D. (1996) The global burden of disease: A comprehensive assessment of mortality and disability from diseases, injuries and risk factors in 1990 and projected to 2020. Summary. Boston: Harvard School of Public Health: World Health Organisation.

Nazroo, J.Y., Edwards, A.C. and Brown, G.W. (1998) Gender differences in the prevalence of depression: artefact, alternative disorders, biology or roles? *Sociology of Health and Illness*, 20(3): 312–330.

Newman, J.P. (1984) Sex differences in symptoms of depression: clinical disorder or normal distress? *Journal of Health and Social Behaviour*, 25: 136–159.

Nicolson, P. (1998) *Post-natal Depression: Psychology, Science and the Transition to Motherhood.* London: Routledge.

Nolen-Hoeksema, S. and Girgus, J.S. (1994) The emergence of gender differences in depression during adolescence. *Psychological Bulletin*, 115: 424–443.

Nolen-Hoeksema, S., Girgus, J.S. and Seligman, M.E.P. (1991) Sex differences in depression and explan-atory style in children. *Journal of Youth and Adolescence*, 20: 233–245.

Nolen-Hoeksema, S., Larson, J. and Grayson, C. (1999) Explaining the gender difference in depressive symptoms. *Journal of Personality and Social Psychology*, 77(5): 1061–1072.

O'Grady, H. (2005) *Woman's Relationship with Herself: Gender, Foucault, Therapy.* London: Routledge.

O'Neil, J.M. (1990) Assessing mans' gender role conflict. In D. Moore and F. Leafgren (eds) *Men in Conflict: Problem Solving Strategies and Interventions.* Alexandria, V.A.: American Counselling Association.

O'Neil, J.M., Helms, B.J., Gable, R.K., David, L. and Wrightsman, L.S. (1986) Gender role conflict scale: college men's fear of femininity. *Sex Roles*, 14: 335–350.

Perugi, G., Musetti, L., Simonini, E., Piagentini, F., Cassano, G.B. and Akiskal, H.S. (1990) Gender medi-ated clinical features of depressive illness. The importance of temperamental differences. *British Journal of Psychiatry*, 157: 435–441.

Perz, J. and Ussher, J.M. (2008) The horror of this living decay: women's negotiation and resistance of medical discourses around menopause and midlife. *Women's Studies International Forum*, 31: 293–299.

Perz, J. and Ussher, J.M. (2009) Connectedness, communication and reciprocity in lesbian relationships: implications for women's construction and experience of PMS. In P. Hammock and B.J. Cohler (eds) *Life Course and Sexual Identity: Narrative Perspectives on Gay and Lesbian Identity*, pp. 223–250. Oxford: Oxford University Press.

Peterson, A.C., Sarigiani, P.A. and Kennedy, R.E. (1991) Adolescent depression: Why more girls? *Journal of Youth and Adolescence*, 20: 247–271.

Pezzini, S. (2005) The effect of women's rights on women's welfare: evidence from a natural experiment. *The Economic Journal*, 115: C208–C227.

Pilgrim, D. and Bentall, R.P. (1999) The medicatisation of misery: a critical realist analysis of the concept of depression. *Journal of Mental Health*, 8(3): 261–274.

Pilgrim, D. and Rogers, A. (1997) Mental Health, Critical Realism and Lay Knowledge. In J.M. Ussher (ed.), *Body Talk: The Material and Discursive Regulation of Sexuality, Madness and Reproduction*, pp. 33–49. London: Routledge.

Pilgrim, D., Kinderman, P. and Tai, S. (forthcoming) Taking stock of the biopsychosocial model in the field of mental health care.

Pomerantz, E.M. and Ruble, D.N. (1998) The role of maternal control in the development of sex differences in child-self-evaluative factors. *Child Development,* 69, 458–478.

Potts, M.K., Burnam, M.A. and Wells, K.B. (1991) Gender differences in depression detection: A comparison of clinician diagnosis and standardized assessment. *Psychological Assessment: A Journal of Consulting and Clinical Psychology,* 3(4): 609–615.

Price, J.S. (1991) Change or homeostatsis? A systems theory approach to depression. *British Journal of Medical Psychology,* 64: 3331–3344.

Rittenhouse, C.A. (1991) The emergence of premenstrual syndrome as a social problem. *Social Problems,* 38(3): 412–425.

Sachs-Ericsson, N. and Ciarlo, J.A. (2000) Gender, social roles and mental health: An epidemiological perspective. *Sex Roles,* 43(9/10): 605–628.

Salokangas, R.K.R., Vaahtera, K., Pacriev, S., Sohlman, B. and Lehtinen, V. (2002) Gender differences in depressive symptoms. An artefact caused by measurement instruments. *Journal of Affective Disorders,* 68: 215–220.

Sayer, A. (2000) *Realism and Social Science.* London: SAGE.

Sirianni, C. and Negrey, C. (2000) Working time as gendered time. *Feminist Economics,* 6(1): 59–76.

Stoppard, J.M. (2000a) *Understanding Depression: Feminist Social Constructionist Approaches.* London: Routledge.

Stoppard, J.M. (2000b) Why new perspectives are needed for understanding depression in women. *Canadian Psychology,* 40(2): 79–90.

Studd, J.M. (1997) Depression and the menopause. *British Medical Journal,* 314: 977.

Sullivan, P.F., Neale, M.C. and Kendler, K.S. (2000) Genetic epidemiology of major depression: review and meta-analysis. *American Journal of Psychiatry,* 157: 1552–1562.

Takeuchi, D.T., Chung, R.C., Lin, K.M., Shen, H., Kurasaki, K., Chun, C.A. et al. (1998) Lifetime and twelve month prevalence rates of major depressive episodes and dysthemia among Chinese Americans in Los Angeles. *American Journal of Psychiatry,* 155(10): 1407–1414.

Tamres, L.K., Janicki, D. and Helgeson, V.S. (2002) Sex differences in coping behavior: A meta-analytic review and an examination of relative coping. *Personality and Social Psychology Review,* 6(1): 2–30.

Taylor, S.E., Klein, L.C., Lewis, B.P., Gruenwald, T.L., Gurung, R.A.R. and Updegraff, J.A. (2000) Biobehavioural responses to stress in females: tend-and-befriend, not fight-or-flight. *Psychological Review,* 107(3): 411–429.

Turner, R.J. and Avison, W.R. (1989) Gender and depression: Assessing exposure and vulnerability to life events in a chronically strained population. *The Journal of Nervous and Mental Disease,* 177(8): 443–445.

Turner, R.J. and Lloyd, D.A. (1995) Lifetime tramuas and mental health: The significance of cumulative adversity. *Journal of Health and Social Behaviour,* 36(4): 360–376.

Ussher, J.M. (1991) *Women's Madness: Misogyny or Mental Illness?* Amherst, MA, US: University of Massachusetts Press.

Ussher, J.M. (1996) Premenstrual syndrome: Reconciling disciplinary divides through the adoption of a material-discursive epistemological standpoint. *Annual Review of Sex Research,* 7: 218–251.

Ussher, J.M. (2000) Women's madness: A material-discursive-intra psychic approach. In D. Fee (ed.) *Psychology and the Postmodern: Mental Illness as Discourse and Experience,* pp. 207–230. London: SAGE.

Ussher, J.M. (2003a) The ongoing silencing of women in families: An analysis and rethinking of premenstrual syndrome and therapy. *Journal of Family Therapy,* 25: 388–405.

Ussher, J.M. (2003b) The role of premenstrual dysphoric disorder in the subjectification of women. *Journal of Medical Humanities,* 24(1/2): 131–146.

Ussher, J.M. (2004) Premenstrual syndrome and self-policing: Ruptures in self-silencing leading to increased self-surveillance and blaming of the body. *Social Theory and Health,* 2(3): 254–272.

Ussher, J.M. (2005) Unravelling women's madness: Beyond positivism and constructivism and towards a material-discursive-intrapsychic approach. In R. Menzies, D.E. Chunn and W. Chan (eds) *Women, Madness and the Law: A Feminist Reader*, pp. 19–40. London: Glasshouse Press.

Ussher, J.M. (2006) *Managing the Monstrous Feminine: Regulating the Reproductive Body*. London: Routledge.

Ussher, J.M. (2010) Are we medicalizing women's misery? A critical review of women's higher rates of reported depression. *Feminism and Psychology*, 20(1): 9–35.

Ussher, J.M. (2011) *Women's Madness: Myth and Experience*. London: Routledge.

Ussher, J.M. and Perz, J. (2008) Empathy, egalitarianism and emotion work in the relational negotiation of PMS: The experience of lesbian couples. *Feminism and Psychology*, 18(1): 87–111.

Ussher, J.M. and Perz, J. (2010) Disruption of the silenced-self: the case of pre-menstrual syndrome. In D.C. Jack and A. Ali (eds) *The Depression Epidemic: International Perspectives on Women's Self-silencing and Psychological Distress*, pp. 435–458. Oxford: Oxford University Press.

Waisberg, J. and Page, S. (1988) Gender role conformity and the perception of mental illness. *Women and Health*, 14(1): 3–16.

Weissman, M.M., Bland, R.C. and Canino, G.J. (1996) Cross national epidemiology of major depression and bipolar disorder. *JAMA*, 276: 293–299.

Weissman, M.M., Leaf, P.J., Holzer, C.E., Myers, J.K. and Tischler, G.L. (1984) The epidemiology of depression: an update on sex differences in rates. *Journal of Affective Disorders*, 7: 179–188.

Whiffen, V.E. (1992) Is postpartum depression a distinct diagnosis? *Clinical Psychology Review*, 12(5): 485–508.

Whiffen, V.E., Foot, M.L. and Thompson, J.M. (2007) Self-silencing mediates the link between marital conflict and depression. *Journal of Social and Personal Relationships*, 24(6): 993–1006.

Whisman, M.A. and Bruce, M.L. (1999) Marital distress and incidence of major depressive episode in a community sample. *Journal of Abnormal Psychology*, 108: 674–678.

Wilhelm, K. and Parker, G. (1994) Sex differences in lifetime depression rates: fact or artifact? *Psychological Medicine*, 24(1): 97–11.

Williams, S. (2003) Beyond meaning, discourse and the empirical world: Critical realist reflections on health. *Social Theory and Health*, 1: 42–47.

Williamson, G.L. (1993) Postpartum depression syndrome as a defence to criminal behaviour. *Journal of Family Violence*, 8(2): 151–165.

Wilson, R. and Cairns, E. (1988) Sex role attributes, perceived competence and the development of depression in adolescence. *Journal of Child Psychology and Psychiatry*, 29: 635–650.

World Health Organisation (2000) *Women's Mental Health: An Evidence Based Review*. Geneva: World Health Organisation.

Yardley, L. (1996) Reconciling discursive and materialist perspectives on health and illness: A reconstruction of the biopsychosocial approach. *Theory and Psychology*, 6(3): 485–508.

7

The Diagnosis of Depression in an International Context

Renata Kokanovic

INTRODUCTION

'Depression' is one of the most extensively described and debated words in the field of mental health. To contribute to this debate, this chapter provides a brief overview of the key academic discussions on depression, with a particular focus on the applicability and relevance of the concept across different cultures. I will consider the role of culture, language and migrant and refugee status in relation to the diagnosis. In addition, this chapter reflects on the debate on the *causes* of depression and on its medicalization.

There has been a proliferation of discourses on depression in contemporary Western societies in recent years, ranging from psychiatry, biomedicine, psychology, social sciences, government policy documents, nutrition studies, consumer guides, websites and media reports. Given the late modern preoccupations with individuality, identity and self-worth, Martin (1999) has described depression as the 'presiding discontent' of contemporary society. In their critical account of the topic Horowitz and Wakefield (2007) outline some processes contributing to the status of depression as a 'major social trend'. They note: the widespread perception that prevalence is increasing; the rise in the number of people in treatment; the manifold increase in prescriptions for antidepressant medications; the explosion of scientific publications on the diagnosis; and media attention on the problem of depression, including the industry of 'evidence-based', and expert produced self-help resources detailing how to cope with and overcome depression.

Among diagnosed mental disorders, depression has been portrayed as the leading global cause of disability (Murray and Lopez, 1996). Depending on the definition employed, depression can afflict as many as *half* of the members of particular population groups, such as female, adolescents and older people (Lavretsky and Kumar, 2002). Horowitz and Wakefield (2007) argue that 'there is widespread perception that depressive disorder is growing at an alarming pace' (Horowitz and Wakefield, 2007: 4).

Many researchers argue that one of the key factors contributing to the rise of the diagnosis of depression is the influence and power of the Diagnostic and Statistical Manual of Mental Disorders (DSM). The latter has attracted much controversy and criticism, largely because with each new revision it has gradually enlarged the list of human behaviours qualified as disorders and as abnormal (Hansen et al., 2003; Newnes et al., 1999, 2001).

Horowitz and Wakefield (2007) argue that the DSM III criteria for depression, 'by distinguishing depressive disorders solely on the basis of symptoms, regardless of their relationship to circumstances' (Horowitz and Wakefield, 2007: 101) are 'largely decontextualized, symptom based criteria [which] stemmed from effort[s] … to develop a common language for psychiatrists with a variety of theoretical persuasions, and to bolster the scientific credentials of the profession' (Horowitz and Wakefield, 2007: 103). They comment that this process, in conjunction with the processes in psychiatry turning to 'heterogeneous conditions of outpatients and community members', have resulted in a 'massive pathologization of normal sadness'(Horowitz and Wakefield, 2007: 103). Such decontextualization, as Horowitz and Wakefield argue, makes the diagnosis of depression less, rather than more scientifically valid. (A fuller account of medicalization is given in Olafsdottir, this handbook.)

The World Health Report (2001) (WHR) offers global prevalence rates for the diagnosis of 1.9 per cent for men, and 3.2 per cent for women, with 5.8 per cent of men and 9.5 per cent of women each year experiencing a depressive episode. Results of many epidemiological and population health studies research have been in accord with WHR data. They differ in rates of depression reported, but it is estimated that around 100 million people have been developing a depressive illness each year as a result of global economic and cultural changes, which may expose people to prolonged psychosocial stressors (Douki and Tabbane, 1996). The rise in psychoactive substance use, mass migrations, growing unemployment in some sectors and uncertain employment in many other industries, breakdown of traditional family structures and poverty are frequently cited among the major contributing factors that generate the increased incidence of 'depressive disorders' (Schwartz, 2000).

The movement throughout the West towards community care and a trend to keep more severely and more visibly 'mentally ill' people outside of institutions and integrate them into the community, has opened the way for more subtle differences in the 'normal' population to become the subject of psychiatric categorization (Pilgrim and Bentall, 1999). Thus, new patient groups have been identified, including children, adolescents and those who differ from the 'norm' in an increasing variety of ways (Turner, 1995). In the process, psychiatry, clinical psychology and medicine has gained increased power to control of the 'lives of others' (Hansen et al., 2003; Newnes et al., 1999, 2001).

Given this recent picture it can be noted that depression has not always been seen as a mental illness in Western societies (Jackson, 1985). Furthermore, the view that we are currently facing a global depression epidemic is a relatively recent phenomenon. Horowitz and Wakefield (2007) comment that:

> What has happened is largely diagnostic inflation, based on a relatively new definition of depressive disorder that is flawed and that, combined with other developments in society, has dramatically expanded the domain of presumed disorder. (Horowitz and Wakefield, 2007: 7)

PROBLEMS WITH DIAGNOSIS

Much of the previous discussion indicates that depression is a complex condition to define and consequently, it is a difficult condition to identify (Horowitz and Wakefield, 2007). Lutz (1985), for example, points out that 'in their discussions of the nature of depression, many Western psychologists place primary emphasis on the depressed person's self-reproach and loss of interest in "pleasurable activity". What is particularly deviant about the depressive is his/her failure to engage in the "pursuit of happiness" or in the love of self that is considered to be normal and basic goal of persons' (Lutz, 1985: 70). Lutz, among others, argues that this desire for happiness is not a natural but culturally constructed goal and should be compared or contrasted with other equally legitimate definitions of normalcy and expressions of natural states. Similarly, Williams (2000) suggests critical questioning of 'ideologies and expert led discourses of personal growth, fulfilment and happiness as themselves (all too often) "unhealthy", promoting rather than mitigating our discontent' (Williams, 2000: 573).

According to Kleinman and Good (1985: 3), 'it seems reasonable to ask to what extent depression itself is a cultural category, grounded both in a long Western intellectual tradition and a specific medical tradition'. Scientific and cultural understandings of depression have changed over time, and there are significant differences in lay understanding and experience and clinical definitions. The psychiatric and clinical psychological literature does not provide a consistent definition of depression but rather identifies its indicators and manifestations. The DSM IV (1994) distinguishes two conditions, major depressive disorder and dysthymic disorder, which have similar symptoms but different severities based on the number of symptoms (e.g. low self-esteem, insomnia, fatigue and feeling of hopelessness) and aetiology.

Qualitative research about the experience of depression provides a different perspective. In Karp's (1996) analysis of 50 interviews, depression emerges as a deep sense of unhappiness described like a 'grief' and resulting in feelings of marginality, neglect and loneliness most often manifesting as frantic anxiety, sleep disturbance and somatic symptoms. Kokanovic et al. (2008) similarly to Karp (1996) found that metaphors are often used to describe the experience of depression ' "a sense of darkness"; "a black hole"; "a heavy black blanket being thrown over you"; "a cancer of your self-esteem" ' (Kokanovic et al., 2008: 457). The effects of depression as described by sufferers include total inertia, social withdrawal, a feeling that they are going to die (Karp, 1996) and as something that consumes and overwhelms the individual (Kokanovic et al., 2008). These phenomenological accounts indicate as well that anxiety symptoms (especially agitation and free floating anxiety or dread) are very common in those with a diagnosis of depression or dysthymic disorder. Given this common mixture, 'depression' may denote the experience of unhappy people less precisely than ordinary language (e.g. 'misery'). Wolpert (1999) in a first hand account describes depression as a combination, among other things, of overwhelming sadness, suicidal thoughts, crying spells, sleeping difficulties, fatigue, lack of energy, inability to concentrate or make decisions, sense of hopelessness, loss of self-esteem and loss of interest and pleasure in any activity.

The problem with the above definitions is that they lack diagnostic clarity. They also reveal how deeply depression is embedded in the cultural and social conditions. For this reason, it is crucial to look at depression in its cultural context and to consider its social determinants. Pilgrim and Bentall (1999) point out that using existing clinical definitions, two individuals with completely different symptoms could be diagnosed with the same condition. This is because depression and its diagnostic criteria overlap with other conditions to such an extent that it is most often impossible to distinguish in a particular case between depression, anxiety or even medical conditions, such as chronic fatigue syndrome (Pilgrim and Bentall, 1999). Some theorists thus see depression as existing on a continuum with 'normal' states (Schwartz, 2000). However, others see it as categorically different and not related to 'normal' states of unhappiness or sadness.

Kleinman and Good (1985) in a study of the relevance of the concept of depression across culture argue that depression differs depending on who identifies and defines it. For clinicians, they comment, 'depression is a common, often severe, sometimes mortal disease with characteristic affective (sadness, irritability, joylessness), cognitive (difficulty concentrating, memory disturbance) and vegetative (sleep, appetite, energy disturbances) complaints which has a typical course and predictable response rates to treatment' (Kleinman and Good, 1985: 9). Following Foucault (1973) and Porter (2002), Bendelow (2009) argues that 'across most of "western" society the growth of scientific medicine in general and psychiatry in particular has meant that medicalization has been the most dominant means of response [to emotional instability] since the nineteen century' (Bendelow, 2009: 81). She states that 'development of biological and neuro-psychiatry has largely dominated therapeutic response[s] to emotional distress' (Bendelow, 2009: 81) providing an obstacle to the notion that mental disorders are still 'illnesses without clear and demonstrable scientific psychopathology' (Bendelow, 2009: 81).

As this brief account of the debates about diagnosis of depression has shown, it is extremely unclear how to accurately *distinguish* between 'normal' feelings of sadness or misery which are a result of distressing life events or everyday disappointments, and 'abnormal' feelings of unhappiness or 'depression'.

Causes of depression

There are a number of theoretical stands about the causes of depression. Here I briefly outline some prevailing psychological, socio-cultural and biomedical perspectives.

Although psychology is a broad, polymorphous discipline, psychological approaches to depression tend to view depression as a mood disorder, which exists on a continuum with 'normal' mental states, often triggered by a stressful life event such as losing one's job or the death of a loved one (Schwartz, 2000). Also, it is often noted that there is a strong correlation between depression and physical illness, such as hormonal disorders or drug and alcohol abuse.

One of the major psychological approaches is a cognitive model which looks at the depressed person as having distorted cognitions, which are biased toward negative attributions. Beck (1976) argues that those suffering from depression see their environment as overwhelmingly negative. They see themselves as bad, hopeless and view the future pessimistically. Such a perception of oneself and one's context is known as the 'cognitive triad' of negative evaluations of the self, world and the future. It is defined as a disorder of the perceptive and interpretive processes (Good et al., 1985; Schwartz, 2000).

Seligman's (1975) learned helplessness theory is often contrasted to Beck's cognitive theory. Seligman argues that people who get depressed as a result of loss or rejection perceive themselves as having no control over everyday events. They usually attribute any failure to their own personality traits. As a consequence they respond to the environment with passivity and helplessness (Schwartz, 2000).

Contrary to the above, qualitative research within anthropology, sociology and critical psychology are critical of the view that psychological distress is the domain of an individual. Work coming from these disciplines argue that social factors and processes are equally if not more significant in naming and identifying patterns of diagnosis and treatment of distress. An early example of this approach is from Brown and Harris (1978) who examined the socio-cultural position of depressed women. They argue that women's social position influences the way they think about the world. Their social environment provides insufficient resources to cope with the lack of opportunity of improved social status, higher education and satisfactory professional career. Brown and Harris identified some socio-cultural factors which leave certain segments of urban population, such as women, more vulnerable to develop mental illness. They conclude that 'no single avenue of intervention is likely to provide the best answer for a condition with such a complex aetiology' (Brown and Harris, 1978: 291).

Many social factors including low educational status, unemployment or low employment, homelessness or insecure housing, inadequate income, poor social support and unsatisfactory interactions are all associated with the increased rates of depression and anxiety and they often interact with one another (Brown and Harris, 1978). One of the major limitations of social causation models such as that put forward by Brown and Harris, according to Bendelow (2009), is that 'although social and cultural factors may create relative risk for a population or a class of people, it is unclear how such factors raise the risk of mental illness for an individual, and the link between social ills and mental illness is more accurately *correlational* rather than causal' (Bendelow, 2009: 100). Also although Brown, Harris and their team discussed criteria for psychiatric caseness, they did not embark on a serious critique of the conceptual validity of diagnostic categories or on the sociological questions surrounding medicalization (cf. Pilgrim and Bentall, 1999).

Thus within sociological debates there remain fundamental differences of position about specific categorizations and the social nature of separating normal from abnormal emotion (Bendelow, 2009; Hansen et al., 2003; Kleinman, 1985; Newnes et al., 1999, 2001; Turner, 1995). Although social-constructivist approaches to understandings of depression include critiques of biological and psychological discourses, advocates of such an approach may still fail to acknowledge that the very definition of the condition has already been socially determined.

Despite the significance of social determinants of depression and an ongoing academic debate about social versus biological causation of this condition, Lock (1997) argues that in the Western biomedical discourses social factors are marginalized while 'efforts to reduce suffering have habitually focused on control and repair of individual bodies. [The social origins of depression] ... are set aside, while effort is expended in controlling disease and averting death through biomedical manipulations' (Lock, 1997: 210).

Traditionally, 'endogenous depression', which was thought to have a biological cause in the diagnosed individual was differentiated from 'exogenous depression', which was thought to be an extreme reaction to external social circumstances. This distinction has recently been officially abandoned in nosological systems but many clinicians maintain the distinction in practice (McPherson and Armstrong, 2006). The biochemical model interprets depression as a physiological malfunction of genes, hormones, chemical imbalances or problems with neurotransmitters (Barlow and Durand, 2002; Healy, 1997, 2004; Schwartz, 2000). Biopsychiatry tends to see social factors mainly as precipitants, emphasizing physiological factors as the ultimate cause. In this context, depression is understood as a biological illness treatable medicinally (Bendelow, 2009; Hansen et al., 2003; Healy 1997, 2004; Horowitz and Wakefield, 2007; Newnes et al., 2001; Schwartz, 2000). Even when within biological discourse social factors are acknowledged as causal components, these are seen as 'triggers' for 'illness' rather than fundamental causes. Treatment is thus generally based around correcting putative physiological imbalances through the use of anti-depressants.

For some diagnosed patients, defining depression as a biologically based condition which manifests itself through a number of physical symptoms such as a lack of sleep, changes to eating patterns and low energy levels may create an impression that their condition is the same as other illnesses and therefore less likely to be stigmatized. Karp (1996) and Lupton (1994), among others, note that some patients are often relieved at being given a medical diagnosis for their distress. It provides them with a label which justifies and explains their feelings and with a legitimate illness identity. They may welcome a biomedical diagnosis, since 'adopting the view that one is victimized by a biochemically sick self constitutes a comfortable "account" for a history of difficulties and failures and absolves one of responsibility' (Karp, 1996: 73). However, it also marginalizes a person diagnosed with depression as suffering from something outside the normal human condition which is a threat to society's emotional equilibrium (Levin, 1987; Lupton, 1994). These contradicting factors place a person who is diagnosed as 'ill' in the role of a patient and a victim. Such a person loses his/her own agency becoming passive, voiceless and aware that they are no longer 'themselves'.

Even though chemical imbalance diagnosed as a cause of depression could be useful strategy for justifying peoples' feelings, Ridge and Ziebland (2006) found in their research that the chemical narrative 'interwove with participant stories, [but] it did not necessarily exclude nonbiological explanations for depression that could coexist with – or even surpass – the biochemical. Instead, there was a complex relationship between the chemical and the social' (Ridge and Ziebland, 2006: 1043).

To conclude, sociologists of health and illness have long recognized the power of the medical profession and medical expertise, which tends to expand its territory by defining human difficulties as essentially medical problems (Foucault, 1967; Turner, 1995). Medical professionals through their expert status have thus become articulators of information about mental conditions and their causes. While it is easy to assume that the biomedical approach will be taken primarily by medical professionals and drug companies in whose interests the use of drugs for depression may be, other social groups confirm its legitimacy (Pilgrim, 2007).

Lay and expert concepts of depression

Definitions of depression are further complicated by the infiltration of expert biomedical discourses of depression into peoples' daily lives and popular discourses. For instance, building on de Swaan's (1990) argument that lay people are increasingly framing their problems in 'proto-professional' terms, Shaw (2002) challenges the notion of lay illness beliefs by arguing that in Western societies lay people are inundated with biomedical discourse throughout their everyday life. The very category of a lay perspective, independent and easily demarcated from professional paradigms of illness, is empirically tenuous

(Kokanovic et al., 2008). Pilgrim and Bentall (1999) suggest a number of similarities and differences between professional (expert) knowledge claims and lay accounts of depression. Lay accounts show that people acknowledge the individuality and uniqueness, rather than generalize their experience; they acknowledge that the ways in which people express their feelings and distress vary across time and place and within different cultures; lay people construct their understandings of emotions in relation to their life history. Experts claim for their understandings a superior epistemological status; they base their legitimacy on the universality of accounts they de-contextualize, historically, culturally and biographically, different understandings of 'mental illnesses' and contexts that produce emotional distress, while at the same time maintain their expert status by producing accounts that seem meaningful enough to be considered credible.

When a lay person defines him/herself as depressed they refer to the subjective and emotional condition. When they relay this to a health professional, depression becomes a depersonalized medical diagnosis. Thus, as Pilgrim and Bentall (1999) argue, depression 'is a professional reification about human misery, not a fact'. They further conclude that, 'If the concept is not working as a coherent pre-empirical notion perhaps we should review its utility instead of generating more and more empirical studies producing more and more ambiguous findings about "depression" ' (Pilgrim and Bentall, 1999: 7).

Culture and depression

The international debate in mental health and cultural diversity discusses whether mental disorders should be considered as universal entities and to what extent they are distinct and therefore different 'cultural realities'. Kleinman and Good (1985) reject the universalist tradition of Euro-American psychiatry and psychology in relation to the experience of depressive illness. They argue that there is significant evidence against the notion of a universal experience of depression. They point to the fact that there are profound differences in:

> the social organization, personal experience, and consequences of such emotions as sadness, grief, and anger, of behaviours such as withdrawal or aggression, and of psychological characteristics such as passivity and helplessness or the resort to altered states of consciousness. (Kleinman and Good, 1985: 492)

Accordingly, these are organized and communicated 'in a wide range of idioms, related to quite varied local contexts of power relations, and are interpreted, evaluated, and responded to as fundamentally different meaningful realities' (Kleinman and Good, 1985: 492).

Culture is the most critical influence determining how individuals perceive and interpret their environment. When Kleinman and Good (1985) posed the question, 'what is cultural about depression?' they initiated a critical debate about the forms of interpretation which determine one's environment as 'normal' or 'disordered'. Such a debate is vital to understandings of the possible universality of depression (Kleinman and Good, 1985). The debate touches upon these complex considerations about:

- whether the concept of depression is relevant across cultures;
- whether its Western biomedical discourse is valid across cultures;
- whether certain cultural groups are at greater risk of depression than others;
- whether the risk of depression is determined by cultural or experiential influences;
- whether culture affects the individual's interpretation of unhappiness and sadness resulting in different responses to emotional distress;
- whether there are cultural variations in the expression, manifestation and experience of depression/unhappiness;
- whether depressive symptoms can take a different course resulting in different health outcomes, and finally;
- how can the diverse needs of people experiencing depression best be met.

This range of overlapping considerations has failed to achieve an interdisciplinary consensus about the universal status and cultural nuances of 'depression'.

An edited volume by Kleinman and Good, published in 1985, presents a significant advancement in how mental illness, including depression, was understood. Kleinman and Good state that:

> the translation of emotional terms required much more than finding semantic equivalents. Describing how it feels to be grieved or melancholy in another society leads straightway into analysis of different ways of being a person in radically different worlds. (Kleinman and Good, 1985: 3)

Articles from around the globe, following this influential work clearly indicated that dysphoric emotions significantly vary in different cultures. In many societies, depression does not have the same 'symptomatology' as in Western Judeo-Christian societies. For Chinese, for example, somatic complaints such as the heart being squeezed or exhaustion of the nerves may be indicated. Migrants from many African societies to the West are unlikely to accept the western, bio-medical model of depression as an explanation for distress. Their understanding may be influenced by cultural variations, value system and linguistic symbols in expressing distress (Kirmayer, 2001; Kleinman, 1998). Many Ethiopians, Somali, Bosnians and Vietnamese for example, do not associate feelings labelled as depression with a classification of 'illness', and therefore are reluctant to use professional services for these problems (Kokanovic et al., 2006, 2010; Kokanovic and Stone, 2010; Papadopolis et al., 2004; Silviera and Allbeck, 2001). Others understand the emotional expression as 'soul loss' (Shweder, 1985). For many cultures, for example Buddhist, unhappiness is not negatively valued. For those from Judeo-Christian traditions, feelings of guilt and sinfulness may be apparent as part of the negative affect, while for other cultures these are missing (Kleinman and Good, 1985). There is also little evidence for separating depression from anxiety and stress that is experienced in other cultures (Beiser, 1985), as we found them in current diagnostic terminology.

At the core of debate about the cross cultural relevance of the idea of depression is the question of the status of emotion-states across cultures. At a fundamental level, it is questionable whether the concept of prolonged unhappiness, which is a key feature of biomedical accounts of depression, exists across cultures. Many cultures do not have words to describe or identify these emotions. Wierzbicka (1999) suggest that simply using English categories of happiness or sadness delimits the available interpretive categories. She points out that the concept of 'feeling' is universal, but that 'emotion' as a concept is culture-bound, as it relies on a combination of three major components – thoughts, feelings and bodily processes. Similarly, Rogers and Pilgrim (2005) argue that the manifestation of emotional distress is endemic across all cultures, although interpretations and responses may vary widely. Wierzbicka suggests a need to identify the semantic equivalent in each language for negative emotions which may be comparable to sadness-like feelings or depression. However, the conceptual linguistic framework will not *necessarily* be congruent across cultures. Therefore, privileging the framework provided by the English language obscures the possibility of other ways of expressing and describing negative emotion.

Others have argued that negative affect is not necessarily negatively valued across cultures. In many cultures, suffering is understood through religious and spiritual concepts rather than through a medical framework. For example, Obeyesekere (1985), when discussing Sri Lankan Buddhism asks:

> How is the Western diagnostic term 'depression' expressed in a society whose predominant ideology of Buddhism states that life is suffering and sorrow, that the cause of sorrow is attachment or desire or craving, that there is a way (generally through meditation) of understanding and overcoming suffering, and the achieving the final goals, cessation of suffering or *nirvana*? (Obeyesekere, 1985: 134)

He notes that Buddhists in Sri Lanka perceive hopelessness, sorrow, meaninglessness and rejecting pleasure not as an illness that could arguably be characterized as depressive symptoms within the DSM definition of depression, but as part of a culturally recognized philosophy of life.

Feelings are experienced and valued differently across cultures. Wierzbicka (1999) further elaborates that the state of happiness as a normal state, is peculiarly an American concept, through which some American psychologists identify the state of being 'happy' as a basic human emotion (p. 249). For some, dysphoric states are part of the emotional goals of a particular culture, for others they are evidence of an illness which requires medical intervention. As Lutz has pointed out:

> In their discussions of the nature of depression, many Western psychologists place primary emphasis on the depressed person's self-reproach and loss of interest in 'pleasurable activities'. What is particularly deviant about the depressive is his failure to engage in the 'pursuit of happiness' or in the love of self that is considered to be the normal and basic goal of persons. This seemingly natural goal is in fact a culturally moulded goal, one that contrasts with other possible definitions of normalcy in which, for example, primary emphasis might be put on taking care of children and other relatives, or on experiencing morally correct but perhaps unpleasant emotions such as shame or righteous indignation. (Lutz, 1985: 70)

Concepts of mental health and illness derive from traditional cultural philosophies, medical discourse, popular culture and the lived experiences of individuals affected by distress. Differences in illness concepts are in a dynamic relation to cultural differences, which include the recognition of experienced illness states, their perception and interpretation, their disclosure and the way this content is communicated within a particular culture. There are diverse understandings in different cultural communities in relation to what constitutes mental health, mental illness and emotional life. Different concepts of emotional and mental distress (e.g. whether emotional distress is conceptualized as an illness or not) may also imply diverse concepts of what constitutes relevant actions to alleviate suffering caused by distress.

Kirmayer (2001) argues that 'culture has effects on neural systems, psychological representations, and interactional patterns that constitute affect throughout the life-span' (Kirmayer, 2001: 22). The context and patterns of reaction and expression of emotions are shaped by ideologies, institutions of society and nature of practices and processes of these constituent cultural elements. Such a complex interactivity provides 'categories and a lexicon for emotional experience [but also] socially acceptable and deviant patterns of emotional expression' (Kirmayer, 2001: 22). This means that culture imposes norms of tolerance on specific emotions, but also influences the sources of distress. In other words, culture shapes 'the form of illness experience, symptomatology, the interpretation of symptoms, modes of coping with distress, help-seeking, and the social response to distress and disability' (Kirmayer, 2001: 22).

Lutz (1985) also points out that the dichotomy of 'emotion' and 'cognition' which underpins biomedical diagnostic categories for depression only make sense in the context of the Euro-American cultural system within which they developed. What we might think of broadly as similar 'transient internal experiences' (such as profound sadness) might in one culture be described as a unity but in another split into thoughts and feelings. This may present significant problems to clinicians in recognizing cultural manifestations of distress that becomes labelled as depression. In addition to these issues, the diagnostic process is affected by the metaphorical linguistic structures used within different cultures and languages to denote and describe subjective experience. Distinguishing between constructs such as 'sensation', 'cognition', 'emotion' and 'behaviour', may be relevant to the description of psychopathology in Western diagnostic systems such as the DSM. But these are not common categories in many other cultures. For example, drawing on the case of the Ifaluk of Micronesia, Lutz (1985) indicates the emotions of *fago* which merges Western categories such as compassion, love and sadness, and *lalomweiu*, which combines feelings of loneliness and sadness. These emotional states may not be readily understood (or empathized with) by outsiders who differentiate between the substrates of these states.

All the above play an important role in the diagnosis of depression in the cross-cultural clinical context. These include: the cross-cultural validity of nosological systems underpinning the diagnostic process, cultural variance in the experience and manifestation of distress, and a lack of common reference in cross-cultural communication and conceptualizing of distress. Culturally shaped experiences and responses to distress may not fit neatly into the diagnostic categories defined within Euro-American nosological systems (Kleinman, 1977, 1987). This presents a marked challenge to the view that dominant diagnostic systems such as DSM should be valid for universal application. The basic issue of validity is whether a diagnostic category such as 'major depressive episode' that is applied to the sense of patient's distress carries sufficient meaning and coherence within the person's cultural context.

Cultural differences generally have a significant impact on the perspective each actor brings to the patient–health practitioner relationship. Disparity between understandings of emotional states between people experiencing distress and health practitioners will significantly affect diagnosis and treatment of distress. In many non-Western cultures, emotional distress is not separated from physical symptoms. Instead, both emotional and physical symptoms are approached in an integrated psychosomatic or somatopsychic way. Somatic illnesses tend to be less stigmatized than those defined as 'mental'. Alternatively, a person may use religious or moral explanations of 'unusual behaviours' that, under a Western diagnostic system, would be regarded as evidence of 'mental illness' (Bentelspacher, 1994; Marmanidis et al., 1994).

Further, it is very difficult to translate Western psychiatric diagnostic instruments into other languages, and to apply them to diverse cultural groups in diverse settings. Good et al. (1985) argue that translating diagnostic instruments which have been developed in one culture into other languages and applying them in other cultures, presumes that experiences and interpretations of symptoms are de-contextualized reflections of physiological states, rather than being local idioms of distress. Taking symptoms which have become part of a constellation of characteristics of a condition simply because they are significant to Americans for example, and translating them to other languages, does little to determine whether the condition as identified in Western societies is actually a valid phenomenon across cultures and in societies not structured on a model of Western societies.

LANGUAGE, TRANSLATING AND INTERPRETING

Emotional distress, as with most other human conditions, is primarily articulated and expressed through verbal and written communication. In spite of a move towards other modes of expression, such as visual and performative communication, both in everyday life and scientific research, in the dominant culture in contemporary industrialized developed societies privileges linguistically based communication. For this reason, linguistic translation presents an additional concern, when attempting to communicate about mental health and emotional distress between different cultures.

Although verbal and written communication is regarded as more precise than other modes of communication, this assumption is only another cultural convention of logo-centric western societies. Language is no less ambivalent than other modes of expression and communication. This only further reveals the complexities of translation and interpreting in communication about depression. Lutz (1985) argues that 'the use of Euro-American ethno theories to guide research has meant that translation had proceeded predominantly in one direction, with American English being the source language, and all others being target languages, that is the languages into which translation is to be achieved' (Lutz, 1985: 89). Werner and Campbell (1970) note that such an approach fails to acknowledge that the worlds of different language speakers are not simply the same worlds with different labels attached. They suggest that translation should not proceed in this 'one-to-many' way, which results in asymmetrical translation, but by providing a set of many equivalent or nearly equivalent statements in each language. They comment that 'the set of statements which provides the context for translating emotion worlds includes the kinds of ethno-psychological premises about person, consciousness, and action' (Werner and Campbell, 1970: 89).

Translation of emotional experience into a form of spoken language represents different concepts in different cultural contexts and significantly varies between cultures. In this process numerous metaphors and other modes of expression of distress are often removed, as in the case of superficial clinical or research interviewing. This contributes to distortion or may obscure the experience of interviewees. It may also lead to diagnostic error, if there is a miscommunication between the two parties. Medical or psychiatric interviewing can carry many uncommon and abstract terms, which may not have a semantic equivalent for different cultural groups. Further, the use of a second language such as English in clinical practice and research can produce distorted results because the interviewee may have an insufficient vocabulary for accurately expressing his or her emotional states (Altarriba and Santiago-Riviera, 1994).

Other difficulties include the potential for dissociation between emotional states and language that is 'saying it without feeling it' (Marcos et al., 1973) and the interviewee's possible guardedness over emotional expression (Del Castillo, 1970). These obstacles may lead to over-diagnosis of psychopathology in members of different cultural groups (Marcos et al., 1973). Additional concern may be the use of interpreters who can contribute to the diagnostic error. Furthermore, the presence of an interpreter can alter important dynamics between the clinician and the patient or a researcher and a research participant. It can introduce new dynamics, which may hinder therapeutic or research goals (Baker and Briggs, 1975; Degotardi, 1995; Westermeyer, 1985).

It is therefore crucial that research aiming to inform clinical practice and produce evidence for the best practice health care for emotional distress explore the full spectrum of local interpretive forms and illness categories (Kleinman, 1982). Another relevant issue is how these interpretive forms are used and what they aim to interpret. In other words, researchers and clinicians need to be aware of the interpretive foci at play in the diagnostic process, for example, how individual life events, spirits, social conditions and physical processes are interpreted. Likewise the semantic networks of symbols and meaningfully related experiences associated with depression should be investigated (Good, Delvecchio Good et al., 1985), particularly in many non-western cultures where there are no distinctive words for depression (Marsella and Pederson, 1981).

FORCED MIGRATION AND MINORITY STATUS AS A RISK FACTOR FOR DIAGNOSED DEPRESSION

In the globalized world where migration occurs on a massive scale, the particular issues faced by immigrant groups, especially those involved in forced migration, are of special concern when developing a culturally sensitive approach to depression and emotional distress. The challenge of understanding and representing the complexity of all who are affected by forced migration across cultures is often underestimated. This requires insight and understanding of the interplay between the individual's social and psychological world, and his or her way of experiencing and verbalizing emotional distress.

DelVecchio, Hyde and Good (2008) call for effort to find new ways to link the social and psychological, to examine how lives of individuals, families and communities are affected by large scale political and economic forces associated with globalization, forced migration and to theorize subjectivity within this larger context. Although there are some positive developments in acknowledging forced migration as impacting on people's emotional state, the 'continued reliance on symptom-focussed [research] methodologies' (Miller et al., 2002) is limiting our understanding of the social and political processes in which impact upon migrants and refugees.

Ahmad and Bradby (2007) comment that historically medicine has tended to pathologize minority cultures. There is often an assumption that migrant and refugee populations are always at a health disadvantage, which is a result of experiences of armed conflicts, prolonged displacement and other traumatic experiences and resulting economic difficulties, adaptation challenges, discrimination, racism and so on. Although these conditions need to be recognized and addressed, it could be said that those who are socio-economically marginalized will be at similar risk. However, immigrants and refugees are a more visible segment of the population and concerns about their health tie into wider agendas for reinforcing their Otherness (Kitzinger and Wilkinson, 1996).

Current research on immigrants and refugees from diverse cultures mainly focus on the influence of pre-migration factors on resettlement and mental health issues after resettlement. This representation often results in the pathologization of forced migration and refugee communities. Miller et al. (2002) argue that research on the mental health of refugees has emphasized the assessment of psychiatric symptomatology, primarily through the use of symptom checklists and structured clinical interviews. Reliance on these methods usually restricts understandings of emotional distress related to voluntary, forced migration and/ or exile. The language of 'trauma' has become widely used and depression, anxiety and other clinical terms for mental distress are used in a number of contexts other than clinical practice. They are employed generically to describe acute suffering, and critically to question the dominance of medicalization over social causal factors. DelVecchio, Hyde and Good (2009: 10) note that such diversity in the use of 'diagnostic language has the potential to reproduce the medicalizing tendencies [and] to assert universal categories without warrant'.

In researching health in culturally different groups of migrants and refugees in host countries, caution is required when assuming that migrants are prone to particular illnesses, including 'depression'. This is an issue highlighted by Ahmad and Bradby (2007):

> Using culture and ethnicity as an explanation of inequality between groups distorts percep-
> tions of how ethnic relations, and the related inequities of power are produced. Defined by
> those in power, the disadvantage of minority ethnic groups too often continues to be seen
> as 'caused' by their diseased genetic and dysfunctional cultural inheritance. (Ahmad and
> Bradby, 2007: 798).

Such a construct places migrants into a marginal position as their 'natural' space, and legitimizes the existing policies and practices of health and care in many Western societies. Further, a special caution needs to be exercised not to homogenize and 'exoticize' diverse cultural groups. People from different cultures (and this applies to majority cultures in Western industrialized countries) experiencing distress should be recognized as social actors with diverse experi-ences and biographies, rather than ascribing to them a common group identity irrespective of differences based on age, gender, socio-economic and cultural backgrounds and general life histories.

Lambert and Sevak (1996) emphasize that health and ill health is 'interpreted in relation to people's life situation and in light of knowledge derived from personal and social experiences' (Lambert and Sevak, 1996: 154). They point out that the very existence of 'cultural differences' in perceptions of health, which predictably correspond to cultural and ethnic affiliations, need to be treated as a research question *per se* and they need to be addressed through empirical inves-tigation. Lambert and Sevak also advocate for a critical appraisal of the concept of 'culturally sensitive' approaches to culture and ethnicity in health care, which are rarely informed by empirical knowledge. Instead, they are based on stereo-types and 'the reification of the culture of minority ethnic groups as static, mono-lithic entities that can be categorized by an index of stereotypical cultural traits and their associated patologization is a consequence of this absent knowledge' (Lambert and Sevak 1996: 155).

FUTURE RESEARCH

It is now 25 years since Kleinman and Good (1985) set out 'to stimulate a new beginning of research into the relation of culture and depression' (Kleinman and Good, 1985: 30). The work in their edited volume has been widely cited and has significantly contributed to the way social researchers and the academic clinical community conceptualize the debate on depression. More recently, DelVecchio, Hyde and Good (2008) in their edited book *Postcolonial Disorders* demonstrate that since 1985 many of the fundamental epistemological and political questions about depression and culture remain unresolved. They also emphasize the necessity of outlining a future research agenda that establishes how to move beyond the reproduction of old knowledge in order to develop new insights.

One of the central questions of cross-cultural debate on depression and disorders highlighted in both Kleinman and Good (1985) and DelVecchio, Hyde and Good (2008) is whether current forms of theorizing have sufficient capacity for an interdisciplinary approach that links social, cultural and psychological understandings of mental 'disorders'. One of the new elements is an increasing use of the terms 'subject' and 'subjectivity' within a broad focus on individualization in a globalized society. Subjectivity in such context denotes a new attention to hierarchy, with a potential to link the most intimate forms of everyday to the national and global economic and political processes. DelVecchio, Hyde and Good (2008) see this as an indicator of change from earlier research of various cultures and psychological experiences into more complex research which 'places the political at the heart of the psychological and the psychological at the heart of the political' (DelVecchio, Hyde and Good, 2008: 2–3).

The concepts of individual, subject and subjectivity include the study of social and personal 'disorders' as well as the ways and modes they intertwine manifesting 'as pathologies, modes of suffering, the domain of the imaginary, or as forms of repression, disordered subjectivity provides entrée to exploring dimensions of contemporary social life as lived experience' (DelVecchio, Hyde and Good, 2008: 2). Similar to the previously commented work of Kleinman and Byron (1985), DelVecchio, Hyde and Good (2008) emphasize the need to develop theoretical models which can facilitate interrelations between studies of individual lives and subjectivity and social analysis. They argue that this could be achieved by 'moving beyond current dichotomization of studies that are either based on poststructuralist writing on agency, clinically influenced writing on trauma and other forms of psychopathology, or ethnographies of social suffering (DelVecchio, Hyde and Good, 2008: 14).

Further, while differences in culture, language and health status must be considered when researching depression across cultures, in growing global migrant populations in particular, it is of crucial importance not to simplify, pathologize and medicalize emotional distress. Discourses of difference and the medicalization of individual experiences shape popular explanations of continued social marginality and contribute to legitimating and perpetuating the social position of marginality of different cultural communities (Eastmond, 1998). Therefore, instead of medicalizing distress as a consequence of the negative outcomes of migration, it is more effective if host countries and community social institutions provide a constructive space to enhance peoples' personal agency in the process of self-reconstruction, adaptation and active participation in a new cultural environment.

It would be useful to consider when researching and diagnosing depression across cultures that this condition is always defined contextually. Fundamentally, people use the term depression as a means to describe ruptures between their subjectivity and their social environment. Some members of minority groups use depression not as a clinical term but rather as a metaphor and a critical view of their actual social, economic and political circumstances and as a descriptive term with which they paint a portrait of life as a member of minority community. As such, depression positions individuals in their social context, and therefore is tied to other social discourses such as those of power, inequality and social exclusion (Kokanovic et al., 2008). As long as distress is treated through palliative means, the need for more complex social change will be obscured. Thus, the dominant explanatory model places responsibility for depression at the level of individuals, who in turn are treated through the individuated lenses of clinical practice focusing on the 'distressed subject' as the object of abnormality (Kokanovic et al., 2008).

In conclusion, formulating a fresh cross cultural research agenda on depression requires particular attention being paid to capturing political and cultural dynamics and the diversity of social experiences behind social constructions and generalized experiences of any kind, including 'refugee experience', 'migrant experience', 'ethnic identity' and 'cultural identity'. Research models need to consider 'the internal variations these categories subsume, the circumstances in which they emerge as relevant and how they interact with other and dominant constructs of identity' (Eastmond, 1998: 179). Social contexts of experiences need a detailed investigation into the ideological frameworks that shape processes of intersection of cultural identity and other discursive domains related to experiences of depression.

REFERENCES

Ahmad, W.I.U. and Bradby, H. (2007) Locating ethnicity and health: exploring concepts and contexts. *Sociology of Health and Illness*, 29(6): 795–810.

Altarriba, J. and Santiago-Riviera (1994) Current perspectives on using linguistic and cultural factors in counselling the Hispanic client. *Professional Psychology: Research and Practice*, 25: 388–397.

American Psychiatric Association (1987) *Diagnostic and Statistical Manual of Mental Disorders,* 4th edn (DSM III). Washington, DC: American Psychiatric Association.

American Psychiatric Association (1994) *Diagnostic and Statistical Manual of Mental Disorders,* 4th edn (DSM IV). Washington, DC: American Psychiatric Association.

Baker, R. and Briggs, J. (1975) Working with interpreters in social work practice. *Australian Social Work* 28(4): 31–37.

Barlow, D. and Durand, M. (2002) *Essentials of Abnormal Psychology.* Australia: Wadsworth/Thomson Learning.

Beck, A.T. (1976) *Cognitive Therapy and the Emotional Disorders.* New York: International Universities Press.

Beiser (1985) A study of depression among traditional Africans, urban north Americans and Southeast Asian refugees. In A. Kleinman and B. Good (eds) *Culture and Depression: Studies in the Anthropology and Cross-Cultural Psychiatry of Affect and Disorder.* Berkeley: University of California Press. pp. 272–298.

Bendelow, G. (2009) *Health, Emotion and the Body.* Cambridge: Polity Press.

Bentelspacher, C.E., Chitran, S. and Rahman, M.B.A. (1994) Coping and adaptation patterns among Chinese, Indian, and Malay families caring for a mentally ill relative. *Families in Society,* 75: 287–294.

Brown, G. and Harris, T. (1978) *Social Origins of Depression.* London: Tavistock.

Degotardi, V. (1995) Vietnamese asylum-seekers in Hong Kong: cultural attitudes to mental illness and health-seeking, behaviour. *Australasian Psychiatry,* 3(2): 93–94.

Del Castillo, L.R. (1970) Effects of interpreters on the evaluation of psychopathology in non-English speaking patients. *American Journal of Psychiatry,* 136(2): 171–174.

DelVecchio Good, M.J., Hyde, S., Pinto, S. and Good B. (2008) *Postcolonial Disorders.* Berkely. CA: University of California Press.

de Swaan, A. (1990) *The Management of Normality: Critical Essays in Health and Welfare.* London: Routledge.

Douki, S. and Tabbane, K. (1996) Culture and depression. *World Health,* 2: 22–25.

Eastmond, M. (1996) 'Luchar y Sufrir' – Stories of life and exile. Reflections on the ethnographic process. *Ethnos,* 61(3/4): 231–250.

Eastmond, M (1998) Nationalist discourses and the construction of difference: Bosnian Muslim refugees in Sweden. *Journal of Refugee Studies,* 2(2): 161–181.

Foucault, M (1967) *Madness and Civilization.* London: Tavistock

Foucault, M (1973) *The Birth of the Clinic.* London: Tavistock.

Good, B. DelVecchio Good, M.J. et al. (1985) The interpretation of Iranian depressive illness and dysphoric affect. In A. Kleinman and B. Good (eds) *Culture and Depression: Studies in the Anthropology and Cross-Cultural Psychiatry of Affect and Disorder.* Berkeley, University of California Press. pp. 369–428.

Good, B., DelVecchio Good, M.J. et al. (2008) Postocolonial Disorders: Reflections on subjectivity in the contemporary world. In M.J. Good DelVecchio et al. (eds) *Postcolonial Disorders.* Berkeley: University of California Press. pp. 1–40.

Gureje et al. (1997) The natural history of somatization in primary care. *Psychological Medicine,* 29: 669–676.

Hansen, S., McHoul, A. and Rapley, M. (2003) *Beyond Help: A Consumer's Guide to Mental Health.* Ross-on-Wye, PCCS Books.

Hawthorne, N. (1970) *The Scarlet Letter.* Penguin: Ohio State University Press.

Healy, D. (1997) *The Anti-Depressant Era.* Cambridge, MA: Harvard University Press.

Healy, D. (2004) *Let Them Eat Prozac.* New York: New York University Press.

Horowitz, A.V. and Wakefield, J.C. (2007) *The Loss of Sadness, How Psychiatry Transformed Normal Sorrow Into Depressive Disorder.* Oxford: Oxford University Press.

Jackson, S. (1985) Acedia, the sin and its relationship to sorrow and melancholia. In A. Kleinman and B. Good (eds) *Culture and Depression: Studies in the Anthropology and Cross-Cultural Psychiatry of Affect and Disorder.* Berkeley, University of California Press. pp. 43–62.

Karp, D. (1996) *Speaking of Sadness: Depression, Disconnection and the Meanings of Illness.* New York: Oxford University Press.

Kelleher, D. and Hillier, S. (eds) (1996) *Researching Cultural Differences in Health.* London: Routledge.

Kessler, B. et al. (2003) The epidemiology of major depressive disorder: Results from the National Comorbidity Survey replication. *Journal of the American Medical Association.* 289: 3095–3105.

Kirmayer, L.J. (2001) Cultural variations in the clinical presentation of depression and anxiety: implications for diagnosis and treatment. *Journal of Clinical Psychiatry,* 62(13): 22–28.

Kitzinger, C. and Wilkinson, S. (eds) (1996) *Representing the Other: a Feminism and Psychology Reader.* London: SAGE.

Kleinman, A. (1977) Depression, somatization and the new cross-cultural psychiatry. *Social Science and Medicine,* 11: 3–10.

Kleinman, A. (1980) *Patients and Healers in the Context of Culture: an Exploration of the Borderland between Anthropology, Medicine, and Psychiatry.* Berkeley: University of California Press.

Kleinman, A. (1987) Anthropology and psychiatry. *British Journal of Psychiatry,* 151: 447–454.

Kleinman, A. (1998) *The Illness Narrative: Suffering, Healing and the Human Condition.* New York: Basic Books.

Kleinman, A. and Good, B. (eds) (1985) *Culture and Depression: Studies in the Anthropology and Cross-Cultural Psychiatry of Affect and Disorder.* Berkeley, University of California Press.

Kleinman, A., Das, V. and Lock, M. (eds) (1997) *Social Suffering.* Berkeley, CA: University of California Press.

Kokanovic, R. and Stone, M. (2010) Doctors and other dangers: Narratives of distress and exile in Bosnian refugees in Australia. *Social Theory and Health* (In press).

Kokanovic, R., Petersen, A. and Klimidis, S. (2006) 'Nobody can help me … I am living through it alone': Experiences of caring for people diagnosed with mental illness in ethno-cultural and linguistic minority communities. *Journal of Immigrant and Minority Health,* 8(2): 125–132.

Kokanovic, R., Dowrick, C., Butler, E., Herrman H. and Gunn, J. (2008) Lay accounts of depression amongst Anglo-Australian and East African refugees. *Social Science and Medicine,* 66(3): 454–466.

Kokanovic, R., May, C., Dowrick, C., Furler, J., Newton, D. and Gunn, J. (2010) Negotiating distress between East Timorese and Vietnamese migrants in Melbourne and their family doctors. *Sociology of Health and Illness* (in press).

Lambert, H. and Sevak, L. (1996) Is 'cultural difference' a useful concept? Perceptions of health and the sources of ill health among Londoners of South Asian origin. In D. Kelleher and S. Hillier (eds) *Researching Cultural Differences in Health.* London: Routledge, pp. 124–159.

Lavretsky, H. and Kumar, A. (2002) Clinically non-major depression: Old concepts, new insights. *American Journal of Geriatric Psychiatry,* 20: 239–255.

Levin, D.M. (ed.) (1987) *Pathologies of the Modern Self: Postmodern Studies on Narcissism, Schizophrenia and Depression.* New York: New York University Press.

Lock, M. (1997). Displacing suffering: the reconstruction of death in North America and Japan. In A. Kleinman, V. Das and M. Lock (eds) *Social Suffering.* Berkeley, CA: University of California Press.

Lupton, D. (1994). *Medicine as Culture: Illness, Disease and the Body in Western Societies.* London: SAGE.

Lutz, C. (1985) Depression and the translation of emotional worlds. In A. Kleinman and B. Good (eds) *Culture and Depression: Studies in the Anthropology and Cross-cultural Psychiatry of Affect and Disorder.* Berkeley, University of California Press. pp. 63–10.

McPherson, S. and Armstrong, D. (2006) Social determinants of diagnostic labels in depression. *Social Science and Medicine,* 62(1): 50–58.

Marcos, L.R., Alpert, M. and Urcuyo, L. (1973) The effect of interview language on the evaluation of psychopathology in Spanish-American schizophrenic patients. *American Journal of Psychiatry,* 130: 549–553.

Marmanidis, H., Holme, G. and Hafner, R.J. (1994) Depression and somatic symptoms: a cross-cultural study. *Australia and New Zealand Journal of Psychiatry,* 28: 274–278.

Marsella, A.J. and Pedersen, P.B. (eds) (1981) *Cross-cultural Counseling and Psychotherapy.* New York: Pergamon Press.

Martin, M. (1999) Depression: Illness, Insight and Identity. *Philosophy, Psychiatry and Psychology* 6(4): 271–286.

Miller, K.E. et al. (2002) Bosinan refugees and the stressors of exile: A Narrative Study. *American Journal of Orthopsychiatry,* 72(3): 341–354.

Murray, C.J.L. and Lopez, A.D. (eds) (1996) *The Global Burden of Disease*. Cambridge, MA: World Health Organization.

Newnes, C., Holmes, G. and Dunn, C. (eds) (1999) *This is Madness: A Critical Look at Psychiatry and the Future of Mental Health Services*. Ross-on-Wye: PCCS Books.

Newnes, C., Holmes, G. and Dunn, C. (eds) (2001) *This is Madness Too: Critical Perspectives on Mental Health Services*. Ross-on-Wye: PCCS Books.

Obeyesekere, G. (1985) Depression, Buddhism and the work of culture in Sri Lanka. In: A. Kleinman and B. Good (eds) *Culture and Depression: Studies in the Anthropology and Cross-cultural Psychiatry of Affect and Disorder*. Berkeley: University of California Press. pp. 134–152.

Papadopolis, I., Lees, S., Lay, M. and Gebrehiwot, A. (2004) Ethiopian refugees in the UK: migration, adaptation and settlement experiences and their relevance to health. *Ethnicity and Health*, 9(1): 55–73.

Pilgrim, D. (2007) The survival of psychiatric diagnosis. *Social Science and Medicine*, 65(3): 536–544.

Pilgrim, D. and Bentall, R.P. (1999) The medicalisation of misery: a critical realist analysis of the concept of depression. *Journal of Mental Health*, 8(3): 261–274.

Porter, R. (ed) (2002) *The Faber Book of Madness*. London: Faber and Faber.

Ridge, D. and Ziebland, S. (2006) 'The Old Me Could Never Have Done That': How people give meaning to recovery following depression. *Qualitative Health Research*, 16: 1038–1052.

Rogers, A. and Pilgrim, D. (2005) *A Sociology of Mental Health and Illness*. Maidenhead, UK; New York: Open University Press.

Schwartz, S. (2000) *Abnormal Psychology*. Mountain View California: Mayfield Publishing Company.

Seligman, M.E.P. (1975) *Helplessness: On Depression, Development and Death*. San Francisco: W.H.Freeman.

Shaw, I. (2002) How lay are lay beliefs? *Health*, 6(3): 287–299.

Shweder, R.A. (1985) Menstrual pollution, soul loss, and the comparative study of emotions. In: Kleinman and B. Good (eds) *Culture and Depression: Studies in the Anthropology and Cross-cultural Psychiatry of Affect and Disorder*. Berkeley: University of California Press. pp. 182–215.

Silveira, E. and Allbeck, P. (2001) Migration, ageing and mental health: An ethnographic study on perceptions of life satisfaction, anxiety and depression in older Somali men in east London. *International Journal of Social Welfare*, 10(4): 309–320.

Turner, B. (with C. Samson) (1995) *Medical Power and Social Knowledge*. London: SAGE.

Werner, O. and Campbell, D.T. (1970) Translating, working through interpreters, and the problem of decentering. In R. Naroll and R. Cohen (eds) *A Handbook of Method in Cultural Anthropology*. New York: The Natural History Press. pp. 398–420.

Westermeyer, J. (1985) Psychiatric diagnosis across cultural boundaries. *American Journal of Psychiatry*, 142: 798–804.

Wierzbicka, A. (1999) *Emotions Across Languages and Cultures: Diversity and Universals*. Cambridge: Cambridge University Press.

Williams, S.J. (2000) Reason, emotion and embodiment: is 'mental' health a contradiction in terms? *Sociology of Health and Illness*, 22(5): 559–581.

Wolpert, L. (1999) *Malignant Sadness: The Anatomy of Depression*. London: Faber and Faber.

World Health Organization (1992) *The ICD-10 Classification of Mental and Behavioural Disorders*. Geneva: WHO.

World Health Organization (2001) *Mental Health: New Understanding, New Hope*. Geneva: WHO.

8

Stressors and Experienced Stress

Susan Roxburgh

INTRODUCTION

In two seminal pieces published in the 1980s, Leonard Pearlin and colleagues outlined a model for understanding the stress process: a heuristic framework designed to facilitate the investigation of the relationship between social stress and well-being (Pearlin et al., 1981; Pearlin, 1989). Since these publications, the stress process framework has become one of the most active areas of research in American medical sociology. Stress process research has been the primary focus of the *Journal of Health and Social Behavior* and is the subject of a section of the American Sociological Association (Section on the Sociology of Mental Health). In her review of the stress process literature, Thoits (1995) noted that over 3,000 articles on stress and health appeared in scholarly journals during the decade preceding her review. Since then the number has risen, with over 6,000 papers on stress and health published in a wide range of medical, psychology, and sociology journals. Some indication of the paradigmatic influence of Pearlin's work is suggested by the fact that the 1981 paper has been cited over 1,800 times and the 1989 piece just under 600 times, with no indication of a decline in the rate of citations in recent years.

The purpose of this chapter is to describe the stress process model and to summarize recent work in this area. Because there are many literature reviews of this field (Aneshensel, 1992; Aneshensel and Phelan, 1999; Coping: Hatch and Dohrenwend, 2007; Mastery: Turner and Roszell, 1994; Social Support: House, 1981; Turner, 1999; Wheaton, 1999), I focus largely, although not exclusively, on the period after Peggy Thoits' influential review (Thoits, 1995). My purpose here is threefold: first, to provide the reader with an introduction to the stress process model and to describe the state of knowledge in the field. A second purpose is to identify gaps in the field and new emerging research directions. Stress process research has largely been an American tradition. Although a discussion of the comparative development of the sociological study of health lies outside the scope of this review, a third aim of this chapter is to describe the many convergences in research on the stress process in the UK and North American context.

WHY STUDY STRESS?

The stress process model is a conceptual framework that delineates the essential elements required to understand the social characteristics and experiences that account for variation in well-being. Extending back to Durkheim (1951), who implicated imbalances in social integration and regulation as responsible for variation in suicide rates, stress researchers have sought to understand how social experience and social location contribute to variation in well-being. In his 1989 paper, Pearlin identified several key factors that motivate stress researchers. First, the study of stress provides a key to understanding how structural arrangements influence variation in well-being and as such, illuminates a fundamental inequality, that of the inequality of happiness. Second, Pearlin argued that variation in distress is an indication of underlying social problems. Unhappiness or misery is not merely an artifact of social experience, but is an accurate reflection of ruptures, disjuncture, and inequity in social organization. Thus, at its roots, stress process researchers have emphasized that their focus should be on the social conditions that generate variation in well-being. A persistent theme in the American tradition of this research has been the relative failure of stress researchers to do just that: to focus on and generate sociological models of stress and well-being (Muntaner et al., 2007; Pearlin et al., 2005).

THE ELEMENTS OF THE STRESS PROCESS MODEL

The stress process model consists of three primary elements: stressors, intervening explanatory variables, and stress outcomes. A stressor is a feature of the environment that requires adaptation, whether in the short-term, as in acute stressors, or in the long-term, in the form of longstanding or persistent adaptive challenges stemming from an actor's social environment. Stressors can also be thought of as threats, demands, or limitations in opportunities and rewards that arise from roles or aspects of social location (Wheaton, 1999). Researchers have distinguished between three broad categories of stressors: life events, chronic strains, and daily hassles. Life events are acute, discrete occurrences such as a divorce or a violent assault. Chronic stressors are persistent life conditions, such as a conflict-ridden marriage or financial hardship (Wheaton, 1983). Daily hassles are defined as quotidian stressors, such as traffic jams or conflicts with teenage children about household chores (Kanner et al., 1981).

The second primary element of the stress process model consists of a large class of intervening variables conceptualized as resources that directly influence well-being, inhibit exposure to stressors, or act as moderators of the impact of stressors that do arise. Resources have been conceptualized as features of the environment, such as social support; as pre-existing cognitive orientations that reduce the exposure and impact of stressors, such as mastery; or as behavioral or cognitive reactions to stressors, such as avoidant coping efforts. The resources that have been the focus of intensive research efforts include social support, psychosocial resources (e.g., self-esteem, mastery), and coping behaviors or attitudes, such as problem-focused coping or avoidant coping. Outcomes, the third element of the stress process model, are defined by Pearlin (1989) as depression and anxiety, with the former consisting of feelings of sadness, demoralization, and alienation; and the latter referring to feelings of tension, restlessness and irritability. Below I describe research regarding each of these elements of the stress process model.

Stressors

Life events

Early research on life events drew on a biological model that characterized any discrete event as representing an adaptive challenge to the organism (Dohrenwend, 1973; Holmes and Rahe, 1967; Selye, 1993). Subsequent research has quite unequivocally demonstrated that it is only negative events that generate stress. There is also widespread consensus that negative life events are associated with distress and depression, particularly in the first 12 months following an event (Brown, 2000; Brown and Harris, 1978; Hatch and Dohrenwend, 2007; Muscatell et al., 2009). Research on the impact of specific events leaves little doubt that life-altering events pose significant challenges that result in depression, anxiety, and alcohol consumption. Events that have been the focus of recent research include parental divorce (Aseltine, 1996; Lorenz et al., 2006), divorce (Lorenz et al., 2006; Sweeney and Horwitz, 2001), death of a parent (Umberson, 2003), and macro-social changes, such as recessions or plant closings (Tausig and Fenwick, 1999).

A number of problems with standard life events inventories have motivated research on life events. One issue concerns the recognition that the social context or the meaning of the life event is influential in shaping variation in adjustment. As Wheaton (1990) demonstrates, the impact of an event on well-being depends on the social context in which the event occurred. Even events with an unequivocal normative valence, such as the death of a spouse or a divorce, are unlikely to be experienced the same way by different individuals or in different social contexts. The departure of a partner can be a positive event if it produces a cessation in physical or emotional abuse. The sudden death of a partner in a car accident is a very different event than a death that was preceded by a long, debilitating illness. In essence, the challenge has been to identify what it is about life events that make them problematic for well-being.

George Brown in the UK and Bruce Dohrenwend in the US have developed narrative rating procedures in order to address this question. Their research shares a common concern for the problem of confounding or "effort after meaning," which is the problem of confounding the subject's mental health status with the retrospective subjective meaning-making that follows life events. Using the Life Events and Difficulties Schedule, Brown and Harris (1978) employed trained raters to assess the contextual threat of life events. Using small samples of largely working-class women followed intensively over time, the work of Brown and colleagues (Brown, 2000; Harris, 2000) showed that a life event is likely to lead to an episode of depression if it negatively impacts a core role, threatens self-worth, and reduces future opportunities. Using a similarly intensive data-collection effort that includes detailed narrative analyses of Vietnam Veterans and external validation methods such as killed-in-action rates of the respondent's military unit, Bruce Dohrenwend and colleagues (2006) identify six dimensions of life events that account for variation in mental health outcomes:

1 The magnitude of the event.
2 Valence of the event.
3 Whether the event was controllable.
4 Whether it was predictable.
5 Whether it was likely to be physically enervating.
6 The likelihood that the event led to the inability to meet other goals.

In a similar effort to specify the stressful nature of life events, another line of research focuses more narrowly on how respondents' evaluation of the meaning of the event influences the impact of the event. Drawing on identity theory, Thoits (1995) focused on how the impact of an event depends on its threat to identity. However, she found limited empirical support for this hypothesis because identity-relevance did not moderate the effect of an event on distress or alcohol/drug use. Using the framework of crisis theory, Reynolds and Turner (2008) argued that the impact of a life event depends on whether the event is a challenge to sense of self and whether it is successfully resolved. Although crisis theory provides an interesting and potentially important way of conceiving of the impact of life events, their results also yielded mixed support for this hypothesis. Although successful resolution of a self-defined crisis was associated with lower depression, successful resolution was not associated with increased mastery, as crisis theory would predict.

Another concern with life events research is the question of non-independence. That is, to what extent do preexisting conditions and dispositional tendencies contribute to exposure to life events? Research on this question suggests that selection effects contribute to the differential probability of exposure to events.

This is especially evident for events that individuals may have caused, such as losing a job (Cue and Vaillant, 1997). For example, Hammen (1991) found that women with recurrent clinical depression were exposed to more stressors in the 12-months prior to their depressive episode, not because they were exposed to more fateful or independent life events (e.g., the death of a parent), but because of their higher rates of exposure to non-fateful or dependent life events (e.g., conflict with others). Even in the case of events to which the individual presumably made little causal contribution, such as the death of a spouse, exposure is not randomly distributed in the general population. Younger individuals, those of low socio-economic status, and African Americans are more likely to report life events (Reynolds and Turner, 2008; Turner and Avison, 1989; Turner et al., 1995). Women are more likely than men to report events to others, although there is mixed evidence that this gender difference explains women's higher depression (Kessler and McLeod, 1985; Turner and Avison, 1989; Umberson et al., 1996).

What this research reveals is that the social characteristics of individuals and the ecological environments in which they are embedded shape exposure to life events. This, in turn, suggests that community surveys that measure life events at one point in time without consideration of the social context in which events occur will fall short of contributing to our understanding of the impact of life events on well-being. In addition, the issue of the non-independence of mental health states and life events remains an important problem. Although some research indicates that the causal relationship that flows from life events to health is as important, if not more important, than the causality that flows from mental health to life events (Turner and Turner, 1999), there is good evidence that prior depression predicts the probability of life events. In response to the non-independence problem, Kessler (2000) argued that a history of depression should be conceived of as a stress modifier. In effect, studies that fail to take into account number of prior episodes of diagnosable depression or history of depressive episodes will substantially misestimate both the relationship between life events and depression and the relationship between other stress modifiers, life events, and depression (Kessler, 1997; Kessler and Magee, 1994b , 2003).

Although life events are the subject of somewhat less recent research within the stress process model, an exception is the study of a sub-set of life events, traumatic or adverse childhood events (Pearlin et al., 2008). This research has focused on developing a better understanding of the extent to which childhood traumas and adversity contribute to lifetime vulnerability to stressors. Research both outside the stress process tradition and within it indicates that specific types of childhood adversity, considered independently, have negative consequences for adult well-being. Sexual and physical abuse and witnessing violence (Kessler et al., 1997; Kessler and Magee, 1994a), parental divorce (Amato and Booth, 1997) and parental death (McLeod, 1991) have all been shown to adversely influence adult well-being. In considering the overall impact of a range of childhood traumas, Turner and Lloyd (2004) showed that childhood adversity was significantly associated with depressive and anxiety disorder among a sample of young adults, irrespective of gender, socio-economic status, and race/ethnicity.

Three important conclusions arise from research on childhood traumatic events. First, age-specific vulnerabilities are an important factor in the consideration of the effects of traumatic exposure. Wheaton et al. (1997) found that parental unemployment was particularly problematic if it occurred during mid-adolescence. Second, some adversities are more context-dependent than others. Foster et al. (2008) reported that childhood neglect was associated with early menarche, a measure of physical weathering, which was in turn linked to adult distress through its impact on subjective weathering (i.e., feeling older than one's age). This conception of the relationship between traumatic childhood events and mental health as a complex chain of stressors is consistent with Pearlin's (1989; Pearlin et al., 1997) concept of stress proliferation, whereby an initial stressor triggers a number of additional or secondary stressors. A third conclusion about life events that can be drawn from the traumatic events literature is that the relationship between trauma and adult outcomes is not linear or consistent with a simple dose–response relationship. Moderately impactful stressors may trigger effective coping strategies at key developmental moments and under some conditions, stressors may facilitate resilience to future adversity (Masten and Coatsworth, 1998). Beyond a particular level of severity, however, or in the face of multiple adverse events, coping efforts are unlikely to be successful and they may create downward cycles of increasing maladjustment (Brown, 2000).

Chronic strains

Chronic strains – enduring difficulties or conflicts – can be either ambient strains that cut across roles/role sets or enduring difficulties that arise within or between roles. A number of typologies of chronic strains have been developed. Wheaton (1983) identified five types of chronic strains:

1   Barriers to achieving goals.
2   An imbalance between the rewards and efforts associated with role activities.
3   Excessive or insufficient demands within roles.
4   Frustrations in role expectations.
5   Eonomic deprivation.

Pearlin (1989) identified five types of chronic strains: role overload, interpersonal conflict within role sets (e.g., conflict with a supervisor), conflict between roles, role captivity, and role restructuring associated with new expectations or norms (e.g., the adult–child adjusting to the demands of caring for aging parents). These formulations share an acknowledgment that chronic strains are embedded in roles and depend on the quality of experience within roles, as well as the suggestion that many chronic strains cut across roles or are pervasive features of the environment. In order to convey something of the depth and range of research on chronic strains in the stress process literature, I review the findings regarding three types of chronic strains that have been the focus of recent research: neighborhood quality, discrimination, and poverty and economic hardship.

Research on neighborhood quality has focused on whether and by what mechanisms the quality of neighborhoods contributes to mental health. This research confirms that high-poverty census tracts are social contexts which generate exposure to other chronic strains. For example, Schulz et al. (2000) found that regardless of race, Detroit residents of high-poverty areas were significantly more likely to be exposed to other stressors (e.g., discrimination, financial stressors) than residents of low-poverty census tracts. Independent of their individual characteristics, the residents of poor neighborhoods were also more distressed than residents of low-poverty neighborhoods (Aneshensel and Sucoff, 1996). Evidence suggests that the experience of neighborhoods independently influences well-being through the subjective experience of disorder (Ross, 2000) and through increased exposure and vulnerability to negative life events (Cutrona et al., 2005). Issues requiring further exploration in the study of neighborhood quality and mental health include better model specification, the role of individual-level variables, the significance of reciprocal effects, and the need to combine qualitative and quantitative approaches (Sampson, 2008).

Discrimination is another chronic strain that has been the focus of recent research. This research indicates that independent of socio-economic status, the experience of racial discrimination is associated with distress (Jackson et al., 1997; Kessler et al., 1999; Pavalko et al., 2003) and with alcohol consumption (Martin et al., 2003). The role of ethnic identity in buffering the impact of discrimination on mental health has also been the focus of considerable recent research. The accumulated evidence on this question suggests that ethnic identity is a buffer for some racial minorities (American Filipino: Mossakowski, 2003), but not for others (Canadian Southeast Asians: Noh et al., 1999; African Americans: Thompson, 1996). Consistent with Wheaton's definition of chronic strains as involving blocked opportunity, researchers have sought to establish an association between subjective discrimination and mental health. Forman (2003) found that perceived workplace racial segmentation (believing that one had a job that "Black people tend to get") was significantly associated with distress, particularly among middle-class African Americans. These studies reinforce the conception of discrimination as a pervasive chronic stressor in the lives of minority individuals, although further work is needed in order to identify the social and socio-historical conditions (e.g., socio-economic status, role occupancy) that modify variation in the discrimination-well-being relationship.

A third line of research on chronic strains, poverty, has benefited from a focus on the trajectories and the timing of poverty experiences (Mirowsky and Ross, 1999). On the one hand, research on poverty and well-being showed that continuous financial hardship is more problematic for health than intermittent experiences of such hardship (Kahn and Pearlin 2006; McLeod and Shanahan, 1996). On the other hand, studies have shown that perceived financial hardship declined with age (Mirowsky and Ross, 2001), as did the anxiety associated with credit-card debt (Drentea, 2000). Frederick Lorenz, K.A.S. Wickrama, and Rand Conger have developed a research agenda that has explored trajectories of chronic stressors, such as parental divorce and unemployment on mental and physical health (Conger and Donnellan, 2007; Wickrama et al., 2005a, b). They have shown that parental rejection is related to depression and early transition events (i.e., early sexual intercourse, early pregnancy and cohabitation, and early departure from the parental home), which in turn, create subsequent cumulative adversity and depression. They conclude that there are "mutually reinforcing reciprocal processes between stressful social pathways and depressive symptom trajectories over the life-course" (Wickrama et al., 2008: 479). This research suggests the more general conclusion that cumulative effect, or allostatic load (Pearlin et al., 2005), is an important influence on well-being, but that some chronic strains, such as financial hardship, may be differentially salient across the life cycle; although whether this is a ceiling effect or a result of adaptation is an unanswered and important question.

Daily hassles

As the name suggests, episodic daily hassles refer to quotidian experiences that represent potential stressors (Kanner et al., 1981). Wheaton (1999) distinguished between daily hassles, which are mundane and unexpected features of daily life, such as having to sit in traffic for an unusually long time, and daily hassles that are regular and expected features of social life that, in their accumulation, may constitute stressors. The latter includes daily experiences, such as caring for one's dog, preparing meals, or being interrupted too often. However, the most widely used measure of daily hassles – the Daily Inventory of Stressful Events (DISE: Almeida et al., 2002) – does not employ this distinction. The DISE measure a wide variety of experiences of daily life (e.g., news that one has not been admitted to a university, conflicts with co-workers) that include both chronic stressors and acute events, creating some conceptual ambiguity regarding the distinction between daily hassles and other types of stressors. In practice, the measurement of daily hassles is relatively uncommon outside the context of daily diary research, in which researchers have tended to focus on quotidian chronic stressors, such as role overloads, and conflicts or arguments with others (Bolger et al., 1989). For example, Grzywacz and colleagues (2004) asked subjects whether, in the course of the day, they had an argument or experienced discrimination. The DISE also asked respondents whether anything else occurred "that most people would consider stressful" (Grzywacz et al., 2004) during the day, an approach that accounts for the criticism that measures of daily hassles confound stressors and outcomes (Dohrenwend et al., 1984). These concerns notwithstanding, the concept of daily hassles captures an important category of stressors – the minor aggravations and unexpected difficulties that constitute such a pervasive feature of modern life. In addition, when researchers select items with the intention of avoiding those that measure life events or chronic strains, research suggests that daily hassles make an independent contribution to variation in distress

(Serido et al., 2004; Wheaton, 1999), although this contribution is relatively small in comparison to the impact of life events and chronic strains.

Research on daily hassles suggests that there is considerable variation in the salience of daily hassles by age, gender, and the social setting in which the daily hassle occurs. For example, in one study women reported more network stressors and men reported more stressors associated with work (Almeida et al., 2002; Almeida, 2005). Daily hassles are not distributed in the same way as chronic stressors and life events, both of which tend to increase as socio-economic status decreases. In contrast, well-educated respondents tend to report a greater number of daily hassles and perceived time pressure. However, individuals of higher socio-economic status but those of higher socio-economic status are less vulnerable to the depressive effects of hassles (Grzywacz et al., 2004; Roxburgh, 2004). Elderly individuals are less likely to be exposed to negative social exchanges (Akiyama et al., 2003; Krause and Shaw, 2002) and are less likely to be depressed by negative social exchanges (Neupert et al., 2007). Thus, research on daily hassles supports the conclusion that negative interactions are a particularly important predictor of mental health. Negative interactions are also more likely and are experienced with greater intensity by low income and poorly educated respondents (Gallo et al., 2006). Thus, daily diary research captures an important dimension of the phenomenology of low-status individuals and it contributes to an understanding of socio-economic variation in health status. As Wilkinson (2005) and others have suggested (Marmot, 2004), a proportion of variation in the relationship between socio-economic status and health is explained by greater exposure to negative interactions that threaten sense of self and reinforce subordinated social status. Daily diary research on the frequency and intensity of negative social interactions has been important in contributing to an understanding of these processes.

The relationship between stressors

As noted above with respect to daily hassles, the relationship between different types of stressors is not without ambiguities. It is difficult, for example, to distinguish the temporality, and hence the relative significance for well-being, of a divorce and the myriad chronic strains that are likely to arise from a divorce, such as having to move to less attractive housing, financial indebtedness, and strains in child–parent relations. In an effort to address this conceptual ambiguity, Pearlin (1989) distinguished between primary and secondary stressors. Primary stressors are the initial event or chronic strain, such as a stroke that incapacitates an elderly relative and the subsequent care requirements that ensue. Secondary stressors are those that arise as a consequence of the initial strain or stressor, such as losing contact with friends because of caregiving responsibilities. In principle, this distinction is compelling as a means of describing the non-independence of many stressful occurrences or ongoing strains, but in practice, it has proven difficult to distinguish between primary and secondary stressors. With the exception of the literature on caregiving (Aneshensel et al., 1995), the distinction has been employed relatively infrequently.

R. Jay Turner and colleagues have contributed to our understanding of the relationship between stressors by emphasizing the importance of specifying the full universe of stressors (Turner et al., 1995). Turner has argued that life events are inadequate measures of the full universe of stressors because life events generally explain a fairly small percentage of variation in mental health (Reynolds and Turner, 2008). Furthermore, without measures of stress that sample the full universe of stressors, estimates of the relationship between stressors and mental health will tend to under-estimate exposure to stress and over-estimate the vulnerability of particular groups to the effect of stressors. This is particularly problematic if stressors are differentially distributed by social characteristics that are themselves related to disadvantage, such as gender, race/ethnicity, and age. Turner and colleagues showed that life events, traumatic life events, and chronic strains were indeed differentially distributed by gender, race/ethnicity, age, and socio-economic status (Turner et al., 1995). With respect to the relationship between chronic strains and life events, Hammen (2003) found that compared with never-depressed women, women with histories of depression experienced chronically stressful life circumstances, manifested in higher rates of conflict with partners and children. Brown and Harris (1989) reported a similar cycle of reciprocal causation, with early traumatic events setting the stage for both depressive episodes and poor relationship quality in adulthood. This research illuminates the complex relationship between adult chronic stressors; life events and mental health; and early childhood conditions and adult mental health.

Resources

In the stress process model, resources are conceptualized as ecological, cognitive, or behavioral arrangements that mediate or moderate the impact of stressors on health. Broadly speaking, resources fall into two broad categories, social support and coping. The question of how different resources influence the stress process has been the focus of a great deal of research. In particular, the question of whether resources buffer (i.e., moderate) or mediate the relationship between stressors and health has been an important one. Stress-buffering refers to the presence of an interaction effect, in which the high resources attenuates the effect of a stressor. Mediating occurs if a resource reduces the direct effect of a stressor on mental health. Ensel and Lin (1991) suggested two major causal pathways by which social resources may influence mental health in the face of stressors: coping and deterring. In their work (Ensel and Lin, 1991; Lin and Ensel, 1999) they argue for greater attention to the variety of causal pathways by which resources can intervene in the relationship between stressors and mental health, as has Blair Wheaton (1985). In spite of these admonitions, research has tended to focus largely on the buffering or moderating effect of resources on the stress process. Below, I review research on the relationship between stressors and coping resources in the two major classes of resources: social support resources and coping resources.

Social support

Years of research has established that social support is an important resource that is significantly associated with mental health, particularly depression (Turner et al., 1983; Turner, 1999). Within the stress process model, there has been significant debate regarding at least two issues. First, how should researchers define social support and what types of social support matter the most for well-being? Second, how does social support operate to reduce stress outcomes?

Defining social support   There are at least three broad classes of social support: perceived support, instrumental support, and structural social support (Turner, 1999). Perceived social support is the perception that one feels loved, needed, and has someone in which to confide. Instrumental or enacted support refers to support resources that are activated in the face of stressors. For instance, the National Health Interview survey, an annual health survey carried out by the US Census Bureau, asks respondents whether they have someone to help them move or someone to care for them in the event of an illness. Structural support refers to characteristics of the social networks in which individuals are embedded. Examples include number of relatives and/or close friends who live close by or measures of the amount and frequency of contact with close friends and/ or relatives. Lin and Ensel (1999) distinguished between social support as a structural property or as a functional property. Within the functional dimension, social support can function to inform, assist in the regulation of emotions, and increase feelings of self-worth (Cobb, 1976). The structural properties of social support can be measured as network size and frequency of contact, or "belongingness," such as how many groups or clubs an individual participates in and the availability of confidant relationships, such as marital partners and close friends. Hartwell and Benson (2007) proposed a multi-dimensional model of social integration, which includes the concept of social capital to refer to resources that arise from the individual's place in the wider community (Putnam, 2000). As these definitions suggest, the concept of social support is best thought of as a multi-dimensional construct that refers to a range of individual, psychological, and community level phenomenon (Turner and Turner, 2000).

Perceived social support and the presence of a close confidant appear to be the most powerful and consistent predictors of well-being (House 1981; Turner, 1999). Studies using structural measures of social support also yielded consistent findings, with the better mental health of the married being one of the most enduring and consistent relationships (Simon, 2002; K. Williams, 2003). Other measures of social network participation, such as number of close friends, involvement in religious institutions or civic activities, and number of roles are in the expected direction (Berkman and Syme, 1979). However, studies of number of roles and mental health tended to observe a curvilinear relationship, such that beyond an optimum number of roles the benefit of additional roles is negligible (Roxburgh, 2004; Thoits, 1986). The relationship between confidants and problem disclosure also tends to be curvilinear, with benefits to well-being of confiding in others diminishing as number of confidants increases (Derlega et al., 1993).

Lin and Ensel (1999) found that number of weekly contacts with social network members, the presence of an intimate tie, and the perception of available expressive support and level of community participation had independent effects on depression. Other research supports a conception of a hierarchical ordering of the relative salience of social support from intimate ties to community participation (Son et al., 2008).

Because it is such a significant resource, it is also important to ask how social support is distributed in the general population and whether the distribution of social support corresponds to the epidemiology of mental health outcomes. Turner's work indicated that social support is distributed in a manner that corresponds to the distribution of well-being, with the more affluent and better-educated reporting higher levels of well-being and higher levels of social support (Turner and Lloyd, 1999; Turner and Marino, 1994). This research contrasts with the qualitative literature on social support, which has emphasized the strength and resilience of the social support networks of poor Americans, particularly Black Americans (Stack, 1974). In exploring this anomaly, Mickelson and Kubzansky (2003) found that perceived social support was inversely related to education and income, but contact with family/friends and frequency of problems disclosure was not differentially distributed by socio-economic status. This research suggests that perceived social support cannot alone account for variation in the distribution of mental health outcomes. It also suggests that other dimensions of the experience of social support, such as quality of social ties, may contribute significantly to variation in well-being. This may be particularly true among groups with cultural norms that encourage affiliation, such as family ties among Hispanics and non-fictive ties among African Americans (Edin and Lein, 1997).

How does Social Support Reduce Stress?   The causal pathways between social support and well-being are fairly well understood. Social support influences mental health through its effect on behavior, emotion-regulations, and through cognition (Cohen et al., 2000). Studies suggest that perceived social support prevents negative life events from occurring (Ensel and Lin, 1991), but also that negative life events deplete social support (Atkinson et al., 1986). This is consistent with the suggestion that social support is eroded and disrupted as the number of life events goes up (House, 1981). Furthermore, since the distribution of social support differs systematically by social characteristics as discussed above, the impact of support intervention may differ across different groups and different types of social support may be consequential for different types of stressors (Pearlin, 1989). In a good examination of these processes, Atkinson and colleagues (1986) followed a small sample of married employed, long-term unemployed, and newly unemployed married men for twelve months. Results indicated that among the recently unemployed men in their sample, social support resource availability was dependent on husbands' distress. In effect, the strain of husbands' response to unemployment reduced marital quality, and, in turn, impaired partner social support. The important insight generated from this paper is that the stress-buffering properties of social support may depend on the nature of the stressor and the source of support. Brown and colleagues made a similar observation in their work, in which they showed that the low quality of social support among low-income women was a function of their limited capacity to form high quality intimate relationships (Brown, 2000; Brown and Harris, 1978).

In summarizing the voluminous literature on social support, Hobfoll and Vaux (1993) concluded that there was mixed evidence regarding the question of whether or not social support buffers or moderates the impact of stressors on well-being (Cobb, 1976; Kessler and McLeod, 1985). Because of its conceptual ambiguity, Hobfoll argued that the concept of buffering itself may have outlived its utility. He also suggested, as have others (Lin, 1986; Wheaton, 1985), that more complex models of the role of social support that take account of the non-independence between stressors and social support are needed (Thoits, 1995). Thus, if stress process models of social support are to go beyond the observation that social support is beneficial for well-being and provide applications to policies, programming, and treatment, more attention needs to be paid to: the predictors of relationship quality (e.g., past experience of trauma may hamper the ability to form quality relationships); the relationship between the stressor and the source and type of social support; the structural constraints that may significantly determine access to high quality social support (e.g., mate selection constraints in poor neighborhoods); and to the context in which social support operates to buffer the impact of life events and/or chronic strains.

Coping
While social support refers to resources available from other actors, networks, and the broader community, coping refers to resources located within the individual. Conceptually, coping and social support are functionally isomorphic (Aneshensel, 1992), although in many studies they are measured without regard for the probable reciprocal relationship between them. Pearlin (1989) identified three functions that coping fulfills. First, coping may function to change the stressful situation. For instance, faced with a hostile supervisor, the individual may apply for a transfer to another department. Second, coping may involve efforts to contain or limit the negative impact of the stressor. An individual faced with the same hostile boss may cope by avoiding the boss as much as possible. Third, coping may involve efforts to change the definition of the situation. For example, an individual faced with an impending divorce may define the new circumstance as an opportunity to improve their lives. The vast literature on this topic can be divided into research that has focused on coping behaviors or cognitions and research on the psychosocial resources that condition the vulnerability of individuals to stressors. The latter refers to relatively stable and enduring personality characteristics that influence adaptation to stress. Examples include self-esteem and mastery. The former refers to the behaviors or cognitions individuals use to respond to stressors such as avoiding thinking about

the problem or responding to a problem by pursuing another activity (Moos and Schaefer, 1993).

Coping cognitions and behaviors   Coping behaviors have been conceptualized in a number of different ways. Pearlin and Schooler (1978) recognized that coping can involve efforts to manage the meaning of the stressor, while other forms of coping involve direct efforts to change the circumstances of the stressor. Folkman and Lazarus (1986) distinguished between emotion-based coping and problem-focused coping. The former involves emotional-responses to a stressor, such as avoiding thinking about a problem. The latter are efforts to change or alter the circumstances of the stressor, such as confronting a co-worker. These typologies recognize that response to stressors includes cognitive and behavioral efforts to manage the consequences and meaning of a stressor (Thoits, 1995). Most research shows that the majority of individuals adopt multiple strategies in the face of stressors and that individuals who adopt problem-focused coping are less depressed than individuals who tend to engage in avoidance coping (Moos and Schaefer, 1993). However, there is a limited consensus regarding which kind of coping is the most efficacious. Mattlin and colleagues (1990) found that positive reappraisal (e.g., thinking about the life event differently) was associated with higher distress if the life event was low-threat or a practical situation, but associated with lower distress if the situation was a problem or strain that could not immediately be remedied, as with a chronic illness, for example. Their results suggest that certain kinds of cognitive coping, such as efforts to see the stressor in a positive light, are ineffective if efforts to change or improve the situation do not accompany the cognitive coping.

Recent assessments of the coping literature suggest that in spite of the vast literature on this topic, surprisingly little is known about whether or not coping actually helps and if so, how (Somerfield and McRae, 2000). This state of affairs is likely because of the complex and dynamic nature of coping responses. As Pearlin (1991) points out, coping strategies and styles are not selected at random, but rather arise systematically as a function of both the specific situation – some kinds of stressors call for certain responses – and as a function of qualities of the individual. Individuals may be differentially effective at utilizing coping efforts to avoid stressors; they may be more or less skillful at selecting coping strategies that are the right ones for the situation; and they may be able to utilize some strategies more effectively than others. Other sources of variation in the coping–stressor–stress chain that are particularly problematic and limit general conclusions about the role of coping include the importance of the timing of the stressor (e.g., a the chronic illness that arises in old age as opposed to in youth), the life history context, and the institutional context in which the stressor arises (e.g., occupation influences the availability of job control). Problems with between-person designs also include the possible temporal ordering of coping efforts. For example, problem-focused coping may precede emotion-focused coping: the latter only being taken up when attempts to address the source of the stress failed (Park and Folkman, 1997).

Interest in coping has tapered off considerably in the sociological literature. In contrast, studies within a psychological framework using clinical or college student samples have proliferated; a recent count noted that there are 13,000 papers on coping behavior (Somerfield and McRae, 2000). Dissatisfaction with the progress of coping research has been registered within the stress process framework (Pearlin, 1991) and by coping researchers working within the psychological tradition (Lazarus, 1999). However, a sociological approach to coping that takes account of the social characteristics of the individual coping and the social context in which coping occurs has not emerged, an issue raised some time ago by Mechanic (1975) and others (Gerhardt, 1979; Thoits, 1995). In her earlier review, Thoits (1995) noted the need for more research on race/ethnicity and socioeconomic differences in coping; this is still a relatively unexplored topic within the stress process framework. Lazarus and colleagues called for better longitudinal idiographic and process-oriented approaches to the study of coping (Lazarus and Folkman, 1984, Lazarus, 2000, Somerfield and McRae, 2000). Research that eschews a between-person design and focuses on within-person variation in adaptation represents one promising direction for future research. For example, Tennen and colleagues have pursued the use of palm-pilot and hierarchical linear modeling to study pain patients and their daily experience of stressors and coping (Davis et al., 2006; Tennen et al., 2000) with interesting results.

Coping resources   In contrast to coping strategies, coping resources are conceptualized as stable dimensions of personality. Coping resources fall into two general categories, beliefs about one's self and beliefs about the nature of the social world. Both concepts share an emphasis on the role that adaptation plays in determining well-being. Self-esteem is an example of the first type of coping resources (Rosenberg, 1986). As one would expect, self-esteem has generally been found to be associated with better mental health (Thoits, 1995). An example of the second type of coping resource is a class of concepts that refer to subjective beliefs about the capacity to exert control. Mastery refers to the beliefs that one is in control of events, able to influence the world, and the belief that one's actions have consequences. Related concepts include self-efficacy (Gecas, 1989), and the inverse of mastery, learned helplessness (Seligman, 1975), alienation (Mirowsky and Ross, 1990), and fatalism (Wheaton, 1980). Wheaton (1980) defined fatalism as a "learned and persistent causal attribution tendency on the part of individuals that directs their perception of the causes of behavioral outcomes either toward external factors (e.g., task difficulty or luck) or toward internal factors (e.g., ability or effort)" (pp.103–104). In hundreds of studies, mastery and self-esteem have been found to be highly associated with mental health (Mirowsky and Ross, 2003; Turner and Roszell, 1994; Turner et al., 2004) and there seems to be little doubt that mastery is a crucial resource associated with mental health.

How mastery operates to influence mental health is less well-established. George (2003) noted: "Despite literally thousands of investigations of sense of control and related constructs, the reasons why internal control beliefs are beneficial remains unanswered … we lack empirical evidence that documents the processes that mediate the effects of control beliefs on outcomes" (p. 39). Coping resources likely operate to improve mental health through a number of mechanisms, such as through generating high-quality social networks and social support (Ensel and Lin, 1991; George, 2003; Krause, 1987); through the higher probability of utilizing efficacious coping actions, such as problem-focused coping (Ross and Mirowsky, 1989; Taylor and Brown, 1988); and because individuals high in mastery having greater resilience in the face of stressors or they possess other skills that can be used to address challenges (Turner and Avison, 1992). There is some evidence that mastery buffers the impact of stressors (Pearlin and Schooler, 1978; Pearlin et al., 1981; Turner and Noh, 1983; Wheaton, 1983), as with job loss (Broman et al., 1990) and care-giving strains (Aneshensel et al., 1995).

Mastery may also increase self-esteem and positive affect (Turner and Roszell, 1994). Wheaton (1980) argued that fatalism may inhibit adaptation by causing individuals to reduce their coping efforts, or by impairing sense of self. Similarly, Brown and colleagues conceived of low self-esteem and low mastery as arising from vulnerabilities experienced in childhood such as the death of a mother. Furthermore, low self-esteem and/or mastery can result from poor quality social support or from occupancy of low quality roles, such as employment that fails to provide a sense of value or validation (Brown, 2001). These contextual factors foster low self-esteem and low mastery, which in turn increases the probability of a generalized sense of hopelessness and helplessness in the face of challenging life events. A similar conception of the life course development of mastery and well-being is provided by American research in community samples in which mastery is suppressed by life experiences that repeatedly suggest to an individual that acting in the world as if one's actions had consequence is largely futile (Avison and Cairney, 2003; Ross and Drentea, 1998; Rotter, 1996).

The social distribution of coping resources   A great deal is known about the social distribution of coping resources. This information contributes to an understanding of how and under what circumstances mastery facilitates well-being and moderates the impact of stressors. Consistent with the life course approach, research suggests that, across the life course, accumulated challenges that are unsuccessful or the strains of the aging process may erode mastery and lower well-being (Mirowsky, 1995; Schieman, 2001) although the relationship between age and mastery may vary as a function of the subjective arena in which the mastery is experienced (Lachman and Prenda Firth, 2004). With respect to gender differences, studies find that women have lower mastery than men have (Lachman and Prenda Firth, 2004; Turner et al. 1999), while others find no difference (Brooks and Roxburgh, 1999; Sastry and Ross, 1998). At least two literature reviews have concluded that there is no compelling evidence to suggest that there are gender differences in mastery (Gore and Colten, 1991; Miller and Kirsch, 1987). However, there is some evidence that mastery may be a particularly important resource for women. Turner et al. (1999) reported that gender moderated the relationship between mastery and depression such that mastery was more salient in reducing depression among women; Brooks and Roxburgh (1999) reported a similar finding in a sample of Americans with diabetes.

With regard to ethnicity, Asians and Asian Americans reported lower levels of perceived control compared with non-Asians and sense of personal control was less salient in accounting for psychological distress (Sastry and Ross, 1998). In addition, Kohn (2006) finds considerable cross-national variation in the relationship between self-directedness and distress. There is a well-established cultural difference in fatalism as a cultural value among Hispanics, but there is evidence that fatalism is not a predictor of distress among Hispanics, perhaps because of high levels of social support among American Hispanics (Ross et al., 1983; Wheaton, 1985). Although at least one study finds that African Americans report lower mastery (Turner et al., 2004), more research regarding the distribution of, and relationship to mental health, of mastery among ethnic and racial minorities, is needed (Ross and Sastry, 1999).

With respect to mastery and socio-economic status, considerable research suggests that mastery is differentially distributed by income and education, with more affluent and better-educated individuals reporting significantly higher mastery (Kohn and Slomczynski, 1990; Lachman and Weaver, 1998; Mirowsky and Ross, 2007; Mirowsky et al., 1996) and self-esteem (Gecas and Seff, 1989). Several studies reported that mastery mediated the relationship between socio-economic status and mental health (Bailis et al., 2001; Turner et al., 1999), which suggests that the differential distribution of mastery is important for explaining and understanding the social class-distress relationship. Ross and Mirowsky (1989) found that lower mastery partially accounted for the distress of those of low SES, but mastery was equally salient, regardless of SES. A number of other studies have confirmed that mastery or sense of control was at least as salient, if not more salient, for mental health among the less affluent (Mirowsky and Ross, 1983; Rosenberg, 1986; Wheaton, 1983). Lachman and Prenda Firth (2004) showed that by domain, the class difference in mastery was due to perceived low control in instrumental resources associated with paid labor, finances, and health, but not within the realm of interpersonal resources (e.g., control associated with sex, marriage, children, life overall). As with age, there is some evidence that the relationship between socio-economic status and mastery is domain-specific and that studies that focus exclusively on a general sense of mastery may miss some of this variation.

Outcomes

As noted earlier, outcomes are defined by Pearlin (1989) as depression and anxiety, with the latter consisting of feelings of sadness, demoralization, and alienation; and the former referring to feelings of tension, restlessness, and irritability. Work within the stress process model has followed this definition, with continuous measures of distress the most frequently employed, and the most commonly used measure being the Center for Epidemiological Studies Depression Scale (CES-D: Radloff, 1977), so much so that Horwitz (2007) has referred to the period of American research on stress after 1970 as the "CES-D Era" (p. 279). However, in spite of the appearance in practice of a consensus, there has been substantial debate about what constitutes appropriate outcome measures. Two issues regarding outcomes have been particularly important sources of debate: first, whether categorical measures of depression designed to identify disorder (e.g., clinical depression) are the most appropriate stress outcome compared with continuous measures of distress and anxiety, and second, the question of what constitutes the appropriate universe of stress outcomes.

Regarding categorical versus continuous measures, the issue has been whether to use a continuous measure or cut-points to distinguish those in the population with clinically-relevant depression from those with no disorder or with symptomatology that is unlikely to require treatment or interfere with daily functioning. In his original paper, Pearlin (1989) was clearly agnostic on the question of outcomes and he encouraged researchers working in the stress process framework to measure a range of outcomes, rather than focus on measuring psychiatric outcomes. Mirowsky and Ross (2002) argued forcefully for a dimensional approach to distress, suggesting that the use of diagnostic categories reifies psychiatric categorizations and undermines the goal of sociology to identify and remedy the social causes of suffering. In defense of dimensionalized measures of distress, many other central figures in the stress process tradition take a similarly humanist stance (Link, 2003; Pearlin, 1989; Wheaton, 2007). For instance, in his Pearlin Award address, Bruce Link (2003) wrote:

> We recognize with Wheaton (2001) that the range of emotions and feelings we study represent the 'ultimate dependent variable' and that when injustices associated with us/ them distinctions cascade downward to these feelings, they deny people what they really want: Happiness and freedom from intense psychic pain. (p. 462)

There are a number of arguments in opposition to this view. First, the use of continuous measures assumes that the association between distress and predictors – chronic stressors, for example – is constant across the range of distress scores (Kessler, 2002). Second, the use of dimensional measures considerably limits the policy and programming applications of stress research. This is because without externally validated measures of clinical conditions, it is not possible to estimate how many respondents need treatment but are not receiving it.

In the UK context, Brown (2000) and colleagues have focused almost exclusively on clinical depression. While acknowledging the dimensional nature of depression and the relatively arbitrary nature of cut-off points, Brown takes the view that such an approach is necessary because what stress researchers should be interested in are the situations in which the response to ordinary life challenges is out of proportion to the effect such challenges would have on a prototypical ordinary person. Horwitz (2007) takes a similar view when he argues that "failure of outcome measures such as CES-D to separate when stressful social arrangements produce distress among non-disordered people and when they cause mental disorder is a fundamental problem in the stress literature" (p. 280). He advocated for methods such as Brown's Life Events and Difficulties Schedule to identify the social circumstances that seek to build a nuanced picture of the magnitude of the stressor, although he noted the practical problems that prevent the application of Brown's methods to large-scale community surveys.

As David Mechanic (2000) has pointed out, Brown's focus on clinical depression was partly a necessity in light of the need to persuade the psychiatric community of the importance of his work. In the American context, funding support for large-scale community surveys has been more readily available and this has facilitated the widespread use of dimensional measures of mental health. Other cultural issues are probably relevant in accounting for the tendency of American stress process researchers to focus on continuous measures of depression and anxiety. The assumption that negative affect captures a fundamental dimension of the human experience is an idea that is particularly resonant in a country that uniquely elevates happiness to the status of a right. Finally, the American tradition of quantitative analysis, in particular, the use of regression techniques may have contributed to a reliance on continuous measures, which are easier to work with using basic regression techniques, compared with diagnostic cut-offs, a methodological bias that Brown and Harris have criticized (Brown et al., 1991).

While it is likely that dimensional measures of distress will continue to dominate community mental health studies, the most productive approach may be to employ both diagnostic criteria and continuous measures; this is the approach that is utilized (e.g., Turner) and/or advocated (e.g., Brown, 2000) by a number of influential figures in the stress process field. Ron Kessler, for example, argued that although studies of the measurement properties of depression and generalized anxiety disorder do not suggest the existence of a latent taxon that would provide a measurement justification for cut-offs, there are still good reasons to use categorical measures along with continuous measures. Measures that integrate both approaches and are relatively less time consuming to administer, such as the Michigan Composite International Diagnostic Interview (Kessler, 2002; World Health Organization, 1997), are now readily available. Such measures, because they do not rely directly on clinical judgments, avoid the objection raised by Horwitz (2002, 2007) that a focus on mental disorders is problematic because it pathologies or stigmatizes "normal" disorder.

The second issue regarding outcomes concerns the question of what constitutes the appropriate universe of stress outcomes. Aneshensel (2000, 2005) argued that a failure to fully sample the mental health universe will lead to an underestimation and/or mis-estimation of the relationship between stressors and well-being. For example, the impact of poverty on children will tend to be under-estimated if researchers only measure problem behavior and ignore the effects of poverty on other dimensions of well-being, such as distress or substance abuse. Anehensel argued that sampling from the universe of outcomes is also important because many of the social effects of stress are non-specific. Conversely, restricted and disorder-specific models will tend to overestimate the social consequences of stressors for some groups but underestimate it for others. This argument has been very influential and as a result, many papers in the stress process tradition, particularly those focused on gender differences, measure multiple outcomes, alcohol and drug consumption and distress (Aneshensel et al., 1991; Roxburgh, 1998, 2006; Umberson et al., 1996). Future research that utilizes measures of alcohol and distress as outcomes would benefit from more refined measures of alcohol consumption, such as a consideration of the drinking context (e.g., alone versus with others) or the use of measures of alcohol dependence, not unit consumption (Lloyd and Turner, 2008).

With respect to other outcomes, Thoits (1995) called for more research on the relationship between stressors and physical health, but this call has been largely unheeded. In her review of *Journal of Health and Social Behavior*, Schwartz (2002), found that 82 percent of papers in the stress process tradition dealt with mental health outcomes compared with 18 percent of studies that dealt with physical health outcomes. More research on physical health outcomes is clearly needed in light of research that shows variation in physical weathering across race and gender (Geronimus, 1992) and in light of the evidence that stress exposure may impair physical health and increase anger, but not depression, among some social groups but not others (e.g., African Americans: Friedman and Booth-Kewley, 1987, Mirowsky and Ross 2003). Anger has also been an outcome of interest for stress process researchers recently (Ross and Van Willigen, 1996; Schieman, 2000). However, as with alcohol consumption, careful consideration needs to be given to the social context in which anger occurs and the extent to which anger is dependent upon gender, social power, and social context (e.g., work vs. home: see Larson and Richards, 1994; Lively and Powell, 2006).

Other outcomes of recent interest include *mattering* – the degree to which individuals feel they matter to others and/or that their lives are meaningful. Hughes (2006) made the point that this outcome may help us understand why highly valued social roles, such as parenthood, tend to be associated with higher distress. Hughes argued that while parenthood increases daily stressors and contributes to depression and anxiety, the role of parent may enhance well-being because parenthood gives life meaning and purpose. His point is that focusing exclusively on negative affect produces a tendency to overlook other aspects of the experience of social roles that influence well-being. Similarly, other researchers have made the case that mattering – feeling needed and wanted by others – is an important and overlooked dimension of well-being (Taylor and Turner, 2004). Keyes (2002) distinguishes between languishing and flourishing in order to capture the relationship between negative affect and positive affect. Social well-being has not been extensively studied, but studies using measures of similar concepts show a significant relationship to health outcomes (Antonovsky, 1979; Mirowsky and Ross, 2003). An interest in social well-being is consistent with the growing literature on civil society in contemporary America (Putnam, 2000). A related focus is American and European work on happiness and quality of life (Phillips, 2006), to which stress process researchers have paid little attention.

FUTURE DIRECTIONS IN STRESS PROCESS RESEARCH

There is no doubt that the stress process framework has been an important impetus for research on stress and mental health. However, the future utility of this framework is less clear. There is some evidence of a diminishment of interest within sociology in the sociology of mental health. A recent assessment of the ratio of American Sociological Association section size and publication in top-tier American journals indicated that articles on mental health are substantially underrepresented in mainstream sociology journals and that the total number of mental health publications in the two top-tier journals, *American Journal of Sociology* and *American Sociological Review*, has declined since 2000 (Pescosolido et al., 2008). Critical self-reflection about the state of the field has not been in short supply (Avison and Gotlib, 1994; Gerhardt, 1979; Pearlin, 1991; Wheaton, 2001) with the problem of developing a model of the stress process that takes account of the agency of social actors being a key issue (Thoits, 2006; William, 2003). As McLeod and Lively (2008) have pointed out, the majority of research on the stress process describes causal process in which individual agency plays a limited role. That is, the contribution that meaning-making and individual agency makes in determining mental health outcomes is generally absent from the vast majority of stress process research. Two recent developments in the field represent promising efforts to address this problem; daily diary research and studies that incorporate the life cycle approach.

The life course perspective

The study of the life course has been an increasingly important perspective for researchers working within the stress process paradigm; Pearlin and Skaff (1996) describe the relationship between the stress process and the life course perspective as a "natural alliance." Interest in the life course is reflected in a number of recent papers focusing on mental health and transitions in and out of roles (Simon and Marcussen, 1999; Turner and Schieman, 2008; Williams and Umberson, 2004) and in the recent interest in research on the relationship between childhood traumas and adult well-being, discussed earlier. Integration of the life course perspective into the stress process offers a number of important correctives to stress process research. First, a focus on trajectories and transitions moves research away from what is often a false distinction between life events, chronic strains, and daily hassles. A second advantage of the life course perspective is that it encourages researchers to take account of the relationship between an individual's past social context and their present social context. Stressors do not occur out of the context of an individual's life, even though they are frequently measured as if this were the case. In a compelling illustration of the importance of this point, Wheaton and Clarke (2003) find that current neighborhood had no effect on mental health, once childhood neighborhood was taken into account. The authors conclude:

> .... adding context to time fundamentally alters our view of how the life course affects mental health, or indeed life changes, by raising the possibility that well-established and familiar relationships at the individual level vary across social contexts, are produced by social contexts, or are events rendered spurious due to the effects of past social contexts. (Wheaton and Clarke 2003: 702)

A third advantage of applying a life course approach to the stress process concern the life course approach emphasis on the intersection of biography and history (Turner and Schieman, 2008). Since Karl Mannheim's (1928/1972) recognition that generational status is as important as socio-economic status in shaping social experience and Glen Elder's (1974) seminal work on the impact of the depression on family structure and fertility, it has been widely recognized that historical events influence individual biography. This important point and its implications for cohort and period variation in the relationship between stressors and outcomes is just beginning to be incorporated into work on the stress process (Mirowsky and Schieman, 2008; Pavalko et al., 2007).

Daily diary research

As noted earlier, research on daily hassles has developed in conjunction with the increasing methodological sophistication of daily diary research. Daily diaries, in which repeated measures are collected from the same subject, either by a daily phone interview or by beeping subjects to respond to a personal data devise, offer a number of advantages. First, the immediacy of the respondent's assessment avoids the memory distortions that occur when subjects are asked to recall their activities and the emotions associated with their activities (Bolger et al., 2003; Almeida, 2005). Second, daily diary measures permit the assessment of within-person variability and processes; the unit of analysis that stress process researchers are presumably the most interested in. An exemplar of this approach is the work of David Almeida and his colleagues. Using the DISE to probe for daily stressors, trained raters are used to score the reported stressor on a number of dimensions including whether the event involved a loss, a danger, frustration, or a challenge. This approach combines the strategy of applying objective evaluations of stressors used by Bruce Dohrenwend and George Brown with daily diary designs that permit the analysis of within-person variation in daily stressors. Almeida and his colleagues are also collecting salivary samples from respondents in order to measure biomarkers such as cortisol and anabolic hormones. This work represents an important new direction in stress process research, one that combines an interest in capturing the meaning of stressors in the stress process with rigorous sampling, design, and methodology.

CONCLUSION

The direction of future work within the stress process framework suggests a growing recognition that this research tradition can be enriched by the insights of life course research and the methodological strategies of daily diary research. Another important way forward involves greater attention to other sub-fields of sociology including social psychology and mixed method approaches that incorporate qualitative data. A final note concerns the need for American stress process researchers to incorporate the insights of their UK and European colleagues, not only those who focus on mental health, but also the rich tradition of research on the relationship between socio-economic status and health. Recent work (Avison et al., 2007; Avison, 2009) suggests the development of a trans-Atlantic and interdisciplinary approach which incorporates the insights of other fields and offers promising directions for research in mental health.

ACKNOWLEDGEMENT

The author thanks Kelly Rhea MacArthur M. A. for her editorial assistance.

REFERENCES

Akiyama, H., Antonucci, T., Takahashi, K. and Langfahl, E.S. (2003) Negative interactions in close relationships across the life span. *Journal of Gerontology. Psychological Sciences*, 58B: 70–79.

Almeida, D.M. (2005) Resilience and vulnerability to daily stressors assessed via diary methods. *Current Directions in Psychological Science*, 14: 64–68.

Almeida, D. M., Wethington, E. and Kessler, R.C. (2002) The Daily Inventory of Stressful Events (DISE): An investigator-based approach for measuring daily stressors. *Assessment*, 9: 41–55.

Amato, Paul R. and Booth, Alan (1997) *Generation at Risk: Growing Up in an Era of Family Upheaval.* Cambridge, MA: Harvard University Press.

Aneshensel, C.S. (1992) Social stress: theory and research. *Annual Review of Sociology*, 18: 15–38.

Aneshensel, C.S. (2002) Answers and questions in the sociology of mental health. *Journal of Health and Social Behavior*, 43: 236–246.

Aneshensel, C. S. (2005) Research in mental health: social etiology versus social consequences. *Journal of Health and Social Behavior*, 46: 221–228.

Aneshensel, C.S., Rutter, C.M. and Lachenbruch, P.A. (1991) Social structure, stress, and mental health: competing conceptual and analytic models. *American Sociological Review*, 56: 166–178.

Aneshensel, C.S., Pearlin, Leonard. I., Mullan, James T., Zarit, Steven H. and Whitlach, C. (1995) *Profiles in Caregiving: The Unexpected Career.* San Diego, CA: Academic Press.

Aneshensel, C.S. and Sucoff, C.A. (1996) The neighborhood context of adolescent mental health. *Journal of Health and Social Behavior*, 37: 293–310.

Aneshensel, C. S. and Phelan, J.C. (eds) (1999) *Handbook of the Sociology of Mental Health.* New York: Kluwer.

Antonovsky, Aaron (1979) *Health, Stress, and Coping.* San Francisco, CA: Jossey-Bass.

Aseltine, R.H., Jr. (1996) Pathways linking parental divorce with adolescent depression. *Journal of Health and Social Behavior*, 37: 133–148.

Atkinson, T., Liem, R. and Liem, J.H. (1986) The social costs of unemployment: implications for social support. *Journal of Health and Social Behavior*, 27: 317–331.

Avison, William R. (2009) Incorporating children's lives into a life course perspective on stress and mental health, paper presented on the occasion of the authors receipt of the Sociology of Mental Health Section's Leonard I. Pearlin Award for Distinguished Contributions to the Study of Mental Health, *American Sociological Association Meetings*. San Francisco, CA.

Avison, William R. and Cairney, John. (2003) Social structure, stress, and personal control. In S.H. Zarit, L.I. Pearlin and K.W. Schair (eds) *Personal Control in Social and Life Contexts*. New York: Springer. pp. 127–164.

Avison, William R. and Gotlib, Ian H. (1994) Introduction and overview. In W.R. Avison and I.H. Gotlib (eds) *Stress and Mental Health: Contemporary Issues and Prospects for the Future*. New York: Plenum Press. pp. 3–14.

Avison, William R., McLeod, Jane D. and Pescosolido, Bernice A. (eds) (2007) *Mental Health, Social Mirror*. New York: Springer.

Bailis, D.S., Segall, A., Mahon, M.J., Chipperfield, J.G. and Dunn, E.M. (2001) Perceived control in relation to socioeconomic and behavioral resources for health. *Social Science and Medicine*, 52: 1661–1676.

Berkman, L.F. and Syme, S.L. (1979) Social networks, host resistance, and mortality: a nine-year follow-up study of Alameda county residents. *American Journal of Epidemiology*, 109: 186–204.

Bolger, N., DeLongis, A. Kessler, R.C and Schilling, E.A. (1989) Effects of daily stress on negative mood. *Journal of Personality and Social Psychology*, 57: 808–818.

Bolger, N., Davis, A. and Rafaeli, E. (2003) Diary methods: capturing life as it is lived. *Annual Review of Psychology*, 54: 579–616.

Broman, C.L., Hamilton, L.V. and Hoffman, W.S. (1990) Unemployment and its effect on families: evidence from a plant closing study. *American Journal of Community Psychology*, 18: 643–659.

Brooks, R. and Roxburgh, S. (1999) Gender differences in the effect of the subjective experience of diabetes and sense of control on distress. *Health: An Interdisciplinary Journal for the Social Study of Health Illness and Medicine,* 3: 399–420.

Brown, G.W. (2000) Some thoughts on the future of social psychiatry. In T. Harris (ed.), *Where Inner and Outer Worlds Meet: Psychosocial Research in the Tradition of George W. Brown*. London: Routledge. pp. 291–231.

Brown, G.W. (2001) Social roles, context and evolution in the origins of depression. *Journal of Health and Social Behavior*, 43: 255–276.

Brown, G.W. and Harris, Tirril O. (1978) *Social Origins of Depression: a Study of Psychiatric Disorder in Women*. New York: Free Press.

Brown, G.W. and Harris, Tirril O. (1989) *Life Events and Illness*. New York: Guilford Press.

Brown, G.W., Harris, Tirril and Lemyre, Louise (1991) Now you see it, now you don't – some considerations on multiple regression. In D. Magnusson, L. R. Bergman, G. Rudinger and B. Torestad (eds) *Problems and Methods in Longitudinal Research: Stability and Change*. Cambridge, MA: Cambridge University Press. pp. 67–94.

Cobb, S. (1976). Social support as a moderator of life stress. *Psychosomatic Medicine*, 38: 300–14.

Cohen, Sheldon., Gottlieb, Benjamin H. and Underwood, Lynn G. (2000) Social relationships and health. In S. Cohen, L.G. Underwood and B.H. Gottlieb (eds) *Social Support Measurement: A Guide for Health and Social Scientists*. London: Oxford University Press. pp. 3–25.

Conger, R.D. and Donnellan, M.B. (2007) An interactionist perspective on the socioeconomic context of human development. *Annual Review of Psychology*, 58: 175–199.

Cui, X. and Vaillant, G.E. (1997) Does depression generate negative life events? *Journal of Nervous and Mental Diseases*, 185: 145–50.

Cutrona, C.E., Russell, D.W., Brown, P.A., Hessling, R.M., Clark, L.A. and Garder, K.A. (2005) Neighborhood context, personality, and stressful life events as predictors of depression among african american women. *Journal of Abnormal Psychology*, 114: 3–15.

Davis, M.C., Affleck, G., Zautra, A.J. and Tennen, H. (2006) Daily interpersonal events in pain patients: applying action theory to chronic illness. *Journal of Clinical Psychology*, 62: 1097–1113.

Derlega, Valerian J., Metts, Sandra, Petronio, Sandra and Margulis, Stephen T. (1993) *Self-Disclosure*. Newbury Park, CA: SAGE.

Dohrenwend, B.S. (1973) Social status and stressful life events. *Journal of Personality and Social Psychology*, 28: 225–235.

Dohrenwend, B.P. (2006) Inventorying stressful life events as risk factors for psychopathology. *Psychological Bulletin*,132: 477–495.

Dohrenwend, B.P., Dohrenwend, B.S., Dodson, M. and Shrout, P.E. (1984) Symptoms, hassles, social supports, and life events: the problem of confounded measures. *Journal of Abnormal Psychology*, 93: 222–230.

Dohrenwend, B.P., J.B. Turner, N.A. Turse, B.G. Adams, K.C. Koenen and R. Marshall (2006) The psychological risks of vietnam for U.S. veterans: A revisit with new data and methods. *Science* 313: 979–982.

Drentea, P. (2000) Age, debt, and anxiety. *Journal of Health and Social Behavior*, 41: 437–450.

Durkheim, Emile (1951) *Suicide: A Study in Sociology*. Translated by John A. Spaulding and George Simpson. New York: Free Press.

Edin, Kathryn and Lein, Laura (1997) *Making Ends Meet: How Single Mothers Survive Welfare and Low-Wage Work*. New York: Russell Sage.

Elder, Glenn H. Jr. 1974. *Children of the Great Depression: Social Change in Life Experience*. Chicago, IL: University of Chicago Press.

Ensel, W.M. and Lin, N. (1991) The life stress paradigm and psychological distress. *Journal of Health and Social Behavior*, 32: 321–341.

Folkman, S. and Lazarus, R.S. (1986) Stress process and depressive symptomatology. *Journal of Abnormal Psychology*, 95: 107–113.

Forman, T.A. (2003)The social psychological costs of racial segmentation in the workplace: A study of African Americans well-being. *Journal of Health and Social Behavior*, 44: 332–352.

Foster, H., Hagan, J. and Brooks-Gunn, J. (2008) Growing up fast: stress exposure and subjective weathering in emerging adulthood. *Journal of Health and Social Behavior*, 49: 162–177.

Friedman, H.S. and Booth-Kewley, S. (1987). The disease-prone personality: A meta-analytic view of the construct. *American Psychologist*, 42: 539–555.

Gallo, L.C., Smith, T.W. and Cox, C.M. (2006) Socioeconomic status, psychosocial processes, and perceived health: an interpersonal perspective. *Annals of Behavioral Medicine*, 31: 109–119.

Gecas, V. (1989) The social psychology of self-efficacy. *Annual Review of Sociology*, 15: 291–316.

Gecas, V. and Seff, M.A (1989) Social class, occupational conditions and self-esteem. *Sociological Perspectives*, 32: 353–365.

George, Linda K. (2003) Commentary: embedding control beliefs in social and cultural context. In S.H. Zarit, L.I. Pearlin and K.W. Schaie (eds) *Personal Control in Social and Life Course Contexts*. New York: Springer. pp. 33–44.

Gerhardt, U. (1979) Coping and social action: theoretical reconstruction of the life-event approach. *Sociology of Health and Illness*, 1: 195–225.

Geronimus, A.T. (1992) The weathering hypothesis and the health of African-Americans and infants: evidence and speculation, *Ethnicity and Disease*, 2: 207–221.

Gore, Susan and Colten, Mary Ellen (1991) Gender, stress, and distress: social-relational influences. In J. Eckenrode (ed.) *The Social Context of Coping*. New York: Plenum Press. pp. 139–163.

Grzywacz, J.G., Almeida, D.M., Neupert, S.D. and Ettner, S.L. (2004) Socioeconomic status and health: A micro-level analysis of exposure and vulnerability to daily stressors. *Journal of Health and Social Behavior*, 45: 1–16.

Hammen, C. (1991) Generation of stress in the course of unipolar depression. *Journal of Abnormal Psychology*, 100: 555–561.

Hammen, C. (2003) Social stress and women's risk for recurrent depression. *Archives of Women's Mental Health*, 6: 9–13.

Hartwell, Stephanie and Benson, Paul R. (2007) Social integration: A conceptual overview and two case studies. In W.R. Avison, J.D. McLeod and B.A. Pescosolido (eds) *Health: An Interdisciplinary Journal for the Social Study of Health Illness and Medicine*, pp. 329–353. New York: Springer.

Hatch, S.L. and Dohrenwend, B.P. (2007) Distribution of traumatic and other stressful life events by race/ ethnicity, gender, SES, and age: A review of the research. *American Journal of Community Psychology*, 40: 313–332.

Hobfoll, Steven E. and Vaux, Alan (1993) Social support: resources and context. In L. Goldberger and S. Breznitz (eds) *Handbook of Stress: Theoretical and Clinical Aspects*, 2nd edition. New York: Free Press. pp. 685–705.

Holmes, T.H. and Rahe, R.H. (1967) The social readjustment rating scale. *Journal of Psychosomatic Research*, 11: 213–218.

Horwitz, A.V. (2002) Outcomes in the sociology of mental health and illness: Where have we been and where are we going?. *Journal of Health and Social Behavior*, 43: 143–151.

Horwitz, A.V. (2007) Distinguishing distress from disorder as psychological outcomes of stressful social arrangements. *Health: An Interdisciplinary Journal for the Study of Health, Illness, and Medicine*, 11: 273–289.

House, James (1981) *Work Stress and Social Support*. Reading, MA: Addison-Wesley.

Hughes, M. (2006) Affect, meaning, and quality of life. *Social Forces*, 85: 611–629.

Jackson, James S., Williams, David R. and Torres, Myriam (1997) *Perceptions of Discrimination: The Stress Process and Physical and Psychological Health*. Washington, DC: National Institute of Mental Health.

Kahn, J.R. and. Pearlin, L.I. (2006) Financial strain over the life course and health among older adults. *Journal of Health and Social Behavior*, pp. 17–31.

Kanner, A.D., Coyne, J.C., Schaefer, C and Lazarus, R.S. (1981) Comparison of two modes of stress measurement: daily hassles and uplifts versus major life events. *Journal of Behavior Medicine*, 4: 1–39.

Kessler, R.C. (1997) The effects of stressful life events on depression. *Annual Review of Psychology*, 48: 191–214.

Kessler, Ron (2000) The long-term effects of childhood adversities on depression and other psychiatric disorders. In T. Harris (ed) *Where Inner and Outer Worlds Meet: Psychosocial Research in the Tradition of George W. Brown*. London: Routledge. pp. 227–244.

Kessler, R.C. (2002) The categorical versus dimensional assessment controversy in the sociology of mental illness. *Journal of Health and Social Behavior*, 43: 171–188.

Kessler, R.C. and Magee, W.J. (1994a) Childhood family violence and adult recurrent depression. *Journal of Health and Social Behavior*, 35: 13–27.

Kessler, R.C. and Magee, William J. (1994b) The disaggregation of vulnerability to depression as a function of the determinants of onset and Reoccurrence. In W.R. Avison and I.H. Gotlib (eds) *Stress and Mental Health: Contemporary Issues and Prospects for the Future*. New York: Plenum. pp. 239–258.

Kessler, R.C. and Magee, W. (2003) Childhood adversities and adult depression: Basic patterns of association in a U. S. national survey. *Psychological Medicine*, 23: 679–690.

Kessler, R.C. and McLeod, J. (1985) Sex differences in vulnerability to undesirable life events. *American Sociological Review*, 49: 620–631.

Kessler, R.C., Gillis Light, Jacquelyn, Story, Amber, Magee, William and Kendler, Kenneth (1997) Childhood adversity and adult psychopathology. In I. H. Gotlib and B. Wheaton (eds) *Stress and Adversity over the Life Course: Trajectories and Turning Points*. Cambridge, MA: Cambridge University Press. pp. 29–49.

Kessler, R.C., Mickelson, K.D. and Williams, D.R. (1999) The prevalence, distribution, and mental health correlates of perceived discrimination in the United States. *Journal of Health and Social Behavior*, 40: 208–230.

Keyes, C.L.M. (2002) The mental health continuum: From languishing to flourishing in life. *Journal of Health and Social Behavior*, 43: 207–222.

Kohn, M.L. (2006) *Change and Stability: A Cross-National Analysis of Social Structure and Personality*. Boulder, CO: Paradigm Publishers.

Kohn, M.L. and Slomczynski, Kazimierz M. (1990) *Social Structure and Self-Direction: A Comparative Analysis of the United States and Poland*. Cambridge, MA: Blackwell.

Krause, N. (1987) Understanding the stress process: Linking social support with locus of control beliefs. *Journal of Gerontology*, 42: 589–593.

Krause, N. and Shaw, B.A. (2002) Negative interactions and changes in functional disability during late life. *Journal of Social and Personal Relationships*, 19: 339–359.

Lachman, M.E., Prenda Firth and Kimberly M. (2004) The adaptive value of feeling in control during midlife. In O.G. Brim, C.D. Ryff and R.C. Kessler (eds) *How Healthy Are We? A National Study of Well-Being at Mid-Life*. Chicago, IL: University of Chicago Press. pp. 320–349.

Lachman, M.E. and Weaver, S.L. (1998) The sense of control as a moderator of social class differences in health and well-being. *Journal of Personality and Social Psychology*, 74: 763–773.

Larson, R. W. and Richards, M. H. (1994). *Divergent Realities: The Emotional Lives of Mothers, Fathers, and Adolescents*. New York: Basic Books.

Lazarus, R.S. (1999) *Stress and Emotion: A New Synthesis*. New York: Springer.

Lazarus, R.S. (2000) Toward better research on stress and coping. *American Psychologist*, 55: 665–673.

Lazarus, R.S. and Folkman, Susan (1984) *Stress, Appraisal, and Coping*. New York: Springer.

Lin, N. (1986) Modeling the effects of social support. In N. Lin, A. Dean and W. M. Ensel (eds) *Social Support, Life Events, and Depression*. Orlando, FL: Academic Press. pp. 173–206.

Lin, N. and Ensel, W.M. (1999) Social support and depressed mood: A structural analysis. *Journal of Health and Social Behavior*, 40: 344–359.

Link, B.G. (2003) The production of understanding. *Journal of Health and Social Behavior*, 44: 457–469.

Lively, K.J. and Powell, B. (2006) Emotional expression at work and at home: Domain, status, or individual characteristics? *Social Psychology Quarterly*, 69: 17–38.

Lloyd, D.A. and Turner, R.J. (2008) Cumulative lifetime adversities and alcohol dependence in adolescence and young adulthood. *Drug and Alcohol Dependence*, 93: 217–226.

Lorenz, F.O., Wickrama, K.A.S., Conger, R.D. and Elder, G.H. Jr. (2006) The short-term and decade-long effects of divorce on women's midlife health. *Journal of Health and Social Behavior*, 47: 111–125.

Mannheim, Karl (1928/1972) The problem of generations. In P. Altbach and R. Laufer (eds) *The New Pilgrims: Youth Protest in Transition*. New York: David McKay and Company. pp. 101–138.

Marmot, Michael (2004) *The Status Syndrome: How Social Standing Affects our Health and Longevity*. New York: Henry Holt.

Martin, J.K., Tuch, S.A. and Roman, P.M. (2003) Problem drinking patterns among African Americans: The impacts of reports of discrimination, perceptions of prejudice and risky coping strategies. *Journal of Health and Social Behavior*, 44: 408–425.

Masten, A. and Coatsworth, J.D. (1998) The development of competence in favorable and unfavorable environments: Lessons from research on successful children. *American Psychologist*, 53: 205–220.

Mattlin, J.A., Wethington, E. and Kessler, R.C. (1990) Situational determinants of coping and coping effectiveness. *Journal of Health and Social Behavior*, 31: 103–122.

McLeod, J.D. (1991) Childhood parental loss and adult depression. *Journal of Health and Social Behavior*, 32: 205–230.

McLeod, J.D. Lively, Kathryn J. (2008) Social psychology and stress research. In W.R. Avison, J.D. McLeod and B.A. Pescosolido (eds) *Mental Health, Social Mirror*. New York: Springer. pp. 275–305.

McLeod, J.D. and Shanahan, M.J. (1996) Trajectories of poverty and children's mental health. *Journal of Health and Social Behavior*, 37: 207–220.

Mechanic, D. (1975) Sociocultural and social-psychological factors affecting personal responses to psychological disorder. *Journal of Health and Social Behavior*, 16: 393–404.

Mechanic, D. (2000) Bringing meaning back into social psychiatric research: Making subjective meanings objective. In T. Harris (ed.) *Where Inner and Outer Worlds Meet: Psychosocial Research in the Tradition of George W. Brown*. London: Routledge. pp. 61–69.

Mickelson, K.D. and Kubzansky, L.D. (2003) Social distribution of social support: The mediating role of life events. *American Journal of Community Psychology*, 32: 265–281.

Miller, Suzanne M. and Kirsch, Nicholas (1987) Sex differences in cognitive coping with stress, in R.C. Barnett, L. Biener and G.K. Baruch. (eds) *Gender and Stress*. New York: Free Press. pp. 278–307.

Mirowsky, J. (1995) Age and the sense of control. *Social Psychology Quarterly*, 58: 31–43.

Mirowsky, J. and Ross, C.E. (1983) Paranoia and the structure of powerlessness. *American Sociological Review*, 48: 228–239.

Mirowsky, J. and Ross, C.E. (1990) The consolation prize theory of alienation. *American Journal of Sociology*, 95: 1505–1535.

Mirwosky, J. and Ross, C.E. (1999) Economic hardship across the life cycle. *American Sociological Review*, 64: 548–569.

Mirowsky, J. and Ross, C.E. (2001) Age and the effect of economic hardship on depression. *Journal of Health and Social Behavior*, 42: 132–150.

Mirowsky, J. and Ross, C.E. (2002) Measurement in the human science. *Journal of Health and Social Behavior*, 43: 152–170.

Mirowsky, John and Ross, Catherine E. (2003) *Social Causes of Psychological Distress*, 2nd edition. Hawthorne, NY: Aldine De Gruyter.

Mirowsky, John and Ross, C.E. (2007) Life course trajectories of perceived control and their relationship to education. *American Journal of Sociology*, 112: 1339–1382.

Mirowsky, John and Schieman, Scott (2008) Gender, age, and the trajectories and trends of anxiety and anger, in H. A. Turner and S. Schieman. (eds) *Stress Process across the Life Course, Advances in Life Course Research*, Volume 13. New York: JAI. pp. 45–74.

Mirowsky, J., Ross, C.E. and Van Willigen, M. (1996) Instrumentalism in the land of opportunity: socioeconomic causes and emotional consequences. *Social Psychology Quarterly*, 59: 322–337.

Moos, Rudolf H. and Schaefer, Jeanne A. (1993) Coping resources and processes: Current concepts and measures. In L. Goldberger and S. Breznitz (eds) in *Handbook of Stress: Theoretical and Clinical Aspects*, 2nd Edition. New York: Free Press. pp. 234–273.

Mossakowski, K. N. (2003) Coping with perceived discrimination: Does ethnic identity protect mental health? *Journal of Health and Social Behavior*, 44: 318–331.

Muntaner, Caroes, Borrell, Carme and Chung, Haejoo (2007) Class relations, economic inequality, and mental health Why social class matters to the sociology of mental health. In W.R. Avison, J.D. McLeod and B.A. Pescosolido (eds) *Mental Health, Social Mirror*. New York: Springer. pp. 127–142.

Muscatell, K.A., Slavich, G.M., Monroe, S.M. and Gotlib, I.M. (2009) Stressful life events, chronic difficulties, and the symptoms of depression. *Journal of Nervous and Mental Disorders*, 197: 154–160.

Neupert, S.D., Almeida, D.M. and Turk Charles, S. (2007) Age differences in reactivity to daily stressors: The role of personal control. *Journal of Gerontology: Psychological Sciences*, 62B: P216–P25.

Noh, S., Beiser, M., Kaspar, V., Hou, F. and Rummens, A. (1999) Perceived racial discrimination, coping, and depression among Asian refugees in Canada. *Journal of Health and Social Behavior*, 40: 193–207.

Park, C.L. and Folkman, S. (1997) Meaning in the context of stress and coping. *Review of General Psychology*, 1: 115–144.

Pavalko, E., Mossakowski, K.N., and Hamilton, V.J. (2003) Does perceived discrimination affect health? Longitudinal relationships between work and discrimination and women's physical and emotional health. *Journal of Health and Social Behavior*, pp. 18–33.

Pavalko, E., Gong, F. and Long, J.S. (2007) Women's work, cohort change, and health. *Journal of Health and Social Behavior*, 48: 352–368.

Pearlin, L.I. (1989) The sociological study of stress. *Journal of Health and Social Behavior*, 30: 241–256.

Pearlin, L.I. (1991) The study of coping: An overview of problems and directions. In J. Eckenrode (ed.) *The Social Context of Coping*. New York: Plenum Press. pp. 261–276.

Pearlin, L.I. and Schooler, C. (1978) The structure of coping, *Journal of Health and Social Behavior*, 19: 2–21.

Pearlin, L.I. and Skaff, M.M. (1996) Stress and the life course: A paradigmatic alliance. *Gerontologist*, 36: 239–256.

Pearlin, L.I., Lieberman, M.A., Menaghan, E.G and Mullan, J.T. (1981) The stress process, *Journal of Health and Social Behavior*, 22: 337–356.

Pearlin, L.I., Aneshensel, C.S. and LeBlanc, A. (1997) The forms and mechanisms of stress proliferation: The case of AIDS caregivers. *Journal of Health and Social Behavior*, 38: 223–236.

Pearlin, L. I., Schieman, S., Fazio, E.M. and Meersman, S.C. (2005) Stress, health, and the life course: some conceptual perspectives. *Journal of Health and Social Behavior*, 46: 205–219.

Pearlin, L.I., Avison,William R. and Fazio, Elena M. (2008) Sociology, psychiatry, and the production of knowledge about mental illness and its treatment. In W.R. Avison, J.D. McLeod and B.A. Pescosolido (eds) *Mental Health, Social Mirror*. New York: Springer. pp. 33–54.

Pescosolido, Bernice A., McLeod, Jane D. and Avison, William R. (2008) Through the looking glass: The fortunes of the sociology of mental health. In W.R. Avison, J.D. McLeod and B.A. Pescosolido (eds) *Mental Health, Social Mirror*. New York: Springer. pp. 3–32.

Phillips, David (2006) Quality of Life: *Concept, Policy, and Practice*. London: Routledge.

Putnam, Robert D. (2000) Bowling Alone: *The Collapse and Revival of American Community*. New York: Simon & Schuster.

Radloff, L.S. (1977) The CES-D scale: A self-report depression scale for research in the general population. *Applied Psychological Measurement*, 1: 385.

Reynolds, J.R. and Turner, R.J. (2008) Major life events, their personal meaning, resolution, and mental health significance. *Journal of Health and Social Behavior*, 49: 223–237.

Rosenberg, Morris (1986) *Conceiving the Self*, 2nd Edition. Melbourne, FL: Academic Press.

Ross, C.E. (2000) Neighborhood disadvantage and adult depression. *Journal of Health and Social Behavior*, 41: 177–187.

Ross, C.E. and Drentea, P. (1998) Consequences of retirement activities for distress and the sense of personal control. *Journal of Health and Social Behavior*, 39: 317–334.

Ross, C.E. and Mirowsky, J. (1989) Explaining the social patterns of depression: Control and problem-solving – or support and talking? *Journal of Health and Social Behavior*, 30: 206–219.

Ross, C.E. and Van Willigan. M. (1996) Gender, parenthood, and anger. *Journal of Marriage and the Family*, 58: 572–584.

Ross, C.E., Mirowsky, J. and Cockerham, W.C. (1983) Social class, Mexican culture, and fatalism: Their effects on psychological distress. *American Journal of Community Psychology*, 11: 383–399.

Ross, C.E. and Sastry, J. (1999) The sense of personal control: Social-structural causes and emotional Consequences. In C.S. Aneshensel and J.C. Phelan (eds), *Handbook of the Sociology of Mental Health*. New York: Kluwer Academic/Plenum Publishers. pp. 369–394.

Rotter, J.M. (1996) *Generalized expectancies for internal vs. external control of reinforcements*. *Psychological Monographs*, 80: 1–28.

Roxburgh, S. (1998) Gender differences in the impact of job stressors on alcohol consumption. *Addictive Behaviors*, 23: 101–107.

Roxburgh, S. (2004) There just aren't enough hours in the day: The mental health consequences of time pressures. *Journal of Health and Social Behavior*, 32: 115–131.

Roxburgh, S. (2006) I wish we had more time to spend together... : The distribution and predictors of perceived family time pressures among married men and women in the paid labor force. *Journal of Family Issues*, 27: 1–25.

Sampson, R.J. (2008) Moving to inequality: neighborhood effects and experiments meet social structure. *American Journal of Sociology*, 114: 189–231.

Sastry, J. and Ross, C.E. (1998) Asian ethnicity and sense of personal control. *Social Psychology Quarterly*, 61: 101–120.

Schieman, S. (2000) Education and the activation, course, and management of anger. *Journal of Health and Social Behavior*, 41: 273–289.

Schieman, S. (2001) Age, education, and the sense of control: A test of the cumulative advantage hypothesis. *Research on Aging*, 23: 153–178.

Schulz, A., Williams, D., Israel, B., Becker, A., Parker, E., James, S.A. and Jackson, J. (2000) Unfair treatment, neighborhood effects, and mental health in the Detroit metropolitan area. *Journal of Health and Social Behavior*, 41: 314–346.

Schwarz, S. (2002) Outcomes for the sociology of mental health: Are we meeting our goals? *Journal of Health and Social Behavior*, 43: 223–235.

Seligman, Martin E. (1975) *Helplessness: On Depression, Development, and Death.* San Francisco, CA: Freeman.

Selye, Hans (1993) History of the stress concept. In L. Goldberger and S. Breznitz (eds) *Handbook of Stress: Theoretical and Clinical Aspects,* 2nd edition. New York: Free Press. pp. 7–17.

Serido, J., Almeida., D.M. and Wethington, E. (2004) Chronic stressors and daily hassles: Unique and interactive relationships with psychological distress. *Journal of Health and Social Behavior*, 45: 17–33.

Simon, R.W. (2002) Revisiting the relationships among gender, marital status, and mental health. *American Journal of Sociology*, 107: 1065–1096.

Simon, R.W. and Marcussen, K. (1999) Marital transitions, marital beliefs, and mental health. *Journal of Health and Social Behavior*, 40: 111–125.

Somerfield, M.R. and McRrae, R.R. (2000) Stress and coping research: methodological challenges, theoretical advances, and clinical applications. *American Psychologist*, 55: 620–625.

Son, J., Lin, N. and George, L.K. (2008) Cross-national comparison of social support structures between Taiwan and the United States. *Journal of Health and Social Behavior*, 49: 104–118.

Stack, Carol S. (1974) *All Our Kin.* New York: Basic Books.

Sweeney, M. and Horwitz, A.V. (2001) Infidelity, initiation, and the emotional climate of divorce: Are there implications for mental health? *Journal of Health and Social Behavior*, 42: 295–309.

Tausig, M. and Fenwick, R. (1999) Recession and well-being. *Journal of Health and Social Behavior*, 40: 1–16.

Taylor, S.E. and Brown, J.D. (1988) Illusion and well-being: A social psychological perspective on Mental Health. *Psychological Bulletin*, 103: 193–210.

Tennen, H., Affleck, G., Armeli, S. and Carney, M.A. (2000) A daily process approach to coping: linking theory, research, and practice. *American Psychologist*, 55: 626–636.

Thoits, P.A. (1986) Multiple identities: examining gender and marital status differences in distress. *American Sociological Review*, 51: 269–272.

Thoits, P.A. (1995) Stress, coping, and social support processes: Where are we? What next? *Journal of Health and Social Behavior*, Extra Issue: 53–79.

Thoits, P.A. (2006) Personal agency in the stress process. *Journal of Health and Social Behavior*, 47: 309–323.

Thompson, Etta L. Sanders (1996) Perceived experiences of racism as stressful life events. *Community Mental Health Journal*, 32: 223–233.

Turner, H.A. and Schieman, S. (eds) (2008) Stress Process across the Life Course. *Advances in Life Course Research*, Volume 13. New York: JAI.

Turner, H.A. and Turner, R.J. (2005) Understanding variations in exposure to social stress. *Health: An interdisciplinary journal for the social study of health. Illness and Medicine*, 9: 209–240.

Turner, R.J. (1999) Social support and coping. In A.V. Horwitz and T.L. Scheid (eds) *A Handbook for the Study of Mental Health: Social Contexts.* Theories, and System. Cambridge, MA: Cambridge University Press. pp. 198–210.

Turner, R.J. and Avison, W.R. (1989) Gender and depression: Assessing exposure and vulnerability to life events in a chronically strained population. *Journal of Nervous and Mental Disease*, 177: 443–455.

Turner, R.J. and Patricia Roszell (1994) Psychosocial resources and the stress process. In W.R. Avison and I.H. Gotlib (eds) *Stress and Mental Health: Contemporary Issues and Prospects for the Future.* New York: Plenum Press. pp. 179–210.

Turner, R.J. and Avison, William R. (1992) Sources of attenuation in the stress-distress relationship: An evaluation of modest innovations in the application of event checklists. In J. Greenley and P. Leaf (eds) *Research in Community and Mental Health.* Greenwich, CT: JAI Press. pp. 265–300.

Turner, R.J. and Lloyd, D.A. (1999) The stress process and the social distribution of depression. *Journal of Health and Social Behavior*, 40: 374–404.

Turner, R.J. and Lloyd, D.A. (2004) Stress burden and the lifetime incidence of psychiatric disorders in young adults. *Archives of General Psychiatry*, 61: 481–488.

Turner, R.J. and Marino, F. (1994) Social support and social structure: A descriptive epidemiology. *Journal of Health and Social Behavior*, 35: 193–212.

Turner, R.J. and Noh, S. (1983) Class and psychological vulnerability among women: The significance of social support and personal control. *Journal of Health and Social Behavior*, 24: 2–15.

Turner, R.J. Turner, J. Blake. (2000) Social integration and support. In C.S. Aneshensel and J.C. Phelan (eds) *Handbook of the Sociology of Mental Health*. New York: Plenum. pp. 301–319.

Turner, R.J., Wheaton, B. and Lloyd, D.A. (1995) The epidemiology of social stress. *American Sociological Review*, 60: 104–125.

Turner, R.J. Frankel, Gail B. and Levin, Deborah M. (1983) Social support: conceptualization, measurement and implications for mental health. In J.R. Greenley (ed) *Research in Community and Mental Health*, Volume 3. Greenwich, CT: JAI Press.

Turner, R.J., Lloyd, D.A. and Roszell, P. (1999) Personal resources and the social distribution of depression. *Journal of Community Psychology*, 27: 643–672.

Turner, R.J., Taylor, J. and Van Gundy, K. (2004) Personal resources and depression in the transition to adulthood: Ethnic comparisons. *Journal of Health and Social Behavior*, 45: 34–52.

Umberson, D. (2003) *Death of a Parent: Transition to a New Adult Identity*. New York: Cambridge University Press.

Umberson, D.M., Chen, M.D., House, J.S., Hopkins, K. and Slaten, E. (1996) The effect of social relationships on psychological well-being: Are men and women really so different? *American Sociological Review*, 61: 837–857.

Wheaton, B. (1980) The sociogenesis of psychological disorder: An attributional theory. *Journal of Health and Social Behavior*, 21: 100–124.

Wheaton, B. (1983) Stress, personal coping resources, and psychiatric symptoms: An investigation of interactive models. *Journal of Health and Social Behavior*, 24: 208–229.

Wheaton, B. (1985) Models for the stress-buffering functions of coping resources. *Journal of Health and Social Behavior*, 26: 352–364.

Wheaton, B. (1990) Life transitions, role histories, and mental health. *American Sociological Review*, 55: 209–223.

Wheaton, B. (1999) The nature of stressors, in A.V. Horwitz and T.L. Scheid (eds) *A Handbook for the Study of Mental Health: Social Contexts, Theories, and System*. Cambridge, MA: Cambridge University Press. pp. 176–197.

Wheaton, B. (2001) The role of sociology in the study of mental health .... and the role of mental health in the study of sociology, *Journal of Health and Social Behavior*, 42: 221–234.

Wheaton, B. (2007) The twain meet: distress, disorder and the continuing conundrum of categories (comment on Horwitz). *Health: An Interdisciplinary Journal for the Study of Health, Illness, and Medicine*, 11: 303–319.

Wheaton, B. and Clarke, P. (2003) Space meets time: Integrating temporal and contextual influence on mental health in early adulthood. *American Sociological Review*, 68: 680–706.

Wheaton, Blair, Roszell, Patricia and Hall, Kimberlee (1997) The impact of twenty childhood and adult traumatic stressors on the risk of psychiatric disorder. In I.H. Gotlib and B. Wheaton (eds) *Stress and Adversity over the Life Course: Trajectories and Turning Points*. Cambridge, MA: Cambridge University Press. pp. 50–72.

Wickrama, K.A.S., Lorenz, F.O., Fang, S., Abraham, W.T. and Elder, G.H., Jr. (2005a) Gendered trajectories of work control and health outcomes in the middle years: A perspective from the rural midwest. *Health and Aging*, 17: 779–806.

Wickrama, K.A.S., Merten, M.J. and. Elder, G.H., Jr. (2006) Community influence on adolescent precocious development: Racial differences and mental health consequences. *Journal of Community Psychology*, 33: 639–653.

Wickrama, K.A.S., Conger, R.D., Lorenz, F. and Jung, T. (2008) Family antecedents and consequences of trajectories of depressive symptoms from adolescence to young adulthood: A life course investigation. *Journal of Health and Social Behavior*, 49: 468–483.

Wilkinson, Richard (2005) *The Impact of Inequality: How to Make Sick Societies Healthier*. New York: New Press.

Williams, G.H. (2003) The determinants of health: structure, context, and agency. *Sociology of Health and Illness*, 25: 131–154.

Williams, K. (2003) Has the future of marriage arrived? A contemporary examination of gender, marriage, and psychological well-being. *Journal of Health and Social Behavior*, 44: 470–487.

Williams, K. and Umberson, D. (2004) Marital status, marital transitions, and health: A gendered life course perspective. *Journal of Health and Social Behavior*, 45: 81–98.

World Health Organization (1997) *Composite Diagnostic Interview* (CIDI, Version 2.1). Geneva, Switzerland: World Health Organization.

9

Religious Beliefs and Mental Health: Applications and Extensions of the Stress Process Model

Scott Schieman

INTRODUCTION

The stress process model provides a guiding framework and a rich set of conceptual tools for the analysis of social causes and consequences of stress, as well as
the psychosocial conditions that function as mediating or moderating resources
(Pearlin, 1999; Wheaton, 1999). Sociologists have tended to focus attention on
the social patterning of stress exposure and/or vulnerability, with a special
emphasis on the distribution across core social statuses and dimensions of stratification (McLeod and Nonnemaker, 1999; Mirowsky and Ross, 2003; Turner
et al., 1995). In analyses of psychosocial resources, research has generally
focused on the sense of personal control or mastery, self-esteem, and social
support (Turner and Roszell, 1994). However, the relevance of religion for these
psychosocial processes and outcomes has received surprisingly less attention
(e.g., see Ellison, 1994; Ellison et al., 2001; Idler, 1987). This is particularly
striking given the relevance of religion in the personal and social lives of many
adults around the world (Stark, 2008; World Values Survey).[1]

The stress process model is a remarkably flexible analytical framework that is
easily able to accommodate conceptual and explanatory extensions (Pearlin,
1999; Wheaton, 1999). I seek to take advantage of these strengths in several ways.

The first main section of this chapter focuses on the relevance of religious beliefs – especially *beliefs about God* – for mental health. I review existing theory and evidence about the overall link between religious beliefs and mental health as well as their role in the association between stressors and well-being. In particular, I examine the ways that the beliefs about God influence the meaning, significance, and consequences of stress. This issue requires an assessment of the ways that beliefs may modify the association between stress and psychological distress or subjective well-being.[1]

In the second main section of this chapter, I identify the ways that these religious beliefs are potentially influential for the core psychosocial resources in the stress process model: the sense of control, self-esteem, and feelings of mattering. Each of these has been identified as an important resource that helps individuals avoid or manage the consequences of stress (Turner, and Roszell, 1994; Wheaton, 1985). My central aim is to document and describe the ways that religious beliefs are associated with these personal resources and whether or not these relationships differ across core social statuses or dimensions of stratification. Among the most influential of these factors are gender, race, age, and social class (Pearlin, 1999; McLeod and Nonnemaker, 1999).

RELIGIOUS BELIEFS AND MENTAL HEALTH

Why focus on religious beliefs?

The three main features of religiosity are *believing*, *behaving*, and *belonging* (Green et al., 1996; Woodberry and Smith, 1998). According to Froese and Bader (2007), *believing* has not received as much attention in either sociological theories or analyses of religion. These authors underscore the importance of addressing this gap – especially given that "at its most fundamental level religion is about belief" (p. 466). However, most research on the links between religion and mental health has examined religious involvement or participation, as indexed by the frequency of attending religious services, praying, or more global measures of religiosity such as salience (see Ellison and Levin, 1998; Ellison et al., 2001; Flannelly et al., 2008; George et al., 2002). So, while there is little doubt that analysis of these forms of religious involvement is a worthwhile aim of mental health research, there has been a surprising lack of emphasis on religious beliefs. Recently, however, several researchers have sought to address that deficit (Flannelly et al., 2006; Pargament, 1997; Schieman et al., 2006). While the complexity, diversity, and varied meanings of religious beliefs presents unique challenges for research, it does seem reasonable to assert that there are several beliefs that represent fairly normative components of the belief systems of major religions – especially Christianity (Prothero, 2007; Smith, 2007). For the most part, I focus on *beliefs about God*, especially the belief in a personal God who is highly involved and influential in everyday life.

The debate: does religion have positive or negative influences on mental health?

There is a long-standing debate about the association between religion and mental health (Ellison, 1994; Glock and Stark, 1965; Hackney and Sanders, 2003; Pargament, 2002). Both sides present provocative, if not equally controversial, arguments. Although the general consensus is that people who report higher levels of *religious involvement* (especially more frequent attendance) report more favorable levels of mental health (Ellison and Levin, 1998; Hackney and Sanders, 2003; Koenig et al., 2001), the specific influence of religious beliefs remains an unresolved issue (George et al., 2002). Two competing hypotheses can be drawn mainly from the religious involvement literature. One view is that religious involvement is related to better psychological adjustment or mental health (Pargament, 2002), some of which may occur via the supportive community that religious participation provides (Ellison and Levin, 1998). A central premise is that religious involvement enhances a sense of meaning and provides a framework for understanding the world (Koenig et al., 2001). Moreover, as Wilson (1982: 32) has observed, "whatever form cultural, local, or personal anxieties may take, religion offers to still these anxieties by recourse to reassuring beliefs, practices, or facilities." He also maintains that that *all* religions have a "vocabulary of suffering" and a "repertoire of methods for their relief." Collectively, these elements of the religious life may contribute to more favorable mental health outcomes – although the association probably depends on the content of specific religious beliefs. Moreover, the potential relevance of stress in these processes is quite explicit.

An alternative perspective argues that religion is associated with more mental health problems. Critics of religion, including a visible crop of proponents of atheism, have long-contended that religious beliefs and practices reflect a delusional form of pathology (Dawkins, 2006; Freud, 1976; Harris, 2004; Hitchens, 2007; Marx and Engels, 1964; Watters, 1992). One of the leading critics, Albert Ellis (1980: 637), has argued that the "emotionally healthy individual is flexible, open, tolerant, and changing, and the devoutly religious person tends to be inflexible, closed, intolerant, and unchanging." In his account of the "pathological characteristics of religiosity," Ellis (1988) also asserts that religion discourages self-directedness and self-acceptance. Particular beliefs, such as divine omnipotence, original sin, and hell, may have especially deleterious psychological consequences (Branden, 1994; Ellis, 1962); in extreme instances, they may play a role in religious-based suicides. The concept of sin, particularly in conservative Christian theology and among individuals who more adamantly adhere to religious teachings and the word of God, may cultivate feelings of shame, guilt, and self-doubt (Ellison, 1993, 1994). Beliefs that integrate God's personal evaluation of the self – and the corresponding rewards and/or *punishments* – may have implications for emotional health. For example, images of "an angry and wrathful God" can increase the awareness of one's own moral inadequacies (Koenig et al., 1993), or they may influence spiritual struggles and their associated risks for poor mental health (McConnell et al., 2006). These views predict that some beliefs may be associated with more psychological distress and disorder.

Collectively, these competing views about the positive and negative consequences of religion and mental health raise questions about the specific *content* of religious beliefs. While there are numerous directions for the analysis of religious beliefs and mental health, I will focus primarily on beliefs about God. In the following section, I outline some of the main conceptual ideas and findings in this area, focusing on studies that have examined the belief in an involved and influential God – especially the belief in God *as a causal agent in everyday life*.

Conceptual and theoretical specifications

Sociologists have long held a scholarly interest in the influence of various forms of religious precepts and practices on the psychological and social functioning of individuals or groups (Durkheim, [1897] 1951; Simmel, 1997; Weber, [1922] 1963). The personal relationship with a divine entity has been a core element in these processes – especially the notion of an omnipotent and omnipresent Supreme Being. For example, William James ([1902] 1999) defined religion as "the feelings, acts, and experiences of individual men in their solitude, so far as they apprehend themselves to stand in relation to whatever they may consider the divine" (p. 36). There is fairly compelling evidence that the *vast majority* of Americans maintain the belief in a highly personal God (Froese and Bader, 2007; Schieman, 2008; Stark, 2008), and these beliefs remain influential in many aspects of American social and political life (Wills, 2007). The question becomes: How are these beliefs relevant for stress and mental health?

Across historical times, societies, and cultures, people have professed a wide array of mental representations of God that typically project human attributes and roles (i.e., "master," "father," "friend") which, in turn, imply an intimate involvement in the everyday lives of people (Armstrong, 1993; Miles, 1995; Sharot, 2001; Stark, 2001, 2007). Core tenets of orthodox Christian theology convey and reinforce the belief that God wishes to maintain a unique bond with each human being and commonly intercedes in their daily affairs (Ellison et al., 2001; Smith, 2007; Watson et al., 1988). The content and intensity of these beliefs, however, likely varies across individuals of different religious affiliations and denominations. For example, some Evangelicals (e.g., Pentecostals) may be more likely than other Christians (e.g., mainline Protestants) to profess the belief that "the Holy Spirit is an active force in the world and that the directives of the Holy Spirit will never contradict the Bible" (Trice and Bjorck, 2006: 284).

The notion of an intimate and personal bond with the divine underscores the ways that many of the faithful sustain divine relations that parallel those with other people (Glock and Stark, 1965; Pollner, 1989). Divine relations of this form may be especially pertinent for mental health because they often encompass the belief that God is a conscious, omnipotent being who has explicit expectations and desires for each human being (Black, 1999; Stark and Finke, 2000). Krause (2002) summarizes these divine relations as a set of themes in which believers have "a sense of trust in God, believe that God is in control of their lives, believe that God knows what is best for them, and believe that God ultimately ensures they will get what they need most" (p. S335). Of all religious beliefs, I argue that beliefs about God's involvement and influence in everyday life are probably among the *most* relevant for stress processes and mental health. Froese and Bader (2007) have recently echoed this sentiment in their analysis of beliefs about God, especially God's *character*:

> Based on theoretical insights of past research and key debates within the philosophy of religion, we hypothesize that two aspects of God's character matter most to the attitudes and behaviors of believers. The first is the extent to which God interacts with the world; for some, God closely guides life on earth by pulling strings like an omnipotent puppeteer, while for others God's presence is not nearly so hands-on. A second important aspect is the extent to which God judges human behavior. For many Americans, God is angered by world affairs and takes sides in human disagreements, while other believers indicate that God mainly views us with love and compassion. Taken together, we argue that these aspects of God's character form the ontological basis of religious attitudes and behavior. (p. 466)

While some people believe that God is involved in the details of their lives, many people also report a belief that God is a *causal* agent in everyday life (Welton et al., 1996). My colleagues and I have referred to this as the belief in "divine control" (Schieman, 2008; Schieman and Bierman, 2007; Schieman, et al., 2005, 2006).[2] The sense of divine control involves the extent that one believes that God exercises a commanding authority over the course and direction of his or her own life. Individuals who profess the belief in divine control perceive that God has a determinative influence on the good and bad outcomes in their lives, that God has decided what their life shall be, and that their fate evolves according to God's will or plan for them. Moreover, they tend to rely on God in their decision-making and more fervently seek His guidance for solutions to problems.[3] This belief has deep theological origins. According to Stark and Glock (1968: 25), "the most universal and basic element in Christian theologies is an elaborate set of assertions about the nature and will of an all-powerful and sentient God." Similarly, Roberts and Davidson (1984) assert that the "theistic or traditional meaning system is the acceptance of God as the primary force governing and explaining life" (p. 340).

Krause (2005) has identified a similar concept – "God-mediated control" – that involves the idea that "problems can be overcome, and goals in life can be reached by working together with God" (p. 137; also see Berrenberg, 1987; Krause, 2007). His index of God-mediated control sums levels of agreement with the following three statements: "I rely on God to help me control my life," "I can succeed with God's help," and "All things are possible when I work together with God." Krause argues that these items were "carefully chosen to reflect working collaboratively with God and not merely believing that God entirely controls all aspects of one's life" (p. 149). These items derive, in part, from Pargament's (1997) research regarding different styles of religious coping. A "deferring" style involves the perception that God has total control over the events and outcomes of life – this implies a highly passive role for the individual. By contrast, the "collaborative" style is indicative of a relationship in which the believer works together with God to avoid or cope with adversities. Pargament contends (and research corroborates) that the collaborative style is more advantageous for psychological adjustment. Collectively, both the divine control and God-mediated control concepts share a basic view of a divine (supernatural) entity or force that maintains an intimate concern with and personal involvement in one's daily affairs and well-being. Unfortunately, however, the link between different styles of coping and these forms of divine control beliefs have yet to be established in population-based research.

The evidence about divine control beliefs and mental health

Few studies have directly examined the association between the beliefs about divine control (or related concepts) and mental health. Those that have done so focus mainly on older adults. For example, my colleagues and I have investigated the link between divine control beliefs and mental health among adults age 65 and older in the metropolitan Washington, DC area (Schieman et al., 2006). Our observations indicate that the association between divine control beliefs and psychological distress *depend* on two other conditions: race and socioeconomic status (SES). Specifically, belief in divine control is associated with lower levels of distress – but that relationship is stronger among African Americans of lower SES. These patterns are consistent with one of the central tenets of the stress process model: social statuses or dimensions of stratification are often influential for stress and mental health (McLeod and Nonnemaker, 1999; Mirowsky and Ross, 2003).

Krause (2005) has also examined the link between God-mediated control and mental health. Using data from a nationally representative sample of adults older than age 65, he found that individuals who believed more strongly in God-mediated control reported, on average, higher levels of life satisfaction, optimism, and a lower level of anxiety about death. His research also exemplifies the relevance of social status variations by documenting that the belief in God-mediated control is associated more positively with levels of life satisfaction and optimism among African-Americans compared to whites. Likewise, the negative association between belief in God-mediated control and anxiety about death is also significantly stronger among African-Americans.

Divine control beliefs and the sense of personal control

As I will discuss in greater detail later, the belief in divine control is conceptually and empirically related to the sense of personal control. Although this is a complicated association, the theory of personal control implies that people who believe in God's causal relevance in everyday life may report a lower sense of personal control (Mirowsky and Ross, 2003; Schieman, 2008). By extension, there is a well-established association between an external sense of control and psychological distress (Ross and Sastry, 1999; Wheaton, 1985). To test the differential association of external attributions and distress, Ross (1990) examined data from a representative sample of Illinois residents. She assessed levels of distress across four different types of external attributions: *luck*, *God*, *good connections*, and *family background*. Ross found that – net of sociodemographic characteristics and emotional expressiveness – the external attributions to luck and good connections are associated with higher levels of distress. By contrast, however, attributions to God and family background are unrelated to distress. In their interpretation of these patterns, Ross and Sastry (1999) speculate that "belief that outcomes are in the hands of God may provide some comfort, hope, and meaning, which counteract the external attribution" (p. 387).

The nature of beliefs about God or other supernatural causes (e.g., Satan or the "Devil") may also be relevant for the perceived causes and the course of mental health or illness. In a study of students of a nondenominational Charismatic Bible training school in the US, Trice and Bjorck (2006) found that "demonic oppression or possession" was one of the highest rated likely causes of depression. With respect to study participants' ratings for the treatment of depression, "reading the *Bible*" was the most highly endorsed item. Given the nature of the sample, this finding may not be surprising. Yet, it does underscore the importance of considering the relevance of religious beliefs not only for levels of mental health problems in the population but also for individuals' perceptions about the causes and treatments. Even more rare are studies of beliefs about God *during* episodes or experiences of mental illness. One in-depth study of 48 young adults diagnosed with schizophrenia or bipolar disorder found that "benevolent religious reappraisals" are linked with more favorable mental health while views of God as punishing or powerful were associated with elevated levels of distress (Phillips and Stein, 2007). These are both areas that are ripe for further investigation in population-based research.

The potential relevance of other religious beliefs: life after death

Although my main focus is on the ways that beliefs about God are influential for mental health, it is also important to consider other types of religious beliefs that may be relevant (and strongly interrelated with beliefs about the divine). *Belief in life after death* seems like an ideal candidate, especially considering the strong links between beliefs about God and life after death. Common phrases like "He's gone to meet his maker" and "She'll have to answer to God when she dies" (an effective social control tactic) imply a strong interrelationship among these ideas and their hypothesized processes. Belief in God is a basic criterion for access to the rewards of the afterlife. Thus, it seems essential to briefly address the following question: Do beliefs in life after death have any influence on peoples' mental health? With the exception of a few recent studies, surprisingly little systematic research has examined this question – especially in large, population-based samples (Flannelly et al., 2006, 2008). Nonetheless, there are compelling theoretical reasons for suspecting that afterlife beliefs should matter for psychological well-being.

First and foremost, afterlife beliefs may be a cornerstone of one's system of faith – an orienting framework that helps people see the larger picture of their own life and their relevance in the material world. By providing a "longer view," this eternal perspective may have important repercussions for the sense of coherence and the capacity to effectively (and positively) appraise everyday events and outcomes – including stressful ones (Antonovsky, 1987; Berger, 1967; Idler, 1987). Taken together, these ideas predict that people who believe in life after death may tend to have a view of this world and their place in it that is "not the end of the road." This is a common theme in the teachings of some of the popular, long-standing religious doctrines (Lindbeck 1984). Perhaps the view that the temporary existence here on earth is only a preview for the eternal life to come is linked to greater tranquility and less worry or fear. Moreover, stressors such as health and financial difficulties may seem less threatening and have fewer actual deleterious consequences for those who sense the promise of greater rewards in the afterlife (Ellison, 1993; Foley, 1988; Idler, 1995). The spiritual may trump the material for these believers, shielding them against exposure to the stressors of life. Moreover, suffering itself may get redefined in ways that dilute its sting.

The belief in life after death may be especially relevant for individuals dealing with loss-related coping and bereavement. Classic indices of stress score the loss of a spouse or partner as among those requiring substantial readjustment (Holmes and Rahe, 1967). This makes the appraisal and coping processes even more relevant for individuals. Some researchers have focused on the impact of afterlife beliefs and the sense of continued attachment with the deceased after death as central elements of appraisal and coping. Religious beliefs may play a critical role in the development of meaning around the loss, coping with loss-related stress, and ultimately avoiding or navigating feelings of distress (Benore and Park, 2004).

Religion has long been seen as a critical part of the coping process, especially when it comes to dealing with loss and the meaning-making processes surrounding it (Park and Folkman, 1997). There are two key ways that afterlife beliefs may be influential for coping and adjustment efforts: (1) these beliefs can help individuals to reappraise the death in a more favorable way; and (2) afterlife beliefs may be part of a package of religious beliefs and practices that afford more coping opportunities. Seeing life after death as associated with rewards and "being in a better place" (especially after a period of suffering) has been linked to less distress among the bereaved. Ultimately, these factors can contribute to efforts to derive meaning from loss and may attenuate the psychological distress that so often occurs after the death of a loved one (Schoenrade, 1989; Schuchte, 1986).

Collectively, the ideas presented above generally predict that beliefs about life after death should be associated with fewer psychological problems or better subjective well-being. While limited, some recent empirical evidence addresses this hypothesis. For example, Ellison and his colleagues (2009) found that individuals who believe in an afterlife report higher levels of life satisfaction, fewer symptoms of anxiety, and a greater sense of tranquility compared to nonbelievers. In a national survey of Americans, Flannelly and his colleagues (2006) observed that people who belief in life after death report fewer symptoms of anxiety, depression, obsessive-compulsion, paranoia, phobia, and somatization. Those authors ruled out the potential influence of sociodemographic variables, stress levels, and social support. However, one study found that individuals who report that *the most important element* of their belief system involves the opportunity for life after death tended to report higher levels of depression and distress (Alvarado et al., 1995). It might be that these individuals placed more emphasis on the rewards of faith and were less intrinsically involved or committed. Collectively, these studies further underscore the importance of considering the psychological health implications of religious beliefs – although much remains unknown about specific features like the nature of afterlife beliefs (e.g., what if one believes that the 'final destination' is hell?) and the influence of beliefs about divine support, involvement, and control in these processes.

Can beliefs about God be stressors?

Is it possible that religious beliefs, especially beliefs about God's involvement and causal relevance in everyday life, sometimes function as stressors? As I noted above, there is a long-standing argument about the deleterious effects of religion on mental health. However, few studies have explicitly identified the ways that beliefs about God can be stressors. Some researchers have sought to establish a link between "spiritual struggles" or "religious doubts" and mental health outcomes. For example, McConnell and colleagues (2006) observe that more frequent spiritual struggles – as indexed by responses to the "Negative Religious Coping" subscale – reported anxiety, phobic anxiety, depression, paranoid ideation, obsessive-compulsiveness, and somatization. The researchers contend that these effects are not attributable to religious involvement indicators or demographic measures and they are "relatively large and robust" (p. 1476). Similarly, Galek and colleagues (2007) found that religious doubt is associated with higher levels of depression, anxiety, phobic anxiety, obsessive-compulsive symptoms, somatization, paranoid ideation, and hostility among a sample of American adults.

It is also highly plausible that the belief in an omnipotent, omnipresent Supreme Being who is not "in your corner" may be psychologically unsettling. If God is deemed a Causal influence in daily adversity, the consequences might be especially deleterious. Scholars have long considered the relevance of religious concepts (e.g., sin) and their implications for well-being (Branden, 1994; Ellis, 1962). The concept of sin, especially in conservative Christian theology and among individuals who more adamantly adhere to religious teachings and the word of God, can cultivate feelings of shame, guilt, and self-doubt (Ellison, 1993, 1994). This constellation of beliefs challenges the integrity and value of the self. The ways that reflected appraisals influence the self-concept are especially relevant here. If one derives a sense of self from divine evaluations, the content of those appraisals can take a serious toll. Beliefs that integrate God's personal evaluation of the self – and the corresponding rewards *or punishments* – may have implications for emotional health. For example, appraisals that include being on the receiving end of "an angry and wrathful God" can increase the awareness of one's own moral inadequacies (Koenig et al., 1993), or they may promote spiritual struggles and erode mental health (McConnell et al., 2006). When combined with the belief in divine involvement and control, this view of God may be particularly deleterious for well-being. These views predict that some religious beliefs may be associated with more psychological distress and disorder. Moreover, these processes may lead some to *doubt* the presence or beneficence of God.

Religious doubts

In a world filled with so much suffering and injustice in the world, how do devoted religious adherents keep the faith? According to Krause (2006: 288), "it may be difficult for some people to believe in a loving and protecting God while at the same time recognizing there is a great deal of pain, suffering, and injustice in the world." This issue underscores one of the most interesting recent directions in understanding the link between religion and mental health: *religious doubt*. Broadly speaking, religious doubt is defined as "a feeling of uncertainty toward, and a questioning of, religious teachings and beliefs" (Hunsberger et al., 1993, p. 28 cited in Krause and Wulff, 2004). Although doubts often involve the nature and content of one's personal relationship with God, they may also extend to broader aspects of the religious life like the credibility of religious texts and other substantive features of religious socialization or practice.

According to Hecht (2003), doubt has long been among the core aspects of the religious life. It is important to not oversimplify this discussion by assuming that religious doubts only have deleterious implications for psychological health. In fact, there are two basic predictions about the psychological consequences of doubt. One is *positive*. According to Paul Tillich (1957), the well-known Protestant theologian, "doubt is not the opposite of faith; it is an element of faith" (p. 57). Others have sought to underscore the value of doubt as a key part of the process of strengthening faith; doubt is an element of a "religious quest" (Batson et al., 1993). While it is certainly plausible that religious doubts can cause personal growth, enhance insights, and foster new ways of viewing one's self and the world, it seems *more* plausible that doubts can have negative consequences for health – especially because of their link to cognitive dissonance (Festinger, 1957). Two opposing ideas often create psychic tension and an array of unpleasant emotions that can undermine well-being.

Taken together, these competing hypotheses about the positive and negative implications of religious doubt are provocative. Unfortunately, evidence is thin. Using a variety of interviewing techniques with older adults, Krause and his team extracted ideas from research participants' own words to generate religious-based concepts (Krause, 2006; Krause et al., 1999; Krause and Wulff, 2004). They then used this information to craft survey questions about religious beliefs, experiences, and practices. Religious doubt was one theme (among many) that emerged. Krause and his team then constructed a set of survey items around this theme, including how frequently individuals have *doubts about* (1) their faith; (2) the things they learn in church (most participants were Christian); (3) whether or not the solutions to problems in life may be found in the *Bible*; and (4) whether or not prayers make a difference.

Krause and his collaborators' discoveries about religious doubt provide clues about the complex nature of relationships with the divine and the ways that relationship may represent a stressor. For example, their studies have documented people who report religious doubts also experience more frequent symptoms of depression, including feeling sad, blue, and depressed (Krause, 2006). They also reported more frequent somatic symptoms of distress, like having difficulty sleeping, having a poor appetite, and feeling low levels of energy (Krause and Wulff, 2004).

Structural location and statuses seem to matter in these processes. Earlier work by Krause and his colleagues (1999) also found that age functions as a contingency such that the link between religious doubt and psychological distress is stronger among younger adults. Krause (2006) has also observed that education functions as an effect modifier such that religious doubt is associated with a *decline* in life satisfaction, self-esteem, and optimism among older adults with lower levels of education. By contrast, religious doubts appear to be unrelated to changes in those indicators of well-being among well-educated older adults. Moreover, Krause found that, "compared to older people with high education, older adults with less education are more likely to feel that having doubts about religion is wrong; they are more likely to try to deny or repress doubts when they arise; and they are less likely to forgive themselves when they encounter doubts about their faith" (pp. 298–299). Collectively, these important preliminary findings reveal that religious doubts seem to matter for mental health and subjective well-being – although as the stress process indicates (McLeod and Nonnemaker, 1999), the patterns are contingent upon core social statuses and dimensions of stratification.

BELIEFS ABOUT GOD AND PERSONAL RESOURCES

The debate: does religion have positive or negative influences on personal resources?

Social and psychological resources – especially those closely aligned with the self-concept like the sense of personal control (or mastery), self-esteem, and the sense of mattering – mediate and/or moderate the links between stressors and psychological functioning (Pearlin, 1999). Numerous studies have established the relevance of these resources for helping individuals avoid or manage the consequences of stress (Taylor and Turner, 2001; Turner and Roszell, 1994; Wheaton, 1985). While these concepts are often related empirically, some evidence suggests that each has important *independent* influences on the stress–distress association (Turner and Lloyd, 1999). Given the relevance of these resources, it is essential to understand the conditions that shape them and their influence on mental health; beliefs about God may be among the most potentially important of those conditions.

Some discussions of the positive mental health benefits of religious involvement underscore the ways that religion may increase feelings of self-esteem and the sense of control (Ellison et al., 2001). One core theoretical aspect of this association entails the nature of individuals' personal relationship with God. As I mentioned above, orthodox Christian theology socializes followers to believe in a God who is personally concerned about and involved in believers' everyday lives (Watson et al., 1988). These beliefs, along with the belief in a loving, personal God who created humans in His image, may enhance the sense of purpose, self-worth, and intrinsic significance (Ellison, 1991; Pollner, 1989).

One hypothesis predicts that religious beliefs mediate the association between religious involvement and personal resources. More specifically, participation in religious activities may encourage the development, maintenance, and enhancement of a personal relationship with God (Ellison, 1991; Pollner, 1989; Wikstrom, 1987). These exchanges with the divine, in conjunction with exposure to religious texts, can provide individuals with support, guidance, and the sense of divine control over future events and outcomes. Across a variety of disciplines, some have speculated about the ways that religious activities and beliefs inculcate the sense of order, meaning, and coherence about the world (Antonovsky, 1987; Berger, 1967; Idler, 1987). Thus, repeated exposure to religious messages in frequent participation may enhance beliefs that, in turn, influence personal resources. As the stress process model suggests, these personal resources have consequences for mental health and well-being.

The sense of personal control

The sense of personal control is a learned, generalized expectancy that is largely shaped by objective social conditions (Mirowsky and Ross, 2003). Individuals who possess a high sense of control perceive that, in general, they determine the positive and negative events and outcomes in their lives. By contrast, individuals with a low sense of control – also referred to as an *external sense of control* – tend to cluster at the other end of the continuum, experiencing higher levels of personal powerlessness, and the sense that chance, luck, fate, or powerful others dictate the direction and outcomes of their lives (Ross and Sastry, 1999). The sense of control shares conceptual ground with other constructs like mastery, self-efficacy, locus of control, and instrumentalism (Pearlin and Schooler, 1978; Rotter, 1966; Wheaton, 1985).

Are beliefs about God associated with the sense of personal control? One of the most provocative issues involves the influence of beliefs in divine control. Two hypotheses help frame the core arguments about that association: the "relinquished control" and the "personal empowerment" hypotheses. The *relinquished control* hypothesis predicts that individuals who profess divine control beliefs should tend to report a *lower* sense of personal control compared to those who do not maintain such beliefs. This hypothesis evolves from a tradition in which, according to Jackson and Coursey (1988: 399), "a common secular perspective on religion assumes that believing God is an active agent in one's life requires relinquishing a sense of personal or internal control." Conceptual specifications of the *external* pole of Rotter's (1966) I–E scale differentiate the "chance" and "powerful other" dimensions from the "God control" dimension (Jackson and Coursey, 1988; Levenson, 1974; Kopplin, 1976). Despite this distinction, Mirowsky and Ross (2003) argue that the external attribution of control to God acts "as a logical opposite of internal control: either I control my life or control rests elsewhere" (p. 201). Ceding control to a powerful other contradicts a central conceptual tenet of personal control theory: The individual – *not a powerful other* – determines the important events, outcomes, and direction of their own lives. If we can assume that the causal attribution to God represents processes similar to attributions to other external forces (e.g., powerful others), then individuals who believe in divine control should tend to report a low sense of personal control. Moreover, the reliance on or deference to God's causal influence may erode feelings of personal agency because it detracts from problem-solving efforts (Ellison, 1993). Pargament (1997) identifies this as deferential coping in which one relies on an omnipotent God to solve their problems for them. Summarizing these ideas, Ellison (1991) has argued that "divine relations may reduce worry or self-blame by encouraging individuals to cede psychological control of problematic situations that appear irreconcilable, or to attribute responsibility for particularly difficult life events to a divine other" (p. 81).

As an alternative to the relinquished control view, the *personal empowerment* hypothesis posits that beliefs about God's involvement and causal relevance enhances the sense of coherence and meaning that, in turn, enables the faithful to more readily reconcile life's uncertainties. These factors should contribute favorably to the sense of control. Central tenets of Judeo-Christian theology socialize that individuals can *collaborate* with God to navigate and solve the adversities of life (Pargament, 1997) – a form of divine interaction that may enhance the sense of personal agency. Common notions that proclaim that "God is my co-pilot" and "All things are possible through Christ" imply personally empowering forms of divine intervention. The highly interactive and exchange orientation embedded in the collaborative coping style suggests that individuals are cognizant of God's personal involvement and guidance (Wikström, 1987). While it is plausible that some individuals rely upon God as an *external* source in order to feel a sense of

personal control, there is evidence that devout religious belief is related positively to feelings of internal control *even if* these processes involve the sense that
God is a highly involved and influential agent (Ellison and Taylor, 1996; Maton,
1989; Pargament et al., 1990). Thus, God's "gift of free will" may be viewed as
the "ultimate enabler" for the sense of personal control (Jackson and Coursey,
1988). As Pargament (1997: 468) observes, the knowledge that believers "can
call on God for help and knowing that God is on their side would not diminish
their sense of efficacy and mastery. It would enhance it." The key distinction is
that, unlike the deferring orientation, individuals who adhere to a collaborative
style perceive God as a partner in navigating life's adversities.

The relinquished control and personal empowerment hypotheses both seem
plausible; to date, most research has generated inconclusive observations. Studies
have documented negative (Pargament et al., 1982), positive (DeVellis et al.,
1988; Jackson and Coursey, 1988; Silvestri, 1979), or null associations (Benson
and Spilka, 1973; Ritzema, 1979) between various measures of God-related
control and the sense of personal control (or similar) measures. These mixed
findings are likely due to wide-ranging differences in methodologies. For example,
many of these studies cited above focus solely on undergraduate students –
sometimes at universities in more conservative Christian regions of the United
States. Others have focused specifically on highly religious samples such as
Baptist fundamentalist African Americans. Moreover, prior studies may be
inconclusive because they do not assess other aspects of the religious role as
contingencies.[2]

In an effort to address these limitations, I recently examined data from a 2005
survey of working Americans (Schieman, 2008). My observations generally support the relinquished control hypothesis: individuals who believe in divine control tend to report significantly lower levels of personal control. However, I also
found that the strength of that association is contingent upon three dimensions of
the religious role: subjective religiosity, the frequency of praying, and the frequency of attending religious services. Specifically, the negative association
between divine control beliefs and personal control is stronger among individuals who report low levels of subjective religiosity and less frequent praying and
attendance activity. By contrast, divine control and personal control are unrelated
among individuals who are more deeply invested in and committed to the
religious role. Thus, individuals who belief that God is a causal agent in their
lives – but who do not simultaneously engage in other core elements of the
religious role – tend to report the lowest levels of personal control.

These findings address Mirowsky and Ross's (2003) claim that the external
attribution of control to God acts "as a logical opposite of internal control: either
I control my life or control rests elsewhere" (p. 200). The mental representations
associated with the sense of divine control contradict a core feature of personal
control theory: The individual – not a powerful other – determines events and
outcomes in his or her own life. Is the causal attribution of life events and
outcomes to God simply the *same* as the attribution to other external forces such

as luck, chance, family background, and other people? If it were, then believers in divine control should have the lowest levels of personal control. My findings suggest some support for this pattern, but only among individuals who were not devoted to other dimensions of the religious role. By contrast, those who profess the sense of divine control and adhere strongly to the participatory features of the religious role report levels of personal control similar to nonbelievers. For them, causal attributions to God may be meaningfully distinct from strictly external attributions and may represent a personally empowering orientation toward God and the adversities of everyday life. These findings parallel those found by Ross (1990): the "belief that one's destiny is in the hands of God had no significant effect on distress" (p. 242).

Self-esteem

Like the sense of personal control, self-esteem is another self-concept that is highly relevant in the stress process model (Pearlin, 1999). Self-esteem is "the evaluation which the individual makes and customarily maintains with regard to himself or herself: it expresses an attitude of approval or disapproval toward oneself" (Rosenberg, 1965: 5). Stress researchers have observed that self-esteem is a personal resource because of its potential to help people avoid or manage stressors (Turner and Roszell, 1994). As Rosenberg (1982) has argued, the self – as a social product – develops through interactions with agents of socialization. Religious institutions, with their associated teachings, symbols, and rituals, have provided a core source of socialization across cultures and societies (Sharot, 2001). Thus, it seems plausible that core features of religious involvement, especially belief systems, are influential in the development and maintenance of self-esteem.

In one of the few studies to assess that claim, Ellison (1993) examines data from the National Survey of Black Americans (1979–1980) to assess the link between religious involvement and self-esteem. He observes that "private religious devotion" – as indexed by the frequency of reading religious books or other religious materials, religious television or radio consumption, and personal prayer – is associated with higher levels of self-esteem. Given my discussion above, it is notable that two of those items directly relate to exposure to the messages of religious texts or media. While Ellison's analyses did not include measures of beliefs about God, it is reasonable to suspect that private religious devotion may contribute to beliefs about God's involvement and influence in everyday life (Schieman and Bierman, 2007); in turn, these factors may contribute to self-esteem. Similarly, Krause (2005) provides a compelling argument for a positive association between belief in *God-mediated control* and self-esteem:

> As social psychologists have argued for decades, feelings of self-worth arise from reflected appraisals provided by significant others (Cooley, 1902). Many Christians believe that God cares for them and wants to help them in their daily lives. If older people believe God is willing to work together with them, then they are also likely to believe that God loves and

values them. And if people believe that God loves and values them, they are likely to have a strong sense of self-worth. Based on this rationale, it is hypothesized that strong feelings of God-mediated control will be associated with a high sense of self-esteem. (p. 142)

Unfortunately, little is known about the link between beliefs about God and self-esteem in population-based studies. In a nationally representative sample of adults aged 66 and older, Krause (2005) found that individuals with a stronger sense of God-mediated control tend to report higher levels of self-esteem compared to those who did not profess those same beliefs. However, that positive association was substantially stronger among older African-Americans compared to whites. Similarly, my colleagues and I observed that the sense of divine control is associated positively with self-esteem among older adults residing in the metropolitan Washington DC area (Schieman et al., 2005). Moreover, that positive association is especially strong among African-American women. Collectively, these findings make two contributions to the literature on the link between religion and self-esteem: (1) they establish a positive association between beliefs about God as an involved and causally relevant force in everyday life and self-esteem; and (2) they concur with a core thesis of the stress process model: Social statuses are associated with personal resources. Moreover, the patterns shed light on the ways social statuses modify the link between beliefs about God and the self-concept. Taken together, these studies underscore the need to consider gender and race differences. Finally, these patterns suggest that future research might seek to assess the extent that religious beliefs, especially the belief in divine control, function as a mediating link between different forms of religious involvement and self-esteem.

The sense of mattering

My colleagues and I have evaluated the possibility that divine control beliefs are associated with the sense of mattering (Schieman et al., forthcoming). Mattering is defined as "the feeling that others depend upon us, are interested in us, are concerned with our fate, or experience us as an ego-extension" (Rosenberg and McCullough, 1981: 165). This "interpersonal attitude of inferred significance" reflects one's assessment of social exchanges, including the attention, importance, dependence and emotional investment that one receives from and gives to others. Mattering is important because it represents "one of the foundation blocks of psychological well-being" (Pearlin and LeBlanc, 2001: 286). A high degree of mattering is a cognitively favorable state in which an individual perceives that his or her thoughts, feelings, and actions are objects of significance and consequence to others (Elliott et al., 2005). It is linked with higher self-esteem, less depression, and reduced suicide ideation (Elliott et al., 2005; Rosenberg and McCullough, 1981; Taylor and Turner, 2001).

Why would beliefs about God be related to the sense of mattering? Scholars have identified the close, personal relationship with God as the core element of religious life (James 1902/1997). As Smith (2007) observes: "In and beyond the cosmic expanse exists a conscious, engaged, remembering, answering Person who cares deeply about the earth and its frail inhabitants … Everything existent is already held in the lovingly cupped hands of a personal, attentive God who listens, who knows, who remembers, who answers, who is coming home and who will in time make all things right" (p. 168). Likewise, ideas from attachment theory suggest that God symbolizes for many people a "secure base" that, in many respects, represents the *ultimate* friend and source of social support (Kirkpatrick, 2005; Taylor et al., 2004). For many, there is an effort to develop and maintain a relationship with God that parallels relations with other people (Ellison and Taylor, 1996; Pollner, 1989).

Numerous scriptural stories and parables in the Christian tradition contain messages about the virtues of helping others and the importance of empathy and compassion (Ellison, 1992, 1993; Krause et al., 2002). As Pargament (1997) has argued, "almost every tradition espouses some form of the Golden Rule that, in one way or another, people must care for the well-being of others just as we care for ourselves because God cares for us all" (p. 57). Individuals may learn about God's expectations for the exchange of socially supportive behaviors through the identification with religious figures in these stories (Ellison and Taylor, 1996; Pollner, 1989). Some research also suggests that individuals who profess a belief in an active, involved God tend to express a more altruistic, prosocial orientation compared to those who do not hold these beliefs (Pargament, 1997). There is a sense that God often works through people. That is, God directs human activity, provides what we need, including social and personal relationships that emerge to offer assistance, information, solace, and so on. God guides prosocial activities within religious communities, and inclines others to be generous and helpful. This belief that God will provide and protect can foster trust in others, within families and congregations (Krause et al., 2002); thus, the faithful may be more prone to experience the good in others, to view their relationships through rose-colored glasses. That may help to explain why some evidence shows that "religious people are nice people" (Morgan, 1983; Ellison, 1992).

Our evidence supports these ideas by showing that divine control beliefs are among the strongest predictors of levels of mattering, net of other forms of religious involvement (Schieman et al., forthcoming). Moreover, divine control beliefs are relevant in linking these forms of religious involvement to mattering. Specifically, among a sample of older adults, our findings indicate indirect effects of religious attendance on mattering through divine control beliefs. Praying increases mattering indirectly only through divine control beliefs. Moreover, divine control beliefs are more strongly associated with mattering among women, African-Americans, and individuals with less education. Collectively, these observations about mattering suggest that beliefs about God's involvement and causal relevance in everyday life has important implications for a key psychosocial resource, although as is the case for self-esteem and mastery, the patterns are contingent upon social statuses and dimensions of stratification.

CONCLUDING THOUGHTS

In this chapter, I have sought to underscore at least two things: (1) the importance of religion's complicated influence on stress, psychosocial resources, and mental health processes; and (2) the ways that discoveries in research on the stress process can stimulate new questions and insights that span beyond the bounds of stress-specific research. In sum, given the clear positive association between being highly devoted and committed to the religious role and the profession of belief in God as a causal agent, I argue that any analyses of the interrelationships among religious involvement, stressors, personal resources, and mental health should attempt to carefully take these religious beliefs into account. Their potential influence will likely be discovered at multiple points in the stress process. According to Linda George and her colleagues (2002), "science cannot tell us whether God heals, but it can tell us whether belief in God affects health" (p. 198). I have sought to provide an overall sketch of these ideas here by drawing more specific attention to the nature or content of individuals' beliefs about God – especially God's involvement and causal influence in everyday life.

NOTES

1 In the World Values Survey (WVS) of more than 50 countries from all continents including Great Britain and the United States, study participants were asked: 'Independently of whether you go to [church] or not, would you say you are *a religious person*?' Collectively, 70 percent of the roughly 80,000 participants worldwide described themselves as a 'religious person', while 25 percent said they were not religious. Only 5 percent self-identified as 'a convinced atheist'. Similarly, the level of religious salience is quite high: 72 percent of WVS participants report that religion is 'very important' or 'rather important' in their lives. In addition, although it is clearly less robust than other indicators, religious practice is also higher than many people might suspect. Study participants were asked: 'Apart from weddings, funerals and christenings, about how often do you attend religious services these days?' Roughly 46 percent of participants reported that they attend religious services at least monthly; 35 percent attend at least weekly. Based on this evidence, I submit that we would be hard-pressed to find *any other form of social activity* that so many people across the globe do as frequently.

2 For example, in highly religious samples it is difficult to delineate the contingent effects of the religious role because these dimensions are mostly invariant. Simply put, the samples are too homogenous with respect to religious role dimensions such as subjective religiosity, frequency of praying, and attendance.

REFERENCES

Alvarado, K.A., Templer, D.I., Bresler, C., and Thomas-Dobson, S. (1995) The relationship of religious variables to death depression and death anxiety. *Journal of Clinical Psychology,* 51: 202–204.

Antonovsky, A. (1987) *Unraveling the Mystery of Health.* San Francisco, CA: Jossey-Bass.

Armstrong, K. (1993) *A History of God: The 4,000-Year Quest of Judaism, Christianity and Islam.* New York: Ballantine Books.

Batson, C.D., Schoenrade, P., and Ventis, W.L. (1993) *Religion and the Individual.* New York: Oxford University Press.

Benore, E.R. and Park, C.L. (2004) 'Death-specific religious beliefs and bereavement: belief in an afterlife and continued attachment'. *International Journal for the Psychology of Religion,* 14: 1–22.

Benson, P. and Spilka, B. (1973) God image as a function of self-esteem and locus of control. *Journal for the Scientific Study of Religion,* 12: 297–310.

Berger, P. (1967) *The Sacred Canopy.* Garden City, NY: Doubleday.

Berrenberg, J.L. (1987) The belief in personal control scale: A measure of God-mediated and exaggerated control. *Journal of Personality Assessment,* 51: 194–206.

Black, H.K. [1999] Poverty and Prayer: Spiritual narratives of elderly African-American women. Review of Religious Research, 40: 357–74.

Branden, N. (1994). *The Six Pillars of Self-Esteem.* New York: Bantam Books.

Dawkins, R. (2006) *The God Delusion.* Boston: Houghton Mifflin.

DeVellis, B.M., DeVellis, R.F., and Spilsbury, J.C. (1988) Parental actions when children are sick: the role of belief in divine influence. *Basic and Applied Social Psychology,* 9: 185–96.

Durkheim, E. ([1897] 1951) *Suicide.* New York: Free Press.

Elliott, G.C., Colangelo, M., and Gelles, R.J. (2005). Mattering and suicide ideation: establishing and elaborating a relationship. *Social Psychology Quarterly,* 68: 223–238.

Ellis, A. (1962) *Reason and Emotion in Psychotherapy.* Secaucus, NJ: Citadel Press.

Ellis, A. (1980) Psychotherapy and atheistic values: a response to A.E. Bergin's 'Psychotherapy and Religious Values'. *Journal of Consulting and Clinical Psychology,* 48: 635–639.

Ellis, A. (1988) Is religiosity pathological?. *Free Inquiry,* 8: 27–32.

Ellison, C.G. (1991) Religious involvement and subjective well-being, *Journal of Health and Social Behavior,* 32: 80–99.

Ellison, C.G. (1992) Are religious people nice people? Evidence from the National Survey of Black Americans. *Social Forces,* 71: 411–430.

Ellison, C.G. (1993) Religious involvement and self-perception among Black Americans. *Social Forces,* 71: 1027–1055.

Ellison, C.G. (1994) Religion, the life stress paradigm, and the study of depression. In J.S. Levin (ed.) *Religion in Aging and Health.* Thousand Oaks: SAGE.

Ellison, C.G. and George, L.K. (1994) Religious involvement, social ties, and social support in a southeastern community. *Journal for the Scientific Study of Religion,* 33: 46–61.

Ellison, C.G. and Sherkat, D.E. (1995) Is sociology the core discipline for the scientific study of religion?. *Social Forces,* 73: 1255–1266.

Ellison, C.G. and Taylor, R.J. (1996) Turning to prayer: Social and situational antecedents of religious coping among African Americans. *Review of Religious Research,* 38: 111–131.

Ellison, C.G. and Levin, J.S. (1998) The religion-health connection: Evidence, theory, and future directions. *Health Education and Behavior,* 25: 700–720.

Ellison, C.G., Boardman, J.D., Williams, D.R., and Jackson, J.S. (2001) Religious involvement, stress, and mental health: Findings from the 1995 Detroit Area Study. *Social Forces,* 80: 215–249.

Ellison, C.G., Burdette, A.M. and Hill, T.D. (2009) Blessed assurance: religion, anxiety, and tranquility among US adults. *Social Science Research,* 38: 656–667.

Festinger, L. (1957) *A Theory of Cognitive Dissonance.* Stanford, CA: Stanford University Press.

Flannelly, K.J., Koenig, H.G., Ellison, C.G., Galek, K., and Krause, N. (2006) Belief in life after death and mental health: Findings from a national survey. *Journal of Nervous and Mental Disease,* 194: 524–529.

Flannelly, K.J., Ellison, C.G., Galek, K. and Koenig, H.G. (2008) Beliefs about life-after-death, psychiatric symptomology, and cognitive theories of psychopathology. *Journal of Psychology and Theology,* 36: 94–103.

Foley, D.P. (1988) Eleven interpretations of personal suffering. *Journal of Religion and Health,* 27: 321–328.

Freud, S. (1976) *The Future of an Illusion,* edited by J. Strachey. New York: Norton, W.W. & Company, Inc.

Froese, P. and Bader, C.D. (2007) God in America: Why theology is not simply the concern of philosophers. *Journal for the Scientific Study of Religion,* 46: 465–481.

Galek, K., Krause, N., Ellison, C.G., Kudler, T., and Flannelly, K.J. (2007) Religious doubt and mental health across the life span. *Journal of Adult Development,* 14: 16–25.

George, L.K., Ellison, C.G., and Larson, D.B. (2002) Explaining the relationships between religious involvement and health. *Psychological Inquiry*, 13: 190–200.

Glock, C.Y. and Stark, R. (1965) *Religion and Society in Tension*. Chicago: Rand McNally and Company.

Green, J.C., Guth, J.L., Smidt, C.E., and Kellstedt, L.A. (1996) *Religion and the Culture Wars: Dispatches from the Front*. Lanham, MD: Rowman & Littlefield.

Hackney, C.H. and Sanders, G.S. (2003) Religiosity and mental health: A meta-analysis of recent studies. *Journal for the Scientific Study of Religion*, 42: 43–55.

Harris, S. (2004) *The End of Faith: Religion, Terror, and the Future of Reason*. New York: W.W. Horton and Company.

Hecht, J.M. (2003) *Doubt: A History*. San Francisco: Harper San Francisco.

Hitchens, C. (2007) *God is not Great: How Religion Poisons Everything*. Toronto: McClelland & Stewart.

Holmes, T.R., and Rahe, R.H. (1967) The social readjustment rating scale. *Journal of Psychosomatic Research*, 2: 213–218.

Hunsberger, B., McKenzie, B., Pratt, M., and Prancer, S.M. (1993) Religious doubt: A social psychological analysis. *Research in the Social Scientific Study of Religion*, 5: 27–51.

Idler, E.L. (1987) Religious involvement and the health of the elderly: Some hypotheses and an initial test. *Social Forces*, 66: 226–238.

Idler, E.L. (1995) Religion, health, and nonphysical senses of self. *Social Forces*, 74: 683–704.

Jackson, L.E. and Coursey, R.D. (1988) The relationship of God control and internal locus of control to intrinsic religious motivation, coping and purpose in life. *Journal for the Scientific Study of Religion*, 27: 399–410.

James, W. ([1902] 1999) *The Varieties of Religious Experience*. New York: Modern Library.

Kirkpatrick, L. A. (2005) *Attachment, Evolution, and the Psychology of Religion*. New York: Guilford.

Koenig, H.G., George, L.K., Blazer, D.G., Pritchett, J.T., and Meador, K.G. (1993) The relationship between religion and anxiety in a sample of community-dwelling older adults. *Journal of Geriatric Psychiatry*, 26: 65–93.

Koenig, H.G., McCullough, M., and Larson, D.B. (2001) *Handbook of Religion and Health*. New York: Oxford University Press.

Kopplin, D. (1976) Religious orientations of college students and related personality characteristics. Paper presented at *American Psychological Association*. Washington, D.C.

Krause, N. (1995) Religiosity and self-esteem among older adults. *Journal of Gerontology*, 50: 236–246.

Krause, N. (2002) Church-based social support and health in old age: Exploring variations by race. *Journal of Gerontology: Social Sciences*, 57B: S332–S347.

Krause, N. (2003) Religious meaning and subjective well-being in late life. *Journal of Gerontology: Social Sciences*, 58B: S160–S170.

Krause, N. (2005) God-mediated control and psychological well-being in late life. *Research on Aging*, 27: 136–164.

Krause, N. (2006) Religious doubt and psychological well-being: A longitudinal investigation. *Review of Religious Research*, 47: 287–302.

Krause, N. (2007) Social involvement in religious institutions and God-mediated control beliefs: a longitudinal investigation. *Journal for the Scientific Study of Religion*, 46: 519–537.

Krause, N. and Wulff, K.M. (2004) Religious doubt and health: Exploring the potential dark side of religion. *Sociology of Religion*, 65: 35–56.

Krause, N., Ingersoll-Dayton, B., Ellison, C.G., and Wulff, K.M. (1999) Aging, religious doubt, and psychological well-being. *The Gerontologist*, 39: 525–533.

Krause, N., Ellison, C.G., and Marcum, J.P. (2002) The effects of church-based emotional support on health: Do they vary by gender?. *Sociology of Religion*, 63: 21–47.

Levenson, H. (1974) Activism and powerful others: Distinctions within the concept of internal–external control. *Journal of Personality Assessment*, 38: 377–383.

Lindbeck, G.A. (1984) *The Nature of Doctrine: Religion and Theology in a Postliberal Age*. Louisville, Kentucky: Westminster John Knox Press.

Maton, K. (1989) The stress-buffering role of spiritual support: Cross-sectional and prospective investigations. *Journal for the Scientific Study of Religion,* 28: 310–323.

Marx, K. and Engels, F. ([1878] 1964) *On Religion*. New York: Schoken Books.

McConnell, K.M., Pargament, K.I., Ellison, C.G., and Flannelly, K.J. (2006) Examining the links between spiritual struggles and symptoms of psychopathology in a national sample. *Journal of Clinical Psychology,* 62: 1469–1484.

McLeod, J.D., and Nonnemaker, J.M. (1999) Social stratification and inequality. In C.S. Aneshensel and J.C. Phelan (eds), *Handbook of the Sociology of Mental Health*. New York: Kluwer Academic/Plenum. pp. 321–344.

Miles, J. (1995) *God: A Biography*. New York: Vintage Books.

Mirowsky, J. and Ross, C.E. (2003) *Social Causes of Psychological distress*, 2nd edition. Hawthorne, New York: Aldine De Gruyter.

Morgan, S.P. (1983) A research note on religion and mortality: Are religious people nice people?. *Social Forces,* 61: 683–692.

Park, C.L. and Folkman, S. (1997) Meaning in the context of stress and coping. *Review of General Psychology,* 1:115–144.

Pargament, K.I. (1997) *The Psychology of Religion and Coping*. New York: Guilford Press.

Pargament, K.I. (2002) The bitter and the sweet: An evaluation of the costs and benefits of religiousness. *Psychological Inquiry,* 13: 168–181.

Pargament, K.I., Sullivan, M.S., Tyler, F.B. and Steele, R.E. (1982) Patterns of attribution of control and individual psychosocial competence: *Psychological Reports*, 51: 1243–1252.

Pargament, K.I., Ensing, D.S., Falgout, K., Olsen, H., Reilly, B., Van Haitsma, K. and Warren, R. (1990) God help me (I): Religious coping efforts as predictors of the outcomes to significant negative life events. *American Journal of Community Psychology*, 18: 793–824.

Pearlin, L.I. (1999) The stress process revisited: Reflections on concepts and their Interrelationships. In C.S. Aneshensel and J.C. Phelan (eds) *Handbook of the Sociology of Mental Health*. New York: Kluwer Academic/Plenum. pp. 105–123.

Pearlin, L.I. and LeBlanc, A. (2001) Bereavement and the loss of Mattering. In T.J. Owens, S. Stryker and N. Goodman (eds) *Extending Self-Esteem Theory and Research*. New York: Cambridge University Press.

Pearlin, L.I. and Schooler, C. (1978) The structure of coping. *Journal of Health and Social Behavior,* 19: 2–21.

Phillips, R. III. and Stein, C.H. (2007) God's will, God's punishment, or God's limitations? Religious coping strategies reported by young adults living with serious mental illness. *Journal of Clinical Psychology*, 63: 529–540.

Pollner, M. (1989) Divine relations, social relations, and well-being. *Journal of Health and Social Behavior,* 30: 92–104.

Prothero, S. (2007) *Religious Literacy: What Every American Needs to Know – and Doesn't*. San Francisco: Harper Collins.

Ritzema, R.J. (1979) Attribution to supernatural causation: An important component of religious commitment?. *Journal of Psychology and Theology,* 7: 286–293.

Roberts, M.K. and Davidson, J.D. (1984) The nature and sources of religious involvement. *Review of Religious Research*, 25: 334–350.

Rosenberg, M. (1965) *Society and the Adolescent Self-Image*. Princeton, NJ: Princeton University Press.

Rosenberg, M. (1982) The self-concept: social product and social force. In M. Rosenberg and R. H. Turner (eds). *Social Psychology: Sociological Perspectives*. New Brunswick, NJ: Transaction Publishers.

Rosenberg, M. and McCullough, B.C. (1981) Mattering: inferred significance and mental health among adolescents. *Research in Community and Mental Health*, 2: 163–182.

Ross, C.E. (1990) Religion and psychological distress. *Journal for the Scientific Study of Religion,* 29: 236–245.

Ross, C.E. and Sastry, J. (1999) The sense of personal control: Social-structural causes and emotional consequences. In Carol S. Aneshensel and Jo C. Phelan (eds). *Handbook of the Sociology of Mental Health.* New York: Kluwer. pp. 369–394.

Rotter, J.B. (1966) Generalized expectancies for internal vs. external control of reinforcements. *Psychological Monographs,* 80: 1–28.

Schieman, S. (2008) The religious role and the sense of personal control. *Sociology of Religion,* 69: 273–96.

Schieman, S. and Bierman, A. (2007) Religious activities and changes in the sense of divine control: dimensions of stratification as contingencies. *Sociology of Religion,* 68: 361–81.

Schieman, S., Pudrovska, T. and Milkie, M.A. (2005) The sense of divine control and the self-concept: a study of race differences in late-life. *Research on Aging,* 27: 165–96.

Schieman, S., Pudrovska, T., Pearlin, L.I., and Ellison, C.G. (2006) The sense of divine control and psychological distress: Variations by race and socioeconomic status. *Journal for the Scientific Study of Religion,* 45: 529–50.

Schieman, S., Alex B., and Christopher G.E., forthcoming. Religious Involvement, Beliefs about God, and the Sense of Mattering among Older Adults. *Journal for the Scientific Study of Religion.*

Schoenrade, P. (1989) When I die .... Belief in afterlife as a response to mortality. *Personality and Social Psychology Bulletin,* 15: 91–100.

Schuchter, S.R. (1986) *Dimensions of Grief: Adjusting to the Death of a Spouse.* San Francisco: Jossey-Bass.

Sharot, S. (2001) *A Comparative Sociology of World Religions: Virtuosos, Priests, and Popular Religion.* New York: New York University Press.

Silvestri, P.J. (1979) Locus of control and God-dependence. *Psychological Reports,* 45: 89–90.

Simmel, G. (1997) *Essays on Religion.* New Haven: Yale University Press.

Smith, C. (2007) Why Christianity works: An emotions-focused phenomenological account. *Sociology of Religion,* 68: 165–78.

Stark, R. (2001) *One True God: Historical Consequences of Monotheism.* Princeton: Princeton University Press.

Stark, R. (2007) *Discovering God: The Origins of the Great Religions and the Evolution of Belief.* New York: Harper.

Stark, R. (2008) *What Americans Really Believe.* Waco, Texas: Baylor University Press.

Stark, R. and Finke R. (2000) *Acts of faith: Explaining the human side of religion.* Berkely, CA: University of California Press.

Stark, R. and Glock, C.Y. (1968) *American Piety: The Nature of Religious Commitment.* Berkeley: University of California Press.

Taylor, J. and Turner, R.J. (2001) A longitudinal study of the role and significance of mattering to others for depressive symptoms. *Journal of Health and Social Behavior,* 42: 310–325.

Taylor, J.T., Chatters, L.M., and Levin, J. (2004) *Religion in the Lives of African Americans: Social, Psychological, and Health Perspectives.* Thousand Oaks: SAGE.

Tillich, P. (1957) *The Dynamics of Faith.* New York: Harper and Brothers.

Turner, R.J., and Lloyd, D.A. (1999) The stress process and the social distribution of stress. *Journal of Health and Social Behavior,* 40: 374–404.

Turner, R.J. and Roszell, P. (1994) Psychosocial resources and the stress process. In William R. Avison and Ian H. Gotlib (eds) *Stress and Mental Health: Contemporary Issues and Prospects for the Future.* New York: Plenum Press. pp. 179–210.

Turner, R.J., Wheaton, B., and Lloyd, D.A. (1995) The epidemiology of social stress. *American Sociological Review,* 60: 104–125.

Trice, P.D. and Bjork, J.P. (2006) Pentecostal perspectives on causes and cures of depression. *Professional Psychology: Research and Practice* 37: 283–294.

Watson, P.J., Morris, R.J., and Hood, R.W. Jr. (1988) Sin and self functioning, part 1: Grace, guilt, and self consciousness. *Journal of Psychology and Theology,* 16: 270–281.

Watters, W. (1992) *Deadly Doctrine: Health, Illness, and Christian God-talk*. Buffalo, NY: Prometheus.

Weber, M. ([1922] 1963) *The Sociology of Religion*. Boston: Beacon Press.

Welton, G.L., Adkins, G.A., Ingle, S.L., and Dixon, W.A. (1996) God control: the fourth dimension. *Journal of Psychology and Theology*, 24:13–25.

Wheaton, B. (1985) Models for the stress-buffering functions of coping resources. *Journal of Health and Social Behavior*, 26: 352–364.

Wheaton, B. (1999) Social stress. In C.S. Aneshensel and J.C. Phelan (eds), *Handbook of the Sociology of Mental Health*. New York: Kluwer Academic/Plenum Publishers.pp. 277–300.

Wikstrom, O. (1987) Attribution, roles, and religion: A theoretical analysis of Sunden's role theory and the attributional approach to religious experience. *Journal for the Scientific Study of Religion*, 26: 390–400.

Wills, G. (2007) *Head and Heart: American Christianities*. New York: Penguin.

Wilson, B. (1982) *Religion in Sociological Perspective*. Oxford: Oxford University Press.

Woodberry, R.D. and Smith, C. (1998) Fundamentalism et al.: Conservative Protestants in America, *Annual Review of Sociology*. Palo Alto, CA: Annual Reviews.

10

Children, Culture and Mental Illness: Public Knowledge and Stigma Toward Childhood Problems

Brea Perry and
Bernice A. Pescosolido

INTRODUCTION

Epidemiological and services research over the last two decades has documented that children's and adolescents' mental health problems are under-recognized and under-treated. Recent estimates indicate that, in any given year, one-fifth of US children have mental health disorders, and one in twenty experience extreme functional impairment. According to the US President's New Freedom Commission on Mental Health (U.S. Department of Health & Human Services, 1999: 58), 'no other illness damages so many children so seriously'. Despite the serious consequences associated with childhood mental disorders, less than one in three children and adolescents with recognizable disorders receive treatment.

Reports suggest relatively equivalent situations in the US and the UK. Both Costello et al.'s (1996) US study and McArdle et al.'s study (2004) Newcastle-upon-Tyne reported a 6–7 per cent rate for severe behavioural disorders. Other statistics from the UK are less dire, but nonetheless troubling since available studies suggest that British children have lower levels of well-being than others in the EU (Cole, 2006) and the Children's Society Report (Layard and Dunn, 2009) expressed concern about reports of rising rates of mental health problems. According to Hitchen (2006) and the 1999 Bristol Child and Adolescent Mental Health Survey (Ford et al., 2003), one in two children in the UK experience some mental health problem, with poorer children at greatest risk (see also Meltzer et al., 2003 on a 10 per cent estimate similar to that in the US). Considerable delay accompanies the use of services (Sayal, 2004) and as Stiffman et al. (2004) document in the US, children enter through many 'gateway' providers (see also Vostanis et al., 2003). According to a House of Commons Report, services and access were both equally inadequate (House of Commons Health Committee, 1997).

There has been a resurgence of research on the public's knowledge and attitudes toward adults' mental health problems in the past decade. Perhaps not surprisingly, the findings from major survey efforts in the Western world revealed many similarities (Angermeyer et al., 1987; Crisp et al., 2000; Pescosolido et al., 2000; Stuart and Arboleda-Florez, 2001). These studies have reported public beliefs on how individuals in the community differentiate between mental health disorders such as schizophrenia, depression and substance abuse; see their under-lying causes as distinct; and call for very different treatments. While a substantial portion of these populations reported adequate knowledge about and recognition of mental health problems, the majority also endorsed stigmatizing attitudes (Pescosolido et al., 2008b). Moreover, study results have often contradicted the commonly-held wisdom that stigma associated with these disorders has decreased in the US (Pescosolido et al., submitted). These findings provided critical new information for major policy statements and on-going stigma reduction campaigns (e.g. the WPA's Open the Doors campaign; Sartorius, 1998).

Unfortunately, a parallel effort has been lacking in providing critical public information on the situation of children's mental health problems in the US and in other countries. British researchers report similar concerns about unmet need among children and adolescents (Singh, 2009), particularly for newly arrived ethnic groups (Dogra et al., 2007), as well as unease about the effectiveness and quality of services in primary care settings (Day and Davis, 2006). However, few studies have targeted community awareness and response.

Concerns about parents' and providers' lack of recognition and treatment referral have resulted in a call to promote public awareness of children's mental health issues. Yet, prior research provides little concrete information to guide those efforts. In particular, it is unclear whether well-described symptom profiles, generally acknowledged to be prototypic of mental disorders, are actually viewed as 'mental illness' by the general public. Are such problems discounted and attrib-uted simply to the problems of growing up, or to physical illnesses? Similarly, we know little about what kinds of advice and treatment the public sees as appropriate for the behavioural problems that children and adolescents confront, whether their reactions are hindered by concerns of stigma, and whether the culture surrounding mental health problems differs across gender, race and education.

In this chapter, we provide information from the first, and to our knowledge, the only nationally representative study of how the public understands, recog-nizes and responds to four different scenarios – children or adolescents meeting criteria for two mental health problems (ADHD and depression), one physical health problem (asthma) and one case of ordinary problems that do not reach clinical criteria. Given the similarity of findings on public reaction to adult mental health problems documented in the US, Canada and the UK, these US data may be useful in a broad sense and, in addition, provide a platform for more research, public discussion and policymaking targeting the mental health concerns facing children, adolescents and their caregivers.

WHY THE LARGER CULTURAL CONTEXT MATTERS

Social science offers an understanding of the community circumstances that surround the onset of mental health problems in children. Research tells us that individuals rarely make decisions about health care on their own. They consult family and friends, neighbours thought to have some relevant expertise, and those in positions of authority (e.g. employers and teachers; Costello et al., 1998; Pescosolido, 1991, 2006; Stiffman et al., 2004). Understanding the larger context in which parents and children/adolescents experience mental health problems, receive advice and decide to seek or avoid treatment is an important first step in addressing the problem of underutilization. It also replaces the often stereotypical assumptions, attitudes and beliefs that practitioners tend to hold unconsciously as members of a society and of a profession that has constructed child health behavioural norms and deviance in a particular way.

   Children with mental illness are susceptible to discrimination and rejection by peers. Evidence suggests that stigmatization begins early. Children as young as five years old report a desire for social distance from people with mental illness relative to other stigmatized groups, and these behavioural tendencies persist through adolescence (Corrigan et al., 2005; Wahl, 2000; Weisz and Weiss, 1991, 1993). Socializing agents like school, media and family also play a key role in attitude development, as negative stereotypes are likely reinforced through interactions with parents, teachers, and peers (Wahl, 1997). Further, children are capable of perceiving symptoms of disorders such as ADHD in same-age peers and recognizing them as abnormal, even in the absence of formal labelling (Bickett and Milich, 1990; Chandra and Minkovitz, 2006; Law et al., 2007; Pelham and Milich, 1984).

   Attitudes toward such children are predominately negative, and these feelings influence peers' willingness to engage in social, physical and academic activities with youth exhibiting symptoms of disorder. Indeed, patterns of nearly immediate peer rejection in youth with psychiatric disorders, particularly ADHD, are well-documented in the psychiatric literature (Milich et al., 1992). Overall, these youth tend to have fewer mutual friends, exhibit difficulty maintaining friendships, and have relationships characterized by high levels of conflict and aggression (Blachman and Hinshaw, 2002). Children tease, avoid and are less friendly toward peers labelled with emotional or behavioural problems, and, in turn, these children reinforce others' dislike by reacting in ways that exacerbate negative attitudes (Milich et al., 1992). In sum, in interactions between children with and without mental illness, negative interpersonal expectancies adversely affect the behaviour and impressions of both participants (Harris et al., 2002).

The data

In the US, a series of stigma studies have been underway since 1996 to provide a representative picture of how the public responds to individuals exhibiting constellations of symptoms aligned with DSM-IV clinical criteria for major mental illness (e.g. schizophrenia, major depression) and substance abuse disorders (e.g. alcohol dependence, drug abuse; see Link et al., 1999; Martin et al., 2000; Pescosolido et al., 1999).

Given the national debates that occurred (and continue to occur) in the United States and Britain surrounding the rise of psychoactive drugs for children and adolescents (Bramble, 2003; McNicholas, 2001; Middleton et al., 2001; Olfson et al., 2003; Safer, 1997; Safer et al., 2003), in 2002 we turned our attention to issues of childhood and adolescent mental health. As before, we chose the US General Social Survey to mount a nationally representative data collection which comprises the National Stigma Study–Children (NSS-C; see text box for technical details).

In order to gauge the public's recognition of mental health disorders, the NSS-C used a vignette strategy, avoiding problems common to stigma research, where it is widely recognized that social desirability interferes with measurement. The public has been sensitized to recognize 'socially acceptable' responses regarding prejudice toward stigmatized groups, including 'those with mental illness'. Thus, in the NSS-C, children's symptoms are described in a story or vignette format, and the child/adolescent is never described as having a mental health problem. Each respondent randomly received only one of the four vignettes. Two vignettes describe children meeting criteria for DSM-IV mental health disorders: (1) Attention Deficit Hyperactivity Disorder (ADHD) and (2) major depression (MD). Two 'control' vignettes describe children with asthma or routine, but subclinical problems (i.e. 'daily troubles' – problems associated with the day-to-day experience of being a child). Asthma was selected both because it is thought to have psychological triggers, and because it does not have clear bodily manifestations (e.g. lesions). The 'daily troubles' vignette provides an analytical baseline.

Results reported may differ marginally from those reported in journal publications due to varying approaches toward handling missing (don't know, refusals) data and rounding differences.

RECOGNITION, ASSESSMENTS OF SEVERITY, AND ATTRIBUTIONS: WHAT DO THEY KNOW?

Figure 10.1 provides data on how the public understands the case scenarios presented to them. Respondents were asked, in separate questions, whether the

THE U.S. NATIONAL STIGMA STUDY – CHILDREN

The NSS-C was fielded as part of the 2002 General Social Survey (GSS) administered by the National Opinion Research Center (NORC) at the University of Chicago. Fielded since 1972, the GSS is one of the premier monitors of American public opinion. To ensure that participants are a nationally representative group, the GSS uses a stratified, multistage area probability sample of clusters of US households. The GSS trains interviewers to visit the selected households and conduct face-to-face interviews. The 2002 GSS included 2,765 non-institutionalized adults living in the contiguous US and was conducted between February and June of 2002. Technically, the GSS segment that makes up the NSS-C is referred to as the 'Children's Mental Health Module'. It included 55 separate questions and occupied 15 minutes on one of the two samples of the 2002 survey for a total of 1,393 individuals who answered NSS-C questions. The response rate for the 2002 GSS was 70 per cent.

In general, GSS samples resemble distribution in the U.S. Census on key socio-demographic variables; the 2002 survey is no exception. Within sampling error, the distribution of GSS NSS-C respondents across demographic categories (race, marital status, place of residence, etc.) is broadly representative of the population of adult Americans. The GSS NSS-C sample mirrors national norms, with an average of 46 years, average education of 13.4 years, an average family income of $50,000, but slightly over-represents women (i.e. 59 per cent women vs. 41 per cent men).

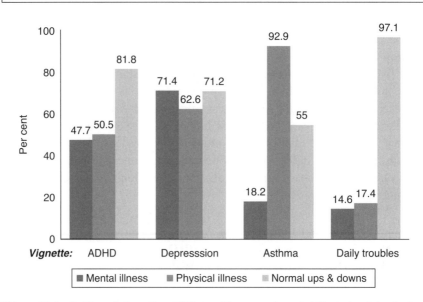

Figure 10.1   Rating of vignette child's problem as a 'mental illness', a 'physical illness' or 'part of the normal ups & downs of childhood', National Stigma Study – Children, 2002

child/adolescent was experiencing a mental illness, a physical illness or just the 'ups and downs' of childhood. Theoretically, they could respond in the affirmative to each possibility. The degree to which they do suggests a lack of clear understanding of the child's situation.

Findings indicate that the public is unclear about the nature of the problem described in the depression vignette. Over 70 per cent (71.4 per cent) of respondents who evaluated the depression vignette defined the child's problem as a mental illness. However, a similarly high proportion saw the problem as nothing more than 'normal ups and downs of childhood' (71.2 per cent), and well over half (62.6 per cent) were willing to characterize this problem as a physical illness. This pattern of uncertainty is less pronounced for those respondents who evaluated the ADHD vignette. In this case, a slight minority (47.7 per cent) described this profile as indicative of a 'mental illness'. A somewhat larger proportion described the ADHD profile as a physical illness (50.5 per cent), while a vast majority (81.8 per cent) of respondents characterized the ADHD child's problems as part-and-parcel of the normal ups and downs of childhood.

The situation is quite different for individuals' characterizations of the two 'control' vignettes. Respondents who were asked to evaluate children described in the asthma and 'daily troubles' conditions were clear and consistent in their assessments of the nature of the problem. Nearly 93 per cent (92.9 per cent) of respondents identified the asthma vignette child as experiencing a physical problem, and 97.1 per cent viewed the 'daily troubles' child as experiencing the normal exigencies of childhood/adolescence. In general, additional analyses (not reported here) indicate that the mental illness label was evoked significantly less frequently by respondents who had achieved higher levels of education (Pescosolido et al., 2007a).

While the public was equivocal on the nature of the scenario, Figure 10. 2 indicates that they were consistent in their assessment of severity. The depression vignette was overwhelmingly seen as a very serious situation (83.6 per cent). While nearly 40 per cent (38.4 per cent) defined the ADHD condition as a very serious problem, a slightly larger proportion (46.0 per cent) viewed this condition as only somewhat serious. The majority of respondents who evaluated the asthma condition defined this as a very serious problem (58.3 per cent). Importantly, only a very small proportion of respondents viewed the 'daily troubles' situation as a very serious problem (3.2 per cent).

The response to these conditions provides some sense that they meaningfully mark how the public understands or does not understand childhood issues, particularly since most viewed the 'daily troubles' case as non-problematic. In a related series of analyses, we found that women and black respondents were significantly more likely to see ADHD and depression as representing a serious problem for the child compared to the 'daily troubles' case. Respondents were also more likely to see ADHD or depression as serious if the condition was described for a younger child, or if they had labeled ADHD or depression as a 'mental illness' (Pescosolido et al., 2007a). Further, and importantly, compared

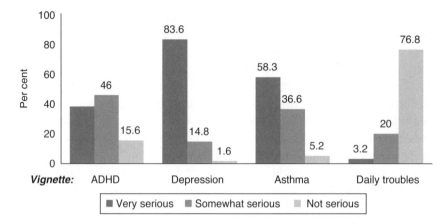

Figure 10.2   Rating of vignette child's problem as 'very', 'somewhat' or 'not serious', National Stigma Study – Children, 2002

to how the public evaluated the severity of depression for adults, depression in children of all ages was viewed as being significantly more serious (Perry et al., 2007).

The NSS-C also asked respondents to endorse the underlying causes or attributions of the behaviours described in the case vignettes. Again, as before, there were no restrictions placed on how many causes the respondents saw at work. As shown in Table 10.1, what is notable in these data is the apparent degree of uncertainty that the US public demonstrated with respect to the causes of the problems experienced by children/adolescents in the ADHD and depression vignettes. While the largest percentage attributed ADHD to stressful circumstances, high percentages of respondents also see ADHD as possibly being the result of a

Table10.1   Percentage of the US public indicating that the vignette child's problem is 'very' or 'somewhat' likely due to each of eight different causes, National Stigma Study – Children, 2002*

	ADHD (%)	Depression (%)	Asthma (%)	Daily troubles (%)
Bad character	40.8	34.5	11.6	33.7
Chemical imbalance	77.7	82.1	38.8	26.3
Stressful circumstances	85.8	96.2	73.5	59.5
Genetics	70.3	70.3	87.0	35.1
Way raised	79.3	79.3	31.4	73.8
TV/Video game Violence	41.5	43.7	14.5	43.1
Lack of discipline	81.3	57.7	17.3	64.4
Allergies	50.2	44.7	85.2	26.1

* Respondents allowed to select more than one possible cause.

lack of discipline (81.3 per cent), the way the child/adolescent was raised (79.3 per cent), and/or a chemical imbalance in the brain (77.7 per cent). Similar levels of uncertainty are evidenced in attributions of the causes of depression. While over 80 per cent (82.1 per cent) attributed depression to a chemical imbalance, nearly 80 per cent (79.3 per cent) pointed to the way the child/adolescent was raised and over 70 per cent (70.3 per cent) also saw genetic bases for depression. Most attributed asthma symptoms to genetic causes (87.0 per cent), and symptoms consistent with 'daily troubles' to the way the child/adolescent was raised (73.8 per cent).

Overall, medical or biological attributions were most likely to be offered as explanations for the depression or asthma conditions. Attributions emphasizing family shortcomings (i.e. lack of discipline, way raised) were likely to be mentioned by more respondents for ADHD. Individual shortcomings, that is, bad character, were also likely to be mentioned by more individuals as the cause of ADHD. In additional analyses not presented in Table 10.1, respondents who labelled ADHD or depression as a 'mental illness' were also at least twice as likely to believe that those behavioural problems were caused by genetic or chemical factors (Pescosolido et al., 2007a).

WHAT WOULD THEY DO?

Following the NSS-C questions on recognition and understanding of the children's case presented to them, respondents were asked about likely outcomes, potential solutions or courses of action. In the US, the public overwhelmingly endorsed the notion that symptoms of ADHD, depression and asthma will improve with medical treatment (Table 10.2). Only in the case of the child/adolescent with 'daily troubles', did they report that the condition will improve on its own. A majority (53.6 per cent) also reported that they believe that the behaviours consistent with ADHD would improve with better discipline. In our other analyses, we found that older respondents and women were significantly more likely to endorse treatment efficacy. Respondents were particularly likely to believe that treatments would be effective when they saw the case as a 'mental illness' or a 'very serious problem' (Pescosolido et al., 2007a).

With the exception of not recommending a hospital visit, the vast majority of the individuals who evaluated cases with symptoms of ADHD and/or depression expressed a willingness to consult any combination of family/friends; teachers; MDs; mental health professionals and/or psychiatrists (Table 10. 3). This pattern does not vary significantly across socio-demographic categories (Pescosolido et al., 2007a).

Because of the central place of the use of psychotropic medications for child and adolescent behavioural and emotional problems, Figures 10.3 and 10.4 focus on a comparison of respondents' support for consulting particular professional and lay 'advisors' with their willingness to accept a medication treatment strategy.

Table 10.2   Percentage of the US public who believe the vignette child's problem is 'very' or 'somewhat' likely to improve under four different scenarios, National Stigma Study – Children, 2002

	ADHD (%)	Depression (%)	Asthma (%)	Daily troubles (%)
Improve on its own	32.9	17.4	27.5	77.1
Improve with discipline	53.6	26.8	13.1	48.4
Improve with diet change	45.4	45.1	70.4	32.6
Improve with medical treatment	75.7	89.8	97.4	29.4

Table 10.3   Percentage of the US public willing to seek help for the vignette child's problem across six alternatives, National Stigma Study – Children, 2002

	ADHD (%)	Depression (%)	Asthma (%)	Daily troubles (%)
Family and friends	70.7	75.0	70.2	54.4
Teachers	88.3	87.8	70.5	76.5
Medical doctor	83.9	88.3	94.9	54.6
MH professional	83.2	95.1	43.7	51.6
Psychiatrists	64.2	86.2	32.9	33.1
Hospital	19.8	44.5	43.0	7.9

According to the NSS-C data, among those respondents who were willing to consult others, a majority would accept recommendations for the use of psychiatric medication to treat ADHD if received from physicians (70.2 per cent) or mental health professionals (68.2 per cent, Figure 10.3). Similar recommendations would be accepted only by a minority of respondents, however, if provided by family (36.4 per cent), teachers (38.1 per cent), psychiatrists (36.3 per cent) or hospital staff (18.8 per cent). For the depression case, a majority of those willing to consult physicians (78.1 per cent), mental health professionals (83.7 per cent) and psychiatrists (79.5 per cent) would accept a recommendation for medication (Figure 10.4). As with the ADHD case, however, only a minority would accept similar recommendations from family (49.7 per cent), teachers (35.6 per cent), or hospital staff (40.5 per cent). For both ADHD and depression, additional analyses indicated that there are few socio-demographic differences among Americans in their reluctance to accept medication recommendations. Only older respondents were more willing to accept the recommendation of physicians. However, importantly for issues of health, black Americans were less willing to accept the recommendation of both teachers and physicians. Lastly, respondents who labeled the vignette child's problem as a 'mental illness' were significantly more likely to accept a medication recommendation from virtually any source (Pescosolido et al., 2007a).

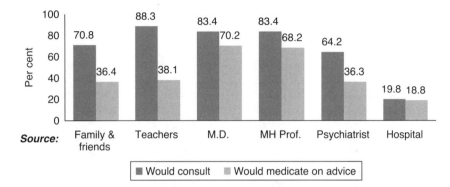

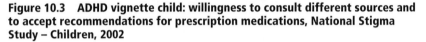

Figure 10.3   ADHD vignette child: willingness to consult different sources and to accept recommendations for prescription medications, National Stigma Study – Children, 2002

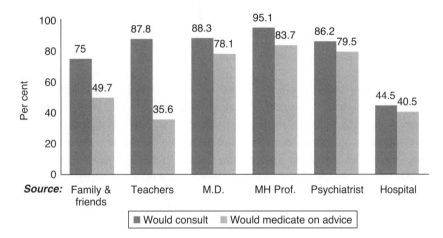

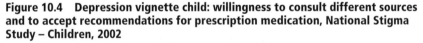

Figure 10.4   Depression vignette child: willingness to consult different sources and to accept recommendations for prescription medication, National Stigma Study – Children, 2002

ARE THEY CONCERNED ABOUT STIGMA AND DO THEY SUPPORT PREJUDICIAL BEHAVIOUR TOWARDS CHILDREN AND ADOLESCENTS WITH MENTAL HEALTH ISSUES?

A central question in the NSS-C and in the research and policy questions surrounding child and adolescent mental health issues revolves around the social implications of diagnosis and treatment. Figure 10.5 suggests a great deal of concern. A majority of the public (57.3 per cent) either 'strongly agreed' or 'somewhat agreed' that, regardless of laws protecting confidentiality, most people in the community would nonetheless know if a child was receiving mental

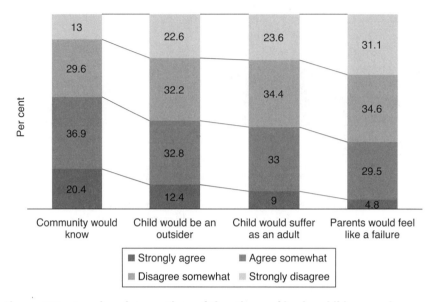

Figure 10.5   Americans' perceptions of the stigma of having children receive mental health treatment, National Stigma Study – Children, 2002

health treatment. Moreover, a significant minority agreed that a child receiving mental health treatment would be an outsider at school (45.2 per cent strongly agreed or somewhat agreed), and would suffer as an adult if others learned that she or he received mental health treatment as a child (42.0 per cent strongly agreed or somewhat agreed). The endorsement of these stigmatizing assessments was, however, significantly lower among women and better educated respondents (Pescosolido et al., 2007b).

Table 10.4 indicates the public's willingness to similarly exclude children with mental health problems, showing the percentage who were either 'definitely' or 'probably' unwilling to have contact with the vignette child and the child's family in four different social settings: as neighbours, as guests, as a friend to their children or as a classmate to their child. According to these estimates, only a minority of Americans expressed a willingness to shun children with these mental health problems. However, across the four settings, the highest levels of rejection were reported for the child with ADHD and depression. In these cases, roughly one of every five Americans reported an unwillingness to interact with the child. Most notably, 22.2 per cent and 29.4 per cent of respondents reported exclusionary preferences for the ADHD and depressed child, respectively. The unwillingness to interact with children with mental health problems was significantly greater among men, and those respondents who attributed the causes of the vignette child's problem to either a lack of discipline or to bad character. Not surprisingly, preferences for social distance were also significantly higher among those respondents who believed children with mental health problems represent a danger to themselves or others (Pescosolido et al., 2007a).

Table 10.4 Percentage of the US public 'definitely' or 'probably' unwilling to interact with the vignette child across four venues, National Stigma Study – Children, 2002

	ADHD (%)	Depression (%)	Asthma (%)	Daily troubles (%)
Neighbour	21.0	18.9	9.7	9.9
Socialize	16.9	17.2	6.8	9.4
Friend	22.2	29.4	4.5	9.5
Classmate	17.8	10.6	2.6	6.1
Vignette mean	19.5	19.0	5.9	8.7

DISCUSSION AND LESSONS FROM SOCIAL SCIENCE TO MEDICINE

This first study of public knowledge of and attitudes toward children with mental health problems suggests both opportunities and challenges. Overall, it appears that the public can discriminate between normal childhood variations in behaviour, physical health problems like asthma, and mental health problems like ADHD and depression. However, while their responses are fairly clear and consistent, there are also uncertainties on a number of issues within mental health problems – including seeing physical illness and 'ups and downs' of childhood as well as mental illness in the profiles that professionals diagnose as ADHD and depression. Overall, the public sees depression as more serious, more in need of treatment and more problematic than ADHD. Our findings suggest that certain groups, including men, older individuals and, in some cases, people of colour, may be most appropriate targets of educational efforts.

Levels of concern and treatment endorsement appear to be higher for children with mental problems than for adults, indicating hope for improvements in services utilization (Perry et al., 2007). However, public attitudes also reveal more prejudice regarding perceptions of dangerousness, which may pose barriers to stigma reduction. Moreover, compared to studies of psychiatric medications in general, the US public reports greater suspicion about the use and efficacy of medications for children and adolescents (Croghan et al., 2003). Most are concerned that receiving mental health treatment will have immediate and long-term negative effects on children's' futures for inclusion and success.

The National Stigma Study – Children represents only a first step in understanding the context in which children, their caregivers and providers respond to the onset of behavioral and emotional problems. We need to know much more from the public, from parents and from those in the treatment and social service systems (see, for example, the work of Regina Bussing and her colleagues on parents of children diagnosed with ADHD; Bussing et al., 1998, 2003). As Davies and Lowes (2006) point out, little evidence is available about how children and adolescents feel about services. Further, cross-national work is critical, particularly on the issue of medications, where national studies (from Germany, for example; Angermeyer et al., 1993) show marked differences from US reports.

However, even at this early stage, sociological research on public views of emotional and behavioral problems among children and adolescents suggest several recommendations that may be useful to the mental health professions (Pescosolido et al., 2008a). Briefly, providers might more successfully confront children's mental health problems by directly asking about and assessing child and caretaker beliefs. This is particularly the case since socio-demographic characteristics provide poor clues and, as a result, mistaken assumptions about what challenges providers need to overcome or address. For example, in the UK, studies of Gujarati families counter typical provider and researcher assumptions since quality of services was given a higher priority by the families than cultural competence (Dogra et al., 2007).

Such an approach would allow providers to offer more targeted and relevant information, increase trust, confront stigma issues directly and debunk typical prejudices, including the fear of psychiatric medications. Finally, findings from the NSS-C (Pescosolido et al., 2008) suggest that a small but significant proportion of people who can identify ADHD or depression reject the label of 'mental illness'. Increasingly, psychiatry has moved to specificity of terms, and our data suggest that this might be useful in the case of children and adolescents.

NOTE

1 Primary funding for the Children's Mental Health Module was provided by the National Science Foundation to the General Social Survey, Eli Lilly & Co., the Indiana Consortium for Mental Health Services Research, and the College of Arts and Sciences at Indiana University-Bloomington. IRB approval for the GSS is held at the University of Chicago (#93216). IRB approval for secondary data analysis of the GSS was given at Indiana University (#04-8885). To see the full public report, *Americans' Views of Children with Mental Health Problems*, as well as the list of scientific publications on which this summary is based, go to http://www.indiana.edu/~icmhsr/ or contact the Indiana Consortium for Mental Health Services Research, Karl Schuessler Institute for Social Research, 1022 E. Third St., Bloomington, IN 47405, tel. 812.855.3841. The website also contains basic information from other studies on public beliefs about psychoactive medication for children; public knowledge and beliefs about the stigma attached to adult mental health problems, and public expectations of medical and mental health care.

REFERENCES

Angermeyer, Matthias C., R. Daeumer and Herbert Matschinger (1993) Benefits and risks of psycho tropic medication in the eyes of the general public: Results of a survey in the Federal Republic of Germany. *Pharmacopsychiatry*, 26: 114–120.

Angermeyer, Matthias C., Bruce G. Link and Alice Majcher-Angermeyer (1987) Stigma perceived by patients attending modern treatment settings: Some unanticipated effects of community psychiatry reforms. *The Journal of Nervous and Mental Disease*, 175: 4–11.

Bickett, L. and R. Milich (1990). First impressions formed of boys with learning disabilities and attention deficit disorder. *Journal of Learning Disabilities*, 23: 253–259.

Blachman, D.R. and S.P. Hinshaw (2002) Patterns of friendship among girls with and without attention-deficit/hyperactivity disorder. *Journal of Abnormal Child Psychology*, 30: 625–640.

Bramble, D. (2003). Annotation: the use of psychotropic medications in children: a British view. *Journal of Child Psychology and Psychiatry and Allied Disciplines*, 44: 169–179.

Bussing, Regina, F.A., Gary, T.L. Mills et al. (2003) Parental explanatory models of ADHD: gender and cultural variations, *Social Psychiatry and Psychiatric Epidemiology*, 38: 563–575.

Bussing, Regina, N. Schoenfield and E.R. Perwien (1998) Knowledge and information about ADHD: evidence of cultural differences among African American and white parents, *Social Science and Medicine*, 46: 919–928.

Chandra, A. and C.S. Minkovitz (2006) Stigma starts early: gender differences in teen willingness to use mental health services. *Journal of Adolescent Health*, 38: 754.

Cole, Andrew (2006) Inquiry opens into state of childhood in the UK. *British Medical Journal* 333: 619.

Corrigan, Patrick W., Barbara Lurie Demming, Howard H. Goldman, Natalie Slopen, Krishna Medasani and Sean Phelan (2005) How adolescents perceive the stigma of mental illness and alcohol abuse. *Psychiatric Services*, 56: 544–550.

Costello, E. Jane, Adrian Angold, Barbara J. Burns, Alaattin Erkanli, Dalene K. Stangl and Dan L. Tweed. (1996). The great smoky mountains study of youth: functional impairment and serious emotional disturbance. *Archives of General Psychiatry*, 53: 1137–1143.

Costello, E. Jane, Bernice A. Pescosolido, Adrian Angold and Barbara J. Burns (1998) A family network-based model of access to child mental health services. In J.P. Morrissey (ed.) *Social Networks and Mental Illness*. Stamford, CT: JAI Press. pp. 165–190.

Crisp, Arthur H., Michael G. Gelder, Susannah Rix, Howard I. Meltzer and Olwen J. Rowlands (2000) Stigmatization of people with mental illness, *British Journal of Psychiatry*, 177: 4–7.

Croghan, Thomas W., Molly Tomlin, Bernice A. Pescosolido, Jack K. Martin, Keri M. Lubell and Ralph Swindle (2003) Americans' knowledge and attitudes towards and their willingness to use psychiatric medications. *The Journal of Nervous and Mental Disease*, 191: 166–174.

Davies, Jane and Lesley Lowes (2006). Development and organization fo child and adolescent mental health services. *British Journal of Nursing*, 15: 604–610.

Day, Crispin and Hilton Davis (2006). The effectiveness and quality of routine child and adolescent mental health care outreach clinics, *British Journal of Clinical Psychology*, 45: 439–452.

Dogra, Nisha, Panos Vostanis, Hala Abuateya and Nick Jewson (2007). Children's mental health services and ethnic diversity: Gujarati families' perspectives of service provision for mental health problems, *Transcultural Psychiatry*, 44: 275–291.

Ford, Tasmin, Robert Goodman and Howard Meltzer (2003). The British child and adolescent mental health survey 1999: The prevalence of DSM-IV disorders, *Journal of the American Academy of Child and Adolescent Psychiatry*, 42: 1208–1211.

Harris, Kathleen Mullan, Greg J. Duncan and Johanne Boisjoly (2002). Evaluating the role of nothing to lose attitudes on risky behavior in adolescence, *Social Forces*, 80: 1005–1039.

Hitchen, Lisa. (2006). Address poverty to reduce mental health problems among children, says BMA, *British Medical Journal*, 332: 1471.

House of Commons Health Committee (1997) *Child and Adolescent Mental Health Services*. 4th report. London: The Stationery Office.

Law, G. Urquhart, S. Sinclair and N. Fraser (2007) Children's attitudes and behavioural intentions towards a peer with symptoms of ADHD: Does the addition of a diagnostic label make a difference? *Journal of Child Health Care*, 11: 98–111.

Layard, Richard and Judy Dunn (2009) *A Good Childhood: Searching for Values in a Competitive Age*. London: Penguin.

Link, Bruce G., Jo C. Phelan, Michaeline Bresnahan, Ann Stueve and Bernice A. Pescosolido (1999) Public conceptions of mental illness: Labels, causes, dangerousness and social distance, *American Journal of Public Health*, 89: 1328–1333.

Martin, Jack K., Bernice A. Pescosolido and Steven A. Tuch (2000) Of fear and loathing: The role of disturbing behavior, labels and causal attributions in shaping public attitudes toward persons with mental illness. *Journal of Health and Social Behavior*, 41: 208–233.

McArdle, Paul, Jonathan Prosser and Izzy Kolvin (2004) Prevalence of psychiatric disorder: With and without psychosocial impairment. *European Child and Adolescent Psychiatry*, 13: 347–353.

McNicholas, F. (2001) Psychotropic prescribing practices of paediatricians in the UK. *Child: Care, Health and Development*, 27: 497–508.

Meltzer, H., R. Gatward, R. Goodman and T. Ford (2003) Mental health of children and adolescents in Great Britain. *International Review of Psychiatry*, 15: 185–187.

Middleton, N., D. Gunnell, E. Whitley, D. Dorling and S. Frankel (2001) Secular trends in antidepressant prescribing in the UK. *Journal of Public Health Medicine*, 23: 262–267.

Milich, R., C.B. McAninch and M. Harris (1992) The effects of stigmatizing information on children's peer relations: believing is seeing. *School Psychology Review*, 21: 400–409.

Olfson, Mark, Marc J. Gameroff, Steven C. Marcus, and Peter S. Jensen (2003) National trends in the treatment of attention deficit hyperactivity disorder. *American Journal of Psychiatry*, 160: 1071–1077.

Pelham, William E. and Richard Milich (1984) Peer relations in children with hyperactivity/attention deficit disorder. *Journal of Learning Disabilities*, 17: 560–567.

Perry, Brea L., Bernice A. Pescosolido, Jack K. Martin, Jane D. McLeod and Peter S. Jensen (2007) Comparison of public attributions, attitudes, and stigma in regard to depression among children and adults. *Psychiatric Services*, 58: 632–635.

Pescosolido, Bernice A. (1991). Illness careers and network ties: A conceptual model of utilization and compliance. In Gary L. Albrecht and Judith A. Levy (eds) *Advances in Medical Sociology*. CT: JAI Press. pp. 61–184.

Pescosolido, Bernice A. (2006). Of pride and prejudice: The role of sociology and social networks in integrating the health sciences. *Journal of Health and Social Behavior*, 47: 189–208.

Pescosolido, Bernice A., Danielle L. Fettes, Jack K. Martin, John Monahan and Jane D. McLeod (2007a) Perceived dangerousness of children with mental health problems and support for coerced treatment. *Psychiatric Services*, 58: 1–7.

Pescosolido, Bernice A. et al. (2008) Public knowledge and assessment of child mental health problems: Findings from the National Stigma Study – Children. *Journal of the American Academy of Child and Adolescent Psychiatry*, 47: 339–349.

Pescosolido, Bernice A., Jack K. Martin, Bruce G. Link, Saeko Kikuzawa, Giovanni Burgos and Ralph Swindle (2000). *Americans' Views of Mental Illness and Health at Century's End: Continuity and Change. Public Report on the MacArthur Mental Health Module, 1996 General Social Survey*. Bloomington, IN: Indiana Consortium for Mental Health Services Research.

Pescosolido, Bernice A., Jack K. Martin, J. Scott Long, Tait R. Medina, Jo Phelan and Bruce G. Link. forthcoming. A Disease Like Any Other? A Decade of Change in Public Reactions to Schizophrenia, Depression and Alcohol Dependence. *American Journal of Psychiatry*.

Pescosolido, Bernice A., Jack K. Martin, Jane D. McLeod, Brea L. Perry, Sigrun Olafsdottir and Francis J. Pescosolido (2008a) Public understanding of child MH: National Stigma Study-Children. *The Brown University Child and Adolescent Behavior Letter*, 24: 3–4.

Pescosolido, Bernice A., John Monahan, Bruce G. Link, Ann Stueve and Saeko Kikuzawa (1999) The public's view of the competence, dangerousness, and need for legal coercion of persons with mental health problems. *American Journal of Public Health*, 89: 1339–1345.

Pescosolido, Bernice A., Sigrun Olafsdottir, Jack K. Martin and J. Scott Long (2008b) Cross-Cultural Aspects of the Stigma of Mental Illness. In Julio Arboleda-Florez and Norman Sartorius (eds) *Understanding the Stigma of Mental Illness: Theory and Interventions*. London: John Wiley & Sons, Ltd.

Pescosolido, Bernice A., Brea L. Perry, Jack K. Martin, Jane D. McLeod and Peter S. Jensen (2007b) Stigmatizing attitudes and beliefs about treatment and psychiatric medications for children with mental illness. *Psychiatric Services*, 58: 613–618.

Safer, Daniel J. (1997) Changing patterns of psychotropic medications prescribed by child psychiatrists in the 1990s. *Journal of Child and Adolescent Psychopharmacology*, 7: 267–274.

Safer, Daniel J., Julie Magno Zito and Susan dosReis (2003) Concomitant psychotropic medication for youths. *American Journal of Psychiatry*, 160: 438–449.

Sartorius, Norman (1998) Stigma: What can psychiatrists do about it? *The Lancet*, 352: 1058–1059.

Sayal, Kapil (2004) The role of parental burden in child mental health service use: Longitudinal study. *Journal of the American Academy of Child and Adolescent Psychiatry*, 43: 1328–1333.

Singh, Swaran P. (2009) Transition of care from child to adult mental health services: The great divide. *Current Opinion in Psychiatry*, 22: 386–390.

Stiffman, Arlene R., Bernice A. Pescosolido and Leopoldo J. Cabassa (2004) Building a model to understand youth service access: The Gateway Provider Model. *Mental Health Services Research*, 6: 189–198.

Stuart, Heather and Julio Arboleda-Florez (2001) Community attitudes toward persons with schizophrenia. *Canadian Journal of Psychiatry*, 46: 245–252.

Vostanis, Panos, Howard Meltzer, Robert Goodman and Tasmin Ford (2003) Service utilisation by children with conduct disorders: Findings from the GB National Study. *European Child and Adolescent Psychiatry,* 12: 231–238.

Wahl, Otto F. (1997) Stigma and mass media. In K. Bernheim (ed.) *Cases and Readings in Abnormal Behavior.* Baltimore, MD: Lanahan Publishers. pp. 357–361.

Wahl, Otto F. (2000) *Telling is Risky Business.* New Brunswick, NJ: Rutgers University Press.

Weisz, J.R. and B. Weiss (1991) Studying the referability of child clinical problems. *Journal of Consulting and Clinical Psychology*, 59: 266–273.

Weisz, J.R. and B. Weiss (1993) *Effects of Psychotherapy with Children and Adolescents.* Newbury Park, CA: SAGE.

11

Stigma and Mental Disorder

Graham Scambler

INTRODUCTION: GOFFMAN'S CLASSIC STUDY

Cultural norms proscribing attributes, traits or conditions regarded as shameful or in some way deviant have a long history. In fact both philosophical and sociological arguments have been invoked to assert the inevitability or omnipresence of such norms. According to the philosopher Wittgenstein (1953), culturally lauded or acceptable behaviour, a staple of enduring sociability, is only possible if the breach of such norms is a realistic and publicly marked possibility. One of the core premises of Durkheim's proto-functionalism is that all social formations have discriminated between the normal and abnormal, insiders and outsiders. There can be no 'normal/acceptable' in the absence of tangible exemplars of the 'abnormal/unacceptable'. As Goffman (1963) puts it, there is a 'self-other, normal-stigmatized unity': stigmatized and non-stigmatized alike are products of the same norms (Falk, 2001).

In this chapter the focus is on mental illness as a mark of abnormality or unacceptability. In a sense this limits the discussion by time and place, since widely recognized and authoritative *psychiatric* labels affirming the presence of mental disorders – if not necessarily the phenomena they depict – are of fairly recent origin and most familiar in Western(ized) cultures. A quite voluminous literature on the 'stigma of mental illness' has nevertheless arisen, much of it postwar and North American. Phelan and colleagues (2008) provide a chronological list of 'stigma models', which is reproduced in Box 11.1. The discussion of this literature here is framed by a broader consideration of the structural, cultural and psycho-social properties of stigma itself, references being made also to chronic physical illness and disability. After all, mental illness represents but one

Box 11.1   Stigma models (in chronological order)

Stigma: notes on the management of spoiled identity (Goffman, 1963). Stigma is 'the situation of the individual who is disqualified from full social acceptance' (preface). The stigmatized individual is 'reduced in our minds from a whole and usual person to a tainted, discounted one' (p. 3). Goffman emphasizes stigma as enacted in 'mixed interactions' between stigmatized and non-stigmatized individuals and how stigmatized individuals manage those interactions.

Social Stigma: the psychology of marked relationships (Jones et al., 1984). 'The stigmatizing process involves engulfing categorizations accompanied by negative affect that is typically alloyed into ambivalence or rationalized through some version of just-world hypothesis' (p. 296). Jones et al. identify six dimensions of stigmatizing 'marks': conceal-ability, course, disruptiveness, aesthetic qualities, origin and peril.

Modified labelling theory of mental disorders (Link et al., 1989). Socialization leads to beliefs about how most people treat mental patients. When individuals enter psychiatric treatment, these beliefs become personally relevant. The more patients believe they will be devalued and discriminated against, the more they feel threatened by interacting with others. They may employ coping strategies that can have negative consequences for social support networks, jobs and self-esteem.

Identity threat models (Crocker et al., 1998; Major and O'Brien, 2005; Steele and Aronson, 1995). Possessing a stigmatized identity increases exposure to potentially stressful, identity threatening conditions. Collective representations (e.g. beliefs about prejudice), situational cues and personal characteristics affect appraisals of the significance of those situations for well-being. Responses to identity threat can can be involuntary (e.g. emotional) or voluntary (i.e. coping efforts). These responses can affect outcomes such as self-esteem, academic achievement and health.

Conceptualizing stigma (Link and Phelan, 2001). Stigma occurs when elements of labelling, stereotyping, cognitive separation into categories of 'us' and 'them', status loss and discrimination co-occur in a power situation that allows these components to unfold.

Evolutionary model (Kurzban and Leary, 2001). 'Phenomena … under the rubric of stigma involve a set of distinct psychological systems designed by natural selection to solve specific problems associated with sociality … Human beings possess cognitive adaptations designed to cause them to avoid poor social exchange partners, join cooperative groups. (for purposes of between-group competition and exploitation) and avoid contact with those differentially likely to carry communicative pathogens' (p. 187).

HIV and AIDS-related stigma and discrimination: a conceptual framework and implications for action (Parker and Aggleton, 2003). 'Stigma plays a key role in producing and reproducing relations of power and control. It causes some groups to be devalued and others to feel … they are superior. Ultimately … stigma is linked to the workings of social inequality' (p. 16).

Goal-directed, self-regulatory coping (Swim and Thomas, 2006). Discrimination threatens core social goals of self-enhancement, trust, understanding, control and belonging. The weighting of these goals, as well as appraisal of one's ability to engage in responses and the ability of a response to address goals, influence choice of coping responses by targets of discrimination.

Moral experience and stigma (Yang et al., 2007). 'Moral experience, or what is most at stake for actors in a local social world' shapes the stigma process for stigmatizers and stigmatized. 'Stigma exerts its core effects by threatening the loss of what really matters and what is threatened' (p. 1524).

Source: Phelan et al. (2008)

enduring way in which normal/insiders can find themselves abnormal/outsiders in the contemporary social world (Scambler, 2009).

It is still to Goffman that sociologists and professionals in health and healing most readily turn for illumination on stigma. For a generation or so his dramaturgical sensitization of the concept in *Stigma: the Management of Spoiled Identity* provided almost unquestioned paradigm and exemplar. A critical appreciation of his approach is therefore essential. It will be argued that while Goffman's contribution retains its insight, subtlety and theoretical perspicacity, it is time to move on, or rather *beyond*: it is not that Goffman was wrong but that there were questions he did not ask. Some of these questions have been put by others, especially those approaching stigma with a firm interest in social structure or political economy.

Goffman's (1963: 13) starting point is to suggest that stigma refers to 'an attribute that is deeply discrediting'; but he insists that it is a 'language of relationships' not attributes that is really required. 'An attribute that stigmatizes one type of possessor', he writes, 'can confirm the usualness of another, and therefore is neither creditable nor discreditable as a thing in itself'. Few sociologists since have disputed this 'relational' anchorage for a concept often deployed outside the discipline with more abandon.

While Goffman's treatise on stigma is frequently cited on the often poignant day-to-day dealings of the 'discredited' (possessors of visible marks of unacceptable difference, whose challenge is to 'manage impressions') and the 'discreditable' (possessors of invisible marks of unacceptable difference, whose challenge is to 'manage information'), it is the symbolic interactionist/dramaturgical basis of his work that invites attention here. His principal interest was in the structure of interaction: 'to describe the rules regulating a social interaction is to describe its structure' (Goffman, 1967: 144). For him the structure of face-to-face interaction in the lifeworld is what steadies and sustains the social order. In many respects, he suggests, people conduct themselves in the everyday world much as actors follow scripts in theatre productions. A number of 'ground rules' specify the means available to individuals to realize their goals; they give normative regulation. One of these ground rules has to do with 'maintenance of face', requiring individuals, like actors on a stage, to present and sustain consistent and positive images of the self and to acknowledge the same process in those with whom they interact. This is accomplished by acting out 'lines': participants in interaction typically act to prevent lines from being discredited, thus avoiding loss of face for all parties. Social life proceeds as smoothly as it tends to because individuals find themselves arriving together at a working definition of the situation. While individuals perform to maintain face through lines in 'front regions' (e.g. hospital clinics), in the absence of an audience they can stop performing, behaving in a manner that contradicts their performance, in 'back regions' (e.g. in the hospital canteen or at home).

Goffman was under no illusion that social life is always cooperative and egalitarian. Definitions of situations can reflect imbalances of power, as is the case in 'total institutions' (Goffman, 1961). In mental hospitals, for example, a person's performed self is discredited and challenged by others positing an alternative definition. The self, in other words, 'is not a property of the person to whom it is attributed, but dwells rather in the pattern of social control that is exerted in connection with the person by himself and those around him' (Goffman, 1961: 168). The self is the product of an institutional nexus of performances, although rarely in the extreme form found in total institutions.

In people's ordinary everyday lives social order is maintained not only by rule-following but by rule-breaking, or 'remedial interchanges' (Goffman, 1971). In fact rule-breaking is pervasive: this is because social interaction is structured primarily to afford individuals opportunities to 'adjust' in pursuit of their own private goals with minimal fuss or stress. Rule-breaking in face-to-face interaction, typically articulated by means of 'accounts, 'apologies' and 'requests', gets the traffic moving again (Goffman, 1971: 108). In other words, it may be more felicitous to overlook someone's rule infraction than to insist on rule-following behaviour. 'Deviance' of this kind is unlikely to be punished.

It has been argued that what is missing from Goffman's account of the structure of interaction is the causal input of social structures more often theorized from outside the symbolic interactionist/dramaturgical fold (Scambler, 2006). These have something of the external and constraining character of Durkheimian 'social facts'. That a synthesis of micro-analyses of the kind favoured by Goffman and familiar in interactionist and phenomenological studies with macro-analyses more often associated with structural-functional or conflict theory can be achieved is evident (Scambler, 2002). This issue features later, but it is to Goffman's immediate legacy that we turn now.

LABELLING AND THE 'PERSONAL TRAGEDY' OF MENTAL ILLNESS

Labelling

What is described as the 'personal tragedy' or 'deviance' orientation to chronic physical and mental illness is not just down to Goffman. It reflects a much broader interactionist perspective. In the USA, as mentioned, a considerable literature has emerged on mental illness. Scheff (1966, 1974) claimed that 'labelling' is the single most important cause of mental illness. His theory has been conveniently broken down into nine constituent propositions by Chauncey (1974: 248) (see Box 11.2). Essentially, Scheff argued that a residue of unusual and incongruous behaviour exists for which culture provides no explicit labels: such forms of behaviour constitute 'residual rule-breaking or deviance'. Most psychiatric symptoms can be categorized as instances of residual deviance. There is a cultural stereotype of mental illness, blunted by sins of omission and commission. When for whatever reason residual deviance comes to public attention, this cultural stereotype becomes the guiding imagery for action. Contact with a

---

Box 11.2   Scheff's 'labelling theory of mental illness'

1 Residual rule-breaking arises from fundamentally diverse sources.
2 Relative to the rate of treated mental illness, the rate of unrecorded residual rule-breaking is extremely high.
3 Most residual rule-breaking is 'denied' and is of transitory significance.
4 Stereotyped imagery of mental disorder is learned in early childhood.
5 The stereotypes of insanity are continually reaffirmed, inadvertently, in ordinary social interaction.
6 Labelled deviants may be rewarded for playing the stereotyped deviant role.
7 Labelled deviants are punished when they attempt to return to conventional roles.
8 In a crisis occurring when a residual rule-breaker is publicly labelled, the deviant is highly suggestible and may accept the proffered role of the insane as the only alternative.
9 Among residual rule-breakers, labelling is the single most important cause of careers of residual deviance.

Source: Chauncey (1974)

---

physician is established, a psychiatric diagnosis made and procedures for hospitalization may follow. Problems of secondary deviance – that is, problems consequent upon the application of a diagnosis – are predictable consequences of authoritative medical labelling.

Chauncey argues that it is propositions 1, 3, 7 and 9 in Box 11.1 that offer most ammunition to his critics. The gist of his own critique is that there is a shortage of supportive evidence for these propositions. He also claims that Scheff fails to respect the 'limits of sociology'. Referring to his 1974 paper, he contends that Scheff 'merely attempts to defend the existence of the social reality while ignoring the question of its relative significance with respect to disease' (Chauncey, 1974: 251). In similar vein, Gove (1970) insists that Scheff neglects the biological and exaggerates every facet of his case, from the nuances of truth and falsity in cultural stereotypes to the ideologies and praxis of professional labellers to differentiated individual coping styles.

Link and his colleagues (1989) are no less vigorous in their criticisms of the anti-labellers. In particular they argue that commentators like Gove, in their enthusiasm to attack Scheff's 'aetiological hypothesis', generally downplay the salience of social factors like stigma and stereotyping. They seek to qualify and extend Scheff's pioneering work by substituting their own 'modified labelling approach'. Even if labelling does not directly produce mental disorder, their argument runs, it can certainly lead to negative outcomes. Processes of socialization induce a set of beliefs about the character and reception of patients with mental illness. When people become patients, these beliefs assume new meanings and import. The more patients believe that they will be negatively evaluated and discriminated against, the more they feel intimidated and threatened by interactions with others. They may in consequence attempt to 'pass as normal' or 'cover', to use Goffman's terms, keeping their treatment secret, withdrawing from potentially troublesome encounters, or trying to educate others. Such strategies can have negative results by undermining support networks, inhibiting performance, for example in job markets, or reducing self-esteem. Representations of Scheff's original labelling approach and Link et al.'s modified approach are to be found in Figure 11.1

In an empirical contribution based on samples of both patients and untreated residents in the community, Link et al. claim sufficient support for their modified labelling approach to promote it over anti-labelling stances. They present evidence that prior to patienthood people have a strong sense of the public rejection of mental patients. In addition, patients endorse strategies of secrecy, withdrawal and education as ways of coping with perceived threat. Moreover, patients' support networks are damaged to the extent that they fear discrimination and adopt coping strategies inimical to everyday sociability. Even if the effects of labelling dissipate over time, as Gove claims, 'the short-term consequences can be powerful and unfortunate – a possibility that most critics deny' (Link et al., 1989: 420).

Current programmes of intervention to reduce psychiatric stigma across developed and developing countries alike typically adopt the premises that better informed publics and sensitized professionals are barriers against virulent cultural stereotypes, likely to reduce both rates of discrimination and the prospects

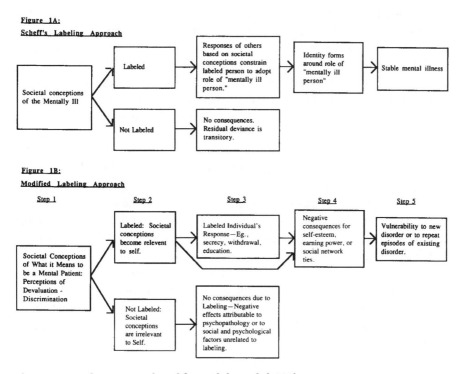

Figure 11.1   Figure reproduced from Link et al. (1989)

for secondary deviance when psychiatric diagnoses are made (see, for example, Putman, 2008). I return to programmes of stigma reduction later.

Personal tragedy

The labelling perspective not only informed American medical sociology but helped define its European progeny, with Freidson's (1970) *Profession of Medicine* being an important catalyst. There followed a plethora of individualistic explorations of the day-to-day accommodation of medically labelled chronic and/or stigmatizing illness (Armstrong, 2003). Significant contributions alluded to the 'biographical disruption' and 'loss of self' occasioned by the onset and diagnosis of physical and mental disorders (Bury, 1982; Charmaz, 1983), as well as to the common need for 'narrative reconstruction' (Williams, 1984). The issue was typically held to be a new and unwelcome deviant – or, for Goffman, 'moral' – career, calling for wholesale readjustment to lives threatened to varying degrees by 'impairment' (body deficit), 'disability' (functional loss) and, at the time of special concern to sociologists, 'handicap' (social cost) (Bury, 1991). It was largely within this framework that studies of the stigma attaching to some but not all medically defined chronic physical and mental disorders blossomed. There was certainly more interest in the labelled than the labellers.

Many conditions and symptoms from nervous ticks and stuttering to tuberculosis and leprosy carry stigmatizing connotations. Before I turn directly to the stigma of mental illness it is worth emphasizing the degree of conceptual and empirical overlap with research on the stigma of physical illness. As a product of their study of epilepsy in the community in the USA, Schneider and Conrad. (1981) produced a typology of modes of adaptation. This built on an underlying distinction between 'adjusted' and 'unadjusted' adaptations. Individuals defined as adjusted were those able to effectively neutralize the negative impact of epilepsy on their lives. They fell into three categories. The 'pragmatic type' downplayed their epilepsy by attempting to pass or cover, only disclosing when strictly necessary and then to a select few. The 'secret type' opted for elaborate tactics to conceal their epilepsy, which they regarded as 'a stigmatizing, negative and "bad" quality of self' (Schneider and Conrad, 1981: 215). The 'quasi-liberated type' went beyond pragmatism by publicly proclaiming their epilepsy in an attempt to sidestep any antagonism and to educate others. Jobling (1977: 83) captured this kind of initiative to 'de-stigmatize' in his study of psoriasis: 'deviance is shown to be no more than difference and discredit is denied'. Schneider and Conrad's identification of quasi-liberated individuals importantly prefigures later rebuttals of the personal tragedy or deviance paradigm, a paradigm epitomized in their remaining category of the unadjusted, comprising people entirely overwhelmed by their epilepsy, for whom it had become a 'master status' or identity, effectively subsuming all others.

Scambler and Hopkins' British study of epilepsy in the community was similarly conceived. It led to a 'hidden distress model of epilepsy', a key distinction being that between 'enacted' and 'felt stigma' (Scambler and Hopkins, 1986; Scambler, 1989). The former refers to overt discrimination against those with epilepsy on the sole grounds of their social unacceptability, while the latter denotes both a sense of shame and a companion fear of encountering enacted stigma. The hidden distress model can be articulated in terms of three propositions. The first asserts that when confronted with a medical diagnosis of epilepsy, state-sanctioned, culturally authoritative and carrying legal weight, individuals develop a 'special view of the world' – or, after Bourdieu (1977), 'epilepsy *habitus*' – characterized by a strong sense of felt stigma and predisposing them to secrecy and concealment. Schneider and Conrad (1980) show how this sense of felt stigma can have its origins in the 'stigma coaching' of others, like over-protective parents and well-intentioned doctors. Second, this first-choice tactic of non-disclosure has the consequence that few others tend to know of a person's epilepsy (four out of five of whom have their seizures well controlled by antiepi-leptic medication). The result, third, is that felt stigma is typically more disrup-tive of the lives of adults with epilepsy than enacted stigma: it is the discredited not the discreditable whose biographies are skewed by enacted stigma.

Scambler and Hopkins, like Schneider and Conrad, recognized among minori-ties of their interviewees a capacity to resist, defy and fight back. While these two studies reflect the personal tragedy orientation of the time, 'infecting' also sig-nificant others through what Goffman (1963) called 'courtesy stigma', a nascent politics of identity can also be discerned. That courtesy stigma can be a signifi-cant phenomenon in its own right is vividly shown in Gray's (2002) study of the parents of children with high functioning autism. He found that most parents experienced both felt and enacted stigma, although these 'types' of stigma were rarely distinguished in their accounts.

Scambler and Hopkins' distinction between enacted and felt stigma is echoed in the literature on mental illness. In their review on mental illness stigma, Rusch and colleagues (2005) deploy the terms public and self-stigma. Public stigma 'comprises reactions of the general public towards a group based on stigma about that group' (p. 530), while self-stigma 'refers to the reactions of individuals who belong to a stigmatized group and turn the stigmatizing attitudes against themselves' (p. 531).

These same authors go on to draw on social psychological research to discern cognitive, emotional and behavioural aspects of public stigma – associated with stereotypes, prejudice and discrimination respectively. Stereotypes are seen as efficient routes to the categorization of information about different social groups: they expeditiously generate impressions and expectations of persons who belong to a stereotyped group. People may not sign up to all the stereotypes they are either aware of or circuitously use. Prejudiced people, on the other hand, endorse negative stereotypes; and prejudice leads to discrimination as a behavioural reaction. In relation to mental illness, prejudice articulated as anger can be an obstacle to help; prejudice in the guise of fear can lead to avoidance. Perceived association between mental illness and 'dangerousness', for example, correlates with social distance. Rusch et al. caution, however, that stereotypes and prejudice are not sufficient for stigma. Anticipating the next section of this chapter, they argue that social, economic and political power is necessary to stigmatize: there is more to the stigma of mental illness than personal tragedy.

Self-stigma too comprises stereotyping, prejudice and discrimination. Those who turn prejudice against themselves tacitly consent to it. This leads to negative reactions, notably low self-esteem and self-efficacy. What the authors call 'self-prejudice' can also elicit behavioural responses: people with mental illness 'may fail to pursue work or independent living opportunities', not because they are mentally ill but because of 'self-discrimination' (Rusch et al., 2005: 531). They continue:

> How does self-stigma arise? Many persons with mental illness know the stereotypes about their group such as the belief that people with mental illness are incompetent. But, as in public stigma, knowledge alone does not necessarily lead to stigma, if persons are aware of the stereotypes but do not agree with them. Thus, fortunately for many persons with mental illness, awareness of stereotypes alone does not lead to self-stigma. (Rusch et al., 2005: 531)

This resonates in many ways with the studies of the stigma associated with epilepsy of Schneider and Conrad and Scambler and Hopkins cited earlier. The principal components of public and self-stigma as defined by Rusch et al. are summarized in Box 11.3.

Rusch et al. conclude their review by asserting that public stigma has a major impact on the lives of people with mental illness, most conspicuously so if it leads to self-stigma. In combination these can disrupt various aspects of life, including work, housing, health care, social life and self-esteem. Predictably,

---

Box 11.3   Elements of public and self-stigma

Public stigma	**Self-stigma**
Stereotype	*Stereotype*
Negative belief about a group such as:	Negative belief about a group such as:
Incompetence	Incompetence
Character weakness	Character weakness
Dangerousness	Dangerousness
Prejudice	*Prejudice*
Agreement with belief and/or	Agreement with belief and/or negative emotional
negative emotional reaction such as:	reaction such as:
Anger or	Low self-esteem or
Fear	Low self-efficacy
Discrimination	*Discrimination*
Behaviour response to prejudice such as:	Behaviour response to prejudice such as:
Avoidance of work and housing	Fails to pursue work and housing
opportunities	opportunities
Withholding help	Does not seek help

Source: Rusch et al. (2005)

thcy join the academic chorus in calling for long-term anti-stigma campaigns to reduce public stigma.

The recognition of coping strategies and styles as well as the lurking hazard of enacted and felt stigma remains salient for the empirical study of accommodating chronic physical and mental illnesses with culturally negative connotations. Nevertheless new paradigms have emerged, most conspicuously in the arena of disability theory/politics. Before these theoretical innovations are reviewed, however, attention should be given to the 'measurement' of stigma conceived as a personal affront.

MEASURING STIGMA AS PERSONAL TRAGEDY

The notion of 'measurement' is itself a controversial one in sociology: one person's operationalization is another's subversion of a complex phenomenon; and stigma relations are complex indeed. Yet as Link and his colleagues (2004) maintain in relation to mental illness, crucial to the scientific understanding of stigma is our capacity to observe and measure it. In his review of the measurement of health-related stigma in 63 published papers covering a wide range of physical and mental conditions, van Brakel (2006: 309) distinguishes between five foci and approaches to measurement. These are annotated in Box 11.4.

Van Brakel recognizes the relevance of a plurality of methods, ranging from qualitative investigations to quantitative studies oriented to operationalization via scales or pre-defined sets of indicators. He considers generic scales/indicators as well as a wide range of instruments addressing particular health conditions, most notably leprosy, HIV/AIDS, tuberculosis, mental illness, epilepsy and physical disability. His conclusions are threefold. First, cross-cultural studies, qualitative and quantitative, suggest that the consequences of stigma are 'remarkably similar

---

Box 11.4   Measuring health-related stigma

1 Surveys of attitudes towards those with certain health conditions conducted with samples of the public or of sub-populations like carers.
2 Assessments or audits of discriminatory and stigmatizing practices:

  • in the community, home or workplace;
  • in healthcare;
  • in legal statutes or practice;
  • in the media;
  • in educational materials in schools.

3 Interviews with those affected by certain health conditions about their actual experience of discrimination and stigmatization.
4 Interviews with those affected by certain health conditions about perceived or felt stigma.
5 Interviews with those affected by certain health conditions about self- or internalized stigma, incorporating feelings of loss of self-esteem and dignity, fear, shame, guilt and so on.

Source: Adapted from Van Brakel (2006)

in different health conditions, cultures and public health programmes' (van Brakel, 2006: 329). Second, most instruments of measurement are condition-specific rather than generic. And third, the *degree of similarity* in the consequences of stigma in different cultural milieu and the 'cross-cutting applicability of many items from stigma instruments' suggest that it might be feasible to develop a 'generic set of stigma assessment instruments' (van Brakel, 2006: 329).

Link et al. (2004) evaluate measurement practices in research on mental illness stigma based on a search (MEDLINE and PSYCHLIT) completed in mid-2003. Like van Brake, they usefully categorize and make accessible a range of measures. Of no less interest, however, is their identification of gaps in the use or availability of measures. They subsume these under five headings. The first is 'structural discrimination', which they define as 'institutional practices that work to the disadvantage of stigmatized groups and that allow extensive disparities in outcomes even when direct person-to-person enactment of discrimination is absent' (Link et al., 2004: 530). They found this area of enquiry 'almost entirely unaddressed' in their log of reviewed papers (although this may in part be a function of their 'gaze'). The second area of neglect is the assessment of the emotional responses of patients/consumers. Only four studies of the shame, humiliation and embarrassment experienced appeared in the reviewers' log. Third is the assessment of children's knowledge, attitudes, beliefs and behaviours, together with their experience of stigma. Once again a mere four studies were discerned. The fourth lacuna is the adoption of 'experimental approaches': there is a shortage, they suggest, of non-vignette experimental studies addressing the stigma of mental illness. And finally, there are surprisingly few cross-cultural studies. Predictably perhaps, there are studies conducted in developing societies that use measures pioneered in the West, and that enhance Western reflexivity, but there remains a scarcity of comparative research designs.

There is a distinction to be drawn between the credibility of, on the one hand, a generic measurement of the consequences of mental health-related stigma and, on the other hand, a generic or cross-cultural *theory of mental health-related stigma*. There is a risk indeed of conflating these two proximal but independent projects. The shame associated with, say, psychosis can have similar sequelae cross-culturally, as captured by a 'generic set of stigma assessment instruments', but be a product of entirely different structural and cultural relations. Another risk associated with measurement *per se* is a reification of the concept of stigma: concepts as subtle and dynamic as this do not readily lend themselves to transmutation into the likes of variables. Certainly as yet it is appropriate to remain sceptical about the possibility of a cross-cultural or 'transfigurational' theory of either mental or physical health-related stigma (Scambler, 2004).

BEYOND PERSONAL TRAGEDY

A divide opened up in the 1980s and 1990s between the sociology of chronic illness and disability and an experientially-endowed and hard-headed 'rival', disability theory/politics. Medical sociology's 'deviance paradigm' was confronted by an 'oppression paradigm' (Thomas, 2007). The *accent was no longer on the labelled but the labellers*. The message implicit in sociology's 1950s and 1960s labelling theory of deviance pioneered by Lemert, Becker, Erikson and consociates, and applied to health and healing by Scheff and others, bore further fruit in the work of disability theorists like Oliver (1990). Why do those licensed and empowered to label act as they do? What else is at stake?

Disability research has as its basic premise the idea that disability involves the social oppression of people whose impairments mark them out, or are discursively constructed as marking them out, as *different*. 'Disablism' is thus appended to sexism, racism, ageism and homophobia as a form of exclusionary and oppressive practice (Thomas, 2007). This premise has often been articulated with reference to the 'social model of disability'. An important catalyst was Hunt's (1966) collection of 12 essays contributed by people with disabilities. Hunt, and later Finkelstein (1980), did the spadework for a social and materialist analysis of disability. As explicated by Oliver (1983), the resultant model was to displace 'individual' models of disability hinging on the notion of personal tragedy; moreover, this displacement was conceived as an urgent political as well as a warranted theoretical project. Disability, it was argued, was not the consequence of impairment but of the social restrictions imposed upon people with impairment, 'ranging from individual prejudice to institutional discrimination, from inaccessible public buildings to unusable transport systems, from segregated education to excluding work arrangements, and so on' (Oliver, 1996: 33). To acknowledge the salience of such oppressive 'social barriers' was to be challenged to politic for change.

Many disability studies scholars subsequently left the materialist fold, turning in particular to non-material or post-structural understandings of culture. Adherence to the pioneering version of the social model of disability is no longer obligatory. Many critics reject the distinction between impairment (characteristics of the body) and disability (social restrictions placed on people with impairments) utilized by Oliver. They dismissed this as another version of biomedical binary and reductionist thinking. Hughes and Paterson (1997: 334–335) advocated a phenomenology of the impaired body drawing on Merleau-Ponty:

> The impaired body is a 'lived body'. Disabled people experience impairment, as well as disability, not in separate Cartesian compartments, but as part of a complex interpenetration of oppression and affliction. The body is the stuff of human affliction and affectivity as well as the subject/object of oppression. The value of a phenomenological sociology of the body to the development of a sociology of impairment is that it embodies the addition of sentience and sensibility to notions of oppression and exclusion. Disability is experienced in, on and through the body, just as impairment is experienced in terms of the personal and cultural narratives that help to constitute its meaning.

There is no space here to trace the nuances of the last decade's re-theorizing of the oppression paradigm. It is relevant, however, to refer to Young's (1990) belatedly influential discernment of five faces of oppression, each one according to Thomas having resonance with ongoing attempts to explicate disablism:

- *Exploitation* draws on Marx and refers to the process by which the products of the labour of one group benefit another;
- *Marginalization* captures the expulsion of people for whom the system of labour has no use and their dispatch to society's margins;
- *Powerlessness* occurs in employment and other settings in which the power and authority of some undermine the autonomy and capabilities of others;
- *Cultural imperialism* arises when the dominant group's beliefs and attitudes are universalized, leaving others – feeling invisible or different – as deviant;
- *Violence* is reflected in systematic attempts to hurt, humiliate or eliminate groups considered beyond the pale.

Young's breakdown of modes of oppression contributes to a more refined conceptual framework for understanding estrangement and outsider status. Disability theory itself demands a sociology of chronic physical and mental illness and disability beyond Goffman-like, personal tragedy-oriented exegeses.

If sociology was slow to position biographical accounts of 'shameful' personal tragedies in wider social and structural contexts, there are indications that this hole is being slowly filled in. Link and Phelan (2001: 363) draw on disability as well as sociological studies to define stigma 'as the co-occurrence of its components – labelling, stereotyping, separation, status loss, and discrimination', critically adding that for stigmatization to occur 'power must be exercised'. Discrimination here does not simply refer to one individual's treatment of another, but to structural (or institutional) discrimination (i.e. a 'disabling environment') and to discrimination one or more steps removed from labelling and stereotyping, as when a loss of status occasioned by stigmatization leads to a spiralling of disadvantage. Link and Phelan (2001: 375) make power central: 'stigma is entirely dependent on social, economic, and political power – it takes power to stigmatize'. This raises a number of pivotal questions:

- do those who might stigmatize have sufficient power to ensure the human difference they recognize and label resonates in the public culture?
- do those who might confer stigma have the power to ensure that the culture 'deeply accepts' the stereotypes they connect to labelled differences?
- do those who might stigmatize possess power enough to underwrite and maintain a separation of 'us' from 'them'?
- do those who might confer stigma have the power to control access to core institutions like schooling, job markets, housing and healthcare in order to 'put really consequential teeth into the distinctions they draw'?

Positive answers to these questions, Link and Phelan (2001) argue, would lead us to expect stigma, while negative answers would seem to preclude stigma.

Parker and Aggleton (2003: 5–6) also insist on the salience of concepts like discrimination and power for understanding stigma. They call for a post-individualist analysis of the stigma associated with HIV/AIDS that acknowledges its functioning 'at the point of intersection between *culture, power and difference*'. Relations of stigma, they contend, are pivotal for the constitution of social order; and the social order 'promotes the interests of dominant groups as well as distinctions and hierarchies of ranking between them, while legitimating that ranking by convincing the dominated to accept existing hierarchies through processes of hegemony'. In similar vein, Rhodes and colleagues (2005) emphasize that 'much of the most needed "structural HIV prevention" is unavoidably political in that it calls for community actions and structural change within a broad framework concerned to alleviate inequity in health, welfare and human rights'.

A post-individualist and post-Goffman sociology of stigma relations must accept that they are part of a nexus of social structures; and, relatedly, that stigmatization (enacted stigma) is rarely the sole ingredient of disadvantage (Scambler, 2004). Returning to a study cited earlier, stigma in the study of epilepsy was designated an *ontological deficit*: picking up on Goffman's (1963) observation that stigma implies an unwitting, non-culpable falling foul of cultural norms, it was suggested that people with epilepsy felt different and experienced shame out of a sense of 'being imperfect' (Scambler and Hopkins, 1986). This led to an analytic distinction between two words with different ancestries – stigma and deviance – which have nevertheless often been treated as synonyms. While stigma denotes an ontological deficit, deviance refers to a *moral deficit*. Stigma invokes 'shame' and deviance 'blame'. This distinction invites empirical consideration of enacted and felt deviance as well as enacted and felt stigma in the health arena.

The point was made earlier that charges of stigma and deviance, even when levelled, are not always internalized or accommodated. This same phenomenon has been highlighted and documented in relation to mental illness by Corrigan and colleagues (2009), who make the point that for some self-stigma is rejected in favour of 'personal empowerment'. This led Scambler and Paoli (2008) to introduce the notions of 'project' stigma and deviance. Project stigma and deviance refer to the conscious rejection of attributions of shame and blame respectively. They signify resistance and/or defiance. These distinctions are outlined in Box 11.5.

The deployment of this conceptual apparatus took place within a frame insisting that the forms of interaction that provided take-off points for Goffman and the labelling theorists can only be explained sociologically if social structures, interpreted as necessary if rarely sufficient conditions of interaction, are empirically exposed. Cultural norms of shame and blame and the labelling processes with which they are bound up never exist in a structural vacuum but invariably arise within a structural nexus. In fact, as Deacon and Stephney (2007) have shown, such norms tend to follow the structural 'fault-lines' of society.

This embeddedness of norms of shame and blame in social structures has been illustrated with reference to the British government's 'welfare-to-work' programmes directed at those with chronic physical and mental disorders (Scambler, 2006: 293-294). Rooted in the premise that the relatively low employment rates amongst these groups contribute to the evils of poverty and social exclusion, these programmes were designed to facilitate the transition from out-of-work benefit receipt to paid employment. The strategies on offer were: education, training and work placements; vocational counselling and support services; in-work benefits; incentives for employers; and the improvement of physical accessibility.

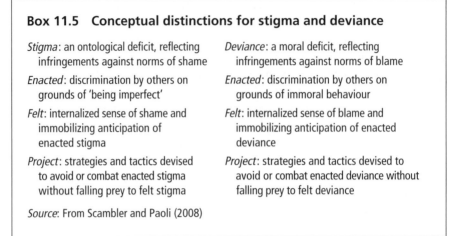

Box 11.5   Conceptual distinctions for stigma and deviance

Stigma: an ontological deficit, reflecting infringements against norms of shame

Deviance: a moral deficit, reflecting infringements against norms of blame

Enacted: discrimination by others on grounds of 'being imperfect'

Enacted: discrimination by others on grounds of immoral behaviour

Felt: internalized sense of shame and immobilizing anticipation of enacted stigma

Felt: internalized sense of blame and immobilizing anticipation of enacted deviance

Project: strategies and tactics devised to avoid or combat enacted stigma without falling prey to felt stigma

Project: strategies and tactics devised to avoid or combat enacted deviance without falling prey to felt deviance

Source: From Scambler and Paoli (2008)

Underpinning these strategies was an insistence on the exercise of 'demonstrable' personal responsibility. Monitoring these initiatives through the 1990s, Bambra and colleagues (2005) conclude that they have 'helped' some with chronic disorders and disabilities get off benefits and into work.

The contention here is that with welfare-to-work schemes, like the philosophy of personal responsibility imported from the USA, any putative gain, or reduction in stigmatization, has to be set against costs in terms of the requirement to actively avoid culpable deviance and in the currencies of exploitation and oppression. What is being maintained is *not* that the stigma associated with chronic illness and disability is never decisive in its own right, nor that stigmatization is now always transmuted into deviance and part and parcel of processes of exploitation and/or oppression. It does seem apparent, however, that stigmatization is rarely the sole ingredient of disadvantage, other notable companions in Britain for example, more conspicuously since the 1970s, being exploitation and oppression. This analysis of an intervention to 'reduce health-related stigma' leads on to a consideration of stigma reduction in mental illness.

REDUCING THE STIGMA OF MENTAL ILLNESS

Accounts of the impact of stigmatizing conditions or labels on individual's lives and coping styles, the personal tragedy approach, should not be condemned out of hand. It is not so much that they are flawed, more than they are limited and, in hindsight, unimaginative and unambitious: they overlooked social structure. Many current interventions to reduce stigma, however, remain obdurately biomedical and individualistic (Heijnders and van der Meij, 2006). In as far as they purport to *empower*, they do so on a 'top-down' basis, emphasizing either information-giving/prevention or self-empowerment (Rhodes et al., 1991). Again, programmes constructed on this basis are not without value (they may be pragmatic best options); but they are likely to be exercises in damage limitation. This is *not* a simple plea for more 'bottom-up' (radical-political or 'social transformatory' (Rhodes et al., 1991)) initiatives, more an exhortation to attend to explanatory adequacy.

Programmes of stigma-reduction in relation to mental illness have long been advocated. One particularly notable example was the initiative of the World Psychiatric Association (WPA) in 1996 to establish an international programme to contest stigma and discrimination in relation to schizophrenia (Sartorius, 1998). Schizophrenia was chosen because it is a serious condition, often of long duration, with symptoms associated in the popular imagination with mental illness. Moreover there is evidence that the rehabilitation of people with schizophrenia is frequently inhibited by stigmatization and related forms of discrimination. The thrust of the WPA programme has been to increase awareness and knowledge of the nature of schizophrenia and treatment options, to improve public attitudes towards individuals with schizophrenia and their families, and to encourage action to eliminate or reduce prejudice and discriminatory behaviour.

The WPA represents one type of intervention. Rusch et al. (2005) discuss stigma-reduction under three headings: 'education', 'contact' and 'protest'. The principal aim of education is to provide information – books, videos and structured teaching programmes for example – to contradict damaging stereotypes. It is well known, however, that education tends to be most effective when directed at those already disposed to assimilate its messages, either because they have a pre-existing awareness or actual experience or contact with mental illness. Messages based on current neurobiological models of mental illness might have either a positive return (if lay persons are encouraged to see mental illness as inherited or biochemical, and thus beyond attributions of shame (stigma), and certainly blame (deviance)); or a negative return (if lay persons come to see those with mental illness as 'almost a different species') (Rusch et al., 2005: 535). The jury is out on theses issues.

Contact with people with mental illness can complement educational initiatives. Familiarity typically mitigates against stigmatization (Angermeyer et al., 2004). There is evidence, however, that the circumstances in which what kind of contact is made with whom may matter a great deal. For example, contact in the workplace with a women with mental illness who is attractive and successful in her professional and personal roles might diminish stigma, but might also lead to a boomerang effect: the woman might be 'subtyped as unusual', re-classified as belonging to 'us' rather than 'them' (Rusch et al., 2005: 536).

Protest interventions can take various forms. In Germany, an alliance comprising people with mental illness (BASTA) deploys email to mobilize members to object to potentially stigmatizing advertisements of media messages. In four out of every five cases it brought BASTA was apparently successful, leading to the withdrawal of offending material and an apology (see Rusch et al., 2005). Similar protests in the USA have also been successful. Corrigan et al. (2005)

suggest, however, that such protests as these might change 'behaviour' while leaving underlying 'attitudes' untouched or even reinforced.

To the trilogy of education, contact and protest might be added two other, related forms of intervention, both of which pick up on points made earlier in this chapter. The first concerns the kind of 'personal empowerment' that can accompany the rejection of any sense of self-stigma and the psychosocial disadvantage likely to accrue from it (Scambler and Paoli's project stigma/deviance). Corrigan et al. (2005, 2009) claim that more effective anti-stigma interventions might eventually be constructed on the basis of an enhanced understanding of personal and social circumstances propitious to the rejection of enacted stigma/deviance on the part of people with mental illness without falling prey to felt stigma/deviance. It is intervention which has as its first premise the avoidance of might, following Bourdieu (1977), be called a *mental illness habitus*.

The second type of intervention is often advocated by social scientists or activists who argue that deeper structural change is a precondition for the effectiveness of anti-stigma campaigns. Personal empowerment, for example, is not viable in the absence of broader institutional and structural change. 'Unintentional' institutional and structural discrimination are the true culprits. This view characterizes many of the disability theorists and activists cited earlier, together with other 'bottom-up' interventionists who stress that it is the labellers not the labelled whose behaviours need to be amended. For many, stigmatization, including that of mental illness, is rarely to be found in the absence of one or more of Young's exploitation, marginalization, powerlessness, cultural imperialism or violence.

On the edge of this camp too are those who question psychiatry's ideological role. Pilgrim and Rogers (2005), for example, see professionally-sponsored anti-stigma campaigns – like the WPA's mentioned earlier, and, specifically, the British Royal College of Psychiatry's 'Changing Minds' campaign in the 1990s – as normative rather than purely scientific. Psychiatry, they insist, 'deals mainly with symptoms (what people say and do during residual rule-breaking) rather than signs (observable bodily changes linked to pain and impairment)' (Pilgrim and Rogers, 2005). Moncrieff (in press) adopts a similar position, proclaiming psychiatry's overriding commitment to social control. Professional ideologies, of course, are deeply embedded in the institutions and structures that constitute a social system.

CONCLUDING COMMENTS: THEORIES AND MODELS

Phelan et al.'s (2008) list of stigma models (see Box 11.1) is illustrative of an imaginative and cumulative enquiry into mental health stigma over half a century. Pescosolido et al. (2008) have recently sought to capture the essence of this enquiry in their 'Framework Integrating Normative Influences on Stigma' (FINIS), which is outlined in Figure 11.2. However, no cross-cultural or 'universal' *theory of stigma or deviance* in relation to mental illness is just around the corner, although adequacy at the level of theory might lead to a worthwhile contextualization, even refinement, of predictions of efficacious stigma reduction programmes of the kind sought by professional advocates and/or activists. In this sense policy sociology cannot be estranged not only from professional but also from critical and public sociologies (Burawoy, 2005). Sociological studies of health-related stigma can no longer afford – Goffman-like – to neglect the social structural underpinnings of cultural norms and individual choice. If Foucault too readily discarded the sociology of domination, his genius was demonstrated in laying bare the seductive properties of power. Enacted stigma and deviance can elide into government, and felt stigma and deviance into governmentality.

It was suggested earlier that work done under the rubric of what came to be called the personal tragedy/deviance paradigm needs to be re-framed and deepened. Stigma and deviance can be inscribed on persons as well as embodied; but they are also – and this is where lessons can be learned from disability theorists and activists promoting an oppression paradigm – 'structured' social relations. Goffman was clear on this but was only a little ahead of his time. Mental health stigma and deviance can be examined from macro- and meso- as well as micro-perspectives, from the vantage point of conflict as well as interactionist sociology.

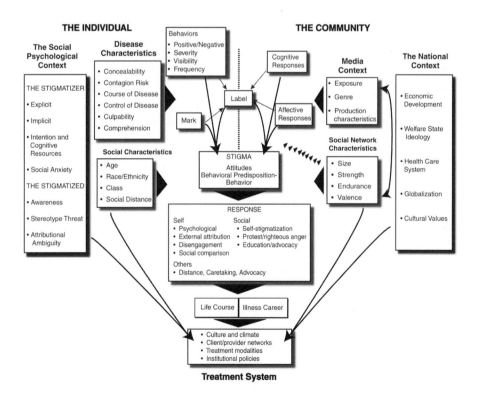

Figure 11.2   Framework integrating normative influence on stigma (FINIS)
Source: Figure reproduced from Pescosolido et al, 2008

As the welfare-to-work example illustrates, stigmatization can be infused with exploitation and oppression. Recalling Young's (1990) modes of oppression – not only exploitation but marginalization, powerlessness, cultural imperialism and violence – there exists a ready conceptual apparatus for the empirical investigation of *why* as well as *how* the dynamic dyad of shame and blame impact on the lives of some individuals and not others.

REFERENCES

Angermeyer, M. Matschinger, H. and Corrigan, P. (2004) Familiarity with mental illness and social distance from people with schizophrenia and major depression: testing a model using data from a representative population survey. *Schizophrenia Research,* 69: 175–182.

Armstrong, D. (2003) The impact of papers in *Sociology of Health and Illness*: a bibliographic study. *Sociology of Health and Illness,* 25: 58–74.

Bambra, C. Whitehead, E. and Hamilton, V. (2005) Does 'welfare-to-work' work? A systematic review of the effectiveness of the UK's welfare-to-work programmes for people with a disability or chronic illness. *Social Science and Medicine,* 60: 1905–1918.

Bourdieu, P. (1977) *Outline of a Theory of Practice.* Cambridge: Cambridge University Press.

Burawoy, T. (2005) For public sociology. *American Sociological Review,* 70: 4–28.

Bury, M. (1982) Chronic illness as biographical disruption. *Sociology of Health and Illness,* 4: 167–182.

Bury, M. (1991) The sociology of chronic illness: a review of research and prospects. *Sociology of Health and Illness,* 13: 167–182.

Chauncey, R. (1974) Comment on 'the labelling theory of mental illness'. *American Sociological Review.*

Charmaz, K. (1983) Loss of self: a fundamental form of suffering in the chronically ill. *Sociology of Health and Illness,* 5: 168–195.

Corrigan, P. Kerr, A. and Knudsen, L. (2005) The stigma of mental illness: explanatory models and methods for change. *Applied and Preventive Psychology,* 11: 179–190.

Corrigan, P. Larson, J. and Rusch, N. (2009) Self-stigma and the 'why try' effect: impact on life goals and evidence-based practices. *World Psychiatry,* 8: 75–81.

Crocker, J. Major, B. and Steele, C. (1998) Social stigma. In D. Gilbert, S. Fiske and G. Lindzey, (eds) *Handbook of Social Psychology* (4th edn), Vol. 2. Boston: McGraw-Hill.

Deacon, H. and Stephney, I. (2007) *HIV/AIDS, Stigma and Children: a Literature Review.* Cape Town: HSRC Press.

Falk, G. (2001) *Stigma: How We Treat Outsiders.* New York: Prometheus Books.

Finkelstein, V. (1980) *Attitudes and Disabled People: Issues for Discussion.* New York: World Rehabilitation Fund.

Freidson, E. (1970) *Profession of Medicine.* New York: Free Press.

Goffman, E. (1961) *Asylums: Essays on the Social Situation of Mental Patients and Other Inmates.* Chicago: Aldine.

Goffman, E. (1963) *Stigma: the Management of Spoiled Identity.* Harmondsworth: Penguin.

Goffman, F. (1967) *Interaction Ritual: Essays on Face-to-Face Behaviour.* New York: Doubleday.

Goffman, E. (1971) *Relations in Public: Microstudies of the Social Order.* New York: Basic Books.

Gove, W. (1970) Societal reaction as an explanation of mental illness: an evaluation. *American Sociological Review,* 35: 873–884.

Gray, D. (2002) 'Everybody just freezes. Everybody is just embarrassed': felt and enacted stigma among parents of children with high functioning autism. *Sociology of Health and Illness,* 24: 734–749.

Heijnders, M. and van der Meij, S. (2006) The fight against stigma: an overview of stigma-reduction strategies and interventions. *Psychology, Health and Medicine,* 11: 353–363.

Hughes, B. and Paterson, K. (1997) The social model of disability and the disappearing body: towards a sociology of impairment. *Disability and Society,* 12: 325–340.

Hunt, P. (ed.) (1966) *Stigma: the Experience of Disability.* London: Chapman.

Jobling, R. (1977) Learning to live with it: an account of a career of chronic dermatological illness. In Davis, A. and Horobin, G. (eds): Medical Encounters: *The Experience of Illness and Treatment.* London; Croom Helm.

Jones, E. Farina, A. Hastorf, A. Markus, H. Miller, D. and Scott, R. (1984) *Social Stigma: the Psychology of Marked Relationships.* New York: Freeman.

Kurzban, R. and Leary, M. (2001) Evolutionary origins of stigmatization: the functions of social exclusion. *Psychological Bulletin,* 127: 187–208.

Link, B. and Phelan, J. (2001) Conceptualizing stigma. *Annual Review of Sociology,* 27: 363–385.

Link, B. Cullen, F. Struening, E. Shrout, P. and Dohnrenwend, B. (1989) A modified labelling theory approach in the area of mental disorders: an empirical assessment. *American Sociological Review,* 54: 400–423.

Link, B. Yang, L. Phelan, J. and Collins, P. (2004). Measuring mental illness stigma. *Schizophrenia Bulletin,* 30: 511–541.

Major, B. and O'Brien, L. (2005) The social psychology of stigma. *Annual Review of Psychology,* 56: 393–421.

Moncrieff, J. (in press) Psychiatric diagnosis as a political device. *Social Theory and Health.*

Oliver, M. (1983) *Social Work with Disabled People.* Basingstoke: Macmillan.

Oliver, M. (1996) *Understanding Disability: From Theory to Practice.* London: Macmillan.

Parker, R. and Aggleton, P. (2003) HIV and AIDS-related stigma and discrimination: a conceptual framework and implications for action. *Social Science and Medicine,* 57: 13–24.

Pescosolido, B. Martin, J. Lang, A. and Olafsdottir, S. (2008) Rethinking theoretical approaches to stigma: a framework integrating normative influences on stigma. (FINIS). *Social Science and Medicine,* 67: 431–440.

Phelan, J. Link, B. and Dovidio, J. (2008) Stigma and prejudice: one animal or two? *Social Science and Medicine,* 67: 358–367.

Pilgrim, D. and Rogers, A. (2005) Psychiatrists as social engineers: a study of an anti-stigma campaign. *Social Science and Medicine,* 61: 2546–2556.

Putnam, S. (2008) Mental illness: diagnostic title or derogatory term? (Attitudes towards mental illness) Developing a learning resource for use within a clinical call centre. A systematic literature review on attitudes towards mental illness. *Journal of Psychiatric and Mental Health Nursing,* 15: 684–693.

Rhodes, T. Holland, J. and Hartnoll, R. (1991) *Hard to Reach or Out of Reach? An Evaluation of Innovative Models of HIV Outreach Health Education.* London: Tufnell Press.

Rhodes, T. Singer, M. Bourgois, P. Freidman, S. and Strathdee, S. (2005) The social structural production of HIV risk among injecting drug users. *Social Science and Medicine,* 61: 1026–1044.

Rusch, N. Angermeyer, M. and Corrigan, P. (2005) Mental illness stigma: concepts, consequences, and initiatives to reduce stigma. *European Psychiatry,* 20: 529–539.

Sartorius, N. (1998) Stigma: what can psychiatrists do about it? *Lancet,* 352: 1058–1059.

Scambler, G. (1989) *Epilepsy.* London: Tavistock.

Scambler, G. (2002) *Health and Social Change: A Critical Theory.* Buckingham: Open University Press.

Scambler, G. (2004) Re-framing stigma: felt and enacted stigma and challenges to the sociology of chronic and disabling conditions. *Social Theory and Health,* 2: 29–46.

Scambler, G. (2006) Sociology, social structure and health-related stigma. *Psychology, Health and Medicine,* 11: 288–295.

Scambler, G. (2009) Review article: health-related stigma. *Sociology of Health and Illness,* 31: 441–455.

Scambler, G. and Hopkins, A. (1986) 'Being epileptic': coming to terms with stigma. *Sociology of Health and Illness,* 8: 26–43.

Scambler, G. and Paoli, F. (2008) Health work, female sex workers and HIV/AIDS: global and local dimensions of stigma and deviance as barriers to effective interventions. *Social Science and Medicine,* 66: 1848–1862.

Scheff, T. (1966) *Being Mentally Ill: A Sociological Theory.* Chicago: Aldine.

Scheff, T. (1974) 'The labelling theory of mental illness'. *American Sociological Review,* 39: 444–452.

Schneider, J. and Conrad, P. (1980) In the closet with illness: epilepsy, stigma potential and information control. *Social Problems,* 28: 32–44.

Schneider, J. and Conrad, P. (1981) Medical and sociological typologies: the case of epilepsy. *Social Science and Medicine,* 15A: 211–219.

Schneider, J. and Conrad, P. (1983) *Having Epilepsy: The Experience and Control of Illness.* Philadelphia: Temple University Press.

Steele, C. and Aronson, E. (1995) Stereotype vulnerability and the intellectual test performance of African-Americans. *Journal of Personality and Social Psychology.* New York: Guilford Press.

Swim, J. and Thomas, M. (2006) Responding to everyday discrimination: a synthesis of research on goal-directed, self-regulatory coping behaviours. In S. Levin and C. Van Laar (eds) *Stigma and Group Inequality.* Mahwah, NJ: Erlbaum.

Thomas, C. (2007) *Sociologies of Disability and Illness: Contested Ideas in Disability Studies and Medical Sociology.* London: Palgrave Macmillan.

Van Brakel, W. (2006) Measuring health-related stigma – a literature review. *Psychology, Health and Medicine,* 11: 307–334.

Williams, G. (1984) The genesis of chronic illness: narrative reconstruction. *Sociology of Health and Illness,* 6: 175–200.

Wittgenstein, L. (1953) *Philosophical Investigations.* Oxford: Blackwell.

Yang, L. Kleinman, A. Link, B. Phelan, J. Lee, S. and Good, B. (2007) Culture and stigma: adding moral experience to stigma theory. *Social Science and Medicine,* 64: 1524–1535.

Young, M. (1990) *Justice and the Politics of Difference.* Princeton, NJ: Princeton University Press.

12

Medicalization and Mental Health: The Critique of Medical Expansion, and a Consideration of How Markets, National States, and Citizens Matter

Sigrun Olafsdottir

INTRODUCTION

Medical innovations and ideologies mirror societal developments and values. The nineteenth century witnessed enormous improvements in health, due in significant part to improvements in social conditions and medicine (McKeown, 1979; McKinlay, 1981). The twentieth century turned to a subsequent reliance on medical solutions for conditions historically not viewed as medical. This increased reliance on medicine, labeled as medicalization, represents a major societal transformation in advanced, industrialized nations (Clarke et al., 2003). It refers to a process in which medical authority has to a large degree replaced religious and legal authority systems (Conrad and Schneider, 1992; Zola, 1972). Social behaviors previously defined as a sin or as a crime are increasingly defined as an illness. Similarly, the sinner and the criminal have been replaced by the patient.

The acknowledgment of human difference is not a new development; in fact, societies have always viewed some individuals as "different." However, the way in which the "difference" is understood and addressed varies over time and context. On the one hand, responses can be inactive, such as ignorance, tolerance, or even appreciation. On the other hand, responses can be active, such as concern, prejudice, or even protection. In any case, these responses involve major social institutions, such as religion, the legal system, or medicine. In fact, the changes from inactive to active responses lie at the heart of medicalization (Conrad and Schneider, 1992). Behavior that previously went unnoticed, was frowned upon, or punished is increasingly viewed through the medical lens, signaling a biological problem that can be fixed with medical solutions. This process of medicalization has been conceptualized as "defining a problem in medical terms, using medical language to describe a problem, adopting a medical framework to understand a problem, or using a medical intervention to 'treat' it" (Conrad, 2000: 322).

Inevitably, the process of medicalization has resulted in a wide array of social behaviors and emotions to be viewed as a medical problem. In some cases, normal biological processes have been medicalized, including childbirth (Oakley, 1980; Rothman, 1982, 1989), fertility (Becker and Nachtigall, 1992; Friese et al., 2006), sexual function (Carpiano, 2001; Conrad, 2007; Graham, 2007), menopause (Bell, 1987, 1990; Meyer, 2001), andropause, (Szymczak, and Conrad, 2006), aging (Downs, 2000; Harding, and Palfry, 1997) and death (Conrad, 1992). Yet, many conditions subjected to medicalization, and importantly, some of the most contested conditions, fall under the mental health jurisdiction, including children's behavioral problems (Conrad, 1975; McLeod et al., 2004), adult ADHD (Conrad and Potter, 2000), alcoholism (Schneider, 1978), sadness (Horwitz and Wakefield, 2007), PMS (Figert, 1996), and gambling (Rosencrance, 1985).

The contested nature of mental health problems makes them ideal to consider in a comparative perspective as they lie at the heart of sociological debates about the social construction of reality (Berger and Luckman, 1966). As early as the 1960s, many prominent scholars, including psychiatrists, argued that mental illnesses were partly or even exclusively a social construction. For example, Scheff (1966) suggested that mental illness was as much a social role as "real illness." Szasz (1961, 1970, 1978) viewed mental illness merely as a myth, and Foucault (1965) illustrated how persons with mental illness were viewed as less acceptable human beings in the seventeenth century. And while later approaches frequently acknowledged the role of biology, they highlighted the role of culture in understanding health, illness, and healing. Here, they pointed out that the categories used to distinguish the sane from the insane are equally constrained by culture and history as biology (Kleinman, 1988; Horwitz, 2002) and interpretations and responses to mental illness are bound by culture (Angel and Thoits, 1987). Further, problems are not merely constructed by others, individuals also use symbols from the larger cultural context to label themselves normal or abnormal (Link and Phelan, 2001; Thoits, 1985). Currently, many social scientists would agree that some mental illnesses have a biological component, yet what is viewed as a mental illness and seen as an appropriate response is, at least in part, socially constructed (Link, 1982; Link et al., 1989; Martin et al., 2000, 2007).

Theories of medicalization are ultimately theories of power: who has the power to define, describe and respond to various social behaviors. Therefore, it is not surprising that researchers interested in medicalization focus on the driving forces of medicalization, often attempting to understand how and why the medical profession became one of the key agents of social control in advanced, industrialized nations during the twentieth century. And as the profession was seen as losing extreme power, looking to the countervailing forces in the present (Conrad and Leiter, 2004; Light, 2000) factors underplayed in the past (Pescosolido, 2006; Pescosolido and Martin, 2004) as well as the ways in which medicalization has been helpful, rather than harmful (Ballard and Elson, 2005; Broom and Woodward, 1996; Williams, 2001). And more recently, they have pointed out the possible influence of the pharmaceutical industry, consumers, and managed care (Ballard and Elston, 2005; Barker, 2008; Conrad, 2005; Conrad and Leiter, 2004; Moynihan and Cassels, 2005), with some even arguing that medicalization has transformed into biomedicalization, driven by technological imperatives (Clarke et al., 2003).

Although medicalization is a broad societal process that has taken place in all advanced, industrialized nations (Conrad, 2007), theories of medicalization have rarely compared medicalization processes across societies, and usually focus on a single society, most frequently the US, and to a less extent the UK. Given the important interplay of cultural understandings and biological realities, I argue that the lack of comparative perspective is problematic resulting in an incomplete, even inaccurate, understanding of medicalization processes. In general, the comparative perspective helps us to identify settings that are associated with particularly low or high levels of phenomena (Martikainen et al., 2004). They are often the only feasible way to evaluate relationships between policies and outcomes and they improve our understanding of the limits and generalizability of sociological theories and research (Martikainen et al., 2004).

Given the unique relationship between the market, the state and medicine in the US, a comparative perspective on medicalization is critical. For example, it has been assumed that medicalization processes have reached greater heights in the US than in any other nation (Conrad, 2007). This can partly be explained by early emphasis among medicalization scholars on the impact of a medical profession that was allowed to operate almost entirely through market dynamics. Consequently, early theories viewed medicalization as being driven by the market and the medical profession. However, this conceptualization may be as much a result of the unique position that the American medical profession found itself in (or forced itself into) as a real reflection of the relationship between the medical profession and medicalization processes. This relationship has always been more complex in other national settings, yet only recently has the potential impact of the state been theorized in medicalization research (Conrad and Leiter, 2004; Olafsdottir, 2007) as well as the changes in the doctor-patient relationship in the

US (McLeod et al., 2004). However, while this focus has broadened from just the medical profession to changes in delivery of health services more generally, most notably through managed care organizations, the fact remains that these relationships have been primarily theorized within one context, rather than comparing across societies.

This chapter begins with a brief overview of US theories and empirical research on the medicalization of mental illness and then examines medicalization as a broad social process applicable cross-nationally. I focus on four key agents of medicalization: the market, the medical profession, the state, and the public. Drawing from my comparative work on medicalization, I offer some insights into how each of these agents may matter for a comparative understanding of medicalization by empirically testing the impact of broader societal factors (e.g., globalization, the welfare state, and the medical profession) on two indicators that signal a medical solution to mental health problems. Centering these analyses in the cultural and political landscape surrounding mental health contexts in the United States, Germany, and Iceland, I focus on how the discourse in these nations views mental illness, ending with an in-depth analysis of how key actors within the mental health field in Iceland conceptualize mental health problems and how they view the medicalization of mental health. While not the only way to look at the medicalization of mental health in a comparative perspective, it does provide new information on how medicalization processes work cross-nationally, representing an early attempt to correct the US-bias in current theories.

MEDICINE, THE MARKETPLACE, AND MEDICALIZATION

The American medical profession was not only able to gain more power within its jurisdiction than medical professions in other nations, it has also been allowed to operate under the law of the market, rather than the principle of health care as a fundamental human right. The United States is the only advanced, industrialized nation that does not provide universal health care to all citizens (Quadagno, 2005). Consequently medicine becomes more of a product in a medical market in the United States than elsewhere. Yet, recent data shows that Americans may have embraced medical solutions to such an extent that they value the product more than the medical expertise. More specifically, they appear to have embraced psychiatric medication as a solution to children's mental health problems, yet they have not simultaneously embraced the exclusive right of medical doctors to prescribe such medication (Olafsdottir and Pescosolido, 2010).

Of course, medicalization has long been a result of technological advances (Conrad, 1975, Wertz and Wertz, 1989), but the relationship between medicalization and technology is changing in a fundamental way. In earlier periods, technology facilitated medicalization, but currently the pharmaceutical industry is becoming a major player supporting medicalization (Angell, 2004; Conrad, 2005, 2007; Clarke et al., 2003; Moynihan and Cassels, 2005). Research in the United States has shown how the relationship between the public and the medical profession has changed with health information and support available on the internet (Barker, 2008; McKinlay and Marceau, 2008) and direct-to-consumer advertisement (Findlay, 2001; Lenzer, 2005; Relman and Angell, 2002; Rosenthal et al., 2002). There are even demonstrated examples of a simultaneous marketing of a disease and a drug to treat that disease; specifically the public was made aware of milder anxiety disorders (e.g., general anxiety disorder) and a specific product (Paxil) that solved the problem (Conrad, 2005; Koerner, 2002).

While the market clearly impacts medicalization in the United States, and likely does the same in other nations, the relationships that emerge are likely to differ. Consequently, the emphasis on the pharmaceutical companies may reflect a US-centered orientation and lack of a comparative perspective. While the transformation from the medical profession toward the market as one of the driving forces of medicalization (Conrad, 2005) may be correct within the American context, the cross-national reality is likely to be more complex. For example, Conrad (2005) argues that the passage of the Food and Drug Administration (FDA) Modernization Act of 1997 changed the rules of the game for the pharmaceutical industry by allowing them to advertise directly to the public. While notable, this is unique to the United States. Direct-to-consumer advertisement is not allowed in most advanced, industrialized nations and the market has not been able to interact with consumers in the same manner in nations other than the US. Yet, research has shown that some nations rival the United States when it comes to prescription of psychiatric medication, while other nations remain with much lower prescription rates (Olafsdottir, 2007). The key question that comparative perspective can answer is: *What explains increased reliance on psychiatric medication within and across nations, and how is this trend impacted by market forces that experience different constrains across different national contexts?*

Insights from a comparative perspective on markets

In what follows, I glean some findings from my own comparative work on medicalization that looks at medicalization in selected countries over selected time-periods. These data provide insight into how medicalization within and across countries may be impacted by markets, the medical profession, the state, and consumers, and begins to answer some of the key questions that a comparative approach to medicalization asks. More specifically, I evaluate the impact of globalization, the welfare state, and the medical profession on two indicators that put mental health problems clearly into the medical jurisdiction: the number of psychiatric beds and prescription of anti-depressants.

While useful, this analysis does not reveal the cultural and political landscape of how groups and societies construct mental illness. To provide insight into the cultural and political landscape of how groups and societies construct mental illness, I draw on data from a discourse analysis of newspapers in three national contexts: the United States, Germany, and Iceland. There is limited comparative research on the relationship between markets and medicalization, and the work that exists largely focuses on the impact of pharmaceutical companies as an important player in the marketplace. Examining trends in prescription of anti-depressants shows that some nations have high prescription rates, while others have low prescription rates. For example, the reliance on antidepressants has increased drastically in Iceland, while remained low in Germany (Olafsdottir, 2007). The question remains if and how this relates to marketing on behalf of the pharmaceutical or if other cultural, political, or institutional factors provide a better explanation.

In the US, newspaper discourse may be expected to attribute responsibility for mental health problems to the market. This is not the case. In fact, only 2 percent of US articles discuss the market explicitly, compared to no articles in Iceland or Germany. A more informative pattern emerges when cross-national differences regarding individual responsibility are considered. In the US, 70 percent of articles locate the responsibility within the individual, compared to 10 percent or less in Germany and Iceland. Individuals should take responsibility for their problems and seek help in the medical marketplace. However, a unique relationship between the market and medicine in the United States is also in evidence. For example, children with mental health problems are referred to as "defective merchandise," the homeless with mental health problems use the street as "place of business," and innovations in medicine are attributed to the market driven nature of American society (Olafsdottir, 2007).

Finally, while the discourse provides insights into the kind of information the public is likely to receive from the media, it does not reveal how decisions about appropriate responses are made. To provide insights into how medicalization of mental health actually takes place, I draw on data with 50 key actors in the mental health field in Iceland, including professionals and policymakers.[1] Although limited to one national context, this last analysis examines how the policymaking process takes place within a context where both the state and the medical profession have significant power in the mental health jurisdiction, and where it is possible to include nearly all key national actors. All respondents acknowledge some market influence, but there is a great variation in terms of how they view its importance. Some respondents view the pharmaceutical industry as inactive, mostly providing information. Conversely, some view the same industry as active in terms of having a great impact on mental health policy and treatment. Not surprisingly, group differences emerge, with almost 90 percent of policymakers believing it to have a direct impact, while only 60 percent of non-medical professionals and advocates and fewer than 10 percent of medical doctors do so. Medical professionals view pharmaceutical companies as important, but inactive, actors that provide information and solutions: "When I look back, I don't think there has ever been an inappropriate pressure from drug companies, over those drugs. This is a new type of drug and of course it had to be introduced and I think they did it well and professionally. Therefore, that is not the reason for all the prescriptions; that is just because they are good." Importantly, all groups except medical doctors view the industry's influence as undesirable, arguing that the companies actually affect what doctors do, resulting in increased medicalization. As some respondents noted, "the pharmaceutical industry has enormous amounts of money and they offer all sorts of education with their own spin," "There is a danger that doctors start to prescribe unusually much of a specific medication, that the drug company that paid for the conference is marketing," and "they are very influential in which drugs are used."

In sum, most national actors agree that the market and more specifically the power and position of the pharmaceutical industry, impacts mental health policy and treatment, although how they view the market forces varies by professional position. While this research was conducted within one national context with high levels of prescription rates and a specific interplay of institutional arrangements, cultural expectations, and health care trajectory, it reveals that the impact of the pharmaceutical companies does not appear to be unique to the United States. Furthermore, the influence was also in effect in the United States prior to direct-to-consumer advertising, with medical doctors as gatekeepers and the pharmaceutical representatives catering exclusively to them, not to the general public.

THE MEDICAL PROFESSION AS A DRIVING FORCE OF MEDICALIZATION

While the market has played some role, the role of the medical profession has always been highlighted. The professional dominance approach was long a leading explanation of medicalization in the United States, yet the focus on the medical profession is problematic in comparative perspective. While the American medical profession was able to obtain high levels of power over its jurisdiction (Freidson, 1970; Starr, 1982), the situation was quite different for medical professions in other countries. The American health care system is also unique in other ways. Most importantly, it is the only system among advanced, industrialized nations that does not provide universal health care for its citizens (Quadagno, 2005) and the private sector, through philanthropy, played a large role in establishing professional power (Pescosolido and Martin, 2004). The particular relationship between medicine and society in the United States makes any generalization outside of its context problematic.

The social organization of health care represents the social contract between society and medicine. Comparative health researchers have categorized national health care systems in multiple ways that partly illustrate how much power the medical profession has within each national context. For example, nations that have adapted the *Insurance Model* allow medical doctors to provide services in an environment where the state only sets and maintains a system of contracts among patients, providers, and insurance. The United States, Germany, Canada, and Japan fall into this category. Contrast this with the *Centralized Model* where all the health care facilities are owned by the state and medical doctors work directly for the state. Countries in this category include Hungary, Czech Republic, Russia, and Poland. In between, the *NHS* system provides universal health care in publicly owned hospitals, but gives more autonomy for the medical profession and, here physicians are allowed to opt out of the system. Nations in this category include Australia, Italy, Sweden, Iceland, and the United Kingdom (Kikuzawa et al., 2008; Lassey et al., 1997; Stevens, 2001).

The different levels of power allocated to the medical profession under different health care systems determine how the profession is able to contribute to the medicalization of social behavior. In general, doctors should be most capable of "pushing" or driving medicalization under the *Insurance model* where most theories of medicalization have focused on (Conrad, 1975; Conrad and Schneider, 1992; Clarke et al., 2003). And not only has the focus been on one type of health care system, it has been on the most unique nation possible, the United States. When theories of medicalization are extended into a comparative perspective, it is clear that medical professions in virtually all other countries have not been given the same freedom to impact issues of health, illness, and healing, as their American counterparts. In each of these nations, medical doctors must engage in negotiations with a state, which either completely controls their work, or controls their work more intensively than in the United States (Hafferty and McKinlay, 1993). However, medical knowledge is frequently viewed as universal, that is medical professionals across national boundaries believe in the same or similar ideas across national boundaries, yet national realities constrain how they can use or even want to use their knowledge (Olafsdottir, 2007). In fact, research from the UK has illustrated that medical doctors may not want jurisdiction over certain health problems and that they are concerned about over-medicalization (Williams and Calnan, 1994). Thus, one of the key questions to generalize medicalization theory for comparative scholars is: *How do medical professionals conceptualize and respond to medicalization and how is their ability to promote a medical framework to understand a wide array of conditions embedded within specific institutional arrangements, cultural expectations, and historical trajectories?*

Insights on mental illness and medicalization from a comparative perspective on the medical profession

While traditional theories of medicalization would assume that the power of the medical profession would increase medicalization, cross-national research has shown that this is not always the case. A quantitative analysis of advanced, industrialized nations indicates that the number of practicing physicians did not increase, but actually decreased the number of psychiatric beds across 19 advanced, industrialized nations from 1960–2000 (Olafsdottir, 2007). While deinstitutionalization clearly became the leading model for mental health treatment across nations, researchers argued that psychiatrists would oppose such development, given their power position within the hospital (Abbott, 1988). This did not happen (Grob, 1991). Similarly, the number of practicing physicians failed to significantly increase the reliance on antidepressants in 10 advanced, industrialized nations from 1990–2005. However, national participation in international psychiatric organization increased the number of beds, indicating that the global ideas of the psychiatric profession were inconsistent with local developments highlighting community services (Olafsdottir, 2007).

Exploring variations in the power of medical ideas, reliance on medical solution and the power of medical doctors across three advanced, industrialized nations (the US, Germany, and Iceland), Olafsdottir (2007) illustrates that there is significant variation in how medicalized mental health is across national context, as well as in the power allocated to medical doctors by national media. This research shows that while the US discourse is more likely to highlight biological explanation for mental health problems and to propose medical solutions for such problems than the discourse in Iceland, the difference is not statistically significant. However, the difference between the US discourse and the German discourse is significant, suggesting that the cultural ideas represented in the US are more medicalized than those represented in Germany (Figure 12.1).

A different picture emerges when exploring the visibility and power given to the medical profession. Here, half of all articles discussing mental health problems in Iceland mention medical doctors, compared to 38 percent of US articles and only 22 percent of German articles. When the analysis is restricted to the profession that most directly controls the mental health jurisdiction, psychiatrists, cross-national differences disappear (Figure 12.2). These results show that it is inaccurate to assume that the US will always have the greatest tendency to medicalize health problems, and underscores the importance of comparative work to fully understand the relationship between medical ideas, the medical profession, and medicalization.

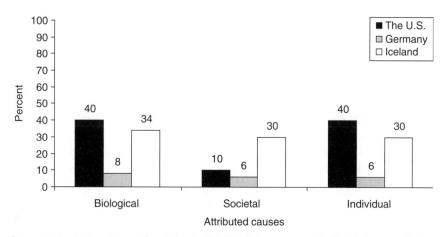

Figure 12.1   Percentage of articles in the US, Germany, and Iceland that attribute causes of mental health problems to biology, society, or individuals

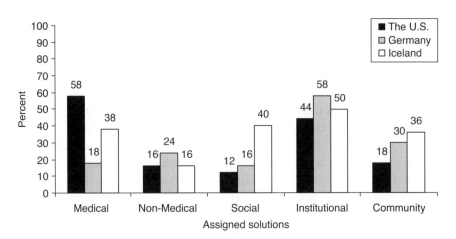

Figure 12.2   Percentage of articles in the US, Germany, and Iceland that assign different types of solutions to mental health problems

What do professionals and policymakers say about medicalization?

Somewhat curiously, scant research on the medical profession as a driving force behind medicalization has looked to the views of medical professionals themselves. The interview study of Iceland, reported here, supports findings from the UK that medical doctors have a complex relationship with medicalization (Williams and Calnan, 1994). Nevertheless, the findings show that medical doctors tend to view medicalization more positively than other key actors in the mental health field. Over 60 percent of medical doctors (general practitioners and psychiatrists) considered medicalization only in positive terms, compared to less than 15 percent of any other group, who either viewed medicalization exclusively as negative, as both positive and negative, or as neutral. Those who view medicalization as a positive process used three arguments to support their position. First, medicalization helps those who suffer; second, it reduces prejudice, and third, it signals a good health care system and an improved system of diagnosis. Interestingly, medical doctors are more likely than other groups to discuss medicalization as a proof of good medical services, arguing that everyone who needs help is receiving help. For example, when discussing the idea of medicalization in Iceland, a psychiatrist pointed out, "General medical doctors are very good in diagnosing depression and we are very good at treating people" (Olafsdottir, 2007).

Although several mental health providers pointed to positive aspects of medicalization, many of those interviewed highlighted the negative aspects. Again, differences between groups emerged. Less than 30 percent of medical doctors view medicalization exclusively in negative terms, compared to almost 40 percent of policymakers and 60 percent or more of non-medical professionals and advocates. The latter respondents gave three reasons for why medicalization is negative. First, that it is a reflection of a culture that demands quick solutions; second, it removes power away from individuals; and third, it signals the lack of other available solutions. A clear conflict appears between medical professionals and other health professionals, where medical doctors view medical solutions as appropriate and other health professionals criticize the overreliance on the medical model. For example, an occupational therapist stated, "This fundamental belief in the medical model, I feel like that is a hindrance in my job and the patients feel it too, it is often viewed as, the one true solution, to take medication and be hospitalized" (Olafsdottir, 2007).

When these key actors were asked which groups have major influence in the mental health field, 74 percent mention medical doctors. Again, interesting differences between groups emerge. Medical doctors themselves are actually less likely to consider themselves to have major impact, than both non-medical professionals and advocates. In fact, approximately 60 percent of policymakers and medical professionals believe the profession of medicine to have major influence, compared to over 80 percent of non-medical professionals and 100 percent of advocates. Not surprisingly, even when national actors in different locations agree that the medical profession has a major impact, their discourse varies by position. Specifically, non-medical professionals, liberal politicians, and advocates are critical of the current system, arguing that there is too great a tendency to frame mental health problems exclusively within a medical framework. Conversely, conservative politicians and medical doctors may acknowledge that medical doctors have a lot of power, but they consider that power to be valid (Olafsdottir, 2007).

These findings suggest that medical doctors may partly drive medicalization, simply because they believe that medicine provides the best solution. Of course, that does not imply lack of concern for their own professional status, rather indicates a more complex relationship, especially within a context that allocates less power to the market. It is equally important to consider the different opinions raised by other actors. While professional conflicts are likely to share some similarities across national context, the unique relationship between the state, the market and medicine impacts national debates and final outcomes of these conflicts. Understanding this in the context of the social organization of health care, the opinions of the medical profession may matter most in the *Insurance Model*, the opinions of state actors may have the most weight under the *Centralized Model*, and that multiple voices may be most likely to be heard under the *NHS Model*.

STATE INTERVENTION IN MEDICALIZATION PROCESSES

Medicalization is a consequence of a specific relationship between the state, the market, and medicine, and does not only take place under specific institutional arrangements. Rather, the relationship between the state, the market, and medicine defines how medicalization takes place and the form it takes. Despite the extensive authority obtained by the American medical profession, the state has long been a key player within the US medical field. Although, the introduction of Medicare and Medicaid in the 1960s was a fundamental change for American medicine, it did not change the relationship between doctors and patients. The changes introduced in the 1980s guided how much doctors could charge for their services. This represented the first state attempt to directly control what doctors could do and what they could charge for their services (Ruggie, 1992). Later, the Clinton health care reform failed but nonetheless spurred the private sector to move to managed care (Jensen et al., 1997). While it would be an overstatement, as some have argued, that physicians lost their power and prestige (Haug, 1973; Ritzer and Walczak, 1988), managed care organizations fundamentally altered the medical landscape. These organizations require approval for medical treatment and set limits on provided care (Goode, 2002; Shore and Beigel, 1996). In turn, these changes within the American medical field resulted in the state receiving increased attention from medicalization scholars (Conrad, 2005, 2007; Conrad and Leiter, 2004). Yet, despite these changes, some continue to argue that the way health policy in the US is conceptualized is fundamentally embedded within a medical framework. This results in an overemphasis on providing equal access to health care while neglecting a focus on equalizing health outcomes (Lantz et al., 2007).

While managed care within the US led to a consideration of how the state impacts medicalization, the fundamental relationship between the state and medicine in other nations has been ignored. Unlike the American medical profession's largely exclusive power, medical professions in other countries had to either negotiate with state actors or in some cases (e.g., Russia), were controlled by state actors. While classifications of nations according to their welfare system traditionally has not paid great attention to health care,[2] these groupings offer an indication of the relationship between the state and the market (including the medical market) in advanced, industrialized nations (Esping-Andersen, 1990; Ferrera, 1996; Huber and Stephens, 2001; Olafsdottir and Beckfield, 2010; Orloff, 1993). As an example, Esping-Andersen (1990) divides nations into three worlds of welfare capitalism: liberal welfare states, conservative welfare states, and social democratic welfare states. The liberal welfare states rely heavily on the market to take care of societal issues and do little to do correct inequalities created in the marketplace. Nations belonging to this regime are the United States, Canada, and the UK. The conservative welfare state prefers solutions outside of the state (e.g., family and charities), yet interfere when these systems fail. Germany, Austria, and Switzerland provide an example of this regime. Finally, the social democratic welfare state explicitly uses state intervention to correct inequalities in the market and generally avoid market solutions to solve societal issues. Sweden, Norway and Iceland are examples of social democratic welfare states (Esping-Andersen, 1990). Even this brief overview of welfare state classification underscores why focusing on the US is problematic. While all advanced, industrialized nations are welfare states, there is a large variation in what they do and how much they interfere with medicine and markets. The liberal welfare states generally provide the least, but the US is an outlier among these countries. Consequently, while it is important to consider cross-national variation in medicalization as a result of different institutional arrangements, the US is likely to be the most unique of all advanced, industrialized nations when it comes to the relationship between the state, the market and medicine.

In the US, the medical profession was able to control virtually every aspect of its work for a long time. In other nations, the state had the ultimate power to define and respond to health problems, although in many nations the medical profession was heavily involved in policymaking. As early as the 1970s, scholars pointed out that medical professionals were the dominant group in health policy, although they had to debate and justify their interest to policymakers and health advocates (Alford, 1975). And while governments, insurers, and large health services delivery organization increasingly challenge the authority of medical professionals (Harrison and Pollit, 1994; Wilsford, 1995), a recent study in Australia finds that the networks and knowledge of medical experts make them extremely powerful in the policy making process (Lewis, 2006). Even the current changes in the US that have led medicalization scholars to pay increased attention to the state, represent yet another case of American exceptionalism (Lipset, 1996). American medicine is moving from a fee-for-service system to a system that is controlled by for-profit insurance companies, rather than the state (Lassey et al., 1997). This uniqueness is reflected in public attitudes toward government intervention in health care. While a large percentage of Americans support government responsibility for health care, the percentage that does so is much lower than in virtually every other advanced, industrialized nation (Kikuzawa et al., 2008). This stands in contrast to other nations, where the recent attacks on large welfare states have led to some retrenchment. Health care, however, remains among the hardest to reduce programs. One of the explanations for this is high public support for these programs (Wilensky, 2002).

Medicalization processes are embedded within institutional arrangements that shape how medicalization happens and what mechanisms are the main forces of medicalization. The key question for understanding the relationship between the state and medicalization in a comparative perspective is: *What role does the state play in medicalization processes, how does it vary between different types of societies, and how do state actors negotiate with other key actors in the health field when defining health problems and responding to illness?*

A comparative look at medicalization and the welfare state

The welfare state can act both as an enabler and constraint on medicalization processes across advanced, industrialized nations. When the welfare state as a whole is considered, high levels of social expenditure decrease institutionalization of individuals with mental health problems. However, nations that have higher public spending on health rely more on both institutions and psychiatric medication (Olafsdottir, 2007). This highlights the importance of considering both the welfare state as a whole and the welfare state as a provider of health care, in attempts to understand how medicalization is impacted by the relationship between the state, the market, and medicine.

Although significant relationships are observed between the welfare state and medicalization in a large sample of nations, a closer look at the cultural aspect of medicalization provides a strong support of how the welfare state shapes national discourses. The analysis of newspaper articles in the US, Iceland, and Germany shows that national discourses, especially in Iceland, both reflect and create welfare state ideology (see Figure 12.3). The Icelandic discourse is most likely to emphasize societal causes for mental health problems, assign social solutions, and assign responsibility to the government and/or society as a whole. The US discourse, in contrast, is more likely to assign causes and responsibility to individuals, representing a view of mental health problems as something that individuals should solve themselves, rather than the state. Overall, discourse produces three cultural regimes, a *Culture of Fear* in the US, a *Culture of Retribution* in Germany, and a *Culture of Solidarity* in Iceland. These patterns show that the extent to which mental health is medicalized within nations is a combination of historical trajectories, cultural traditions, and institutional arrangements (Olafsdottir, 2007).

Adding to this, the interview data from Iceland show that over 60 percent of key actors in the mental health field consider the state as having major impact on responses to mental health problems. Medical doctors and policymakers are more likely to highlight the importance of the state than non-medical professionals and advocates. The findings illustrate a clear conflict between state actors and medical professionals. While policymakers view it as essential that decisions about medical issues are political decisions, medical professionals criticize policymaking for relying too little on medical expertise. For example, a medical doctor states, "I think about those who rule within the health care system that make all

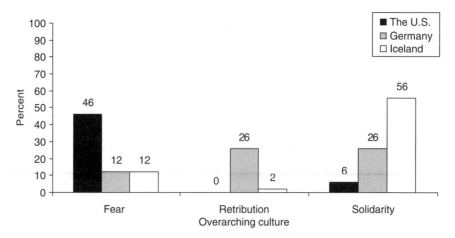

Figure 12.3   Percentage of articles in the US, Germany, and Iceland representing the culture of fear, retribution, or solidarity

sorts of decisions against what professional thinks." Similarly, policymakers high-light their own role, yet underscore the importance of decision making outside of the medical field, partly because of tendency of medical doctors to over-medicalize (Olafsdottir, 2007).

Thus, the state represents a key actor defining and responding to mental health problems in advanced, industrialized nations. While important US research has highlighted the role of managed care (Conrad and Leiter, 2004) and the state as one of countervailing powers in the health field (Light, 2000), the history of the relationship between the state and the medical profession is clearly different in other countries. Outside the US, the medical profession has a long history of negotiating with the state within the medical jurisdiction, and even more impor-tantly they are negotiating with a state that is primarily concerned with providing health services to the entire population.

THE PUBLIC AS A DRIVING FORCE FOR MEDICALIZATION

Medicalization theories have always acknowledged the potential role of the public in medicalization processes. Early insights viewed the power of the public as possible through creation of social movements fighting for medicalization (or de-medicalization) of specific illnesses (Fox, 1989; Halpern, 1990; Kroll-Smith and Floyd, 1997; Pawluch, 1983; Scott, 1990; Wertz and Wertz, 1989). However, with the changing US medical system, "patients" have been transformed to "consumers." The provision of health care is increasingly open to market forces with medical care beginning to resemble other products and services. Individuals and families select health insurance plans, select between providers, and hospitals compete for patients (Conrad, 2007).

In the United States, the public generally endorses a wide variety of medical explanations and solutions to mental health problems, signaling that a large proportion of Americans have accepted medical definitions and solutions to mental health problems (Link et al., 1999, McLeod et al., 2004; Olafsdottir and Pescosolido, 2010; Pescosolido et al., 1999; Schnittker et al., 2000). Further, even where the medical profession resists medicalization, it has been pursued by patient groups (Asbring and Narvanen, 2003; Barker, 2008; Barsky and Borus, 1999). Because the American public appears to be less tolerant of mild symp-toms than before (Barsky and Boros, 1995; Schnittker, 2009), these changes have also been referred to as the medicalization of everyday life (Szasz, 2007).

Although higher levels of education, increased access to information, and more emphasis on quality of life (Inglehart, 1997) represent general trends in advanced, industrialized nations, the relationship between the public and medi-cine varies substantially between the US and other nations. In the US, citizens have grown accustomed to viewing medicine as a product that can be bought and sold in the marketplace, rather than as a social citizenship right provided by the state (Lassey et al., 1997; Olafsdottir and Beckfield, 2010). In fact, research has shown that Germans are likely to utilize services for minor problems, simply because they view medical care as an inherent social right (Lassey et al., 1997). These differences have implication for medicalization and the demands citizen make on the health care system and policymakers regarding medical definitions and treatments. The key question for the relationship between the public and medicine in a comparative perspective becomes: *What is the extent to which the public in different nations embraced medicine and with what consequences?*

Public demands in a comparative perspective

While the US arguably does most to "sell" medicine to the public (Conrad, 2007), it appears that citizens in other nations have embraced the medical model as well and even to a greater extent. For example, results from the Stigma in Global Context Study (SGC-MHS) indicate that despite significant cross-national variation, the public in other Western nations (e.g. Germany, Iceland and Spain) has embraced medicine as a key solution to mental health problems (Pescosolido et al., 2008). And somewhat surprisingly, for medicalization theories, the American public is not more supportive of psychiatric medication than the Icelandic public. In fact, Icelanders appear to be slightly more likely to embrace such medication (Olafsdottir and Pescosolido, n.d.). These findings illustrate that while medical solutions are available to the American public as a consumer good, this does not necessarily translate into higher endorsement of medical solutions in the US. It appears that some forces, other than the law of the market, operate in an effort to make the public in other nations generally supportive of medical innovations and consequently, willing to medicalize various conditions.

Although the public clearly includes a larger group of individuals than those experiencing mental health problems and their social networks, how these groups are perceived provides insights into the relationship between the public and medicine within and across nations. The three nation discourse analysis shows that individuals experiencing health problems are mentioned in 60 percent of newspaper articles in the US, 68 percent in Germany, and 52 percent in Iceland. Yet, the results also show that while the German articles are most likely to discuss patients, they are least likely to give them voice in the media, depicting them as inactive patients, rather than active participants in their own illness experience. But in the US, 34 percent of all articles discuss individuals experiencing mental health problems as criminals, compared to less than 20 percent in both Iceland and Germany. Theories of medicalization imply a historical process, moving social problems from a sin, to a crime, to an illness (Conrad and Schneider, 1992). Combined, these findings may indicate that the US is trailing behind regarding this development, still more likely to view individuals as criminals than patients (Olafsdottir, 2007).

About 60 percent of key actors in the mental health field in Iceland believe that consumers have a major impact in the medical field and an interesting group difference emerges. All advocates and 80 percent of policymakers believe that the voice of consumers really matters, compared to 50 percent or less among medical and non-medical providers. When elaborating on the role of the consumer, most agree that the key contribution has been to open up the mental health discourse, more specifically to change mental illness from something that was shameful to something that could happen to everyone. This is illustrated in the words of a politician, "We have started to see very smart people who are willing to come forward and say, yes, I am mentally ill but that does not mean that I am not a part of society." Importantly, for medicalization theories, respondents explicitly mention how pressure from interest groups changed mental health treatment in Iceland, moving it from institutions to the community. While that does not imply demedicalization, living in the community with assistance from a wide range of professionals represents a less direct medical intervention than living in a hospital monitored by medical professionals (Olafsdottir, 2007).

TOWARD A COMPARATIVE RESEARCH AGENDA ON MEDICALIZATION

Individuals, groups, and societies conceptualize and respond to variations in social behavior, emotions, and feelings in different ways. It is clear that Western societies have increasingly witnessed medicalized definitions and responses, yet less is known about how these definitions and responses vary across societies and what explains this variation. In this chapter, I have provided insights from comparative work on medicalization that clearly illustrates the importance of institutional arrangements, cultural traditions, and historical trajectories for understanding how and why mental health has been medicalized in advanced, industrialized nations.

Current work on medicalization has powerfully demonstrated how and why specific conditions have become medicalized within a specific context, and theorized about the factors that are likely to increase and perhaps decrease medicalization. Comparative work provides insights into both these processes. Here, the question is twofold: Are there conditions that are medicalized within one context but not another? If the condition is medicalized in both contexts, was the process similar or different? Second, a comparative approach allows us to empirically test the factors that impact medicalization, both quantitatively and qualitatively. The former can be used to test whether factors such as the pharmaceutical industry or the power of the medical profession has impacted various indicators of medicalization and the latter can evaluate whether the factors that mattered in the medicalization within one country also matter in another context.

While an understanding of medicalization in a comparative perspective adds to our understanding of the interplay between social construction and biological realities, it also has implications for individuals living with mental health problems (or variations in mental health) across societies. The ways in which mental health problems are presented in society matters for the lived experience of individuals in that society. For example, it is likely that an Icelander diagnosed with mental illness may have a different view of what is happening than an American. The Icelander would be used to seeing mental illness conceptualized as a societal problem, rather than an individual problem. Further, changes in how we view mental illness provide the public with new stereotypes of the "mentally ill," which shapes both responses toward the individual as well as the internal process that takes place once a person is diagnosed (Link and Phelan, 2001). The increased tendency of viewing mental illness as a genetic disorder in the US, has not only resulted in the public believing mental illness to be more serious and persistent, it has also resulted in increased social distance on the domains of family, marriage and children (Phelan, 2005). Sociological theories of the twentieth century have clearly demonstrated that medical knowledge is not neutral and not always based on discovering new and "better" truths. A cross-cultural perspective lays bare the differences, providing an important counterpoint to an image of medical absolutes.

NOTES

1 More specifically, medical doctors, psychiatrists, psychologists, social workers, occupational therapists, nurses, policymakers, and consumers.

2 For example, including only sickness benefits in an index measuring decommodification, for detail see Olafsdottir and Beckfield (2010).

REFERENCES

Abbott, Andrew Delano (1988) *The System of Professions: An Essay on the Division of Expert Labor.* Chicago, IL: University of Chicago Press.

Alford, Robert R. (1975) *Health Care Politics: Ideological and Interest Group Barriers to Reform.* Chicago, IL: University of Chicago Press.

Angel, Ronald and Peggy A. Thoits (1987) The impact of culture on the cognitive structure of illness. *Culture, Medicine, and Psychiatry,* 6: 465–494.

Angell, Marcia (2004) *The Truth about the Drug Companies: How They Deceive Us and What To Do About It.* New York, NY: Random House.

Asbring, Pia and Anna-Liisa Narvanen (2003) Ideal versus reality: physicians perspectives on patients with chronic fatigue syndrome (CFS) and fibromyalgia. *Social Science and Medicine,* 57: 711–720.

Ballard, Karen and Mary A. Elston (2005) Medicalisation: a multi-dimensional concept. *Social Theory and Health,* 3: 228–241.

Barker, Kristin K. (2008) Electronic support groups, patient-consumers, and medicalization: the case of contested illness. *Journal of Health and Social Behavior,* 49: 20–36.

Barsky, Arthur J. and Jonathan F. Borus (1995) Somatization and medicalization in the era of managed care. *Journal of the American Medical Association,* 274: 1931–1934.

Becker, Gay and Robert D. Nachtigall (1992) Eager for medicalisation: the social production of infertility as a disease. *Sociology of Health and Illness,* 14: 456–471.

Bell, Susan E. (1987) Changing ideas: the medicalization of menopause. *Social Science and Medicine,* 24: 535–542.

Bell, Susan E. (1990) Sociological perspectives on the medicalization of menopause. *Annals of the New York Academy of Sciences*, 592: 173–178.

Berger, Peter L. and Thomas Luckmann (1966) *The Social Construction of Reality: A Treatise in the Sociology of Knowledge*. Garden City, NY: Doubleday.

Broom, D. and Woodward, R. (1996) Medicalisation reconsidered: a collaborative approach to care. *Sociology of Health and Illness*, 18: 357–378.

Carpiano, Richard M. (2001) Passive medicalization: the case of viagra and erectile dysfunction. *Sociological Spectrum*, 21: 441–450.

Clarke, Adele E., Laura Mamo, Jennifer R. Fishman, Janet K. Shim, and Jennifer Ruth Fosket Fosket (2003) Biomedicalization: technoscientific transformations of health, illness, and U.S. biomedicine. *American Sociological Review*, 68: 161–194.

Conrad, Peter (1975) The discovery of hyperkinesis: notes on the medicalization of deviant behavior. *Social Problems*, 23: 12–21.

Conrad, Peter (1992) Medicalization and social control. *Annual Review of Sociology*, 18: 209–232.

Conrad, Peter (2000) Medicalization, genetics, and human problems. In C.E. Bird, Peter Conrad, and Allen M. Fremont (eds). *Handbook of Medical Sociology*. Upper Saddle River, NJ: Prentice Hall. pp. 322–333.

Conrad, Peter (2005) The shifting engines of medicalization. *Journal of Health and Social Behavior*, 26: 3–14.

Conrad, Peter (2007) *The Medicalization of Society: On the Transformation of Human Conditions into Treatable Disorders*. Baltimore, MD: Johns Hopkins University Press.

Conrad, Peter and Valerie Leiter (2004) Medicalization, markets and consumers. *Journal of Health and Social Behavior*, 45: 158–176.

Conrad, Peter and Deborah Potter (2000) From hyperactive children to ADHD adults: observations on the expansion of medical categories. *Social Problems*, 47: 559–582.

Conrad, Peter and Joseph W. Schneider (1992) *Deviance and Medicalization: From Badness to Sickness*. Philadelphia, PA: Temple University Press.

Downs, Murna (2000) Dementia in a socio-cultural context: an idea whose time has come. *Ageing and Society*, 20: 369–375.

Esping-Andersen, Gøsta (1990) *TheThree Worlds of Welfare Capitalism*. Princeton, NJ: Princeton University Press.

Ferrera, Maurizio (1996) The 'Southern Model' of welfare in social Europe. *Journal of European Social Policy*, 6: 17–37.

Figert, Anne E. (1996) *Women and the Ownership of PMS: The Structuring of a Psychiatric Disorder*. New York, NY: Aldine De Gruyter.

Findlay, S.D. (2001) Direct-to-consumer promotion of prescription drugs: economic implications for patients, payers and providers. *PharmacoEconomics*, 19: 109–119.

Foucault, Michel (1965) *Madness and Civilization: A History of Insanity in the Age of Reason*. New York, NY: Pantheon Books.

Fox, Patrick (1989) From senility to Alzheimer's disease: the rise of the Alzheimer's disease movement. *The Milbank Quarterly*, 67: 58–102.

Freidson, Eliot (1970) *Profession of Medicine: A Study of the Sociology of Applied Knowledge*. New York, NY: Harper and Row.

Friese, Carrie, Gay Becker, and Robert D. Nachtigall (2006) Rethinking the biological clock: eleventh-hour moms, miracle moms and meanings of age-related infertility. *Social Science and Medicine*, 63: 1550–60.

Goode, Erica (2002) Psychotherapy shows a rise over decade, but time falls. *New York Times*, p. 421.

Graham, Cynthia A. (2007) Medicalization of women's sexual problems: a different story? *Journal of Sex and Marital Therapy*, 33: 443–447.

Grob, Gerald N. (1991) *From Asylum to Community: Mental Health Policy in Modern America*. Princeton, N.J.: Princeton University Press.

Hafferty, Frederic W. and John B. McKinlay (1993) *The Changing Medical Profession: An International Perspective*. New York, NY: Oxford University Press.

Halpern, Sydney A. (1990) Medicalization as professional process: postwar trends in pediatrics. *Journal of Health and Social Behavior*, 31: 28–42.

Harding, Nancy and Colin Palfrey (1997) *The Social Construction of Dementia: Confused Professionals?* London, UK: Jessica Kingsley Publishers.

Harrison, Stephen and Christopher Pollitt (1994) *Controlling Health Professionals: The Future of Work and Organization in the National Health Service*. Buckingham, UK: Open University Press.

Haug, Marie R. (1973) Deprofessionalization: an alternative hypothesis for the future. *Sociological Review Monograph*, 20: 195–211.

Horwitz, Allan V. (2002) *Creating Mental Illness*. Chicago, IL: University of Chicago Press.

Horwitz, Allan V. and Jerome C. Wakefield (2007) *The Loss of Sadness: How Psychiatry Transformed Normal Sorrow into Depressive Disorder*. Oxford, UK: Oxford University Press.

Huber, Evelyne and John D. Stephens (2001) *Development and Crisis of the Welfare State: Parties and Policies in Global Markets*. Chicago, IL: The University of Chicago Press.

Inglehart, Ronald (1997) *Modernization and Postmodernization: Cultural, Economic, and Political Change in 43 Societies*. Princeton, NJ: Princeton University Press.

Jensen, Gail A., Michael A. Morrisey, Shannon Gaffney, and Derek K. Liston (1997) The new dominance of managed care: insurance trends in the 1990s. *Health Affairs*, 16: 135–136.

Kikuzawa, Saeko, Sigrun Olafsdottir, and Bernice A. Pescosolido (2008) Similar pressures, different contexts: public attitudes toward government intervention for health care in 21 nations. *Journal of Health and Social Behavior*, 49: 385–399.

Kleinman, Arthur (1988) *Rethinking Psychiatry: From Cultural Category to Personal Experience*. New York, NY: Free Press.

Koerner, Brendan I. (2002) Disorders, made to order. *Mother Jones*, 27: 58–63.

Kroll-Smith, J. Stephen and H. Hugh Floyd (1997) *Bodies in Protest: Environmental Illness and the Struggle over Medical Knowledge*. New York, NY: New York University Press.

Lantz, Paula M., Richard L. Lichtenstein, and Harold A. Pollack (2007) Health policy approaches to population health: the limits of medicalization. *Health Affairs*, 26: 1253–1257.

Lassey, Marie L., William R. Lassey, and Martin J. Jinks (1997) *Health Care Systems around the World: Characteristics, Issues, Reforms*. Upper Saddle River, NJ: Prentice Hall.

Lenzer, Jeanne (2005) American medical association rejects proposal to ban consumer adverts for prescription medicines. *British Medical Journal*, 331: 7.

Lewis, Jenny M. (2006) Being around and knowing the players: networks of influence in health policy. *Social Science and Medicine*, 62: 2125–2136.

Light, Donald W. (2000) The medical profession and organizational change: from professional dominance to countervailing power. In C.E. Bird, P. Conrad, and A.M. Fremont (eds). *Handbook of Medical Sociology*, 5th edition. Upper Saddle River, NJ: Prentice Hall.

Link, Bruce (1982) Mental patient status, work, and income: an examination of the effects of a psychiatric label. *American Sociological Review*, 47: 202–215.

Link, Bruce G. and Jo C. Phelan (2001) Conceptualizing stigma. *Annual Review of Sociology*, 27: 363–385.

Link, Bruce G., Francis T. Cullen, Elmer Struening, Patrick Shrout, and Bruce P. Dohrenwend (1989) A modified labeling theory approach in the area of mental disorders: an empirical assessment. *American Sociological Review*, 54: 400–423.

Link, Bruce G., Jo C. Phelan, Michaeline Bresnahan, Ann Stueve, and Bernice A. Pescosolido (1999) Public conceptions of mental illness: labels, causes, dangerousness, and social distance. *American Journal of Public Health*, 89: 1328–1333.

Lipset, Seymour Martin (1996) *American Exceptionalism: A Double-Edged Sword*. New York, NY: W.W. Norton.

Martikainen, Pekka, Eero Lahelma, Michael Marmot, Michikazu Sekine, Nobuo Nishi, and Sadanobu Kagamimori (2004) A comparison of socioeconomic differences in physical functioning and perceived health among male and female employees in Britain, Finland and Japan. *Social Science and Medicine*, 59: 1287–1295.

Martin, Jack K., Bernice A. Pescosolido, and Steven A. Tuch (2000) Of fear and loathing: the role of 'disturbing behavior', labels, and causal attributions in shaping public attitudes toward persons with mental illness. *Journal of Health and Social Behavior*, 41: 208–223.

Martin, Jack K., Bernice A. Pescosolido, Sigrun Olafsdottir, and Jane D. McLeod (2007) The construction of fear: Americans' preferences for social distance from children and adolescents with mental health problems. *Journal of Health and Social Behavior*, 48: 50–67.

McKeown, Thomas (1979) *The Role of Medicine: Dream, Mirage, or Nemesis?* Princeton, NJ: Princeton University Press.

McKinlay, John B. (1981) Refocusing upstream. In P. Conrad and R. Kern (eds). *The Sociology of Health and Illness*. New York: St. Martin's Press.

McKinlay, John and Lisa Marceau (2008) When there is no doctor: reasons for the disappearance of primary care physicians in the US during the early 21st century. *Social Science and Medicine*, 67: 1481–1491.

McLeod, Jane D., Bernice A. Pescosolido, David T. Takeuchi, and Terry Falkenberg White (2004) Public attitudes toward the use of psychiatric medications for children. *Journal of Health and Social Behavior*, 45: 53–67.

Meyer, Vicki F (2001) The medicalization of menopause: critique and consequences. *International Journal of Health Services*, 31: 769–792.

Moynihan, Ray and Alan Cassels (2005) *Selling Sickness: How the World's Biggest Pharmaceutical Companies are Turning us All into Patients*. New York, NY: Nation Books.

Oakley, Ann (1980) *Women Confined: Towards a Sociology of Childbirth*. New York, NY: Schocken Books.

Olafsdottir, Sigrun (2007) Medicalizing mental health: a comparative view of the public, private, and professional construction of mental illness. *Sociology*. Bloomington, IN: Indiana University.

Olafsdottir, Sigrun and Jason Beckfield (2010) Health and the social rights of citizenship: integrating welfare state theory and medical sociology. In B.A. Pescosolido, J.K. Martin, J.D. McLeod, and A. Rogers (eds). *Handbook of Sociology of Health, Illness, and Healing*.

Olafsdottir, Sigrun and Bernice Pescosolido (2010) Professional boundaries and public responses: how lay preferences for child mental health care support and counter struggles in the medical division of labor. In *Annual Meeting of the Eastern Sociological Society*. Boston, MA.

Olafsdottir, Sigrun and Bernice Pescosolido (eds) (forthcoming) Compassion or expertise: comparing trust toward doctors in the US and Iceland. Unpublished manuscript.

Orloff, Ann Shola (1993) Gender and the social rights of citizenship: the comparative analysis of gender relations and welfare state. *American Sociological Review*, 58: 303–328.

Pawluch, Dorothy (1983) Transitions in pediatrics: a segmental analysis. *Social Problems*, 30: 449–465.

Pescosolido, Bernice A. (2006) Professional dominance and the limits of erosion. *Society*, 43: 21–29.

Pescosolido, Bernice A., John Monahan, Bruce G. Link, Ann Stueve, and Saeko Kikuzawa (1999) The public's view of the competence, dangerousness, and need for legal coercion of persons with mental health problems. *American Journal of Public Health*, 89: 1339–1345.

Pescosolido, Bernice A. and Jack K. Martin (2004) Cultural authority and the sovereignty of American medicine: the role of networks, class, and community. *Journal of Health Politics, Policy and Law*, 29: 735–756.

Pescosolido, Bernice A., Sigrun Olafsdottir, Jack K. Martin, and J. Scott Long (2008) Cross-cultural issues on the stigma of mental illness. In J. Arboleda-Florez and N. Sartorius (eds). *Understanding the Stigma of Mental Illness: Theory and Interventions*. West Sussex, England: John Wiley and Sons.

Phelan, Jo. (2005) Geneticization of deviant behavior and consequences for stigma: the case of mental illness. *Journal of Health and Social Behavior*, 46: 307–322.

Quadagno, Jill S. (2005) *One Nation, Uninsured: Why the U.S. has no National Health Insurance*. Oxford, UK: Oxford University Press.

Relman, Arnold S. and Marcia Angell (2002) America's other drug problem. *New Republic*, 227: 27–41.

Ritzer, George and David Walczak (1988) Rationalization and the deprofessionalization of physicians. *Social Forces*, 67: 1–22.

Rosecrance, John (1985) Compulsive gambling and the medicalization of deviance. *Social Problems*, 32: 275–284.

Rosenthal, Meredith B., Ernst R. Berndt, Julie M. Donohue, Richard G. Frank, and Arnold M. Epstein (2002) Promotion of prescription drugs to consumers. *New England Journal of Medicine*, 346: 498–505.

Rothman, Barbara Katz (1982) *In Labor: Women and Power in the Birthplace*. New York, NY: Norton.

Rothman, Barbara Katz (1989) *Recreating Motherhood: Ideology and Technology in a Patriarchal Society*. New York, NY: Norton.

Ruggie, Mary (1992) The paradox of liberal intervention: health policy and the American welfare state." *American Journal of Sociology*, 97: 919–944.

Scheff, Thomas J. (1966) *Being Mentally Ill: A Sociological Theory*. Chicago: Aldine Publishing Company.

Schneider, Joseph W. (1978) Deviant drinking as disease: alcoholism as a social accomplishment. *Social Problems*, 25: 361–372.

Schnittker, Jason (2009) Mirage of health in the era of biomedicalization: evaluating change in the threshold of illness, 1972–1996. *Social Forces*, 87: 2155–2182.

Schnittker, Jason., Jeremy Freese, and Brian Powell (2000) Nature, nurture, neither, nor: black-white differences in beliefs about the causes and appropriate treatment of mental illness. *Social Forces*, 78: 1102–32.

Scott, Wilbur J. (1990) PTSD in DSM-III: A case in the politics of diagnosis and disease. *Social Problems*, 37: 294–310.

Shore, Miles F. and Beigel Allan (1996) The challenges posed by managed behavioral health care. *New England Journal of Medicine*, 334: 116–119.

Starr, Paul (1982) *The Social Transformation of American Medicine*. New York, NY: Basic Books.

Stevens, Fred (2001) The convergence and divergence of modern health care systems. In W.C. Cockerham (eds). *The Blackwell Companion to Medical Sociology*. Malden, MA: Blackwell Publishers Inc.

Szasz, Thomas S. (1961) *The Myth of Mental Illness: Foundations of a Theory of Personal Conduct*. New York, NY: Dell Publishing Company.

Szasz, Thomas S. (1970) *The Manufacture of Madness: A Comparative Study of the Inquisition and the Mental Health Movement*. New York, NY: Harper & Row.

Szasz, Thomas S. (1978) *The Myth of Psychotherapy: Mental Healing as Religion, Rhetoric, and Repression*. Garden City, NY: Anchor Press/Doubleday.

Szasz, Thomas S. (2007) *The Medicalization of Everyday Life: Selected Essays*. Syracuse, NY: Syracuse University Press.

Szymczak, Julia E. and Conrad, Peter (2006) Medicalizing the aging male body: andropause and baldness. In D. Rosenfeld and C. Faircloth (eds) *Medicalized Masculinities*. Philadelphia: Temple University Press.

Thoits, Peggy A. (1985) Self-labeling processes in mental illness: the role of emotional deviance. *American Journal of Sociology*, 91: 221–249.

Wertz, Richard W. and Wertz, Dorothy C. (1989) *Lying-in: A History of Childbirth in America*. New Haven, CT: Yale University Press.

Wilensky, Harold L. (2002) *Rich Democracies: Political Economy, Public Policy, and Performance*. Berkeley, CA: University of California Press.

Williams, Simon R. (2001) Sociological imperialism and the profession of medicine revisited: where are we now? *Sociology of Health and Illness*, 23: 135–158.

Williams, Simon R. and Calnan, Michael (1994) Perspectives on prevention: the views of general practitioners. *Sociology of Health and Illness*, 16: 372–393.

Wilsford, David (1995) States facing interests: struggles over health care policy in advanced, industrial democracies. *Journal of Health Politics, Policy and Law*, 20: 571–613.

Zola, Irving K. (1972) Medicine as an institution of social control. *Sociological Review*, 20: 487–504.

13

Danger and Diagnosed Mental Disorder

David Pilgrim and Anne Rogers

INTRODUCTION

This chapter deals with a contentious and ambiguous topic. It is contentious because when mental disorder has been deemed to be a recurring source of danger, it has provoked extensive debates about evidence and prejudice. It is ambiguous because the commonly held belief, which the title of the chapter connotes for many in advanced societies, is that mental disorder is a *source* not an *outcome* of danger. This is an example of what Bourdieu called 'doxa': a self-evident belief in society, in this case about mental disorder. In order to query doxa in relation to our topic, this chapter will examine the relationship between danger and diagnosed mental disorder, with an emphasis on a two way, not a one way, relationship.

An immediate challenge in relation to violence and doxa is our ingrained tendency to view violence purely as a matter of individual victims and perpetrators. And in the case of mental disorder the latter overwhelmingly predominates in the public imagination and in 'mental health policy' formation. This pulls our attention away from hidden or systemic violence and so a pacifist like Ghandi could insist legitimately in protest at this seduction that 'the deadliest form of violence is poverty'.

This highlights that terms such as 'symbolic violence' or 'systemic violence' are useful in reminding us that sociological accounts need to look beyond the micro-politics of violence to its wider context of inequalities and their political maintenance (Zizek, 2007). For example, as we will see later, individuals who use street drugs are at a higher risk of being violent. But their acts pale into insignificance compared to the violence implicated in maintaining and resisting an illicit drug trade. In 1993 this point was made in the USA by the National Academy of Science in its deliberations on drug misuse: 'For illegal psychoactive drugs, the illegal market itself accounts for far more violence than pharmacological effects' (Reiss and Roth, 1993). If individual drug use is criminalized then there will be violent consequences from both the state and from organized crime, which will spiral into widespread victimization.

In this chapter, these background assumptions need to be borne in mind as we examine the micro-politics of danger. We use the term 'danger' rather than 'violence' for two reasons. First, much of the risk assessment and management of mental disorder is based on the *prospect or possibility* of violence, rather than proven past violent acts (which may or may not be taken into consideration case by case). Second, 'danger' as a broader term points to topics, which include, but also lie beyond proven violence to the self or others. These include notions of 'threat' and 'nuisance' in relation to third party risk, as well as emotional abuse, symbolic violence and the insecure settings which affect mental health.

The chapter will first look at the empirical evidence and legal contention surrounding danger as a basis for the social control of those deemed to be mentally disordered. In the second half of the chapter, we then move to the dangerous contexts which increase the probability of mental disorder appearing in our midst as a socially negotiated state.

DANGER TO SELF AND OTHERS

Legal assumptions and challenges

'Mental health legislation' is not about mental health but focuses only on a sub-population of those deemed to be *mentally disordered*. The existence of such legislation is considered by those like the World Health Organization and most governments in developed countries to be an unambiguous sign of socio-political progress. However, this assumption has not gone unchallenged. Libertarians have argued now for over forty years that the medicalization of psycho-social problems is an offence to human freedom, when coercive powers of the state are invoked to control deviance (Szasz, 1963).

In the UK in the run up to the development of the Mental Health Act of 2007, these fundamental debates were evident. Opponents, including for example the British Psychological Society, argued that the previous Mental Health Act (of 1983) should be abandoned and replaced by a law about *dangerousness,* which was not focused on mental state *per se* and which could be complemented by extant legislation on disability rights. Such a scenario was ruled out of court in advance by the government but the fact that the policy was debated at all indicates that we now live in a period when taken for granted paternalism and discrimination is being challenged and disrupted. For example, it is now recognized in reviews of mental health law that its existence is inherently discriminatory because it separates out one risky group in society and not others for special legal consideration (Department of Health, 1999). For example, we know actuarially that young intoxicated males are at high risk of perpetrating violence against others every weekend in city centre streets, on the roads and in the home but there is no dedicated law to detain them as a group without trial or advocacy for their freedom.

Thus the existence of so called 'mental health law' is about the lawful control of some (but not all) those deemed to be mentally disordered and some (but not all) of all those manifesting risky action in society. Despite this, the more benign justification of such law refers not to social control but to beneficence; it might ensure that people in need receive the benefits of medical interventions (Pols, 2001). Given these different readings about the very point of legal arrangements about mental disorder, the field is mired in mystification and contention, with paternalists defending it as a self-evident necessity to do good and civil libertarians attacking it as a form of State sanctioned violence.

In the latter regard, with the exception of anti-terrorism legislation, mental health law imposes coercive control on adults without trial and with regard to speculations about prospective risks rather than proven danger to date. Certainly in any other circumstances, many of the actions associated with the enforced detention and treatment of some mentally disordered people would leave perpetrators open to charges of abduction, false imprisonment and assault. The existence of 'mental health law' protects agents of the state from these charges.

Suicide and self harm

In those countries in which suicide is not illegal, then those making suicidal attempts or gestures might still be controlled coercively using mental health law. The same applies to those who are distressed and self-harming but not intending to end their life (e.g. those with heavy blood loss, who cut themselves). It also applies at times to those starving themselves; low weight anorexic patients might be detained and force fed. Thus mixed cultural messages are common in those countries, which permit suicide but also contain mental health law.

For example, patients discharged from psychiatric facilities are immediately at high risk of completed suicides, with those detained compulsorily being at particular risk (Hunt et al., 2009). This suggests that even though suicide may not be illegal (implying that it is a matter a citizen's choice) in most countries, psychiatric patients are constrained, albeit not always successfully, from making a decision to end their life. Amongst other things, coercive psychiatric containment would seem to defer, if not always prevent, suicide.

In the case of suicide and intended suicide, contingencies are always important. Those apprehended in the act, or those who insistently tell those around them that they are going to end their life, will invite the attention of mental health professionals but those acting more discreetly will not, implicating different outcomes.

An important implication of suicide and self-help attracting professional attention is that the expertise of the latter is then invoked and legitimized.

For example, 'psychological autopsies' by psychiatry have now framed suicide as a form of obvious mental disorder under the posthumous clinical gaze, even though, since Durkheim, social science has been sensitized to a range of non-pathological possibilities. Similarly, self-harm in society is highly variegated and exists on a continuum, with a wide range of motivations implicated (from norms of religion, drug use and fashion). However, under some contingencies but not others it is deemed to be clear evidence, or an expression, of mental disorder. (This is an example of a more general point explored by Olafsdottir, this handbook, in relation to medicalization.)

As an example of the challenge of sense-making about a world, in which risks to the self are part of daily life, take the high risk of completed suicide by people regularly intoxicated. If habitual intoxication is deemed to be a mental disorder (which it is under DSM and ICD) then 'substance misuse' *as a psychiatric condition* predicts suicide (Schnieider, 2009). On the other hand, if regular intoxication is not deemed to be a symptom, or type, of a mental disorder, which it was not prior to the psychiatric nosologies of the mid-twentieth century, it still remains a predictor of suicide. However, both suicide and drunkenness might alternatively be understood in variegated social-existential, not specific clinical, terms. The role of substances in risking harm to others, rather than the self is discussed later.

A final point to make is that the failure to seek treatment can be grounds for psychiatric detention and forced intervention. In other words, some people who do not enter the patient role voluntarily are deemed to be putting themselves at risk in a range of ways, which then invoke a 'duty of care' and a 'right to treat' on the part of psychiatric professionals. Thus a dynamic process ensues in which illness without insight is the basis for rationalizing coercive acts on the part of agents of the state. The forced re-admission of psychotic patients known to services and who are observed becoming more symptomatic or who are deemed to 'decompensate' in their community settings is an example of this point.

Once more, in socio-legal terms, this makes psychiatric patients different from physically ill patients. Many of us in the latter category fail to seek treatment or have habits which are injurious to our health and yet it is very rare for legal statute to be invoked to force treatment upon us, let alone justify our deprivation of liberty without trial. For example, obesity is common in developed countries and it increases the risk of morbidity and premature death but there is not legal provision to lock up and treat manifestly over-weight people for the good of their health or to alter patterns of healthcare utilization and tax burden (which is a logical policy option). Thus the existence of mental health law ensures in a pointed and discriminatory way that acts of agents of the state, which would otherwise be deemed to be forms of violence against others, are rendered lawful and legitimate *about some forms of personal risk and not others*.

The tension between restrictions on citizenship and paternalistic risk management are at their most evident when legal measures are used to control mental disorder, when the latter implies risk to self or others (Dennis and Monahan, 1996; Szmukler and Appelbuam, 2001). As with the use of the death penalty, here there is an ironic scenario: the state offers violence as a response to violence, rendering one form legitimate and the other illegitimate.

Madness and violence to others

The association in the public imagination between madness and violence dates back to antiquity and changed little with modernity (Rosen, 1968). This assumption remains so deeply ingrained that it has inevitably maintained a form of policy formation, in which risk to others is a recurring concern not of the criminal justice system alone but also of the 'mental health system'. However, the empirical justification for this is dubious and contestable. This is not to say that some people with mental health problems are not dangerous – they are. But given that most violent crimes are committed by people with no psychiatric diagnosis, the degree of overlap between patient and non-patient populations is important to ascertain. As we will see in the next section, this exercise is clouded though by the increasing designation of anti-social conduct as forms of mental disorder.

With these points in mind, we can turn to what is known about the link between madness and dangerousness. Early studies of the relationship between 1925 and 1965 suggested that people with mental health problems were actually *less violent* than the general population (Rabkin, 1979). However, this was the very period in which most psychiatric patients were warehoused semi-permanently in institutions, which created a structural impediment to potential violence in open society (see Scull this handbook).

Later studies suggested that indeed a relationship did exist. Link et al. (1992) found that after 1965 the median ratio was one of 3:1, with patients being more violent than non-patients. A number of factors could account for this reversal. The first was just noted about institutional containment. The second is that when patients were discharged, this was very often into risky community settings. In the latter, socially disorganized, neighbourhoods crime rates were high, so patients were at increased risks of becoming both perpetrators and victims. A third ecological factor relates to base rates of substance abuse in those localities. Access to disinhibiting substances was very limited in the asylum system.

Reviewing this small positive relationship, Monahan (1992: 510) noted that:

> None of the data give any support to the sensationalized caricature of the mentally disordered served up by the media ... Compared with the magnitude of risk associated with the combination of male gender, young age, and lower socio-economic status for example, the risk of violence presented by mental disorder is modest. Compared with the magnitude of risk associated with alcoholism and other drug abuse, the risk associated with major mental disorders such as schizophrenia and affective disorder is modest indeed. Clearly, mental health status makes at best a trivial contribution to the overall level of violence in society.

Subsequent reviews of the literature revealed a complicated inter-relationship between clinical, personality and social contextual factors (Blumenthal and

Lavender, 2000; Pilgrim and Rogers, 2003). An increasing number of studies began to address specific aspects of the relationship between mental state and violence.

In community settings Swanson et al. (1990) found that psychotic patients who did not abuse substances were three times more dangerous than their non-patient equivalents over a period of a year. By contrast, Steadman et al. (1998) found that psychotic patients who did not abuse substances were no more likely to be violent than their neighbours. Given that violent acts are quite rare it is also worth noting that even in the Swanson et al. study, their findings only pointed to 7 per cent of violent compared to 93 per cent non-violent patients. This is why the summary of the small aggregate relationship by Monahan above refers to a 'trivial contribution'.

When examining the specific role of psychosis this triggering or synergistic impact of substance misuse became an important factor to consider. Substances that create behavioural disinhibition were thus firmly implicated in violent action – a finding that is true for *all in the population*. However, when a psychotic patient has a history of violence, is grudge bearing or is obsessed by a particular victim (e.g. in stalking) then they do become more dangerous than others who abuse substances, when intoxicated (Hambracht and Hafner,1996; Soyka, 2000; Steadman et al., 1998).

Some specific symptoms also seem to increase the risk of violence, such as command hallucinations with violent content and delusions involving hostile threat from others (Junginger, 1995; Taylor, 1985). Substance abuse plus violent ruminations also increase the risk of violence (Grisso et al., 2000). However, there is not a *general* demonstrable relationship between the simple presence of psychotic symptoms and violent action. The *particular* content, rather than the general presence, of symptoms is the key nuance.

Moreover, broad diagnostic categories, other than that of 'personality disorder' (see next section), are of little use as a risk predictor (Appelbaum et al., 1999, 2000; Monahan, 2000). For example, even after the reversal of the pattern of violence noted after 1965, studies continued to find that a diagnosis of 'schizophrenia' indicated no increased risk of violence (Teplin et al., 1994) and in some cases found that this diagnostic group was actually *less* likely to commit aggressive acts, than those in the general population (Rice and Harris, 1995).

In the light of these findings two others are relevant for any understanding of why some psychotic patients are violent but not others. The first relates to personality factors and substance misuse, just mentioned. 'Dual diagnosis' or 'co-morbidity' in those psychotic patients who do manifest a violent pattern is very common. The second relates to ecological variables. These were noted already in relation to accounting for the reversal of findings about the association between mental disorder and violence before and after 1965. When patients are discharged into richer areas they are less dangerous than in poorer areas (Silver et al., 1999). The latter areas of 'concentrated poverty' contain what Hiday (1995) calls the 'violence inducing social forces', we noted earlier. Hiday's multi-factorial model only places mental illness as one amongst many variables in accounting for violent action in society.

This reminds us that the clinical and lay discourses, which focus on clinical variables alone, are clearly reductionist. However, this is not to say that individual variables are irrelevant. They account, for example, for why some psychotic patients are very dangerous and some are not dangerous at all. For example, does this patient enjoy using disinhibiting substances? Do they have a history of violence? Are their symptoms hostile in content? Might they be described as having a 'personality disorder', in addition to psychotic symptoms? However, individual considerations are more than clinical considerations – they take into account particular personal contexts not just evidence of psychopathology.

The medicalization of anti-social action

One of the most controversial implications of some criminal acts being framed as mental disorder is the reputation it creates for that wide range of people with mental health problems, who are no more, or maybe even less, violent than the general population. At the centre of the complex interaction of mental state, personality features and temporary drug-induced disinhibition, noted in the previous sections, lies a socio-historical trend and source. 'Moral insanity' was noted in the early nineteenth century in the asylums. For example, Prichard (1835) noted the following about some residents:

> The moral principles of the mind are strongly perverted or depraved; the power of self government is lost or greatly impaired and the individual is found to be incapable not of talking or reasoning upon any subject proposed to him, but of conducting himself with decency and propriety in the business of life. (Prichard 1835)

Later in the nineteenth century, others like Lombroso and Havelock Ellis did *not* make a clear distinction between the impervious moral sensibility of some asylum inmates, who were unlike the type of lunatic habitually observed, and the mind of the common career criminal. However, a variant of Prichard's view was championed by Mercier (1905/2006) inside psychiatry and it was to emerge in a fuller fashion later in the work of Cleckley and Hare (see below). This created a discourse about individual psychopathology to explain some anti-social action but not others.

This medical emphasis diverted one type of deviance from the jurisdiction of the courts, with their lay, common-sense, judgements about morality and culpability in the juror system, into a special medically-codified realm of expertise about some violent people in society. However, it was not until the first part of the twentieth century that immorality and fecklessness were medicalized in earnest. For example, in the Netherlands, legislation was introduced about 'psychopathy' in 1925 to set out the conditions under which (non-psychotic) prisoners could receive psychiatric treatment.

In other countries, such as England, criminal lunatic asylums became high security or 'special' hospitals, which contained psychotic patients, those with learning difficulties who had acted criminally or dangerously in open settings, as well as 'psychopaths'. The latter group was articulated in British law under the 1959

Mental Health Act as 'a persistent disorder or disability of mind … which results in abnormally aggressive or seriously irresponsible conduct'.

This type of definition highlighted a more general dilemma about functional descriptions in psychiatry about tautology. How do we know this man is a psychopath? Answer – because he rapes children and shows no sign of remorse. Why does he do such terrible things? Answer – because he is a psychopath. Thus that part of the criminal population which is habitually violent and is not constrained by normal expectations of shame and anticipatory guilt can be framed as being mentally disordered, warranting treatment rather than punishment. At the time of writing, we find the following contention about the medicalization of violence:

The first contention has just been noted about the weaknesses of *policies justified tautologically.* The criteria offered by the World Health Organization (1992) for what it calls 'dissocial personality disorder' are as follows:

- callous unconcern for the feelings of others;
- gross and persistent attitude of irresponsibility and disregard for social norms, rules and obligations;
- incapacity to maintain enduring relationships, though having no difficulty in establishing them;
- very low tolerance to frustration and a low threshold for discharge of aggression, including violence;
- incapacity to experience guilt and to profit from experience, particularly punishment;
- marked proneness to blame others, or to offer plausible rationalizations, for the behaviour that has brought the patient into conflict with society.

The list signals that what starts as an attempt to define defective individuals must appeal ultimately to a tautological judgement about incorrigible rule trans-gression in relation to norms of emotions and conduct. A further complication is that criteria offered by the WHO (with similar ones appearing as 'anti-social per-sonality disorder' under DSM IV (American Psychiatric Association, 1994)) are elaborated in the clinical discourse about 'psychopathy', which refers to the work of Cleckley (1941). For example, the Canadian psychologist Robert Hare (Hare and Neumann, 2008) offers a more elaborate description which includes histri-onic and narcissistic features, not just those proposed by the APA and WHO:

- Glibness/superficial charm
- Grandiose sense of self-worth
- Need for stimulation/proneness to boredom
- Pathological lying
- Cunning/manipulative
- Lack of remorse or guilt
- Shallow affect
- Callous/lack of empathy
- Parasitic lifestyle
- Poor behavioural controls
- Promiscuous sexual behaviour
- Early behavioural problems

- Lack of realistic, long-term goals
- Impulsivity
- Irresponsibility
- Failure to accept responsibility for own actions
- Many short-term marital relationships
- Juvenile delinquency
- Revocation of conditional release
- Criminal versatility

Again, even with this more elaborate description of the psychopath in our midst, each criterion refers to an expectation about emotional expression and moral probity – they refer to consideration for others, conformity to legal action and 'emotion rules' in society. (However, arguably this process of inferring individual pathology from social deviance could be attributed to all other functional psychiatric diagnoses).

What Hare's contribution highlights though is that 'psychopathy' reflects a continuum, as we are all more or less egocentric and manipulative of others. And if there is a category, it is not 'natural' but it is constructed by the cut-off agreed by professionals who reflect and mediate social norms. Hare also suggests that the term 'psychopathy' should not be limited to criminal populations, when he notes that many of the above characteristics can be found in those operating within the law (such as scheming politicians and those with high status management roles in organizations) (Babiak and Hare, 2000).

This proposal might suggest that the *most* successful psychopaths achieve their egocentric ends but evade a criminal trajectory: they are 'sub-criminals'. 'Psychopathy' thus signals an egocentric orientation towards life, which necessitates a lack of socially-shared emotions (a lack of empathy for others or guilt or shame about rule transgressions). This deviant emotional connotation is distinguished by Hare in a North American context in which the term 'sociopath' can be used to describe *conformity* to sub-cultural anti-social norms; the individuals themselves are not (necessarily) emotionally abnormal. For example, 'sociopaths' may be capable of warmth and compassion in relationships outside of their criminal activity. This introduces a potential distinction between violent 'career criminals', traceable to delinquent socialization on the one hand and abnormal personality development on the other, whether or not the latter is expressed in a criminal or non-criminal way.

This returns us to the distinction made originally by Prichard and Mercier in the nineteenth century and at odds with others like Lombroso and Ellis. That tension remains though in the ongoing disputes about criminal culpability – if personality disorders are mental disorders, do those diagnosed lack the capacity to make moral judgements because of their emotional abnormality? This question still brings opposing answers in both lay and professional circles.

The second contention to be noted is that there remains *a lack of professional consensus on whether having labelled habitual violence as 'personality disorder', it is 'treatable'*. As with the psychiatric response to most forms of mental abnormality, treatment specificity and effectiveness are open to considerable question. Indeed if 'personality' means anything, it refers to *enduring or persistent* characteristics of an individual. Why should 'abnormal' personalities be expected to buck that general expectation? Is the 'successful treatment of personality disorder' an oxymoronic aspiration? Not surprisingly, given these questions, this sort of statement is typical in the literature: 'there is no convincing evidence that psychopaths can or cannot be successfully treated' (Dolan and Coid, 1993). This may be no more than saying that old habits die hard, including anti-social habits. (See Manning, this handbook.)

Contention even remains about whether 'treatment' may make this anti-social group in society worse, for example by encouraging more psychological skills to aid deception and manipulation of others. Indeed one study found this outcome (Rice et al., 1992). However, a later review of the evidence found that only three of all the studies reviewed were sufficiently sound methodologically to draw conclusions of any sort (D'Silva et al., 2004) but what evidence there is about effectiveness is weak.

Salekin (2002) reported that improvements can be demonstrated between control and treatment groups but the latter require intense and prolonged intervention. Pro-social outcomes are slow to achieve and accurate risk prediction is difficult to ascertain for particular individuals. That is, even where therapeutic benefits are proven (and this is variable), these are only at the *aggregate* level. Thus, whilst it may be better to treat than not treat overall, clinical and judicial decision-making about risk habitually refers to *individuals not groups.* Consequently, where open-ended detention is permissible (as in secure psychiatric facilities) there is a tendency towards a false positive decision-making bias; professionals are rarely criticized for detaining those not at risk but are criticized for the reverse of this error.

The third contention relates to *the separation of some criminals for purposes of open-ended preventative detention.* In Britain in the recent past, this has been reflected in the invention of a political rather than clinical category of offender (those with 'Dangerous and Severe Personality Disorder') and British legislation now allows for people with a diagnosis of personality disorder to be detained using mental health law, with proof of treatability not necessarily required. This signals that governments can be keen to use the psychiatric option of open-ended preventative detention, as an alternative to the risks entailed in defined sentencing. This points to a more general criticism of mental health law: its use to justify *no estimated date of release* for those deemed to be risky.

Thus the medicalization of violence offers a particular risk management strategy for politicians. In this context, it is misleading rhetoric to claim a therapeutic paradigm for anti-social action, when in truth the dominant driver of policy is preventative detention. It would be less mystifying if open-ended preventative detention was singularly a criminal justice matter but permitted all-comers to be evaluated not just those deemed to be mentally disordered. Hence there could be the possible scenario of legislation about *dangerousness,* discussed earlier in the chapter, replacing mental health law in a less discriminatory way. At present the criminal given a defined sentence (even if it is for a long time or even life) knows where they are in relation to the future but the psychiatric detainee does not.

The fourth contention relates to *the conflation of incorrigible violent criminality with 'psychopathy'*. Although the term 'psychopath' is at the centre of the overlapping discourse about violent criminality and mental disorder, even those accepting the legitimacy of psychiatric diagnoses in principle consider that there is a complex picture. Blackburn (1998) notes that from empirical studies of criminal populations and those detained in secure psychiatric facilities, we find a very wide range of personality problems amongst offenders. For example, in the case of female offenders, the diagnosis of 'borderline personality disorder' predominates. Also, indicating cultural differences, the invocation of 'dissociative identity (or multiple personality) disorder', to explain violent conduct and, controversially, to exculpate perpetrators at times, has been a particular feature of the US criminal justice system. However, it is a far less common legal and clinical matter outside of North America (Owens et al., 1997; Saks and Behnke, 1997). The emphasis on the connection between these other diagnoses of personality disorder is an empirical caution against conflating non-psychotic criminality in offenders deemed to be mentally disordered with 'psychopathy'.

The ambiguity is amplified when we look at the literature on offender rehabilitation. Given the extensive utilization of therapeutic technologies (from chemical castration to cognitive-behavioural therapy) it is noteworthy that in prisons this (quasi) psychiatric or clinical psychological approach is applied to many sex and violent offenders, who are not formally designated as being 'mentally disordered' (McGuire, 1995). This reminds us that the medicalization of anti-social action has been quite elastic in its character and this has blurred substantially the discursive boundary between mental abnormality and criminality.

DANGER AS A SOURCE OF MENTAL DISORDER

In this part of the chapter we offer a corrective to the notion that the relationship between danger and mental disorder is a 'one way street'. When we examine the wider literature about violence and threat in all its societal expression, it soon becomes evident that mental disorder is an outcome not just (or even predominantly) a source. To demonstrate this point we will provide brief case studies in relation to warfare, current interpersonal violence and child abuse and neglect. These demonstrate the way in which danger and threat impact upon vulnerable individuals to increase the risk of mental health problems (also see Hermann, this handbook).

Warfare as a danger to mental health

By the end of the nineteenth century, the system of large asylums was defining the stable present and likely future of psychiatry. This institutional containment of madness, on behalf of civil society, was at the centre of this policy emphasis. All this was to change with the First World War.

The eugenic emphasis in the asylums was out of sync with what was emerging in conditions of war. Working class volunteers and officers and gentleman ('England's finest blood') broke down with predictable regularity during the 'Great War' between 1914 and 1918 (Stone, 1985). 'Shell-shock' duly morphed into 'war neurosis', 'battle fatigue' or 'post-traumatic stress disorder' and it could not be accounted for readily within the eugenic framework preferred by the medical superintendents of the civilian asylums.

The 'shellshock' doctors began to raise the prospect that some form of interaction, between extreme external stress and inner psychological vulnerability, accounted for the symptoms evident in the casualties of the trenches (Salmon, 1917). These patients were not the assumed degenerates of the asylum system but decent, ordinary and, in civilian life, apparently mentally stable people. They had broken down under conditions of extreme adversity and this suggested, in an open ended way, that any of us in the right conditions might become mentally abnormal (Keane, 1998).

In the first half of the twentieth century large scale warfare brought other lessons. For example it created an insight about 'institutional neurosis', which was also called 'institutionalism' or 'institutionalization'. A medical student volunteer with the Red Cross observed the opening of the concentration camps. Barton (1958) watched as skeletal inmates in unsanitary conditions paced around with their arms folded. When asked to move to more fresh and clean conditions by the liberating forces, they strangely resisted. Barton subsequently noticed that psychiatric patients in the large asylums manifested similar stereotypical conduct and an irrational dependency on the institution.

But probably the most important point about warfare for our purposes here relates to the common governmental and lay discourse about individual violence. If all of the criminal acts of violence committed by individuals, globally, in the last 100 years (whether or not they were considered to be mentally disordered) were added together, the total would pale into insignifance in the context of warfare. The latter has been responsible for the recurrent mass killing of swathes of the civilian population by the military wing of the State in many countries during the same period. Also its traumatized survivors as civilians or combatants attend mental health services in disproportionate numbers.

Between 1945 and 1990 there were 150 wars leading to the deaths of 22 million people (Goldson, 1993); our Western notions of 'First' and 'Second' 'World Wars' are thus misleading as global warfare is persistent. Since 1990 there have been wars in the Balkans, the Middle East and in Africa, which have continued this trend of state sponsored mass killing. Moreover the trend of modern warfare has been less and less about military casualties and more and more about the annihilation, persecution and traumatization of millions of unarmed civilians. The psychological consequences for survivors are now immeasurable, as they extend into subsequent generations (Solkoff, 1992). Apart from post-traumatic symptoms of distress, explosive anger may also be common in civilian victims of warfare (Silove et al., 2009). The scale of this state sanctioned military violence and its negative psychological consequences for innocent civilians reminds us of the point, noted at the outset made by Zizek (2007), about systemic violence and the risk of tunnel vision in relation to offensive individual dangerous acts. A narrow, personalistic, frame creates a de-contextualized ethical and social framework for understanding violence.

Current interpersonal violence and mental health

A number of studies have now demonstrated that exposure to current violence increases the risk of adults developing mental health problems. The most obvious example of this just discussed refers to traumatization of combatants and civilian victims of warfare. However, the violent context of civilian peacetime existence is also a source of similar mental health consequences.

Mental health problems are correlated with the prevalence of neighbourhood violence. Victims are traumatized when attacked and the anxiety levels of prospective victims are affected. This pattern of direct contextual impacts of threat and violence in the immediate environment begins in school, with bullying and harassment having adverse consequences for young victims (Abada, et al., 2008). The evidence about the positive aspects of social support and social capital on mental health (see Secker and Pescosolido, this handbook) is the opposite side of the same coin as evidence about interpersonal traumatization. For example, poor mental health is predicted by neighbourhoods, which are both low in social support and high in violent crime (Stockdale et al., 2007). Thus neighbourhoods can be more or less benign in their character and affect all living in them accordingly.

The contemporary exposure to external threats, pressure and insults may implicate a range of stressors, which can act separately, additively or synergistically. These include, violent victimization, being witness to the latter or knowing of its local occurrence. A range of stressors, from harassment and bullying to sexual and non-sexual violence can co-occur in the workplace, on the streets or in the home and so current traumatic victimization in adulthood needs to be considered as a multi-factorial phenomenon (Kaminer et al. 2008). When we turn to the empirical data on intimate partner violence, we find a picture in which a number of debates are emerging and findings are contested. Below this contention is briefly summarized:

- Sexuality, gender, age and patriarchy Intimate or partner violence is now a well documented source of psychological trauma in both same sex and heterosexual partnerships (Burke and Follingstad, 1999; Gwat-Yong and Gentlewarrier, 1991; Kelly and Washafsky, 1987; Lehman, 1997; Lhomond and Surel-Cubizolles, 2006). This has created a debate about the full or modified role of patriarchy (Dutton and Nichols, 2001; Strauss, 2008). Commenting on same sex relationships, Roe (2010) notes that age also has to be taken into consideration when examining crime survey data:

   People who were lesbian/gay or bisexual were more likely to have experienced any domestic abuse in the past year compared with heterosexual/straight people (13 per cent compared with 5per cent). The higher level of domestic abuse amongst lesbians/gays or bisexuals may be due, at least in part, to the younger age profile of individuals identifying themselves as in this group. Nearly two-fifths (37per cent) of those reporting to be lesbian/gay or bisexual were aged 16 to 24 compared to just over one-fifth (21per cent) who identified as hetero-sexual/straight (data not shown). Previous analysis has shown that risk of intimate violence is higher amongst 16 to 24 year olds compared with older age groups.... (Roe, 2010)

In societies where gender inequalities are marked, the rates of male to female violence are much higher (Ferguson et al., 2004). Thus the probability of inter-personal violence is bound up, to some extent, with structural power discrepancies between social groups and so gendered violence rates will vary accordingly (Archer, 2004).

- *The role of mental state*. Given that the purpose of this half of the chapter is to focus on danger as a source of mental health problems, the discussion of mental state in the literature is another complicated consideration. Dutton (2007) emphasises personality disorder rather than gender as the central matter in intimate violence. However, this is possibly a tautological code for people who are in recurrent violent relationships (as victims, perpetrators or both) as both 'anti-social personality disorder' and 'borderline personality disorder' emerge more often in biographical contexts of trauma and violence. Thus male perpetrators might be disproportionately deemed to be suffering from 'anti-social personality disorder' (Muftic and Bouffard, 2007), with a similar possibility for women of 'borderline personality disorder'. Also, both male and female perpetrators have a high incidence of intoxication at the time of offending, suggesting that substance misuse might be a key pathological source of abusive action, a well proven point more generally in relation to violence in society (Hester, 2009). Thus whilst unreasonable psychological reductionism might be implicated in Dutton's account, it is also obvious that there are important biographical correlates that increase or decrease the risk of perpetration. Thus social structure and social group membership alone cannot explain particular acts. It may be possible in the future to document this psycho-social complexity as a dynamic one in contextualised relationships, rather than it being about either psychological or sociological explanations alone.
- *Reporting rates and police action*. Most of the literature based upon criminal justice system records suggests that women remain at most risk of serious injury or death. In the UK for example, most (over 90 per cent) arrested perpetrators are male and most victims (over 90 per cent) female (Hester and Westmarland 2005; Romito and Grassi, 2007; Sorenson and Taylor, 2005; Westmarland & Hester 2007). However meta-analyses, including community sampling, suggest that male and female perpetrators exist in about equal measure (around 7 per cent in hetero-sexual couples) (Archer, 2004), with some studies claiming that women, not men, are more prone to initiating violence in domestic settings (Stets and Straus, 1992). According to Roe (2010) reviewing British Crime Survey data:

Women were more likely than men to have experienced intimate violence across all the different types of abuse... In contrast, men, particularly young adults, are at greater risk of experiencing any violent crime... Overall, more than one in four women (28per cent) and around one in six men (16 per cent) had experienced any domestic abuse since the age of 16 ... These figures are equivalent to an estimated 4.5 million female victims of domestic abuse and 2.6 million male victims. (Roe, 2010)

- *Cautions about data interpretation*. Given the above picture, sociological interpretations must be provisional, as must hypotheses about the psychological nature of intimate abuse. Compared to other social problems, intimate violence has been investigated in depth only relatively recently and findings and interpretations are in flux as we write. For example, Hester (2009) comments in relation to this survey data, men tended not to report partner abuse to the police because they considered the incident 'too trivial or not worth reporting' (ibid.: 67). In another example, Kernsmith (2005) proposes that some women use violence to retaliate against violent male partners, whereas males are more prone to creating chronic pressure in a planned pattern of partner entrapment (Hamberger 1997; Hester 2009). Whilst arrests of female perpetrators have increased over time, this might be interpreted as a result of actual increased incidence, changes in policing policies or efforts of male perpetrators to manipulate police action, by calling them to make a pre-emptive accusation; or some combination or some other explanations yet to be determined (DeLeon-Granados et al., 2006; Miller, 2001).

* *Ideological tension in the field and the role of selective methodology*. The debates above implicate ideology in a post-feminist social science context, as well as many unresolved methodological questions about comparability of samples. For example, some of the material on gay relationships does not ask the same questions of heterosexual samples. Also as was clear above, numerical estimates seem to vary both in terms of prevalence reported and in relation to gender correlations, from equal incidence to a high predominance of male perpetrators in heterosexual relationships. It is not easy to separate the chicken from the egg- do empirical findings inform ideological reflection or does ideology determine which empirical questions are asked and not asked, as well the interpretations offered of data? An example of the ideological tension implicated in this field here, DeKeseredy (2007) reviewing Dutton's 'gender neutral' view notes that:

> … it is not likely to influence many progressive sociologists to rethink their own positions on the plight of abused women. Even so, in a current political economic climate characterized by an intense right-wing assault on feminism, there is an enormous audience for this book and it undoubtedly will be used to justify erroneous claims such as "women are as violent as men" and to challenge feminist efforts to reduce all forms of gender inequality.

More is said on intimate violence and sexuality in the chapter by Ussher in this volume. We now move to childhood adversity, within which family violence is an important consideration as children can be both secondary victims (if they have warring parents) and primary victims when violence is directed at them.

Child abuse and neglect as a danger to mental health

Adaptations of Bowlby's attachment theory have triggered empirical research into the short term and long term consequences of childhood adversity (Alexander, 1992; Bowlby, 1951; Cichetti, 1987; cf. Rutter, 1981; Wurtele, 1998). Childhood maltreatment implicates dysfunctional parent–child–environment transactions. Also, neuro-developmental delays impact upon psychological health in the growing child. For example, children who are physically abused or neglected are more likely to show intellectual impairment, as a result of poor stimulation, poor diet, emotional withdrawal and sometimes direct neurological damage from trauma. They show significant delays in comprehension and in expressed language and they go on to manifest a range of behavioural problems of impulsivity, aggression, oppositional challenges to authority and later criminality.

The risk of abuse of the next generation is also increased by these responses to the victim's maltreatment. These children show a range of post-traumatic symptoms including depression, anxiety, nightmares and flashbacks. The psycho-social presentation of adult victims of neglect and physical abuse is complex. It is often variable within the same individual over time, with some acting out their difficulties, possibly in an anti-social manner and others showing various forms of distress.

The sexual victimization of children impacts predictably on later mental health. As well as manifesting post-traumatic symptoms, victims may become sexually precocious ('traumatic sexualization') and they are often prone to later sexual dysfunction and confusion about their sexuality (Kendall-Tackett et al., 1993). When the abuse is intra-familial there is an increased risk of chaotic adult behaviour involving suicidal action, self-harm, substance misuse, mood swings, dissociation (hysterical fugue states) and dramatic panic about abandonment in intimate relationships (Browne and Finkelhor, 1986). The diagnosis of 'borderline personality disorder' in adulthood may be linked to such histories.

The survivors of childhood victimization are over-represented in statutory mental health services. For example, Polusny and Follette (1995) found that childhood sexual abuse predicts a range of later psychiatric diagnoses including eating disorders, major depression, anxiety disorders, substance misuse, somatization and personality disorders. Most of the work linking early adversity and later mental health problems has been retrospective. However, prospective studies also demonstrate the link (e.g. Spataro et al., 2004).

The child sexually victimized by a relative is not just traumatized, they are also personally betrayed. This impacts on their confidence in subsequent intimate relationships. This has lead researchers such as Finkelhor (1988) to argue that trauma need may well lead not just to the symptoms of post-traumatic stress disorder (PTSD) but also to distorted attachment behaviour. Whereas PTSD can arise from impersonal traumatization (e.g. a car crash), intra-familial abuse is dramatically personalized. The meanings attached to the experience are predictably different for the survivor. One large survey of female survivors found that 'a range of long-term psychological effects was significantly related to ... abuse perpetrated by father or step-father, abuse which was repeated or prolonged, presence or threats of violence, blaming the child, saying that disclosure would split the family and a younger age of onset' (Ussher and Dewberry, 1995: 177).

Most of the focus on the traumatic consequence of childhood adversity refers to neurotic symptoms or dysfunctional acting out by survivors (e.g. Bifulco and Moran, 1998). However, there is also evidence that psychotic symptoms are predicted by early trauma and confused communications in families. Retrospective studies have confirmed that psychotic patients report high levels of trauma, including sexual abuse, during their early lives (Goodman et al., 1997; Neria et al., 2002), and these findings have been supported by prospective investigations (Jannsen et al., 2004). Also, adverse interpersonal influences have been identified as predicting psychosis, especially parental 'communication deviance' – vague and unstructured communications between the parent and the child (Wahlberg et al., 1997).

Several large scale studies have reported a specific association between childhood sexual abuse and hallucinations (Read et al., 2003; Hammersley et al., 2003; Shevlin et al., 2007). Given that post-traumatic stress is associated with intrusive thoughts and images, their may be a common mechanisms in hallucinations and PTSD. Communication deviance, on the other hand, has been specifically associated with thought disorder (Wahlberg et al., 1997) Returning to the question of disrupted attachments, the risk of psychosis is raised if children experience early separation from their parents (Morgan et al., 2007).

This emphasis on the predictive aspects of the childhood environment needs to be complemented by other evidence about the influence of *current* conditions. For example, in an early study by Brown (1958), it was found that psychotic patients returning to parents or spouses were more likely to be readmitted to hospital than patients leaving to live with sibs or in hostels. Subsequent research identified the 'high-expressed emotion' characteristics of family members that are linked to relapse in terms of criticism, hostility and over-protectiveness (Brown and Rutter, 1966; Butzlaff and Hooley, 1998). Self-esteem may be a mediator between expressed emotion and symptom-exacerbation (Barrowclough et al., 2003) and high-expressed emotion relatives are likely to have experienced insecure attachment to their own parents (Paley et al., 2000).

These findings about adverse intra-familial conditions and mental health are also complemented by evidence about abuse by adults of children in other settings. For example, at the time of writing the Catholic Church is struggling to maintain its legitimacy in the face of extensive evidence over many years and across the world that its priests and nuns have been found guilty of widespread child abuse (Fortune and Longwood, 2003). There have been reports of national significance in Australia, Canada, Austria, the Czech Republic, France, Peru, the Phillipines, Mexico, New Zealand and the USA (with the largest claims from surviving victims against the church). In the Republic of Ireland since 2000 no less than three large government commissioned inquiries have been conducted into child abuse in the Irish Church and all of them are damning of both the Church and State authorities.

In the most recent (*The Murphy Report* (2009)) it was found that the Church knowingly covered up the abuse. The investigation team was prevented from seeing nearly 5,000 files by a named Cardinal in 2008. The report summarizes the accumulation of over thirty years of investigation into the matter and offers a critical analysis of the role of Archbishops, Bishops, the Irish police force, health authorities and the Director of Public Prosecutions. No less than four Archbishops in Dublin had, one after another, been aware of the abuse but done nothing to ensure investigation and public justice.

Also police connivance with the abuse was evident, with complaints to them not being recorded or being passed on uncritically to the Church hierarchy who failed to investigate or take action. The victims were faced with the expectations of trust and the experience of awe in relation, not only to a daily secular world of adult power, but also of a spiritual power, claimed and believed. These children experienced both physical and spiritual entrapment (McLaughlin, 1994), often creating a special 'trauma bond' constantly implicating the victim's allegiance and sense of responsibility (Rosetti, 1995).

CONCLUSION

This chapter has demonstrated that the relationship between danger and mental disorder is a complex topic. That very complexity alerts us to the prejudicial view, which at times has guided social policy, that the matter is singularly one of threat from those with mental health problems. We have argued that whilst the empirical evidence about the latter still deserves serious consideration, a rounded view of our topic leads to a number of conclusions.

A few psychotic symptoms predict violence but many do not – and certainly global diagnoses such as 'schizophrenia' have no predictive value. When psychotic patients are prone to violence this risk is largely accounted for by other variables – especially intoxication and personality problems identified by past anti-social acts, as well as the risky living settings of many psychiatric patients. Moreover, the latter factors are strong predictors of violence in the general population. The medicalization of substance misuse and personality problems, which occurred in the early part of the twentieth century, has left us now with a legacy in which mental disorder is very broad in its scope. As a result, the framing of anti-social action as mental disorder now legitimizes unfair public prejudice about *all* psychiatric patients being assumed sources of danger.

When we shift the focus away from whether or not that source of danger exists and look instead at danger being a source of mental disorder, then this re-frames patients from being perpetrators to being victims. We have offered summaries of the evidence for this being a reasonable shift of focus in relation to warfare, multi-factorial stressors in peacetime impacting on adult citizens and in the light of the evidence of the impact of child abuse and neglect. This re-framing, as much as the need to look closely at the empirical evidence about mental disorder and dangerousness, is important if we are to develop a comprehensive sociological description about this chapter's topic.

(Note from the authors – The authors are grateful to Pat Cox, Helen Spandler and Nicky Stanley, University of Central Lancashire and Suzanne Martin, University of Kent for their advice on the section on intimate violence in this chapter.)

REFERENCES

Abada, T., Hou, F. and Ram, B. (2008) The effects of harassment and victimization on self-rated health and mental health among Canadian adolescents. *Social Science* and *Medicine,* 67(4): 557–567.

Aldarondo, E. (1998) Perpetrators of domestic violence. In A.S. Bellack & M. Hersen (eds) *Comprehensive Clinical Psychology,* vol 9. London: Pergamon.

Alexander, P. (1992) Application of attachment theory to the study of sexual abuse. *Journal of Consulting and Clinical Psychology,* 60: 185–95.

American Psychiatric Society (1994) *Diagnostic and Statistical Manual of Mental Disorders (Fourth Edition).* Washington DC: APA.

Appelbaum, P.S., Robbins, P.C. and Roth, L.H. (1999) A dimensional approach to delusions: comparisons across delusional type and diagnosis. *American Journal of Psychiatry,* 156: 1938–1943.

Appelbaum, P.S., Robbins, P.C. and Monahan, J. (2000) Violence and delusions: data from the MacArthur Violence Risk Assessment Study. *American Journal of Psychiatry,* 157(4): 566–572.

Archer, J. (2004) Sex differences in aggression in real-world settings: A meta-analytic review. *Review of General Psychology,* 8: 291–322.

Babiak, P. and Hare, R. (2000) *Snakes in Suits: When Psychopaths Go To Work.* New York: Harper Collins.

Barrowclough, C., Tarrier, N., Humphreys, L., Ward, J., Gregg, L. and Andrews, B. (2003) Self-esteem in schizophrenia: The relationship between self-evaluation, family attitudes and symptomatology. *Journal of Abnormal Psychology,* 112: 92–99.

Barton, W. R. (1958) *Institutional Neurosis,* Bristol: Wright and Sons.

Bifulco, A. and Moran, P. (1998) *Wednesday's Child: Research into Women's Experience of Neglect and Abuse in Childhood, and Adult Depression.* London: Routledge.

Blackburn, R. (1998) Psychopathy and the contribution of personality to violence. In T. Millon, E. Simonsen and M. Birket-Smith (eds) *Psychopathy: Anti-Social Violent and Criminal Behaviour.* New York: Guilford Press.

Blumenthal, S. and Lavender, T. (2000) *Violence and Mental Disorder.* London: Zito Trust.

Bowlby, J. (1951) Maternal care and mental health. *Bulletin of the World Health Organization* (Monograph), 3: 355–534.

Brown, G.W. (1959) Experiences of discharged chronic schizophrenic patients in various types of living groups. *Millbank Memorial Fund Quarterly,* 37: 105.

Brown, G.W. and Rutter, M. (1966) The measurement of family activities and relationships: A methodological study. *Human Relations,* 19: 241–263.

Browne, A. and Finkelhor, D. (1986) The impact of child sexual abuse: a review of the research. *Psychological Bulletin,* 99: 66–77.

Burke, L.K., and Follingstad, D.R. (1999) Violence in lesbian and gay relationships: theory, prevalence, and correlational factors. *Clinical Psychology Review,* 19(5): 487–512.

Butzlaff, R.L. and Hooley, J.M. (1998) Expressed emotion and psychiatric relapse. *Archives of General Psychiatry,* 55: 547–552.

Cicchetti, D. (1987) Developmental psychopathology in infancy: illustration from the study of maltreated youngsters. *Journal of Consulting and Clinical Psychology,* 55: 837–845.

Cleckley, H. (1941) *The Mask of Sanity.* St Louis: Mosby.

DeKeseredy, W.S. (2007) Review of *Rethinking Domestic Violence* by D.G. Dutton (2007) *Canadian Journal of Sociology Online,* November–December.

DeLeon-Granados, W., Wellsa, W. and Binsbacher, R. (2006) Arresting developments, trends in female arrests for domestic violence and proposed explanations. *Violence Against Women,* 12(4): 355–371.

Dennis, D.L. and Monahan, J. (eds) (1996) *Coercion and Aggressive Community Treatment.* New York: Plenum Press.

Department of Health (1999) *Report of the Expert Committee: Review of the Mental Health Act (1983).* London: Stationery Office.

Dolan, B. and Coid, J. (1993) *Psychopathic and Antisocial Personality Disorders. Treatment and Research Issues.* London: Gaskell.

Dutton, D.G. (2006) *Rethinking Domestic Violence.* Vancouver: UBC Press.

Dutton, D.G. and Nichols, T.L. (2005) The gender paradigm in domestic violence research and theory: part 1 the conflict of theory and data *Aggression and Violent Behavior,* 10(6): 680–714.

D'Silva, K., Duggan, C. and McCarthy, L. (2004) Does treatment really make psychopaths worse? A review of the evidence. *Journal of Personality Disorders,* 18(2): 163–177.

Ferguson, H., Hearn, J., Gullvag Holter, O., Jalmert, L., Kimmel, M., Lang, J. and Morrell, R. (2004) *Ending Gender Based Violence: A Call for Global Action to Involve Men* (SIDA). Available at www.sida.se/shared/jsp/download.jsp?f=SVI34602.pdf&a=3108

Ferns Report (2005) *Report Presented to the Minister for Health and Children.* Dublin: Government Publications.

Finkelhor, D. (1988) The trauma of child sexual abuse: two models. In G. Wyatt and G. Powell (eds) *The Lasting Effects of Child Sexual Abuse.* Newbury Park CA: Sage.

Fortune, M.M. and Longwood, W. (eds) (2003) *Sexual Abuse in the Catholic Church: Trusting the Clergy.* New York: Haworth Pastoral Press.

Goldson, E. (1993) War is not good for children. In L.A. Leavitt and N.A. Fox (eds) *The Psychological Effects of War and Violence on Children*, Hillsdale, NJ: Erlbaum.

Goodman, L.A., Rosenberg, S.D., Mueser, K. and Drake, R.E. (1997) Physical and sexual assault history in women with serious mental illness: Prevalence, correlates, treatment, and future research directions. *Schizophrenia Bulletin,* 23: 685–696.

Grisso, T., Vesselinov, R., Appelbaum, P.S. and Monahan, J. (2000) Violent thoughts and violent behaviour following hospitalization for mental disorder. *Journal of Consulting and Clinical Psychology,* 68(3): 388–398.

Gwat-Yong, L. and Gentlewarrier, S. (1991) Intimate violence in lesbian relationships. *Journal of Social Service Research,* 15(1/2): 41–59.

Hamberger, L.K. (1997) Female offenders in intimate partner violence: A look at actions in their context. *Journal of Aggression, Maltreatment and Trauma,* 1: 117–130.

Hambracht, M. and Hafner, H. (1996) Substance abuse and the onset of schizophrenia. *Biological Psychiatry,* 40: 1155–1163.

Hammersley, P., Dias, A., Todd, G., Bowen-Jones, K., Reilly, B. and Bentall, R.P. (2003) Childhood trauma and hallucinations in bipolar affective disorder: A preliminary investigation. *British Journal of Psychiatry, 182*: 543–547.

Hare, R.D. and Neumann, C.S. (2008) Psychopathy as a clinical and empirical construct. *Annual Review of Clinical Psychology,* 4: 217–246.

Hester, M. (2009) *Who Does What to Whom? Gender and Domestic Violence Perpetrators*, Bristol: University of Bristol in association with the Northern Rock Foundation.

Hester, M. and Westmarland, N. (2005) *Tackling Domestic Violence: Effective Interventions and Approaches.* Home Office Research Study 290, London: Home Office.

Hiday, V. (1995) The social context of mental illness and violence. *Journal of Health and Social Behaviour,* 36: 122–137.

Hunt, I.M., Kapur, N., Webb, R., Robinson, Burns, J., Shaw, J. and Appleby, L. (2009) Suicide in recently discharged psychiatric patients: a case-control study. *Psychological Medicine,* 39(3): 443–449.

Janssen, I., Krabbendam, L., Bak, M., Hanssen, M., Vollebergh, W., De Graaf, R. and van Os, J. (2004) Childhood abuse as a risk factor for psychotic experiences. *Acta Psychiatrica Scandinavica,* 109: 38–45.

Junginger, J. (1995) Command hallucinations and the prediction of dangerousness. *Psychiatric Services,* 46: 911–914.

Kaminer, D., Grimsrud, A., Myer, L., Stein, D.J. and Williams D.R. (2008) Risk for post-traumatic stress disorder associated with different forms of interpersonal violence in South Africa. *Social Science and Medicine* 67(10): 1589–1595.

Keane, T.M. (1998) Psychological effects of human combat, in B.P. Dohrenwend (ed.) *Adversity, Stress and Psychopathology.* Oxford: Oxford University Press.

Kelly, C.E. and Washafsky, L. (1987) Partner abuse in gay and lesbian couples. Paper presented at the 3rd National Family Violence Research Conference. Durham, NH.

Kendall-Tackett, K.A., Williams, I.M. and Finkelhor, D. (1993) Impact of sexual abuse on children. A review and synthesis of recent empirical studies. *Psychological Bulletin,* 113: 164–180.

Kernsmith, P. (2005) Treating perpetrators of domestic violence: gender differences in the applicability of the theory of planned behaviour. *Sex Roles,* 52: 11/12.

Lehman, M. (1997) At the end of the rainbow: a report on gay male domestic violence and abuse. Minnesota Center Against Violence and Abuse. http://www.mincava.umn.edu/documents/rainbow/At%20The%20End%20Of%20The%20Rainbow.pdf.

Lhomond, D. and Surel-Cubizolles, M.J. (2006) Violence against women and suicide: the neglected impact of same-sex sexual behaviour. *Social Science and Medicine* 62(8): 2002–2013.

Link. B.G., Andrews, H.A. and Cullen, E.T. (1992) The violent and illegal behaviour of mental health patients reconsidered. *American Sociological Review,* 57: 275–292.

McGuire, J. (ed) (1995) *What Works? Reducing Re-offending, Guidelines for Research and Practice.* London: Wiley.

McLaughlin, B. (1994) Devastated spirituality: the impact of clergy sexual abuse on the survivor's relationship with God and the church. *Sexual Addiction and Compulsivity: The Journal of Treatment and Prevention,* 1: 145–158.

Mercier, C. (1905/2006) *Sanity and Insanity.* London: Hesperides Press.

Miller, S.L. (2001) The paradox of women arrested for domestic violence. *Violence Against Women,* 7: 1339–1376.

Monahan, J. (1992) Mental disorder and violent behavior perceptions and evidence. *American Psychologist* 47(4): 511–521.

Monahan, J. (2000) Clinical and actuarial prediction of violence. In D. Fagman, D. Kaye, M. Saks and J. Sanders (eds) *Modern Scientific Evidence: The Law and Science of Expert Testimony.* St Paul MN: West Publishing Company.

Morgan, C., Kirkbride, J., Leff, J., Craig, T., Hutchinson, G. and McKenzie, K. (2007) Parental separation, loss and psychosis in different ethnic groups: A case-control study. *Psychological Medicine,* 37: 495–503.

Muftic, L.R. and Bouffard, J.A. (2007) Evaluation of gender differences in the implementation and impact of a comprehensive approach to domestic violence *Violence Against Women,* 13(1): 46–69.

Neria, Y., Bromet, E. J., Sievers, S., Lavelle, J. and Fochtmann, L. J. (2002) Trauma exposure and post-traumatic stress disorder in psychosis: Findings from a first-admission cohort. *Journal of Consulting and Clinical Psychology,* 70: 246–251.

Owens, S., Parry, J.W. and Lichtenstein, E.C. (1997) *Criminal Responsibility and Multiple Personality Defendants.* Chicago: American Bar Association.

Paley, G., Shapiro, D.A. and Worrall-Davies, A. (2000) Familial origins of expressed emotion in relatives of people with schizophrenia. *Journal of Mental Health,* 9: 655–663.

Pilgrim, D. and Rogers, A. (2003) Mental disorder and violence: an empirical picture in context. *Journal of Mental Health,* 12(1): 7–18.

Pols, J. (2001) Enforcing patients' rights or improving care: the interference of two modes of doing good in mental health care. *Sociology of Health and Illness,* 25(4): 325–347.

Polusny, M. and Follette, V. (1995) Long-term correlates of child sexual abuse: theory and review of the empirical literature. *Applied and Preventive Psychology,* 4: 143066.

Rabkin, J. (1979) Criminal behaviour of discharged psychiatric patients: a critical review of the research. *Psychological Bulletin,* 86: 1–27.

Read, J., Agar, K., Argyle, N. and Aderhold, V. (2003) Sexual and physical abuse during childhood and adulthood as predictors of hallucinations, delusions and thought disorder. *Psychology and Psychotherapy: Theory, Research and Practice,* 76: 1–22.

Reiss, A. and Roth J.A. (eds) (1993) *Understanding and Preventing Violence.* Washington, D.C.: National Academy Press.

Regier, D.A., Farmer, M.E., Rae, D.S., Locke, B.J., Keith, S.J., Judd, L.L. and Goddwin, F.K. (1990) Comorbidity of mental disorders with alcohol and other drug use: results from the epidemiologic catchment area (ECA) study. *Journal of the American Medical Association,* 264: 2511–2518.

Rice, M.E. and Harris, G.T. (1995) Psychopathy, schizophrenia, alcohol abuse and violent recidivism. *International Journal of Law and Psychiatry,* 18: 333–342.

Rice, M.E., Harris, G.T. and Cormier, C.A. (1992) Evaluation of a maximum security therapeutic community for psychopaths and other mentally disordered offenders. *Law and Human Behaviour,* 16: 399–412.

Roe, S. (2010) Intimate violence: 2008/09 BCS. In K. Smith and J. Flatley (eds) *Homicides, Firearm Offences and Intimate Violence 2008/09 Supplementary Volume 2 to Crime in England and Wales 2008/09.* London: Home Office.

Romito, P. and Grassi, M. (2007) Does violence affect one gender more than the other? The mental health impact of violence among male and female university students. *Social Science and Medicine,* 65: 1222–1234.

Rosen, G. (1968) *Madness in Society.* New York: Harper.

Rossetti, S. (1995) The impact of child sexual abuse on attitudes toward God and the Catholic Church. *Child Abuse and Neglect,* 19: 1469–1481.

Rutter, M. (1981) *Maternal Deprivation Reassessed.* Middlesex: Penguin Books.

Saks, E.R. and Behnke, S.H. (1997) *Jekyll on Trial: Multiple Personality Disorder and Criminal Law.* New York: New York University Press.

Salekin, R.T. (2002) Psychopathy and therapeutic pessimism. Clinical lore or clinical reality? *Clinical Psychology Review,* 22(1): 79–112.

Salmon, T.W. (1917) The care and treatment of diseases and War neuroses: 'shellshock' in the British army *Mental Hygiene,* 1: 509–575.

Schneider, B. (2009) Substance use disorders and risk for completed suicide. *Archives of Suicide Research,* 13(4): 303–316.

Shevlin, M., Dorahy, M., and Adamson, G. (2007). Childhood traumas and hallucinations: An analysis of the National Co-morbidity Survey. *Journal of Psychiatric Research,* 41: 222–228.

Silove, D., Brooks, R., Steel, C.R.B., Steel, Z., Hewage, K., Rodger, J. and Soosay, I. (2009) Explosive anger as a response to human rights violations in post-conflict Timor. *Social Science and Medicine* 69(5): 670–677.

Silver, E., Mulvey, E.P. and Monahan, J. (1999) Assessing violence risk among discharged psychiatric patients: towards an ecological approach. *Law and Human Behavior,* 23: 237–255.

Solkoff, N. (1992) Children of survivors of the holocaust: a critical review of the literature, *American Journal of Orthopsychiatry,* 62: 342–358.

Sorenson, S.B. and Taylor, C.A. (2005) Female aggression toward male intimate partners: an examination of social norms in a community-based sample. *Psychology of Women Quarterly,* 29: 79–96.

Soyka, M. (2000) Substance misuse, psychiatric disorder and violent and disturbed behaviour. *British Journal of Psychiatry,* 176: 345–350.

Spataro, J., Mullen, P.E., Burgess, P.M., Wells, D.L. and Moss, S.A. (2004) Impact of child sexual abuse on mental health: prospective study in males and females. *British Journal of Psychiatry,* 184: 416–421.

Steadman, H.J., Mulvey, E.P., Monahan, J., Robbins, P.C., Applebaum, P.S., Grisso, T., Roth, L.H. and Silver, E. (1998) Violence by people discharged from acute psychiatric facilities and by others in the same neighbourhood. *Archives of General Psychiatry,* 55: 109.

Stets, J. and Strauss, M.A. (1992) *The Marriage License as a Hitting License: Physical Violence in American Families.* New York: Transaction Publishers.

Stockdale, S.E., Wells, K.B., Tang, L., Belin, T.R., Zhang, L. and Sherbourne, C.D. (2007) The importance of social context: neighbourhood stressors, stress buffering mechanisms and alcohol, drug and mental disorders. *Social Science and Medicine,* 65: 1867–1881.

Stone, M. (1985) Shellshock and the psychologists. In WF. Bynum, R. Porter and M. Shepherd (eds) *The Anatomy of Madness* (Volume II). London: Tavistock.

Strauss, M. A. (2008) Dominance and symmetry in partner violence by male and female university students in 32 nations. *Children and Youth Services Review,* 30: 252–275.

Straus, M.A. (1999) The controversy over domestic violence by women. A methodological, theoretical and sociology of science analysis. In X.B. Arriaga and S.D. Oskamp, S. (eds) *Violence in Intimate Relationships.* Thousand Oaks, CA: SAGE.

Swanson, J.W., Holzer, C.E., Ganju, V.K. and Jono, R.T. (1990) Violence and psychiatric disorder in the community: evidence from the catchment area surveys. *Hospital and Community Psychiatry,* 41: 761–770.

Szasz, T.S.(1963) *Law, Liberty and Psychiatry.* New York: Macmillan.

Szmukler, G. and Appelbaum, P. (2001) Treatment pressures, coercion and compulsion. In G. Thornicroft and G. Szmukler (eds) *Textbook of Community Psychiatry.* Oxford: Oxford University Press.

Taylor, P.J. (1985) Motives for offending among violent psychotic men. *British Journal of Psychiatry,* 147: 491–498.

Teplin, L.A., Abram, K.M. and McClelland, G.M. (1994) Does psychiatric disorder predict violent crime among released jail detainees? A six-year longitudinal study. *American Psychologist,* 49: 335–342.

Ussher, J. and Dewberry, C. (1995) The nature and long-term effects of childhood sexual abuse: a survey of adult women survivors in Britain. *British Journal of Clinical Psychology,* 34: 177–192.

Wahlberg, K.-E., Wynne, L. C., Oja, H., Keskitalo, P., Pykalainen, L., Lahti, I., Moring, J., Naarala, N., Sorri, A., Seitamaa, M., Laksy, K., Kolassa, J. and Tienari, P. (1997). Gene–environment interaction in vulnerability to schizophrenia: Findings from the Finnish Adoptive Family Study of Schizophrenia. *American Journal of Psychiatry,* 154: 355–362.

Westmarland, N. and Hester, M. (2007) *Time for Change.* Bristol: University of Bristol.

WHO (1992) *The ICD-10 Classification of Mental and Behavioural Disorders.* Geneva: WHO.

Wurtele, S.K. (1998) Victims of child maltreatment. In A.S. Bellack and M. Hersen (eds) *Comprehensive Clinical Psychology* (341–358, Volume 9) New York: Pergamon.

Zizek, S. (2007) *Violence.* London: Profile.

Clinical and Policy Topics

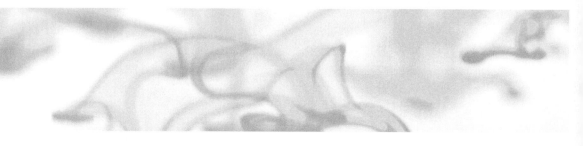

Editors' Introduction

In this section of the book discussions of the general social context addressed earlier will shift to a clinical and policy focus. Phil Thomas examines the strong biomedical tradition, when madness has been considered in the recent past. He does this by focusing on the most common form of diagnosed 'severe mental illness': 'schizophrenia'. He is concerned to establish the ways in which bio-reductionism in Anglo-American psychiatry have led us into a cul-de-sac of understanding. Thomas is not 'anti-biological' but is concerned that the blinkered focus on the skin-encapsulated processes favoured by his own profession, as well as the drug companies (see Pilgrim, Rogers and Gabe in the first section of the book) have distracted us from an honest understanding, or necessary humility, about understanding madness in its social context. Also, the strong and simple expectation that a genetic account of madness is in the offing, considered by Clarke in the first chapter of the book, is a matter that Thomas returns to in conclusion.

The next contribution comes from a clinical psychologist Richard Bentall, who looks at the ways in which what appear to be extraordinary and difficult to fathom phenomena, like hallucinations and delusions, might be understood. Starting with the assumptions asserted by Emil Kraepelin in the late nineteenth century, he traces the implications of a categorical approach to madness and offers a different way of thinking about it. This is about psychological processes, which are implicated in the way all of us think and feel. This is a profound political move because it does not divide sanity and insanity into two separate camps of humanity These forms of understanding have been made possible by a shift from a bio-reductionist view of madness to one based upon some notion of interaction, between stress and vulnerability or nature and nurture. These points connect with the explorations of Clarke and Roxburgh in the first section of the book.

If madness has dominated the concerns of specialist mental health services, it is also the case that those who have regular service contact often receive a diagnosis of personality disorder, either on its own or combined with others ('dual diagnosis', 'co-morbidity' or 'complex cases'). Nick Manning considers how wider sociological questions might inform our understanding of personality disorder. Starting with an ontological question about it as an object of inquiry, he moves onto the perspective of sociology in relation to other questions about its diagnosis and treatment. How is it distributed within the population and how effective are interventions to deal with it? These questions also emerge in other chapters (see Olafsdottir on medicalization and Pilgrim and Rogers on danger and mental disorder in the first part). Personality disorder is about people recurrently acting in ways others do not like, with distress being distributed, in some ratio, between identified patients and those around them. It is about a form of incorrigibility in a moral order.

If the incorrigibility associated with 'personality disorder' reflects one way in which mental health services are involved in the social control of deviance, the closely associated topic of 'substance misuse' is also relevant to consider. During the 1930s the jurisdiction of psychiatry began to extend to other forms of rule breaking beyond madness. Recurrent intoxication and its associated personal and social difficulties now came within the ambit of psychiatric authority and accordingly 'substance misuse' is now considered to be a form of mental disorder and is often associated with chronic service utilization in psychotic patients (back to 'co-morbidity' or 'dual diagnosis'). Michael Bloor and Alison Munro provide a sociological account of 'substance misuse', starting with an overview of drug use and market factors. They then move on to investigations of drug-dependency treatment programmes, as well as looking at the prospects of relapse and recovery in the 'untreated' user of substances. They conclude their discussion by noting the uncertain impact of research on policy and the role of sociology in an overlapping area – the understanding of how to combat the HIV/AIDS epidemic.

The term 'substance misuse' implies the notion of 'substance use' and that patients may, as it were, take the 'wrong' kinds of drugs (or the 'right' ones in the 'wrong' context). Jonathon Gabe joins two of us (Pligrim and Rogers) to explore the ambiguities involved in these distinctions. Prescribed psychotropic medication not only may be 'abused' (for example it may be sold as a 'street drug'), it has also been subjected to extensive user criticism and professional critique, within its assumed framework of legitimate use. Much of this contention has arisen since strong claims began to emerge in the 1950s, from both the pharmaceutical industry and the medical profession, about drugs as a technological fix for psycho-social problems. The chapter focuses on two main aspects of this so called 'pharmacological revolution': the chemical management of madness and the treatment of misery in primary care, which links to the next chapter.

Anti-depressant medication is now the stock-in-trade of general practitioners (superseding discredited drugs, like the barbiturates and benzodiazepines). Primary care is the first port of call for a range of psycho-social problems and so, within this, the 'management of depression' is a common part of the medical discourse. An academic primary care physician, Carolyn Chew-Graham, writes about the treatment of depression in the setting of the British NHS. The frequent occurrence of primary care consultations for diagnosed depression or 'common misery' is a springboard to address social context. Can we treat problems of individuals which are enmeshed so strongly with that context (implicating inter-personal and supra-personal factors)? Is depression under-recognized in primary care (and does this matter)? What does common misery tell us about social inequalities?

If primary care remains the first line of engagement between those with 'common mental health problems' and specialist services (now rarely managing those problems), it has also been looked to at times, by policy-makers, as a site of primary or secondary prevention and health promotion. In the next chapter, Helen Hermann, an academic psychiatrist who has worked closely with the World Health Organization, considers the bigger picture of mental health promotion and considers the need to look beyond healthcare. She examines the definition of mental health and the development of mental health promotion, in a context of wider public health policies internationally. This ensures that our attention is drawn to the intersecting influences of education, employment and community or social development. Mental health cannot be the singular remit of responsibility for healthcare services; there must be an inter-sectoral and inter-agency approach to both social policy and social analysis.

The promotion of mental health and wellbeing is currently a priority for mental health policy makers. However, in the subsequent chapters, attention is paid to policies related to what are now often called those with 'severe and enduring' mental health problems. In the days of the large asylum system most of these patients would have been warehoused permanently outside of civil society, until their death. Andrew Scull, a social historian, considers the ramifications of moving from institutionalization to one of de-institutionalization (or 'decarceration'). As a critic of both the asylum as a physical institution itself and the false dawns of 'community care', Scull returns to an important current and unresolved matter for many of us involved in mental health debates. Is there a place for true 'asylum' for any of us if we need it and if so how might it be achieved? Certainly disaffected service recipients even today still ask for support and asylum when in acute crisis, as an alternative to coercion and imposed iatrogenic treatment which takes us to the next chapter.

In the wake of large hospital rundown, the voice of the service user has been heard more often than previously (though objections by the mad about their treatment and social position are not completely new). Diana Rose and Peter Campbell have both been long term users of mental health services and they provide a summary account of user campaigning in the British context. The term 'user' and 'survivor' remain ambiguous. Other terms such as 'client' or 'consumer' are used in the Anglophone world, as well as the more traditional 'patient' or 'ex-patient'. (In the North American context, 'user' is generally eschewed, probably because of its connotations of 'narcotics'.) The term 'survivor' is even more open-textured, possibly connoting the survival of psychiatric attention (coercion and iatrogenic treatment), the survival of stigma and social exclusion, the survival of the primary impairment of mental disorder and maybe the survival of extreme childhood adversity (possibly in some combination). The term 'psychiatric survivor' or 'survivor of mental health services' may indicate that there remains a particular focus on the oppressive character of the mental health services system.

Currently it is a matter of contention whether recovery from mental health problems actually arose from survivor demands for citizenship or it is being insinuated by politicians and professionals for other reasons. Now for whatever reason, it is noteworthy that there is an increasing expectation that people will recover from their mental health problems. Reviews this recent policy consensus in the social and historical context of other innovations and fashions in mental health work. 'Recovery' has clear resonances with therapeutic optimism (which has waxed and waned) as well as emerging in a context of structural changes, such as de-institutionalization (see chapter by Scull, this section) and wellbeing (see chapter by Brogge in section 1). McCrain concludes with an agenda for sociological inquiry into this important recent policy consensus about recovery from mental health problems.

The final two chapters return to themes considered in those on user campaigning and recovery. The first, from Jenny Secker, provides a British perspective on social inclusion and social exclusion and their ambiguous relationship. She examines the ways in which 'social exclusion' is assumed to be rectified by 'social inclusion', as a policy and service aspiration, especially in mental health policies. Particular attention is paid to black and ethnic minority patients in the British context (returning us to the topic addressed by Nazroo and Iley in the first section of the book). Also Secker emphasizes that 'social inclusion' is not always embraced by service users and nor is it self-evidently a progressive policy option (or if it is, the case must be made rather than assumed).

The final chapter of the book from one of us (Pescosolido) takes a sociological look at the role of social networks in the lives of people with mental health problems. This might appear at first glance like a straightforward task (as commonsense tells us that relationships maintain mental health, account often for its breakdown and underpin recovery, when it occurs). However, complexity has arisen in conceptualizing and investigating social networks in relation to mental health, with much empirical work still implied rather than completed. Much is now known about the basic empirical point that having social networks matters, but much less about how they work, where they come from and how they interact with a wide range of psychological, biological and clinical factors. The programmatic implications are for now not completely clear.

14

Biological Explanations for and Responses to Madness[1]

Philip Thomas

Schizophrenia is an idea whose very essence is equivocal, a nosological category without natural boundaries, a barren hypothesis. Such a blurred concept is not a valid object of scientific enquiry ... it is a cloak for ignorance and exposes psychiatry to ridicule. As a model of psychosis it is an oversimplification, which serves the interests of neither scientists nor patients. It is time to abandon this concept with its history of semantic wrangling. (Brockington, 1992)

These words come not from a left-wing sociologist, or an angry and disaffected survivor of mental health services, but from a professor of psychiatry who devoted his professional life to investigating the classification of psychoses in the second half of the twentieth century, a time when biological accounts of madness dominated professional, public and governmental thought. Biological accounts of madness dominate mental health policy in Britain and America. The National Service Framework for Mental Health (Department of Health, 1999) and George W. Bush's plans to screen the entire US population for mental disorders linked to the Texas Medical Algorithm Project (Lenzer, 2004) confirm this. Biomedical models of madness have always featured prominently in British academic psychiatry (Moncrieff and Crawford, 2001). American academic psychiatry on the other hand, which was once an eclectic mix of psychoanalytic, sociological and biological discourse, is now dominated by the biological (Pincus et al., 1993). On the 17 June, 1990 in Presidential Proclamation 6158, George Bush Senior declared the new decade the 'Decade of the Brain' to '... enhance public awareness of the benefits to be derived from brain research through appropriate programmes, ceremonies and activities (Bush, 1990). Much has been written about the rise of biological explanations of madness, and although it is not my intention to dwell on this in any detail, a short overview of the origins of the approach may be helpful in understanding its current status. It is also important to avoid simple dualisms that maintain that biological models are bad, and non-biological models are good simply by virtue of their non-biological nature. This was an unhelpful feature of some aspects of anti-psychiatry, and elsewhere Pat Bracken and I (Bracken and Thomas, 2008) have argued against the reductionism that is implicit in certain forms of dualism. However, we must also be very careful about the status accorded to biological explanations because of the foundational claims that are made for them.

Caveats issued, it is time to move on. In this chapter I will focus exclusively on the condition known as schizophrenia. There are two reasons for this. First, schizophrenia exemplifies the use of biology by psychiatry to account for all forms of madness. The broad approach outlined here has been used by psychiatry to explore all areas of human subjectivity that are identified with madness. Second, schizophrenia as a diagnostic category has played a particularly important historical role in the origins and growth of psychiatry. In some ways it has come to symbolize the power and medical authority of the profession[2]. For this reason I will first briefly consider the historical origins of modern biological accounts of madness. Then, I will review recent biological theories about madness, focussing on genetic, psychopharmacological and neuro-developmental. This is not meant to be a systematic review. Rather, I want to draw attention to particular theories and areas of activity because of their therapeutic implications. Third, I shall consider the implications of these theories for biological interventions. I will conclude with a brief account of some of the problems of biomedical accounts. Presenting evidence for the biological basis of schizophrenia should not be taken to indicate that the phenomenon is unproblematic; there are in any case many excellent and detailed critiques of the concept (Boyle, 1993; Bentall, 2003; Johnstone, 2000).

ORIGINS OF BIOLOGICAL PSYCHIATRY

It is worth pointing out that there are two very different approaches to the history of psychiatry. The first is a feature of the writings of those firmly encamped within the tradition of biological psychiatry (e.g. Torrey and Miller, 2001; Panksepp, 2004), which sees the scientific understanding of madness as little more than the inevitable march of progress. In this view the truth about madness exists as part of the natural world, independently of human concerns and interests. It is inevitable, given sufficient time and resources, that science will ultimately reveal all there is to know about psychosis. The second is exemplified by the work of Michel Foucault, whose writings about the history of psychiatry (Foucault, 2006, 2006a) paint a very different picture. Foucault sees the origins of psychiatric knowledge in nineteenth century social policy and legislation that granted authority to the infant profession over the insane. Thus psychiatric theories about madness are not an inevitable outcome of the march of science, but are contingent upon social policy, and ultimately politics and the exercise of power. The implication of this view is that how we understand psychosis is to a large extent historically and culturally contingent.

Although the influence of what Porter (1997) calls rational or empirical medicine has waxed and waned at different periods in Western history, the most significant developments in understanding contemporary biomedicine began with that period of history known as the European Enlightenment, or the Age of Reason. Historians differ as to what exactly the Enlightenment was, how it started, when it began and ended, but there is broad agreement that the period from the seventeenth century through until the end of the eighteenth century had a great impact on Western thought across the humanities, politics, science and medicine, and helped to establish contemporary ways of thinking about the world. There are three aspects of contemporary psychiatry that can be traced back to the Enlightenment (Bracken and Thomas, 2005). These are the role played by psychiatry in social control (maintaining an 'orderly' society), the belief that human problems would ultimately yield to technological and scientific solutions (tied to the value of 'progress') and a preoccupation with interiority, the view that human subjectivity has depth and is contained within the inner recesses of the mind. In this chapter I am primarily concerned with the second of these – the role of (medical) science and technology in understanding madness. This initially became possible through the body-mind dualism implicit in Descartes' philosophy, and then through the rapid expansion of the natural sciences that followed the Enlightenment. What had been metaphysical specula-tions about humors was replaced by a new materialism. The late Roy Porter writes:

> The Enlightenment secured the triumph of a radical new rendering of the very constitution of Nature. After 1660, the Aristotelian metaphysics of elements, humours, substances, qualities and final causes … were finally superseded by models of Nature viewed as matter in motion, governed by laws capable of mathematical expression. This enthronement of the mechanical philosophy, the key paradigm switch of the 'scientific revolution', in turn sanctioned the new assertions of man's rights over Nature so salient to enlightened thought. (Porter, 2000: 138–139)

It follows, of course, that a 'scientific revolution' that asserted man's rights over nature meant that it became possible through science to assert our right to study human experience *as part of nature*. This study took off in earnest in the nineteenth century in Germany, and is exemplified by the work of Hermann von Helmholtz, the physicist and physician, who applied theories from mathematics and physics to human perceptual processes, thus setting out the basis for a new science of experimental psychology. Also in nineteenth century Germany the proto-psychiatrists were involved in work that became immensely influential in the twentieth century. Wilhelm Griesinger, the neurologist and proto-psychiatrist, became the founder of the modern discipline of academic psychiatry. Marx (1970) describes three aspects of Griesinger's work that are relevant to contemporary psychiatry. First, he believed that mental disorders were brain disorders related to the presence of cerebral pathology. Thus the psychiatrist was best thought of as a physician. Second, he maintained that psychopathology had to be based in an empirical, scientific psychology. Mental processes were a matter for scientific investigation not philosophical speculation. Third, he applied theoretical models developed by neurologists to psychopathology, in the belief that ultimately, mental disorders would be understood in terms of neurological processes.

If Griesinger set out some of the basic priorities and key assumptions of biomedical psychiatry, Kraepelin set out the basis of classification that continued to dominate twentieth century psychiatry. In the fourth edition of his textbook published in 1893, he described an illness which he called dementia praecox, under the heading of 'Psychic Degenerative Processes'. This group of illnesses, subsequently renamed schizophrenia by Bleuler, was characterized by a progressive and irreversible deterioration of intellectual function, typically beginning in adolescence. It is important to remember that in Kraepelin's time medicine had achieved considerable success in understanding the pathological basis of common causes of insanity such as neuro-syphilis. Late nineteenth century asylums contained a wide mix of people, many of whom were suffering from organic brain syndromes associated with syphilis, tuberculosis, malnutrition, alcoholism and epilepsy. Consequently, the proto-psychiatrists believed that medical science would reveal the cause of all forms of insanity. Kraepelin's system of detailed case descriptions, which included study of the outcome of individual cases, led him to the view that although people generally recovered from manic-depressive psychosis, this was not so for dementia praecox, which was characterized by a progressive and irreversible deterioration of intellectual function and social function. However, basic sciences such as bacteriology and neuropathology that had so successfully revealed the cause of neurosyphilis, failed to do the same for dementia praecox.

The importance of Kraepelin's work is not limited to its historical role. In recent years it has become highly influential in biomedical research, as can be seen in the growth of what has been called neo-Kraepelinism. Wilson (1993) describes the increasing preoccupation of academic psychiatrists, from the 1970s on, with the reliability of psychiatric diagnosis in DSM-III and the revisions that followed as a rejection of psychoanalytic theories in favour of a return to scientifically rigorous approaches to the problems of psychiatric diagnosis. This trend may also be partly understood as part of the response of the profession of psychiatry to the attacks of the anti-psychiatrists. At about the same time, other academic psychiatrists, particularly in Britain, were renewing their interest in a core Kraepelinian feature of schizophrenia – dementia. This can be seen in an influential paper titled *The Dementia of Dementia Praecox* (Johnstone et al., 1978). An important outcome of this work was research into the distinction between positive symptoms (unusual beliefs, hallucinations and some forms of thought disorder) and negative symptoms (blunting of affect and poverty of speech). Positive symptoms form the basis of many contemporary systems of classification such as DSM-IV, but negative symptoms are thought to correspond more closely to the core 'deficit' syndrome associated with poor-prognosis schizophrenia. The problematic relationship between the two remains unresolved, something we will return to later in this chapter.

THE BIOMEDICAL MODEL IN THE TWENTIETH CENTURY

Twentieth century biomedical psychiatry can be seen as a quest for the biological basis of schizophrenia. This has been taken forward on three main fronts; genetic studies, biochemical studies and neuropathological studies.

Genetic studies

In the first half of the twentieth century, genetic research into the cause of schizophrenia was largely epidemiological, focused on estimates of the heritability (risk) of the condition in affected families, and more specifically the concordance rates for identical and non-identical twins[3]. Gottesman et al. (1987) summarized the results of all published European family and twin studies of schizophrenia, over the preceding sixty years. If you have a relative suffering from schizophrenia, then your chances of being affected increases as your relationship to the sufferer becomes closer. If we take the general population risk to be about 1 per cent, then it is claimed that the risk increases to 1.5 per cent for first cousins, 12 per cent for non-identical twins and 44 per cent for identical twins. There have been many studies of concordance rates (CR) for schizophrenia in identical and non-identical twins. Gottesman and Shields (1982) summarised the results of earlier studies that yielded risks of 47 per cent in identical twins and 12 per cent for non-identical twins. This suggests that genetic factors make a significant contribution to the risk of developing schizophrenia, but if the condition were entirely genetically determined, one would expect a much higher CR in identical twins. This is not so. In over 50 per cent of identical twins only one of the pair is affected. This suggests that environmental factors must play an important role. One way of disentangling the contribution of heredity and environment is through adoption studies, which examine the prevalence of schizophrenia in the children of affected parents who are adopted by non-schizophrenic families. If these children carry a genetic risk it is argued that they will subsequently develop schizophrenia, even though they have been brought up in 'normal' families. Heston (1966) found a high rate of schizophrenia in the children of schizophrenic mothers reared in foster homes. However, he also found a wide variety of other conditions in these children, including personality disorders, neurotic disorders and learning disabilities. Rosenthal et al. (1971) failed to find a significant excess of children who subsequently developed schizophrenia, if strict criteria were used to diagnose schizophrenia in the biological parents. The most comprehensive adoptive study was undertaken by Tienari et al. (1987), who identified over 164 Finnish women suffering from schizophrenia, and who had adopted away 179 children. Only 10 per cent of the children of affected mothers subsequently developed psychotic illnesses, and of these only 50 per cent suffered from schizophrenia. This suggests that the mechanisms of genetic transmission in schizophrenia are far from clear, and, if anything, favour some sort of interaction between genetic and environmental factors.

The failure of early studies to demonstrate a clear pattern of inheritance has forced those working in the field to reconsider the evidence. First, it has been argued that the single gene theory can hold for schizophrenia if the condition has what is called variable penetrance. This means that in some relatives who possess the 'gene' its effect is not fully apparent in the phenotype (i.e. the behavioural or physical characteristics of the individual that are thought to be genetically determined). For example, some individuals rather than developing schizophrenia may have schizotypal personalities, or other psychiatric conditions such as depression or substance misuse. Second, polygenic theory holds that schizophrenia is the final outcome of the combined effect of a number of different genes. One implication of this idea is that the liability to develop schizophrenia exists on a continuum in the general population. This view sits reasonably comfortably with recent critiques of the categorical model of schizophrenia by psychiatric epidemiologists (van Os, 2003) and psychologists (Bentall, 2003), but it isn't popular with psychiatric geneticists because it is much more difficult to test empirically, especially using the newer linkage studies. Finally, genetic heterogeneity theory proposes that schizophrenia consists of a group of conditions some of which may have a genetic basis with different patterns of inheritance, associated with some non-genetic forms. Again such a model is extremely difficult to test empirically given the current state of knowledge.

Molecular genetics

Recent advances in technology have shifted the focus of genetic studies from epidemiology to laboratory-based scientific investigation. Earlier linkage studies relied on the identification of a 'marker' gene in affected families that 'co-segregated' with schizophrenia. In other words those members of the family who developed schizophrenia also showed phenotypical evidence of the marker gene. Molecular genetic studies use broadly similar techniques of subject identification, but shift the search into the laboratory by attempting to identify the specific changes in gene sequence that are associated with the condition under investigation. Such studies have been successful in identifying the gene responsible for Huntington's disease, but this condition has a very clear pattern of inheritance, and so far similar studies in schizophrenia have yielded mixed results. Craddock et al. (2005) recently reviewed molecular genetic studies in schizophrenia and bipolar disorder. Although there appear to be some promising areas, the results of these studies are far from clear. They examined studies that used a variety of methods commonly used in contemporary genetics research, including linkage studies, and studies examining functional candidate genes as well as those of chromosomal abnormalities. The findings of these studies are mixed, and at present the precise nature of the genetics of schizophrenia remains unclear. Several candidate sites on a number of chromosomes have been identified in individual studies, but there have been problems in replicating these findings. Szatmari et al. (2007) have reached broadly similar conclusions in their review of studies of the molecular genetics of schizophrenia.

A slightly different approach involves the attempt to relate molecular genetics not to schizophrenia but to features of psychosis that are thought to be related to the underlying pathophysiology. These so-called endophenotypes include cognitive deficits, as well as neurophysiological and neurodevelopmental features. Recent work, reviewed by Gur et al. (2007) has identified a number of neurobiological markers, such as measures of attention, verbal and working memory and facial processing that appear to be good candidates for endophenotypes of psychosis. Although this appears to be a potentially fruitful area, the authors conclude that much work remains to be done if evidence for the role of genetic effects in schizophrenia is to be forthcoming. Braff et al. (2007) point out that one of the problems of contemporary molecular genetic studies is that they generate enormous amounts of data that require very sophisticated statistical and mathematical modelling. The interpretation of such data becomes an extremely complex task when dealing with conditions that like psychosis that have multifactorial determinants.

Biochemical theories

In the logic of biomedical psychiatry it follows that a genetic basis for schizophrenia were it to be discovered, means that at some level a biochemical disturbance must exist. But the biochemistry of the brain is complex, and there have been many biochemical theories of schizophrenia over the years, most of which have been rejected because of lack of supporting evidence. The most enduring of these, the dopamine theory (Carlsson and Lindquist, 1963; Snyder, 1976), holds that positive symptoms of schizophrenia arise from over-activity in dopaminergic pathways that extend from the mid-brain to the temporal and frontal lobes. There are two indirect strands of evidence to support this. Amphetamine use occasionally leads to an acute psychosis, which is claimed to be indistinguishable from acute paranoid schizophrenia (Angrist and Sudilovsky, 1978). Amphetamines are known to increase the turnover of dopamine in the brain, so, it is argued, the clinical features of schizophrenia arise as a result of dopaminergic excess. However, the similarity of the amphetamine psychosis and schizophrenia is debatable. According to Snyder (1972) the symptoms of the former commonly include visual hallucinations and hypersexuality, both of which are uncommon in schizophrenia. The second strand of evidence concerns the mode of action of neuroleptics widely used to treat schizophrenia[4], which block dopamine transmission (Seeman et al., 1976). This stimulated much research into central dopaminergic systems, including animal studies, post-mortem studies of the brains of people who had suffered from schizophrenia in life, and a search for biochemical evidence of increased dopamine activity in cerebrospinal fluid or other body tissues. Wyatt's (1986) review of these studies concluded that the results were conflicting. There do not appear to be convincing replicable differences in dopaminergic activity between psychiatrically healthy control subjects and those suffering from schizophrenia. Indeed, some studies suggest that increased dopamine turnover may be an artefact of neuroleptic drug treatment (Clow et al., 1980; Reynolds et al., 1981).

Neither has the recent introduction of new brain imaging techniques clarified the situation unequivocally. Dopaminergic activity can now be examined more or less directly by positron emission tomography (PET). Subjects are given a small dose of chemicals labelled with a radioactive marker, which is selectively taken up by dopamine systems. The evidence from these studies is equivocal. Laruelle and Abi-Dargham (1999) used PET and single positron emission tomography to study dopaminergic transmission in D_2 receptors. They found evidence of hyperactivity associated with the presence of acute psychosis that was not present when the psychosis had stabilized. These changes were present too in people who had never had prior exposure to neuroleptic drugs. Wong et al. (1986) used similar technologies and found increases in dopamine receptors in medication-free subjects, although Farde et al. (1987) failed to confirm this finding. Carlsson (1990) has argued that the failure to replicate these findings casts doubt on the durability of the dopamine hypothesis.

The psychopharmacologists Iverson and Iverson (2007), who studied dopamine for many years note that unlike Parkinson's disease, where an understanding of the key role played by dopamine in the condition came from research advances in basic science, the dopamine theory of schizophrenia arose from the serendipitous discovery that neuroleptics also happened to block dopamine receptors. Writing from different perspectives Richard Bentall (2003) and Joanna Moncrieff (2008) have drawn broadly similar conclusions about the limitations of the dopamine theory in schizophrenia. Of course this does not invalidate the dopamine theory, but it does throw its provenance into question. Setting aside this little difficulty, there remain several substantial problems with the theory.

First, many people who have a diagnosis of schizophrenia fail to respond to neuroleptics. Curson et al. (1988) found that almost 50 per cent of a sample of long-stay psychiatric patients with a diagnosis of schizophrenia had persistent delusions and hallucinations, despite years of vigorous treatment with neuroleptics. In addition to this, one PET study found that medicated people with a diagnosis of schizophrenia who had not responded to neuroleptics showed just as much evidence of dopaminergic receptor blockade on PET scan as people who had responded (Coppers *et al.*, 1991). These findings are difficult to reconcile with the notion that the mode of action of neuroleptics is specifically related to their ability to block dopaminergic transmission.

The second problem concerns the apparent delayed mode of onset of neuroleptic drugs. Although dopaminergic blockade starts in the brain very shortly, usually an hour or so, after taking neuroleptics, clinical experience indicates that patients have to wait two or three weeks before they experience any benefit from taking these drugs. This observation is difficult to reconcile with the view that the 'antipsychotic' properties of these drugs relates to their ability to block dopamine transmission. However, a meta-analytic study by Ajid *et al.* (2003) suggests that if neuroleptic drugs are going to be effective, this is apparent in the first week or so of starting the medication. They identified over forty double-blind placebo controlled trials published between 1980 and 2001, which reported treatment response in the first four weeks of treatment. After standardizing the clinical measures (different rating scales were used in these studies) and taking into account the extent of the placebo response, they found mean significant improvements in overall clinical symptom ratings from week one to week two. It is worth noting, however, that there are serious difficulties in the interpretation of meta-analyses. Ajid *et al.* make no reference to the problems of publication bias (multiple publication of positive results and the failure to report negative findings) described by Melander *et al.* (2003). Nevertheless, the results of this study provide some support for the idea that neuroleptics have an early mode of onset.

A third problem concerns the precise role of dopaminergic activity in relation to positive and negative symptoms. The distinction between the two is of fundamental importance in understanding the origins of the clinical features of some neurological disorders, and can be traced back to the neurologist Hughlings Jackson (1889), who compared the symptoms of mental illness with those found in conditions such as epilepsy. He concluded that negative symptoms arose directly from the effects of pathology on the brain, whereas positive symptom arose through the release of healthy activity in the lower levels of the central nervous system by the pathological process. Negative symptoms are very difficult to fit in to the theory that schizophrenia is caused by dopaminergic excess. Davis *et al.* (1991) tried to surmount this by suggesting that there may be *reductions* in dopaminergic activity in areas associated with the frontal cortex thought to be important in emotional activity and social behaviour, and *excessive* activity in subcortical areas associated with positive symptoms. This idea remains current (Abi-Bergham, 2004), but as Joanna Moncrieff (2008) points out, precisely how a single disease process can elevate dopamine activity in one brain system and suppress it in another remains to be established.

Finally, there is the problem of the relationship between neurochemical theories of schizophrenia and the psychological and phenomenological features of the condition. Put bluntly, what difference does it make if dopamine transmission is abnormal? How does this finding, even if it were robust, stand in relation to the psychological and clinical features of the condition? Cohen and Servan-Schreiber

(1993) attempted to answer this question by turning to connectionism and artificial intelligence theory. They suggested that we can liken the brain to a computer that functions as a parallel distributed processing (PDP) system in understanding how it processes information. PDP systems (or neural networks) consist of a group of interconnected processing units, each of which is responsible for a particular computation. Each unit is widely connected to other units, receiving both excitatory and inhibitory influences. The balance of excitation and inhibition governs the level of activity in a single unit. They propose that in the brain these units may correspond to single nerve cells and fibres, or larger groups of these. Information is represented by the pattern of activity between units, and information processing is represented by the spread of activity (or change of pattern in activity) amongst units. They (Cohen and Servan-Schreiber, 1992) have also proposed that dopamine plays a key role in modulating the level of activity in systems responsible for processing information, by regulating the signal to noise ratio. The frontal lobes have an important role in representing environmental context, as well as maintaining our attention. Overactivity of dopaminergic systems associated with the frontal cortex means that subjects are less well able to modify their responses to environmental signals. More recently, Kapur (2003) has focused on the role of dopamine in mediating the 'salience' of environmental events and the internal representations of these. He proposes that at the 'brain' level dopaminergic overactivity leads to the aberrant allocation of salience at the mental level. In this model delusions occur as a result of the subject's attempts to make sense of the aberrant experiences that arise. Hallucinations, on the other hand, are a direct experience of the aberrant salience of internal representations[5]. In this model, neuroleptics are thought to act by damping down aberrant salience in dopaminergic systems.

Moncrieff (2008) has proposed that the reason there is so much conflicting evidence in relation to the role of dopamine and neuroleptic drugs is because we rely on a disease-centred model of neuroleptic action. Her analysis has thrown into question the idea that neuroleptics are a specific treatment for schizophrenia. This is difficult to accept for those who are committed to the medical model, because it strikes right at the heart of the model. She proposes instead that the actions of neuroleptic drugs are better understood through a drug-centred model. This refers to the non-specific effects these drugs have in damping down all spontaneous cognitive and emotional activity, and inducing a state of indifference. She notes that the range of effects of neuroleptics on mood and cognition are so profound that it is hardly surprising that clinical trials reveal them to be effective in a wide range of conditions.

Neurodevelopmental model of schizophrenia

This model lies closest to the Kraepelinian view that schizophrenia is a neurodegenerative disorder. It holds that schizophrenia is a disease caused by a yet to be identified abnormality of brain development. Although this abnormality may have a genetic basis, environmental events are necessary for it to become apparent. In recent years there have been hundreds of studies suggesting that structural abnormalities are common in the brains of some people suffering from schizophrenia (Cannon and Marco, 1994). Early post-mortem studies found a reduction in weight and volume of the brains of people who suffered from schizophrenia (e.g. Brown et al., 1986; Pakkenberg, 1987; Bruton et al., 1990), compared with people suffering from other psychiatric disorders and non-psychiatric groups. Histological examination of brain tissue removed at post-mortem has also revealed abnormalities in the organisation of cells in the cerebral cortex. For example, Jakob and Beckman (1986) found that some cells had failed to migrate to their expected position in the temporal lobes. Murray (1994) has argued that these findings could arise from a failure of pre or postnatal cerebral development.

The introduction of computerised axial tomography (CT) scanning in the 1970s, and more recently nuclear magnetic resonance (NMR) scanning, made it possible to study brain structure non-invasively. One of the earliest CT studies found that some people with a diagnosis of schizophrenia had enlarged ventricles (Johnstone et al., 1976), a finding that has been repeated. Subsequent studies suggest that this abnormality may be present in the earliest stages of the illness (Weinberger et al., 1980; Lewis, 1993) and related to the presence of abnormalities of personality prior to the onset of symptoms. Similar findings have emerged from NMR scan studies. Harvey et al. (1993) found a small but significant reduction in total cerebral volume in people suffering from schizophrenia. These reductions were not apparent in the brains of people diagnosed with serious depression (Harvey et al., 1994). Others have found that these changes are prominent in certain areas, especially the temporal lobes and related structures (Suddath et al., 1989; Bogerts et al., 1990).

There is also evidence that some people diagnosed with schizophrenia are more likely to show evidence of childhood developmental delay. Done et al. (1994) identified 40 people suffering from schizophrenia via the National Child Development Study, all of whom had had assessments of socialisation and language development on three occasions in childhood. They compared this group with people suffering from a variety of other psychiatric disorders and control NCDS subjects with no psychiatric disorders. At the age of 7 years, children who subsequently developed schizophrenia were considered by their teachers to show more evidence of social maladaptation. This particularly applied to boys. The same group (Crow et al., 1994) found that academic impairments were more common in the pre-schizophrenic children at ages 7, 11 and 16. These children were slow in reading and had speech difficulties. Jones et al. (1994) reported similar findings in a group of nearly 5,000 children followed up into adulthood.

There are two main problems with these earlier studies[6]. First, they fail to account for the confounding effects of treatment and institutionalization. Many were carried out on patients who had been on neuroleptic medication for many years, and who had also been exposed to other physical treatments, such as ECT or psychosurgery, which are known to be associated with cognitive impairment and structural brain changes. Recent work has exposed neuroimaging studies to more critical scrutiny. Steen et al.'s (2006) review and meta-analysis of earlier magnetic resonance brain imaging studies focused specifically on studies of either first-episode schizophrenia, or those of subjects not previously exposed to neuroleptic medication. They found relatively few such studies, most of which had relatively small sample sizes. Those with the smallest sample sizes tended to report higher levels of statistical significance where differences between patients and control subjects were found. Overall, relatively few significant differences in brain volume were found between patients and control subjects when first onset and neuroleptically naïve subjects were involved. Where volumetric differences were found, these findings were not well-replicated, and '... few findings [were] robustly significant, in either cross-sectional or longitudinal studies' (Steen et al., 2006: 513).

A second difficulty in interpreting the results of brain imaging studies concerns the use of volumetric measures based in magnetic resonance imaging techniques. According to Steen et al. (2006), these are at best imprecise. The magnitude of the changes measured in longitudinal studies is of the order of 4 per cent per annum, which is close to the limits of detection of the technique. In any case, such changes are very small, so although they may reach statistical significance, interpreting their clinical significance is extremely difficult in individual cases. At the end of his review of neuroimaging and other neurobiological indices of schizophrenia, Waddington (2007) writes:

> At this stage in our understanding of the biology of schizophrenia over its life time trajectory, the inconsistency and extent of variability in essentially all such measures still precludes the generation of predictive models that are utilitarian for individual patients. (Waddington, 2007: 56)

Finally, cortical structure may either not be correlated with brain functions, or only weakly so (Uttal, 2001). This casts further doubt on the possible relevance of these studies in understanding what exactly schizophrenia is.

IMPLICATIONS FOR THERAPY

The use of chlorpromazine, the first neuroleptic used as a treatment in schizophrenia, did not follow on rationally from new insights into the nature of schizophrenia delivered by biological science. It was originally introduced as an aid to anaesthesia by the French surgeon, Laborit. His description of the drug's effects on patients led two psychiatrists, Delay and Deniker, to wonder if it might be useful in schizophrenia (Moncrieff, 2008: 65-66). Since then many early studies investigated the effectiveness of neuroleptics in acute schizophrenia. In general, they found that these drugs were effective in keeping people out of hospital in the short-term, but there were problems with their long-term efficacy. Many patients who had been successfully treated and discharged from hospital were re-admitted months later, often more acutely ill than they had been when they first presented.

It soon became clear that this was in part because they had stopped taking medication[7] (Crumpton, 1967; Engelhardt and Freeman, 1969). This resulted in the introduction of long-acting injectable neuroleptic medication to ensure that people would not forget to take it. However, the question of the long-term effectiveness of these drugs in preventing relapse remains unanswered. The issue at stake here is the Kraepelinian view that schizophrenia is a chronic condition from which recovery is unlikely, and that the social functioning of many people who experience the condition deteriorates over time. If neuroleptic medication has specific actions in rectifying whatever underlying biochemical disturbance is responsible for the condition, then this medication should improve the long-term prognosis. This has formed the basis for the argument that once on medication it would be necessary to remain on it for a long period of time, not only to prevent relapse, but also to maintain social function.

The key issue here is the relationship between medication use, symptom control and outcome. There is evidence that a significant proportion of people do not respond to neuroleptics. The proportion varies depending on study design, definitions of symptom control, and subject selection (e.g. whether acutely ill or long-stay institutionalised subjects are studied), from 25 per cent (Davis and Caspar, 1977), 30 per cent (Davis, 1980), 20 per cent (Kane et al., 1988) and 46 per cent (Curson et al., 1988). Indeed, Kane and Freeman's (1994) review raises serious doubts as to whether medication has any beneficial effect on outcome in schizophrenia; 'It remains debatable whether or not long-term neuroleptic treatment substantially alters the course and outcome of this disorder...' (Kane and Freeman, 1994:22). Of course, this and similar evidence provided the impetus for the introduction of so-called 'novel' neuroleptics[8] such as clozapine, rather than being used to question the value of the dopamine theory as a disease model for schizophrenia. Moncrieff (2008) argues that it is impossible to conclude that long-term treatment with neuroleptics has advantages over placebo in terms of relapse prevention, because entry into a randomised controlled trial means taking people off active medication and placing them on placebos. This in itself carries the risk of triggering withdrawal effects that may be interpreted as relapse, but which in reality is an iatrogenic effect.

PROBLEMS WITH THE BIOMEDICAL APPROACH

We have already considered some of the limitations of specific areas of investigation, but I will end this chapter by stepping back and considering some of the broader problems of schizophrenia as a biomedical concept. There are three main areas; the problem of validity, the problem of outcome and finally the problem of harm.

The problem of validity

Earlier, we saw that over the last fifty years, partly in response to the criticisms of antipsychiatrists like Thomas Szasz (1972), who denied the existence of mental illness, psychiatric research became preoccupied with the problem of reliability. Until DSM-III psychiatric diagnosis was notoriously unreliable. It was extremely difficult to get psychiatrists to agree on definitions of symptoms and diagnoses. DSM-III attempted to rectify this, but the problem of validity remains. The issue of validity in psychiatry was examined by the philosopher Carl Hempel (1961). He argued that the validity of a concept like schizophrenia depended upon the extent to which it represents a naturally occurring category. If it does, then there should be an identifiable biological property of individuals who have the diagnosis that makes them unique and distinct from those who don't. In other words the category schizophrenia should 'carve nature at the joint'. The failure so far of basic science research to reveal a specific biological abnormality that distinguishes those who are categorized as having schizophrenia from other people has led some biological psychiatrists to argue that categorical diagnostic systems such as DSM-IV and ICD-10 have outlived their usefulness, and should be replaced by more sophisticated systems. Owen et al. (2007) have argued that genetic studies of schizophrenia are limited by current taxonomic systems. This raises the need to consider different approaches to classification that presumably do not rely on a late nineteenth century concept. They also suggest that in future molecular genetics will contribute to the reclassification of psychosis, and thus lead to improved diagnostic systems that have greater predictive validity in terms of prognosis and treatment response. There are now strong claims being made by psychologists (Bentall, 2003) and psychiatrists (van Os, 2003) to replace categorical approaches to diagnosis with a more sophisticated approach that recognizes that psychosis is distributed on a continuum throughout the population.

The problem of prognosis

We have seen that in the classical view, schizophrenia is a condition associated with poor outcome and deterioration in social function. The resurgence of interest in the idea of 'deterioration' and 'deficits' as a core feature of schizophrenia, together with the widely held clinical view that insidious onset in schizophrenia is associated with a poor prognosis, has had a significant influence on recent thinking about treatment and the organization of services, especially for young people in their first episode. The view has gained ground that the longer the duration of untreated psychosis (DUP), the greater the risk of poor outcome, and to reduce this risk it is necessary to commence treatment with neuroleptic medication at the earliest signs of symptoms. In Australia, the Early Psychosis Prevention and Intervention Centre (EPPIC) (McGorry et al., 1996) was set up to ensure early treatment with neuroleptics, to minimize the DUP with the objective of improving long-term outcome in schizophrenia. In Britain the Department of Health's National Service Framework for Mental Health has seen the introduction of early intervention services, based in the EPPIC model.

We have already seen that there is scant evidence that neuroleptics improve the prognosis of schizophrenia and minimise 'deficits'. In any case, there is evidence

Table 14.1   Results of four long-term outcome studies in schizophrenia

Author(s)	Number of Subjects	Follow-up (years)	% Improved
Bleuler (1978)	200	22	53
Huber (1979)	>500	21	57
Ciompi (1980)	300	37	49
Harding (1987)	262	32	68

that the prognosis of schizophrenia is much better than Kraepelin's work would have us believe. In his original study, Kraepelin (1913) reported that only 13 per cent of his patients suffering from dementia praecox recovered. Table 14.1 summarizes the results of four recent long-term outcome studies of people diagnosed with schizophrenia, which show that in broad terms 50 per cent or more of people improve significantly.

It is worth noting that many of Kraepelin's subjects suffered from what today would be identified as organic psychoses. Comprehensive health care was not a feature of nineteenth century medicine. In addition, many of the subjects included in the studies in Table 14.1 became ill before the introduction of neuroleptics, and were unlikely to have received them during the early stages of their illnesses. Richard Warner (1994) reviewed the results of outcome studies of schizophrenia in Western societies. He found that despite the introduction of pharmacotherapy, outcome has remained relatively constant. Indeed, the most powerful influence on the outcome of schizophrenia in the West appears to be the economic situation at the time that studies were undertaken. Those carried out in prosperous times reported better long-term outcomes for people diagnosed with schizophrenia. Warner also examined the results of the World Health Organisation's International Pilot Study of Schizophrenia carried out in nine countries in the 1970s. In general the outcome for schizophrenia was better in economically disadvantaged countries like Nigeria than in economically advantaged countries (WHO, 1973; 1979).

Recent work in Singapore and Madras confirms this. Kua et al.(2003) found that two thirds of their patients in Singapore had good or fair outcome at 20 years. In Madras, Thara et al. (2004) found that only 5 out of their 61 subjects followed up over 20 years had been continuously ill. More than three quarters were in employment. This evidence throws doubt on the view that schizophrenia is of necessity a condition that has a poor prognosis. It suggests that economic and cultural factors arguably have a greater influence on the outcome of schizophrenia than medication or early intervention.

Harmful aspects of diagnosis

It is extremely difficult for mental health professionals who attach great importance to the value of beneficence to accept that on occasions aspects of their work may cause harm. Service user led research indicates that some people find diagnosis and medical interventions helpful (Rogers et al., 1993; Faulkner and

Layzell, 2000), but many do not. Some find psychiatric diagnosis and treatment oppressive and harmful, as some of the personal narratives in Read and Reynolds (1996) indicate. The most direct evidence for the harmfulness of the diagnosis of schizophrenia comes from recent work on stigma and mental illness. Sayce (2000) has explored in detail the implications of stigma, particularly the loss of citizenship associated with being a psychiatric patient. A label of 'chronic schizophrenia' is especially apt to have a negative effect on a person's social identity.

It is widely believed in professional circles that attempts to improve public understanding of schizophrenia in biomedical terms will improve public attitudes towards people who experience the condition, and thus reduce stigma. This view is based on the assumption that if the public can be educated to accept that the causes of psychosis are attributable to biological factors over which the person has no control, then the individual cannot be blamed or held responsible. Angermeyer and Matschinger (2005) tested this assumption by subjecting two representative population surveys of public attitudes to psychiatric patients (using vignettes of schizophrenia), conducted in the Länder of the former German Federal Republic in 1990 and 2001 to a trend analysis. Over the period of the study they found an increase in public acceptance of biomedical explanations of psychosis, associated with public desire for increased distance from people with a diagnosis of schizophrenia. These time trends did not hold for major depressive disorder. Read et al., (2006) have recently subjected the literature on stigma and schizophrenia to a comprehensive review to assess whether the 'schizophrenia is an illness like any other' approach helps reduce prejudice and stigma towards those with the diagnosis. They found a recent increase in biological causal beliefs across Western countries, suggesting that this approach is gaining hold. However, biological attributions for psychosis were overwhelmingly associated with negative public attitudes in 18 of 19 studies, whereas psychosocial attributions were associated with positive attitudes in 11 of 12 studies. Biological attributions are thus strongly linked to negative public attitudes, or stigma. This appears particularly to be the case for the diagnosis of schizophrenia.

CONCLUSIONS

Although biomedical explanations of psychosis have become extraordinarily influential over the last fifty years, they have yet to yield convincing evidence that biological differences between people with a diagnosis of schizophrenia actually exist, or that they may lead to more rational interventions. No less an authority than the clinical neuroscience and genetics research agenda group for DSM-V has recently concluded that:

> Although the past two decades have produced a great deal of progress in neurobiological investigations, the field has thus far failed to identify a single neurobiological phenotypic

marker or gene that is useful in making a diagnosis of a major psychiatric disorder or for predicting response to psychopharmacological treatment. (First, 2004)

It is difficult to avoid the conclusion that the commercial interests of the pharmaceutical industry and the political interests of a small number of highly influential academic psychiatrists keep the biological model in psychiatry afloat. At the same time, for many people psychosis is an intensely distressing and disabling experience. Yet others learn to live with, cope with and recover from the experience. They achieve this by themselves, with the help and support of their families and other survivors or service users, and also with the help and support of psychiatrists, psychologists and other mental health workers. The rise of expertise and technical skill over the last fifty years has meant that we tend to overlook the value of what have been called non-specific factors (Bracken et al., 2010) such as the quality of the therapeutic relationship and the meaning response (Moerman, 2002). The best quality care for people who experience psychosis arises when we find the right balance between science and non-specific factors. We still have a long way to go.

NOTES

1 The word madness is used here because it makes no assumption about how we might best understand the phenomenon. The word mad and its derivative, madness, are old words whose origins can be traced back to Middle English and Old High German (Shorter Oxford English Dictionary), that is more than 1000 years.

2 The late Robert Barrett, dually trained as a psychiatrist and anthropologist, has written a first class account of role that the concept of schizophrenia has in the power and authority of the profession of psychiatry (Barrett, 1996).

3 It is worth commenting in passing that early twentieth century genetics played an important role in the development of eugenic theories that led to the deaths of thousands of psychiatric patients in Nazi Germany, and which were a prelude to the Holocaust. Ernest Rudin, described by Lifton (1986) as a '…fanatical genetecist…' was a pupil of Emil Kraepelin. Rudin played a key role in the scientific legitimation of the Nazi regime's racial policies.

4 The word neuroleptic is used here in preference to antipsychotic because as will be seen, there is no evidence that these drugs are specifically antipsychotic in the sense that their mode of action in schizophrenia relates to their pharmacological properties in rectifying an underlying disturbance in dopamine transmission.

5 Both Kapur's and Cohen and Servan-Schreiber's models take us into deep waters. Without dwelling on the philosophical issues raised here in any detail, they presuppose that it is possible to account for experience either in physical (i.e. neurochemical), or mental terms (i.e. in terms of mental representations). In other words they are characterized by body-mind, or ontological, dualism whose origins can be traced back to the philosophy of Descartes. We have examined in detail the implications and limitations of this view in relation to psychiatry and medicine. Although beyond the scope of this chapter, interested readers are referred to Thomas and Bracken (2010) for a detailed examination of body-mind dualism in psychiatry.

6 These problems are of relevance to many other studies of the biological substrate of psychosis, but here they are particularly important because of the aetiological claims that are made for changes in brain structure, which may be confounded by long-term physical treatments and institutionalisation.

7 Recent work reviewing the relationship between 'relapse' and the discontinuation of medication suggests that the long-term use of neuroleptic medication may alter the way that schizophrenia presents over time (Moncrieff, 2006). Specifically, rapid discontinuation of these drugs results in a more florid form of 'relapse' that differs in its clinical features from the original episode of psychosis. This may be evidence of a so-called supersensitivity syndrome similar to a drug withdrawal state.

8 'Novel' in the sense that they are thought to act on a variety of neurotransmitter systems, such as 5-hydroxytryptamine, in addition to dopamine.

REFERENCES

Abi-Dargham, A. (2004) Do we still believe in the dopamine hypothesis? New data bring new evidence. *International Journal of Neuropsychopharmacology.* 7(suppl. 1): S1–S5.

Agid, O., Kapur, S., Arenovich, T. and Zipursky, R. (2003) Delayed-Onset Hypotheis of Antipsychotic Action: A Hypothesis Tested and Rejected. *Archives of General Psychiatry.* 60, 1228–1235.

Angermeyer, M. and Matschinger, H. (2005) Causal beliefs and attitudes to people with schizophrenia: Trend analysis based on data from two population surveys in Germany. *British Journal of Psychiatry,* 186, 331–334.

Angrist, B. and Sudilovsky, A. (1978) Central nervous system stimulants: historical aspects and clinical effects. In Iversen, L. et al. (eds), *Handbook of Psychopharmacology,* 11: 99–165. New York: Plenum Press.

Barrett, R. (1996) *The Psychiatric Team and the Social Definition of Schizophrenia: An Anthropological Study of Person and Illness.* Cambridge: Cambridge University Press.

Bentall, R. (2003) *Madness Explained: Psychosis and Human Nature.* London: Allen Lane.

Bleuler, M. (1978) *The schizophrenic disorders: Long-term patient and family studies.* New Haven: Yale University Press.

Bogerts, B., Ashtari, M., Degreef, G. et al. (1990) Reduced temporal limbic structure volumes on magnetic resonance images in first episode schizophrenia. *Psychiatry Research, Neuroimaging,* 35: 1–13.

Boyle, M. (1993) *Schizophrenia: a scientific delusion.* London, Routledge.

Bracken, P. and Thomas, P. (2005) *Postpsychiatry: Mental health in a postmodern world.* Oxford, Oxford University Press.

Bracken, P. and Thomas, P. (2008) From Szasz to Foucault: On the Role of Critical Psychiatry. In Press February 2010, *Philosophy, Psychiatry and Psychology.*

Bracken, P., Thomas, P. and Timimi, S. (2010) Kuhn, Evidence-Based Medicine and Psychiatry. In preparation, for submission to *Philosophy, Psychiatry and Psychology.*

Braff, D., Freedman, R., Schork, N. and Gottesman, I. (2007) Deconstructing schizophrenia: an overview of the use of endophenotypes in order to understand a complex disorder. *Schizophrenia Bulletin,* 33: 21–32.

Brockington, I. (1992) Schizophrenia: yesterday's concept. *European Psychiatry,* 7: 203–207.

Brown, R., Colter, N., Corsellis, J.A.N. et al. (1986) Post-mortem evidence of striatal brain changes in schizophrenia. *Archives of General Psychiatry,* 43: 36–42.

Bruton, C.J., Crow, T., Frith, C.D. et al. (1990) Schizophrenia and the brain. *Psychological Medicine,* 20: 285–304.

Bush, G. (1990) *Project on the Decade of the Brain: Presidential Proclamation 6158.* Accessed at http://www.loc.gov/loc/brain/proclaim.htpl (accessed 10 April, 2008).

Cannon, T.D. and Marco, E. (1994) Structural brain abnormalities as indicators of vulnerability to schizophrenia. *Schizophrenia Bulletin,* 20: 89–101.

Carlsson, A. and Lindquist, M. (1963) Effects of chlorpromazine or haloperidol on the formation of 3-methoxytyramine and normetanephrine in mouse brains. *Acta Pharmacologica,* 20: 140–144.

Carlsson, A. (1990) Early psychopharmacology and the rise of modern brain research. *Journal of Psychopharmacology,* 4: 120–126.

Ciompi, L (1980) The natural history of schizophrenia in the long term. *British Journal of Psychiatry,* 136: 413–420.

Clow, A., Theodorou, A., Jenner, P. and Marsden, C.D. (1980) Changes in rat striatal dopamine turnover and receptors activity during one year's neuroleptic administration. *European Journal of Pharmacology,* 63: 135–144.

Cohen, J.D. and Servan-Schreiber, D. (1992) Context, cortex and dopamine: a connectionist approach to behaviour and biology in schizophrenia. *Psychological Review,* 99: 45–77.

Cohen, J.D. and Servan-Schreiber, D. (1993) A theory of dopamine function and its role in cognitive deficits in schizophrenia. *Schizophrenia Bulletin,* 19: 85–104.

Coppens, H., Sloof, C., Paans, A., Wiegman, T., Vaalburg, W. and Korf, J. (1991) High central D2-dopamine receptor occupancy as assessed with positron emission tomography in medicated but therapy-resistant patients. *Biological Psychiatry.* 29: 629–634.

Craddock, N., O'Donavan, M. and Owen, M. (2005) The genetics of schizophrenia and bipolar disorder: dissecting psychosis. *Journal of Medical Genetics.* 42: 193–204.

Crow, T.J., Done, D.J. and Sacker, A. (1994) Childhood precursors of psychosis as clues to its evolutionary origins. *European Archives of Psychiatry and Neurological Sciences,* 245(2): 61–69.

Crumpton, N. (1967) Maintaining patients in the community. The role of drugs. *British Journal of Geriatric Practice,* 4: 186–192.

Curson, D., Patel, M., Liddle, P.F. and Barnes, T.R. (1988) Psychiatric morbidity of a long-stay hospital population with chronic schizophrenia, and implications for future community care. *British Medical Journal,* 297: 818–822.

Davis, J.M. and Casper, R. (1977) Antipsychotic drugs: clinical pharmacology and therapeutic use. *Drugs,* 14: 260–282.

Davis, J.M., Schaffer, C.B., Killian, G.A. et al. (1980) Important issues in the drug treatment of schizophrenia. *Schizophrenia Bulletin,* 6: 70–87.

Davis, K., Kahn, R., Ko, G. and Davidson, M. (1991) Dopamine in schizophrenia: a review and reconceptualization. *American Journal of Psychiatry,* 148: 1474–1486.

Department of Health (1999) *Modern Standards and Service Models: Mental Health National Service Frameworks.* London, Department of Health.

Done, D.J., Crow, T.J., Johnstone, E.C. and Sacker, A. (1994) Childhood antecedents of schizophrenia: social adjustment at ages 7 and 11. *British Medical Journal,* 309: 699–703.

Engelhardt, D.M. and Freedman, N. (1969) Maintenance drug therapy: the schizophrenic patient in the community. In Kiev (ed.), *Social Psychiatry,* 1: 256–282. London: Routledge and Kegan Paul Ltd.

Farde, L., Wiesel, F-A., Hall, H., Halldin, C., Stonelander, S., Sedvall, G. (1987) No D2 receptor increase in PET study of schizophrenia. *Archives of General Psychiatry.* 44: 671–672.

Faulkner, A. and Layzell, S. (2000) *Strategies for Living: A report of user-led research into people's strategies for living with mental distress.* London: Mental Health Foundation.

First, M (2004) A research agenda for DSM-V: Summary of the DSM-V preplanning white papers published in May 2002. On http://www.dsm5.org/whitepapers.cfm (accessed 26 October, 2006).

Foucault, M. (2006) History of Madness. Murphy J, Khalfa J (translators). London: Routledge.

Foucault, M. (2006a) Psychiatric Power: Lectures at the Collège de France 1973-1974. In J. Jagrange (ed.), trans G. Burchell (trans.). Basingstoke: Palgrave Macmillan.

Gottesman, I. and Shields, J. (1982) *Schizophrenia: the epigenetic puzzle.* Cambridge: Cambridge University Press.

Gottesman, I., McGuffin, P. and Farmer, A. (1987) *Genetics and Schizophrenia – Current State of Negotiations in Human Genetics.* Eds. Vogel, F. and Sperling, K. Berlin. Springer-Verlag.

Gur, R., Calkins, M., Gur, R., Horan, W., Nuechterlein, K., Seidman, L. and Stone, W. (2007) The Consortium on the Genetics of Schizophrenia: neurocognitive endophenotypes. *Schizophrenia Bulletin,* 33: 49–68.

Harding, C. M., G. W. Brooks, et al. (1987). The Vermont longitudinal study of persons with severe mental illness: I. Methodology, study sample, and overall status 32 years later. *American Journal of Psychiatry,* 144(6): 718–726.

Harvey, I., Ron, M., Du Boulay, G. et al. (1993) Diffuse reduction of cortical volume in schizophrenia on magnetic resonance imaging. *Psychological Medicine,* 23: 591–604.

Harvey, I., Persaud, R., Ron, M. et al. (1994) Volumetric MRI measurement in bipolars compared with schizophrenics and healthy controls. *Psychological Medicine,* 24: 689–699.

Hempel, C. (1961) Introduction to problems of taxonomy. In J. Zubin (ed.) *Field Studies in the Mental Disorders.* New York: Grune and Stratton. pp. 3–22.

Heston, L.L. (1966) Psychiatric disorders in foster home reared children of schizophrenic mothers. *British Journal of Psychiatry,* 112: 819–835.

Huber, G., G. Gross, et al. (1975). A long-term follow-up study of schizophrenia: Psychiatric course of illness and prognosis. *Acta Psychiatrica Scandinavica*, 52: 49–57.

Iverson, S. and Iverson, L. (2007) Dopamine: 50 years in perspective. *Trends in Neurosciences*, 30: 188–193.

Jackson, J.H. (1889) On post-epileptic states: A contribution to the comparative study of the insanities. *Journal of Mental Science*, 34: 490–500.

Jakob, H. and Beckman, H. (1986) Prenatal development disturbances in the limbic allocortex in schizophrenics. *Journal of Neural Transmission*, 65: 303–326.

Johnstone, E.C., Crow, T.C., Frith, C.D. et al. (1976) Cerebral ventricular size and cognitive impairment in chronic schizophrenia. *Lancet*, ii: 924–926.

Johnstone, E., Crow, T., Frith, C., Stevens, M., Kreel, J. and Husband, J. (1978) The dementia of dementia praecox. *Acta Psychiatrica Scandinavica*, 57: 305–324.

Johnstone, L. (2000) *Users and abusers of psychiatry.* (2nd edition) London, Routledge.

Jones, P., Murray, R.M. and Rodgers, B. (1994) Child development preceding adult schizophrenia. *Schizophrenia Research*, 11: 97.

Kane, J., Honigfeld, G., Singer, J. et al. (1988) Clozapine for the treatment resistant schizophrenic. Archives of General Psychiatry, 45: 789–796.

Kane, J.M. and Freeman, H.L. (1994) Towards more effective antipsychotic treatment. *British Journal of Psychiatry.* 165(suppl. 25): 22–31.

Kapur, S. (2003) Psychosis as a State of Aberrant Salience: A Framework Linking Biology, Phenomenology, and Pharmacology in Schizophrenia. *American Journal of Psychiatry*, 160:13–23.

Kraepelin, E. (1913) *Psychiatrie, ein Lehrbuch fur Studierende und Artzt* (Psychiatry, a textbook for students and practitioners) (8th edition), Vol. 3. Leipzig: Barth.

Kua, J., K. E. Wong, et al. (2003). A 20-year follow-up study on schizophrenia in Singapore. *Acta Psychiatrica Scandinavica*, 108(2): 118–125.

Laruelle, M. and Abi-Dargham, A. (1999) Dopamine as the wind of the psychotic fire: new evidence from brain imaging studies. *Journal of Psychopharmacology*, 13: 358–371.

Lenzer, J. (2004) Bush plans to screen entire US population for mental illness. *British Medical Journal*, 328: 1458.

Lewis, S. (1993) A controlled quantitative study of computed X-ray tomography in functional psychoses. MD thesis, University of London.

Lifton, R. (1986) *The Nazi Doctors: Medical Killing and the Psychology of Genocide.* New York: Basic Books.

Marx, O. (1970) Nineteenth-Century Medical Psychology: Theoretical Problems in the Work of Griesinger, Meynert, and Wernicke. *Isis*, 61: 355–370.

McGorry, P. D., Edwards, J., Mihalopoulos, C., et al. (1996) EPPIC: An evolving system of early detection and optimal management. *Schizophrenia Bulletin*, 22: 305–326.

Melander, H., Ahlqvist-Rastad, J., Meijer, G., Beermann, B. (2003) Evidence biased medicine— selective reporting from studies sponsored by pharmaceutical industry: review of studies in new drug applications. *British Medical Journal*, 327: 1171–1176.

Moerman, D. (2002) *Meaning, medicine and the 'placebo effect'.* Cambridge: Cambridge University Press.

Moncrieff, J. and Crawford, M. (2001) British psychiatry in the twentieth century: Observations from a psychiatric journal. *Social Science and Medicine*, 53: 349–356.

Moncrieff, J. (2006) Why is it so difficult to stop psychiatric drug treatment? It may be nothing to do with the original problem. *Medical Hypotheses*, 67: 517–523.

Moncrieff, J. (2008) *The Myth of the Chemical Cure: A critique of Psychiatric Drug Treatments.* Basingstoke, Palgrave Macmillan.

Murray, R.M. (1994) Neurodevelopmental schizophrenia: the rediscovery of dementia praecox. *British Journal of Psychiatry*, 165(suppl. 25): 6–12.

Owen, M., Craddock, N. and Jablensky, A. (2007) The genetic deconstruction of psychosis. *Schizophrenia Bulletin*, 33: 905–911.

Pakkenberg, B. (1987) Post-mortem study of chronic schizophrenic brains. *British Journal of Psychiatry*, 151: 744–752.

Panksepp, J. (2004) Biological psychiatry sketched – past, present, future. In J. Panksepp (ed.) *Textbook of Biological Psychiatry*. New York: John Wiley. pp. 3–32.

Pincus, H., Henderson, B., Blackwood, D. and Dial, T. (1993) Trends in research in two general psychiatric journals in 1969 – 1990: Research on research. *American Journal of Psychiatry*, 150: 135–142.

Porter, R. (1997) *The Greatest Benefit to Mankind: A Medical History of Humanity from Antiquity to the Present.* London: Harper Collins Publishers.

Porter, R. (2000) *Enlightenment: Britain and the Creation of the Modern World.* Harmondsworth, Allen Lane: The Penguin Press.

Read, J. and Reynolds, J. (eds) (1996) *Speaking Our Minds: An Anthology.* London, Macmillan: Open University.

Read, J., Haslam, N., Sayce, L., Davies, E. (2006) Prejudice and schizophrenia: a review of the 'mental illness is an illness like any other' approach. *Acta Psychiatrica Scandinavica,* 114: 303–318.

Reynolds, G.P., Riederer, P. Jellinger, K. et al. (1981) Dopamine receptors and schizophrenia: the neuroleptic drug problem. *Neuropharmacology*, 20: 1319–1320.

Rogers, A., Pilgrim, D. and Lacey, R. (1993) *Experiencing Psychiatry: User's views of services.* London: MIND/MacMillan.

Rosenthal, D., Wender, P., Kety, S.S. et al. (1971) The adopted-away offspring of schizophrenics. *American Journal of Psychiatry*, 128: 307–311.

Sayce, L. (2000) From *Psychiatric Patient to Citizen: Overcoming Discrimination and Social Exclusion.* London: Macmillan Press.

Seeman, P., Lee, T., Chau-Wong, M. and Wong, K. (1976) Anti-psychotic drug doses and neuroleptic/dopamine receptors. *Nature*, 261: 717–719.

Snyder, S. (1972) Catecholamines in the brain as mediators of amphetamine psychosis. *Archives of General Psychiatry*, 27: 169–179.

Snyder, S. (1976) The Dopamine Hypothesis of Schizophrenia; focus on the role of the dopamine receptor. *American Journal of Psychiatry*, 133: 197–202.

Steen, R., Mull, C., McClure, R., Hamer, R., Lieberman, J. (2006) Brain volume in first episode schizophrenia: Systematic review and meta-analysis of magnetic resonance imaging studies. *British Journal of Psychiatry*, 188: 510–518.

Suddath, R.L., Christison, G., Torrey, E.F. et al. (1989) Quantitative magnetic resonance imaging in twin pairs discordant for schizophrenia. *Schizophrenia Research*, 2: 129.

Szasz, T. (1972) *The Myth of Mental Illness.* London: Paladin.

Szatmari, P., Maziade, M., Zwaigenbaum, L., Merrette, C., Roy, M-A., Joobher, R. and Palmour, R. (2007) Informative phenotypes for genetic studies of psychiatric disorders. *American Journal of Medical Genetics*, 144: 581–588.

Thara, R. (2004). Twenty-Year Course of Schizophrenia: The Madras Longitudinal Study. *Canadian Journal of Psychiatry,* 49(8): 564–569.

Thomas, P. and Bracken, P. (2010) Dualisms in *The Myth of Mental Illness*: A Critical Analysis Using the Philosophy of Merleau-Ponty. In J. Moncrieff (ed.), *Demedicalising Misery* forthcoming), Basingstoke: Palgrave Macmillan.

Tienari, P., Lahti, I. and Sorri, A. (1987) The Finish adoptive family study of schizophrenia. *Journal of Psychiatric Research,* 21: 437–445.

Torrey, E. and Miller, J. (2001) *The invisible plague: the rise of mental illness from 1750 to the present.* New Brunswick New Jersey: Rutgers University Press.

Uttal, W. (2001) *The new phrenology: The limits of localising cognitive processes in the brain.* Cambridge: Cambridge University Press.

van Os, J. (2003) Is there a continuum of psychotic experience in the general population? *Epidemiologiae Psychiatria Sociale*, 12(4): 242–252.

Waddington, J. (2007) Neuroimaging and other neurobiological indices in schizophrenia: relationship to measurement of functional outcome. *British Journal of Psychiatry*, 191(suppl. 50): 52–57.

Warner, R. (1994) *Recovery from Schizophrenia: Psychiatry and Political Economy*. New York, Routledge.

Weinberger, D.R., Cannon-Spoor, E., Potkin, S.G. et al. (1980) Poor premorbid adjustment and CT scan abnormalities in chronic schizophrenia. *American Journal of Psychiatry*, 137: 1410–1413.

Wilson, M. (1993) DSM-III and the Transformation of American Psychiatry: A History. *American Journal of Psychiatry*, 150: 399–410.

Wong, D.R., Wagner, H.N., Tune, L.E., et al. (1986) Positron emission tomography reveals elevated D2 dopamine receptors in drug-naive schizophrenics. *Science*, 234: 1558–1563.

World Health Organization (1973) *International pilot study of schizophrenia*. Geneva: World Health Organization.

World Health Organization (1979) *Schizophrenia: an international follow-up study*. Chichester, Wiley.

Wyatt. R.J. (1986) The dopamine hypothesis: variations on a theme (II). *Psychopharmacology Bulletin*, 22: 923–927.

15

The Psychology of Psychosis

Richard Bentall

INTRODUCTION

The psychoses are a family of psychiatric conditions, usually characterized by hallucinations (the perception of stimuli that are actually absent; in the case of patients with psychosis, a voice or several voices are typically heard, but visual hallucinations are also common) and delusions (bizarre and apparently irrational beliefs) in which the patient, when most severely ill, in some sense seems to lose touch with reality. These conditions, which roughly correspond to the popular understanding of madness, are usually regarded as the most severe types of mental illness, often resulting in the patient receiving a diagnosis of *schizophrenia* or *bipolar disorder* (although other diagnoses may apply). They are often contrasted with the neuroses (more common and less severe types of mental illness in which the individual, although very anxious or depressed, is aware of being ill and does not experience hallucinations and delusions) and the personality disorders (life-long dysfunctional patterns of relating to other people).

The psychoses are the source of considerable distress to patients and families, and concern to health agencies and governments. Estimates of the annual incidence rate (the number of new cases each year) of schizophrenia from different parts of the world range from about 7 to about 40 new cases per 100,000 population (McGrath, 2005) and similar figures have been reported for bipolar disorder (Lloyd et al., 2005). The number of people who receive a diagnosis of schizophrenia at some point in their lives certainly exceeds 0.5 per cent (Jablensky, 1995) and, again, about the same can be said for bipolar disorder (Goodwin and Jamison, 1990). Taking a broader perspective and including those individuals who do not meet the full criteria of either of these diagnoses, it has been estimated that the lifetime risk of being diagnosed as suffering from any kind of psychosis may be as high as 3 per cent (Perala et al., 2007) which, if extrapolated to the population of the world, amounts to over 200 million people. Long-term impairment is common – in one study of schizophrenia patients it was estimated that over a quarter remained socially and occupationally disabled after 15 years (Wiersma et al., 2000). In the developed world, about 5 per cent of schizophrenia patients (Palmer et al., 2005) and an even more bipolar patients die by suicide (Marangell et al., 2006).

The direct cost of caring for people diagnosed as suffering from schizophrenia in the USA has been estimated at $2.3 billion (Blomqvist et al., 2006), which does not take into account the indirect costs accrued through, for example, loss of economic productivity by patients and their carers. For example, in 2002 it was estimated that the British National Health Service spent £199 million caring for patients with bipolar disorder, but that the annual cost to the country attributable to the condition was £1.8 billion (Gupta and Guest, 2002).

Not surprisingly, the psychoses have been subjected to sustained research efforts over many decades. Nevertheless, outcomes have little improved since the Victorian period and are at least as good in the developing world as in the industrialized nations (Bentall, 2009; Warner, 1985). In this chapter I will focus on attempts to understand the psychoses within a psychological framework, and trace the evolution of the three main approaches to psychosis – the Kraepelinian paradigm, stress-vulnerability models, and symptom-based models – from the nineteenth century to the present day.

A word of caution about language is required at the outset. Many of the concepts that are widely used to describe psychotic problems – especially *schizophrenia* – have been contested, because they have been said to be unscientific and/or because they are believed to be stigmatizing. This leaves me with a dilemma, because some kind of brief label is needed to indicate the kinds of patients involved in the various studies that I will consider. To describe someone as 'schizophrenic' or 'bipolar' is, I think, unacceptable to most people today. However, the terms 'persons diagnosed as suffering from schizophrenia', although accurate and neutral in most instances, is a bit of a mouthful. In the earlier parts of this chapter I will therefore use the terms 'schizophrenia patient' or 'bipolar patient', as short hand for 'person in receipt of the relevant diagnosis'. This approach reflects the mainstream view that the terms schizophrenia and bipolar disorder are unproblematic, an assumption which, we will see towards the end of this chapter, does not survive careful scrutiny.

EMIL KRAEPELIN AND HIS FOLLOWERS

Psychiatry as a medical discipline was an invention of the nineteenth century Germany-speaking world (Shorter, 1997). Early researchers, assuming from the outset that psychiatric disorders were brain diseases, focused much of their effort on basic research in neuroscience and, in the clinical domain, were mainly concerned with classification and diagnosis. Undoubtedly, the psychiatrist of this period whose influence proved most enduring was Emil Kraepelin, a man who (although hardly a household name) shaped the way that his profession developed much more decisively than Freud (Engstrom and Weber, 2007; Jablensky, 2007).

Kraepelin took inspiration from his older brother, a distinguished botonist who worked on the classification of plant species. He argued that researchers in the field should use a wide range of methodologies, including studies in psychopharmacology and neuroanatomy, cross-cultural investigations and investigations with psychological tests. However, he assumed that progress could only be achieved following the development of a meaningful system of diagnosis. To this end, he collected detailed data on the symptoms and outcomes of his patients, eventually using this evidence to justify three key clinical concepts, which remain in use today (Kraepelin, 1899, 1990). Kraepelin argued that *dementia praecox* (literally, senility of the young), which typically began in late adolescence, was the consequence of profound cognitive impairment, particularly in the domain of attention, resulting in intellectual deterioration accompanied by hallucinations and delusions. By contrast, *manic depressive illness* (under which heading Kraepelin included what we now know as unipolar depression) was characterized by extreme mood states and usually had a benign course. Finally, *paranoia* was a condition in which the individual experienced delusional beliefs in the absence of any impairment of consciousness or cognitive functioning. Despite informing most subsequent research into psychosis, this typology later underwent a number of revisions.

Eugene Bleuler (1911, 1950) disliked the term dementia praecox, arguing that it was not really a dementia (partial recovery was possible) or necessarily praecox (although early onset was typical, it could take hold later in life) and proposed, instead the term *schizophrenia* (by which he meant a shattering of the mental faculties, rather than a split-mind). Influenced by Freud's theories (although declining to embrace them wholeheartedly) he emphasized the importance of subtle emotional and cognitive difficulties rather than gross cognitive deterioration. Later, Kurt Schneider (1959) proposed a list of eleven first-rank symptoms of schizophrenia, which were all types of hallucinations or delusions. Although Schneider's intention was purely pragmatic – he was simply attempting to identify those symptoms which were diagnostically useful and certainly did not intend them to be regarded as the core of the illness – his efforts led to the modern conception of schizophrenia, which emphasizes *positive symptoms* (hallucinations and delusions) over *negative symptoms* (apathy, anhedonia and flat affect, in which there is absence of normal function).

A second innovation followed the recognition that some patients exhibited a mixture of schizophrenia and manic depressive symptoms. This observation led to the introduction of the concept of *schizoaffective disorder*, first proposed by Kasanin (1933). Finally, the concept of manic depression underwent a series of transformations, most notably when Klaus Leonhard (1957, 1979) argued for a distinction between *unipolar depression*, in which the individual experiences repeated episodes of depression, and bipolar disorder, in which the individual experiences also experiences episodes of *mania* (periods of extreme excitement, which often begin with pleasant and grandiose ideas, but which often spiral out of control into panic and agitation accompanied by delusional ideas).

The extent to which these changes have preserved Kraepelin's clinical concepts remains moot. Boyle (1990), for example, has argued that many of Kraepelin's dementia praecox patients were probably suffering from neurological infections and would not meet modern criteria for schizophrenia. Of his three major diagnostic concepts, paranoia perhaps remained the least revised, although the term *delusional disorder* is used to describe this condition today. Nonetheless, Kraepelin's general approach has undoubtedly been the most dominant paradigm within psychiatry throughout the last century.

One feature of this paradigm has been a preoccupation with explanations of psychosis that focus on genetics and neuroscience. Indeed some of the earliest research in psychiatric genetics, which involved studies of the inheritance of schizophrenia, were conducted in the Munich research centre where Kraepelin ended his career (Joseph, 2003). The psychiatrists who conducted these studies have been criticized for taking the idea that schizophrenia was inherited as an axiom rather than a hypothesis (Marshall, 1990). Certainly, their interpretations of their data – which resulted in very high heritability estimates – have seemed untrustworthy when carefully scrutinized by modern researchers (Joseph, 2003; Rose et al., 1985).

However, genetic data was not the only kind of biological evidence that seemed to support the Kraepelinian paradigm. The adventitious discovery of the first effective antipsychotic drug chlorpromazine after the Second World War (Healy, 2004), and the subsequent demonstration that all effective antipsychotics block dopamine D_2 receptors in the midbrain (Seeman et al., 1976) seemed, to many, incontrovertible evidence that the psychoses were brain diseases. This idea also seemed to be supported by a large volume of psychological research apparently demonstrating that psychotic patients perform poorly on various neurocognitive tests presumed to be sensitive to brain malfunction. The apparent success of this endeavour has led some leading American psychologists to insist that schizophrenia should be considered a neurocognitive disorder (Green and Nuechterlein, 1999).

Later, we will consider some limitations of the Kraepelinian paradigm in detail. Before proceeding, however, it is important to note that it has not survived without being challenged from within psychiatry. During the middle years of the twentieth century, for example, many American psychiatrists were very sceptical about the value of medical-style diagnoses. They took their inspiration from the work of Adolf Meyer who, ironically, had been largely responsible for the introduction of Kraepelin's ideas to the United States. After his appointment as director of the prestigious Phipps Clinic at Johns Hopkins University, Meyer increasingly advocated a pragmatic approach based on individual formulations of each patient's difficulties (Marx, 1993). Famously, in a comment that was perhaps meant to be reference to Kraepelin's brother, 'We should not classify people as plants'.

For a later generation of psychiatrists, it was the inhumane conditions in the asylums that provided a motive for questioning the Kraepelinian approach. It was a South African psychiatrist practicing in London, David Cooper (1967) who coined the term *anti-psychiatry* to describe an approach based on a radical rejection of everything that Kraepelin stood for. Prominent critics from within psychiatry who were associated with 'anti-psychiatry' included Ronald (R.D.) Laing and Thomas Szasz, although both ultimately rejected the label, and had quite different reasons for opposing conventional practice. For Laing, psychotic experiences were meaningful reactions to the human condition (Laing, 1960). At different times, he saw psychosis as the consequence of victimizing family dynamics (Laing and Esterson, 1969) or as a transcendental journey from which the individual could later emerge healed (Laing, 1967). Szasz (1960), by contrast, has always objected to the way that conventional practice infringes human rights, arguing that mental illness is a myth used to justify the ill-treatment of society's misfits.

In the end, these critiques failed to have a lasting impact on psychiatry because their authors failed to develop a viable alternative to conventional treatment. Laing's therapeutic community at Kingsley Hall in London collapsed under the weight of his organizational incompetence (although a more sensibly organized trial of a non-medical therapeutic community conducted in the United States obtained good results; Mosher, 1999; Mosher and Menn, 1978). At the same time, progress in the neurosciences, for example the observation of reduced ventricular volume in the brains of schizophrenia patients as measured with newly available CT scans (Johnstone et al., 1976), seemed to hold the promise of genuine advances in the medical understanding of severe mental illness.

This last development was accompanied by renewed interest in psychiatric diagnoses, particularly amongst psychiatrists in the United States, culminating in the publication of the influential third edition of the American Psychiatric Associations Diagnostic and Statistical Manual (DSM-III; American Psychiatric Association, 1980). Many of the psychiatrists who were involved in the design of the manual styled themselves as neo-Kraepelinians. One of their number, Gerald Klerman (1978) published a manifesto, which articulated, in ten propositions, the main assumptions of the neo-Kraepelinian approach. Klerman argued that, 'there is a boundary between the normal and the sick' (proposition 4), that 'there are discrete mental illnesses' (proposition 5) and that 'there should be an explicit and intentional concern with diagnosis and classification' (proposition 7).

STRESS-VULNERABILITY MODELS

From the 1960s onwards, a number of psychological researchers proposed modifications to the Kraepelinian paradigm, leading to a series of models that emphasized the continuum between psychosis and normal functioning. An influential model introduced by the American psychologist Paul Meehl (1962) took as its starting point the observation that schizophrenia fails to follow simple Mendelian patterns of inheritance. The children of patients were known to have a high risk of mental illness, but at most only 10 per cent became schizophrenic and by far the majority failed to develop psychosis. Based on twin and adoption studies, genetic researchers such as Gottesman and Shields (1982) still insisted that the heritability of the disorder was as high as 70–80 per cent (although, as we will see later, this statistic is often misunderstood) but it seemed most likely that disorder was polygenic (many genes involved) with genes of low penitrance (individuals with the implicated gene do not always become ill) and expressivity (individuals inheriting the relevant genes have symptoms of varying severity). Hence, it seemed that many people must inherit a tendency towards schizophrenia without actually becoming ill. (See Clarke in this handbook.)

Meehl's speculative model proposed that perhaps 10 per cent of the population at large inherits a vulnerability to schizophrenia, which he called schizotaxia. Schizotaxic individuals have subtle cognitive and affective characteristics, which Meehl characterized as 'cognitive slippage' and 'anhedonia' (the inability to experience pleasure). Such individuals would only become schizophrenic if exposed to unspecified environmental stressors; otherwise in adulthood they would show *schizotypal personality traits*, such as odd beliefs and other forms of eccentricity.

This model was embraced by many neo-Kraepelinians, partly because it seemed to account for the results of a series of adoption studies conducted by a team of American and Danish investigators. In these studies, adoption records in Denmark were used to identify mothers with a diagnosis of schizophrenia who had given up their children to adoption at an early age. The children were followed up into adulthood to see whether they had a high risk of schizophrenia compared to adopted children whose biological mothers had not been diagnosed with schizophrenia. In a parallel series of investigations, the adoption records were used to work backwards and find the biological parents of adopted children who either had or had not been diagnosed as suffering from schizophrenia. The researchers expected that the biological mothers of the schizophrenia patients would also have high rates of schizophrenia when compared to the biological mothers of mentally-well adoptees.

Although hailed as definitive evidence that schizophrenia is inherited, the results were disappointing from a genetic perspective: few definite cases of schizophrenia were found, either in the adopted-away children of mothers with psychosis, or amongst the biological mothers of adoptees who had been diagnosed with schizophrenia (Kety et al., 1975; Rosenthal et al., 1971). The researchers, believing that they could often observe more subtle abnormal personality characteristics in their samples, argued for a broader concept of schizophrenia spectrum disorder which, they claimed, was over-represented in the key groups. This move proved controversial amongst critics who, to this day, continue to insist that the findings from the Danish–American studies were essentially negative (Joseph, 2003; Rose et al., 1985). However, the notion of a schizophrenia spectrum was adopted in DSM-III, which included the diagnosis of *schizotypal personality disorder* (American Psychiatric Association, 1980).

Psychologists who subsequently explored this notion of schizotypal personality included Gordon Claridge (1985, 1987, 1990) at Oxford in the UK and Jean and Loren Chapman at Wisconsin in the United States (Chapman and Chapman, 1980; Chapman et al., 1994, 1976, 1980). Using simple questionnaires, these researchers found that it was surprisingly easy to measure hallucinatory-like experiences, odd beliefs and other schziotypal characteristics in ordinary people, typically samples of university students. As a consequence, schizotypal personality has become a major area of psychological and biological investigation in its own right (Raine, 2006).

Claridge insisted that a disease model of schizophrenia could survive the apparent continuity between psychosis and normal functioning, and drew a parallel with systemic physical diseases such as essential hypertension (Claridge, 1990). Just as blood pressures are distributed normally, so that the line at which we decide that blood pressure is high is necessarily arbitrary, so too schizotypal traits might be distributed normally, but high scores might still be a cause for concern. Just as high blood pressure is asymptomatic, until some kind of additional factor causes a heart attack or a stroke, so too high levels of schizotypy may be tolerable until stress causes de-compensation into illness. Importantly, Claridge argued that highly schizotypal but mentally well individuals might have positive traits such as high levels of creativity (Claridge, 1998). This reminds us that behavioural and experiential deviations from norms may be viewed pathologically or positively.

In the United States, Zubin and Spring (1977) proposed a simple framework in which it was assumed that vulnerability varied continuously and interacted with stress so that, for example, a highly vulnerable person could be plunged into illness by a comparatively minor stressor whereas a major stressor would be required to make a less vulnerable person ill. This idea was developed further by researchers at UCLA, who sought to identify information processing deficits which, they believed, might be markers of vulnerability (Nuechterlein et al., 1994) and who proposed more complex models in the hope of explaining what happens when a recovered patients has a relapse (Nuechterlein and Dawson, 1984; Nuechterlein and Subotnik, 1998). These developments, without a doubt, constituted an advance on earlier theories but had a number of important limitations.

First, this approach assumed that cognitive deficits – problems of memory and attention – play a crucial role in conferring vulnerability to illness, an assumption that is consistent with Kraepelin's original conception of dementia praecox. Consistent with this account, data from a number of birth cohort studies (in which children have been followed up into adulthood) have been used to show that future schizophrenia patients often do poorly on early indices of cognitive ability (Jones et al., 1994) (e.g. measures of early language development or performance at school). However, although patients, on average, score poorly on a wide range of psychological tests, as the celebrated case of John Forbes Nash demonstrates (Nasar, 1998) it is possible to be a Nobel Prize winning psychotic patient. Moreover, research has consistently failed to find a relationship between deficits and the severity of positive symptoms (Keefe et al., 2007).

In both schizophrenia and bipolar patients, cognitive deficits seem to predict social functioning (the ability to get on with friends, to maintain a job, etc.) rather than the kind or severity of illness (Green, 2006). In the face of these observations, some researchers have insisted that cognitive deficits are the core feature of schizophrenia, and that positive symptoms are of lesser importance (Green, 1998). Others have suggested that it is the impaired inter-connectivity between different brain regions that confers vulnerability to psychosis, rather than impairments to specific cognitive functions (Dickinson and Harvey, 2009).

A second limitation of the stress-vulnerability models is that they have largely remained silent about the types of environmental events that might precipitate illness. The only type of stress to be subjected to sustained investigation during the 1970s and 1980s was family atmosphere. This line of research was prompted by the surprising observation that patients discharged from hospital to the care of their spouses or parents were more likely to relapse and be readmitted than patients discharged to hostels (Brown et al., 1958). Subsequent investigations discovered that patients were most likely to relapse if living with relatives who were critical, hostile and/or over-controlling (Vaughn and Leff, 1976); such relatives were said to exhibit high expressed emotion (EE). The effect was worst, the greater time spent with the high EE relative. Although this finding has been replicated many times (Butzlaff and Hooley, 1998), many EE researchers (perhaps reacting to an earlier period in which psychoanalysts and antipsychiatrists blamed schizophrenia on 'schizophrenogenic' families) continue to insist that family atmosphere affects the course of illness but not whether an individual becomes ill in the first place.

POST-KRAEPELINIAN APPROACHES

The stress-vulnerability models developed from the 1960s onwards challenged the neo-Kraepelinian paradigm in only one respect, claiming a continuity between psychosis and normal functioning. These models accepted the fundamental validity of Kraepelinian diagnoses such as schizophrenia and bipolar disorder. More recent challenges to the Kraepelinian approach have, however, questioned whether these concepts are useful at all.

In an early attempt to address this issue, British psychologist Don Bannister (1968) pointed out that the diagnosis of schizophrenia is a disjunctive category, so that two patients with the diagnosis (one with hallucinations and thought disorder, the other with paranoid delusions and negative symptoms) might have no symptoms in common. Later, in a speculative but highly influential paper, the British psychiatrist Tim Crow (1980) argued that not one but two discrete disease processes were responsible for schizophrenia symptoms. According to Crow, the positive symptoms (hallucinations and delusions) were the consequence of some kind of dysfunction in brain circuits that utilized the neurotransmitter dopamine (these symptoms were exacerbated by dopamine agonists such as amphetamine but responded to D_2-blocking antipsychotic drugs) whereas the negative symptoms (apathy, anhedonia and flat affect, in which there is absence of normal function) were associated with neurodegeneration as revealed by enlarged cerebral ventricles measured on CT scans.

Peter Liddle (1987) was the first researcher to use modern statistical techniques (factor analysis) to examine the extent to which the symptoms of psychotic cluster together. However, instead of finding a single 'factor' of highly inter-correlated symptoms (corresponding to Kraepelin's account) or two independent factors (corresponding to Crow's model), he found three: positive symptoms, negative symptoms and symptoms of cognitive disorganization. This discovery launched a large number of similar investigations, which have usually found at least three factors and sometimes more. Interestingly, when schizotypal questionnaire data collected from healthy individuals has been factor-analysed similar dimensions have usually been observed (Bentall et al., 1989; Claridge et al., 1996). Moreover, similar results have also been reported when the symptoms of psychotic patients with non-schizophrenia diagnoses have been analyzed (Toomey et al., 1998). Indeed, it has been suggested that all of the symptoms of psychosis can be accommodated in a five-factor, dimensional model, with, in addition to the positive, negative and cognitive disorganization dimensions, two further dimensions of depressive and manic symptoms (van Os and Kapur, 2009). According to this account, the standard Kraepelinian diagnoses correspond to different configurations of these five dimensions (see Figure 15.1).

The discovery that the same factor structure can be used to describe patients with schizophrenia, bipolar disorder and schizoaffective disorder is consistent with other evidence that these conditions are not discrete and separable in the way that Kraepelin supposed. For example, as we saw earlier, Kraepelin argued that schizophrenia patients could be distinguished from bipolar patients by their poor outcome. However, although it is certainly true that patients who have predominantly affective symptoms have, on average, a better outcome than those with purely schizophrenic symptoms, both groups of patients experience the full range of possible outcomes (from full recovery to unremitting illness) (e.g. Ciompi, 1984; Goodwin and Jamison, 1990) as do schizoaffective patients, whose average outcome falls somewhere in between those of the two extreme groups (Kendell and Brockington, 1980).

Similarly, whereas most researchers have argued that Kraepelin's taxonomy was validated by the fact that diagnoses ran 'true' in families (schizophrenic patients tended to have relatives who suffered from schizophrenia but not bipolar disorder, whereas the converse was true for bipolar patients), recent epidemiological evidence has shown that the family histories of psychotic patients fail to segregate in the way that the Kraepelinian paradigm would imply (the relatives

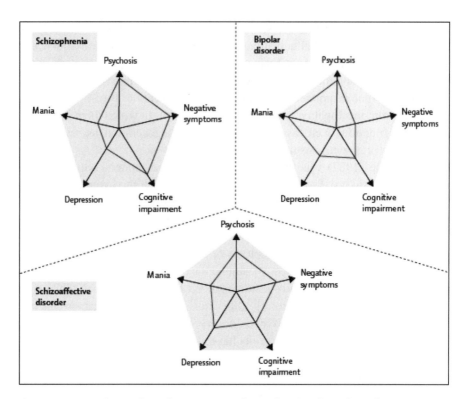

Figure 15.1   Dimensional structure of psychosis, showing the symptoms experienced by schizophrenic, schizoaffective and bipolar patients (reproduced from van Os and Kapur, 2009)

of psychotic patients, whatever their diagnoses, are at increased risk of experiencing symptoms across the psychotic domain) (Crow, 1991; Lichtenstein et al., 2009).

Finally, it seems that Kraepelinian diagnoses fail to predict which treatments patients will respond to (their whole point, from a clinical perspective). Following the discovery of chlorpromazine it became widely believed that antipsychotic drugs are anti-schizophrenic, whereas other drugs, for example lithium carbonate (a naturally occurring salt which was found to quell agitation) are anti-manic or mood-stabilizing drugs. It was Crow who first carried out the obvious experiment of randomly assigning psychotic patients to antipsychotics and/or lithium carbonate, finding that diagnosis was a poor predictor of drug response whereas specific symptoms were (patients with hallucinations and delusions tend to respond to antipsychotics, whatever their diagnosis, whereas patients with mood disturbance tend to respond to lithium carbonate, again irrespective of diagnosis) (Johnstone et al., 1988). Even two decades later, some researchers still express surprise that antipsychotics are effective in the treatment of patients with diagnoses other than schizophrenia (Tamminga and Davis, 2007).

Hence, at the end of the first decade of the twenty-first century, we can say with some certainty, that Kraepelin's classification of the psychotic disorders enjoys almost no empirical support and, indeed, is refuted by much of the evidence that has become available in the past few decades. However, although there is widespread (albeit often reluctant) acceptance of this conclusion, there is less agreement about what should replace the Kraepelinian system. Many psychiatrists hope that a better diagnostic system will eventually emerge. However, a more radical approach would be to abandon psychiatric diagnoses altogether (Bentall, 2003).

It is sometimes assumed that such a comprehensive rejection of the Kraepelinian system entails a post-modern rejection of the project of developing a scientific account of mental illness. However, there is no reason why patients should not be grouped together for research in terms of their complaints (particular classes of behaviour and experience described by patients and their carers; what psychiatrists call *symptoms*) or why this approach might not be extended to provide a coherent account of mental illness (Bentall, 2003).

HALLUCINATIONS

To illustrate the complaints-based approach it will be helpful to consider some specific examples. *Hallucinations* are a very common psychotic complaint, and are most often experienced in the auditory modality, although visual, tactile and olfactory hallucinations are also common (Slade and Bentall, 1988). The rules embodied in modern diagnostic systems ensure that most patients with hallucinatory experiences are diagnosed as suffering from schizophrenia, but they are also reported by a minority of patients with other diagnoses, for example bipolar disorder (Goodwin and Jamison, 1990). Moreover, epidemiological studies have revealed that a surprising proportion of the population experience them at some point in their lives. For example, Tien (1991) estimated that, of 18,000 participants in a US population study, between 11 and 13 per cent had experienced hallucinations at some time in their lives. In a similar Dutch study, it was found that 1.7 per cent of the 7,000 participants interviewed had experienced clinically relevant hallucinations, but that a further 6.2 per cent had experienced hallucinations that were judged clinically irrelevant because they were not associated with distress (van Os et al., 2000).

Auditory hallucinations vary in linguistic complexity (from simple words to whole conversations) and location (some located outside the body, some being sensed as occurring within the head) (Stephane, 2003). Patients may experience one or more voices, which may comment on the patient's actions, talk directly to the patient or issue commands (Leudar and Thomas, 2000). Clinicians often gain the impression that voices are negative in content, for example because they deride the patient or issue distressing commands. However, even patients seeking treatment may experience voices as friendly and supportive, to the point that some patients would rather that they not be removed (Miller et al., 1993). Unsurprisingly, the voices of those who do not seek treatment tend to be more positive than those of people who become psychiatric patients.

In patients who hallucinate the self is often experienced as weaker than the voices whereas, in non-patients, the opposite is often the case (Honig et al., 1998). Indeed, psychiatric patients' beliefs that their voices are omniscient and omnipotent has been identified as an important cause of distress, and therefore a potential target for psychotherapeutic intervention (Chadwick and Birchwood, 1994). Interestingly, hallucinating patients often have dysfunctional metacognitive beliefs (that it is catastrophic if thoughts cannot be controlled) that are quite similar to those reported by patients with obsessional thoughts (Morrison and Wells, 2003).

The normal phenomenon of 'inner speech' provides a clue to the psychological mechanisms involved in auditory hallucinations. The ability to regulate one's behaviour by means of self-directed speech develops in early childhood, when children first talk out aloud to themselves before learning to internalize this process, culminating in adulthood in the capacity for mature, verbal thought (Vygotsky, 1962). Even in adulthood, this kind of thought is accompanied by 'subvocalization' – covert activations of the speech muscles that can by detected by electromyography. It has been known for many years that auditory hallucinations are also accompanied by subvocalization (e.g. Gould, 1948) and more recent neuroimaging studies have shown that they are also accompanied by activations of the speech areas of the brain (McGuire et al., 1993). These findings have inevitably suggested to many researchers that auditory hallucinations occur when inner speech is misattributed to an external source (Bentall, 1990; Hoffman, 1986).

This account implies that people with hallucinations should be impaired in their ability to distinguish between self-generated thoughts and externally presented stimuli. This has been demonstrated experimentally. For example, using signal detection paradigms, some investigators have shown that people who hallucinate, or whose questionnaire responses suggest that they are vulnerable to hallucinations, have an abnormal response bias, leading to 'false positive' responses, when asked to detect an externally presented voice against a noisy background (Barkus et al., 2007; Bentall and Slade, 1985).

More complex experiments, in which people with and without hallucinations have been compared in their ability to discriminate between things they have thought and things they have heard have also yielded evidence in support of the defective source monitoring hypothesis (Ditman and Kuperberg, 2005; Johns et al., 2001; Laroi, et al., 2005). Some investigators have studied the physiological processes underlying source monitoring. For example, in a series of electrophysiological investigations, Ford and Mathalon (2004) found that, when ordinary people think in words, the auditory perception areas in the temporal lobes of the brain become less sensitive to sounds because they are suppressed by a corollary discharge from the speech generating areas in the left frontal cortex.

This mechanism apparently reduces the risk that self-generated speech will be mistaken for an external voice. Ford and Mathalon found that this mechanism was absent in hallucinating patients.

Although the defective source monitoring hypothesis provides a convincing framework for understanding hallucinations, many questions remain unanswered. For example, there is evidence that, in patients with hallucinations, source monitoring is more impaired for emotionally salient than emotionally non-salient material (Johns et al., 2001; Morrison and Haddock, 1997) and patients' hallucinations tend to worsen during periods of negative mood (Norman and Malla, 1991) but the role of emotional disturbance in hallucinations is poorly understood.

PARANOID DELUSIONS

Paranoid beliefs are probably even more commonly experienced by psychotic patients than hallucinations; it has been estimated that some 90 per cent of patients with a diagnosis of schizophrenia experience persecutory delusions (Moutoussis et al., 2007). However, like hallucinations, these beliefs are also found in a substantial minority of ordinary people (van Os et al., 2000) and it has been claimed, therefore, that they exist on a continuum with less pathological forms of suspiciousness (Freeman et al., 2005). However, Trower and Chadwick (1995) argued that it is important to distinguish between: 'bad-me' paranoia in which the individual feels persecuted for good reason (because of some terrible crime they have committed) and the more typical 'poor-me' paranoia in which the individual feels unjustly persecuted. Although patients tend to fluctuate between poor-me and bad-me, they most often express poor-me beliefs (Melo et al., 2006) whereas paranoid but non-psychotic people are usually bad-me (Melo et al., 2009).

The core of paranoia is the over-anticipation of threats from other people (Bentall et al., 2009). Two main kinds of theories have been proposed to explain this tendency. Some theories have implicated impaired reasoning processes. For example, Garety et al. (1991) found that deluded patients tend to 'jump to conclusions' (JTC) on probabilistic reasoning tasks in which they are given the choice of making a guess or seeking more information to test their hypotheses, and this finding has been widely replicated (Dudley and Over, 2003). The JTC bias appears to be more marked when patients reason about personally salient material (Dudley et al., 1997).

However, in a version of Garety's task in which participants were first presented with evidence favouring one hypothesis before being presented with evidence favouring another, Garety et al. (1991) reported that deluded patients changed their minds more readily than healthy controls, a finding that seems paradoxical, given the apparent incorrigibility of delusional beliefs. Recent studies have shown that the JTC bias is probably closely related to more general measures of intellectual ability (Bentall et al., 2009). One possibility that it reflects a general impairment of executive functioning that affects the ability to evaluate the plausibility of hypotheses.

A second class of theories implicates motivational factors. Researchers inspired by psychoanalysis have suggested that paranoid beliefs arise from dysfunctional attempts to maintain self-esteem (Colby, 1977) or that paranoia is a form of camouflaged depression (Zigler and Glick, 1988). Following the observation that paranoid patients tend to assume that negative events in their lives are caused by external (not caused by self), stable (unchangeable) and global (likely to affect all aspects of life) causes, Bentall et al. (1994) argued that beliefs about persecution arise from patients' attempts to avoid explanations for their experiences that are self-blaming.

One objection to this kind of account is that paranoid patients often have low self-esteem (Freeman et al., 1998). However, both population studies (Thewissen et al., 2007) and studies of patients (Thewissen et al., 2008) have shown that paranoia is associated with self-esteem that is highly unstable over time. Moreover, self-esteem is higher in those patients with poor-me beliefs than in those with bad-me beliefs (Chadwick, et al., 2005).

In all probability, both motivational factors and reasoning biases are important in paranoia. Coltheart (2007) has suggested that a comprehensive explanation of any kind of delusional system would have to explain first, where delusional ideas come from, and second, why delusional individuals are unable to reason their way out of their beliefs. Motivational factors seem to be relevant to the first of these issues, whereas reasoning problems seem to address the second.

SOCIAL ADVERSITY AND PSYCHOSIS

One conclusion that can be drawn from the research on complaints is that both cognitive and affective processes are important in psychosis. Previous research within the Kraepelinian paradigm has tended to over-estimate the importance the former and neglect the latter. Consistent with this new emphasis on affect, epidemiological research has begun to reveal strong associations between psychosis and different kinds of social adversity.

Much of this research was stimulated by the discovery that Afro-Caribbean immigrants to the UK have an unexpectedly high rate of psychosis (Harrison et al., 1988). Subsequent studies has shown that the same is true of immigrant populations elsewhere (Selten et al., 2001) and that migrants are especially at risk if they went to live in predominantly indigenous neighbourhoods (Boydell et al., 2001; Veling et al., 2008). Other studies demonstrating an association between psychosis and victimization (Janssen et al., 2003) and bullying (Schreier et al., 2009) have suggested that experiences of social defeat play an important causal role in psychosis. Interestingly, there is evidence from animal studies that social defeat results in sensitization of the dopamine system (Selten and

Cantor-Graae, 2005), which is consistent with neuropharmacological evidence that the dopamine system plays an important role in the anticipation of threat (Moutoussis et al., 2008).

Despite widespread scepticism about an earlier generation of theories which implicated family dynamics in psychosis (e.g. Laing and Esterson, 1969) recent studies have implicated disruption of attachment relationships (Myhrman et al., 1996), and early separation from parents (Morgan et al., 2007) in conferring risk of illness. There is also consistent evidence that individuals who have experienced abuse in childhood have an elevated risk of psychosis (Bebbington et al., 2004; Neria et al., 2002; Shevlin et al., 2007). Interestingly, some of these effects may be complaint-specific, as hallucinations appear to be associated with early trauma (perhaps because this kind of experience somehow disrupts source monitoring) and paranoid beliefs appear to be associated with attachment difficulties and more chronic forms of victimization (Bentall and Fernyhough, 2008).

NEUROSCIENCE AND GENETICS IN THE POST-KRAEPELINIAN WORLD

Although the complaints-orientated approach to psychosis has become more mainstream over the last decade or so, the idea that a completely adequate account of psychosis can be developed this way remains controversial. Some psychological researchers, while carrying out research on particular complaints, still feel that it is fruitful to propose models of psychosis as more broadly conceived (for an influential attempt to do this, see Garety et al., 2001). An important issue that is only just beginning to be addressed is the relationship between psychological models and neuroscientific and genetic research into psychosis.

As I have already indicated, there is no contradiction between studying biological variables and a focus on complaints. Indeed, we have seen that some neuroscientists have begun to study the functional neuroanatomy underlying the various cognitive and affective processes that have been implicated. Just as crucially, it is important to recognize that there is no contradiction between the observation of neurobiological abnormalities in patients and the idea that social factors may play a causal role (Read et al., 2001). We have already seen that oversensitivity of the dopamine system, long implicated in psychosis, may be a consequence of experiences of social defeat (Selten and Cantor-Graae, 2005) and the observation of profound neuroanatomical and neurobiochemical changes in the brains of victims of sexual abuse (Teicher et al., 2006) raises the possibility that the abnormal structural characteristics observed in psychotic patients' brains on CT and MRI scans may be, at least partially, explained in the same way.

These observations obviously do not preclude the involvement of genetic factors and most researchers continue to believe that some kind of hereditary vulnerability is required for the development of psychosis. Perhaps the best evidence for this remains the increased concordance for psychosis in monozygotic compared to dizygotic twins (Torrey et al., 1994) although recent research has given much lower estimates for these rates (22.4 per cent vs. to 4.5 per cent) than earlier studies (Joseph, 2003). The high heritability rates often calculated from these kinds of data (estimates of 80 per cent are not uncommon) have often been misunderstood as indicating that psychosis is nearly entirely caused by genes but, for a variety of technical reasons, heritability calculations tend to underestimate the significance of environmental influences or of gene x environment interactions (Bentall, 2009; Clarke, this). Moreover, attempts to identify specific genes associated with psychosis have been disappointing (Crow, 2008; Sanders et al., 2008). Recent research suggests that there are no genes of major effect for psychosis, that perhaps a thousand genes each play a minor role (The International Schizophrenia Consortium, 2009), and that many of these effects are common to patients with a range of diagnoses (Craddock et al., 2005).

Some researchers have attempted to clarify the relationship between genetic vulnerability and psychosis by investigating *endophenotypes* – variables associated with psychosis which might be more amenable to genetic analysis (Cannon and Keller, 2006) – and the mechanisms identified by psychological researchers are obvious candidates for this approach. Further progress in understanding the origins of severe mental illness will require a much more sophisticated understanding of the interplay between genetic, environmental and psychological processes than has been typical of research in the past.

REFERENCES

American Psychiatric Association (1980) *Diagnostic and Statistical Manual of Mental Disorders,* 3rd Edition. Washington, DC: Author.

Bannister, D. (1968) The logical requirements of research into schizophrenia. *British Journal of Psychiatry,* 114: 181–188.

Barkus, E., Stirling, J., Hopkins, R., McKie, S. and Lewis, S. (2007) Cognitive and neural processes in non-clinical auditory hallucinations. *British Journal of Psychiatry,* 191(suppl. 51): 76–81.

Bebbington, P., Bhugra, D., Bhugra, T., Singleton, N., Farrell, M., Jenkins, R., et al. (2004). Psychosis, victimisation and childhood disadvantage: Evidence from the second British National Survey of Psychiatric Morbidity. *British Journal of Psychiatry,* 185: 220–226.

Bentall, R.P. (1990) The illusion of reality: A review and integration of psychological research on hallucinations. *Psychological Bulletin,* 107: 82–95.

Bentall, R.P. (2003) *Madness Explained: Psychosis and Human Nature.* London: Penguin.

Bentall, R.P. (2009) *Doctoring the Mind: Why Psychiatric Treatments Fail.* London: Penguin.

Bentall, R.P., Claridge, G.S. and Slade, P.D. (1989) The multidimensional nature of schizotypal traits: A factor-analytic study with normal subjects. *British Journal of Clinical Psychology,* 28: 363–375.

Bentall, R.P. and Fernyhough, C. (2008) Social predictors of psychotic experiences: Specificity and psychological mechanisms. *Schizophrenia Bulletin,* 34: 1009–1011.

Bentall, R.P., Kinderman, P. and Kaney, S. (1994) The self, attributional processes and abnormal beliefs: Towards a model of persecutory delusions. *Behaviour Research and Therapy,* 32: 331–341.

Bentall, R.P., Rowse, G., Shryane, N., Kinderman, P., Howard, R., Blackwood, N., et al. (2009) The cognitive and affective structure of paranoid delusions: A transdiagnostic investigation of patients with schizophrenia spectrum disorders and depression. *Archives of General Psychiatry,* 66: 236–247.

Bentall, R.P. and Slade, P.D. (1985) Reality testing and auditory hallucinations: A signal-detection analysis. *British Journal of Clinical Psychology,* 24: 159–169.

Bleuler, E. (1911/1950) *Dementia Praecox or the Group of Schizophrenias* (E. Zinkin, Trans.). New York: International Universities Press.

Blomqvist, A.G., Leger, P.T. and Hoch, J.S. (2006) The cost of schizophrenia: Lessons from an international comparison. *Journal of Mental Health Policy and Economics,* 9: 177–183.

Boydell, J., van Os, J., McKenzie, J., Allardyce, J., Goel, R., McCreadie, R. G., et al. (2001) Incidence of schizophrenia in ethnic minorities in London: Ecological study into interactions with environment. *British Medical Journal,* 323: 1–4.

Boyle, M. (1990) *Schizophrenia: A Scientific Delusion.* London: Routledge.

Brown, G.W., Carstairs, M. and Topping, G. (1958) Post hospital adjustment of chronic mental patients. *Lancet,* ii: 685–689.

Butzlaff, R.L. and Hooley, J.M. (1998). Expressed emotion and psychiatric relapse. *Archives of General Psychiatry,* 55: 547–552.

Cannon, T.D. and Keller, M.C. (2006) Endophenotypes in the genetic analyses of mental disorders. *Annual Review of Clinical Psychology,* 2: 267–290.

Chadwick, P. and Birchwood, M. (1994) The omnipotence of voices: A cognitive approach to auditory hallucinations. *British Journal of Psychiatry,* 164: 190–201.

Chadwick, P., Trower, P., Juusti-Butler, T.-M. and Maguire, N. (2005) Phenomenological evidence for two types of paranoia. *Psychopathology,* 38: 327–333.

Chapman, L.J. and Chapman, J.P. (1980) Scales for rating psychotic and psychotic-like experiences as continua. *Schizophrenia Bulletin,* 6: 477–489.

Chapman, L.J., Chapman, J.P., Kwapil, T.R., Eckblad, M. and Zinser, M.C. (1994) Putatively psychosis-prone subjects 10 years later. *Journal of Abnormal Psychology,* 103: 171–183.

Chapman, L.J., Chapman, J.P. and Raulin, M.L. (1976) Scales for physical and social anhedonia. *Journal of Abnormal Psychology,* 85: 374–382.

Chapman, L.J., Edell, E.W. and Chapman, J.P. (1980) Physical anhedonia, perceptual aberration and psychosis proneness. *Schizophrenia Bulletin,* 6: 639–653.

Ciompi, L. (1984) Is there really a schizophrenia?: The longterm course of psychotic phenomena. *British Journal of Psychiatry,* 145: 636–640.

Claridge, G., McCreery, C., Mason, O., Bentall, R.P., Boyle, G. and Slade, P.D. (1996) The factor structure of 'schizotypal' traits: A large replication study. *British Journal of Clinical Psychology,* 35: 103–115.

Claridge, G.S. (1985) *The Origins of Mental Illness.* Oxford: Blackwell.

Claridge, G.S. (1987) The schizophrenias as nervous types revisited. *British Journal of Psychiatry,* 151: 735–743.

Claridge, G.S. (1990) Can a disease model of schizophrenia survive? In R.P. Bentall (ed.) *Reconstructing schizophrenia.* London: Routledge. pp 157–183.

Claridge, G.S. (1998) Creativity and madness: Clues from modern psychiatric diagnosis. In A. Steptoe (ed.) *Genius and the Mind.* Oxford: Oxford University Press.

Colby, K.M. (1977) Appraisal of four psychological theories of paranoid phenomena. *Journal of Abnormal Psychology,* 86: 54–59.

Coltheart, M. (2007) The 33rd Sir Frederick Bartlett Lecture: Cognitive neuropsychiatry and delusional beliefs. *The Quarterly Journal of Experimental Psychology,* 60: 1041–1062.

Cooper, D. (1967) *Psychiatry and antipsychiatry.* London: Tavistock Press.

Craddock, N., O'Donovan, M.C. and Owen, M.J. (2005) The genetics of schizophrenia and bipolar disorder: Dissecting psychosis. *Journal of Medical Genetics,* 42: 193–204.

Crow, T.J. (1980) Molecular pathology of schizophrenia: More than one disease process? *British Medical Journal,* 280: 66–68.

Crow, T.J. (1991) The failure of the binary concept and the psychosis gene. In A. Kerr and H. McClelland (eds) *Concepts of Mental Disorder: A Continuing Debate.* London: Gaskell. pp 31–47.

Crow, T.J. (2008) The emperors of the schizophrenia polygene have no clothes. *Psychological Medicine,* 38: 1679–1680.

Dickerson, F.B., Boronow, J.J., Stallings, C., Origoni, A.E., Cole, S.K. and Yolken, R.H. (2004) Cognitive functioning in schizophrenia and bipolar disorder: comparison of performance on the Repeatable Battery for the Assessment of Neuropsychological Status. *Psychiatry Research,* 129: 45–53.

Dickinson, D. and Harvey, P.D. (2009) Systemic hypotheses for generalized cognitive deficits in schizophrenia: A new take on an old problem. *Schizophrenia Bulletin,* 35: 403–414.

Ditman, T. and Kuperberg, G.R. (2005) A source-monitoring account of auditory verbal hallucinations in patients with schizophrenia. *Harvard Review of Psychiatry,* 13: 280–299.

Dudley, R.E.J. and Over, D.E. (2003) People with delusions jump to conclusions: A theoretical account of research findings on the reasoning of people with delusions. *Clinical Psychology and Psychotherapy,* 10: 263–274.

Dudley, R.E.J., John, C.H., Young, A.W. and Over, D.E. (1997) The effect of self-referent material on the reasoning of people with delusions. *British Journal of Clinical Psychology,* 36: 575–584.

Engstrom, E.J. and Weber, M.M. (2007) Making Kraepelin history: A great instauration? *History of Psychiatry,* 18: 267–273.

Ford, J.M. and Mathalon, D.H. (2004) Electrophysiological evidence of corollary discharge dysfunction in schizophrenia during talking and thinking. *Journal of Psychiatric Research,* 38: 37–46.

Freeman, D., Garety, P., Fowler, D., Kuipers, E., Dunn, G., Bebbington, P., et al. (1998) The London–East Anglia randomized controlled trial of cognitive-behaviour therapy for psychosis IV: Self-esteem and persecutory delusions. *British Journal of Clinical Psychology,* 37: 415–430.

Freeman, D., Garety, P.A., Bebbington, P.E., Smith, B., Rollinson, R., Fowler, D., et al. (2005) Psychological investigation of the structure of paranoia in a non-clinical population. *British Journal of Psychiatry,* 186: 427–435.

Garety, P.A., Hemsley, D.R. and Wessely, S. (1991) Reasoning in deluded schizophrenic and paranoid patients. *Journal of Nervous and Mental Disease,* 179(4): 194–201.

Garety, P.A., Kuipers, E., Fowler, D., Freeman, D. and Bebbington, P.E. (2001) A cognitive model of positive symptoms of psychosis. *Psychological Medicine,* 31: 189–195.

Goodwin, F.K., and Jamison, K.R. (1990) *Manic-depressive Illness.* Oxford: Oxford University Press.

Gottesman, I.I. and Shields, J. (1982) *Schizophrenia: The Epigenetic Puzzle.* Cambridge: Cambridge University Press.

Gould, L.N. (1948) Verbal hallucinations and activity of vocal musculature. *American Journal of Psychiatry,* 105: 367–372.

Green, M.F. (1998) *Schizophrenia from a Neurocognitive Perspective: Probing the Impenetrable Darkness.* Boston: Allyn and Bacon.

Green, M.F. (2006) Cognitive impairment and functional outcome in schizophrenia and bipolar disorder. *Journal of Clinical Psychiatry,* 67(supp 9): 3–8.

Green, M.F. and Nuechterlein, K.H. (1999) Should schizophrenia be treated as a neurocognitive disorder? *Schizophrenia Bulletin,* 25: 309–319.

Gupta, R.D. and Guest, J.F. (2002) Annual cost of bipolar disorder to UK society. *British Journal of Psychiatry,* 180: 227–233.

Harrison, G., Owens, D., Holton, A., Neilson, D. and Boot, D. (1988) A prospective study of severe mental disorder in Afro-Caribbean patients. *Psychological Medicine,* 18: 643–657.

Healy, D. (2004) *The Creation of Psychopharmacology.* Boston, Mass: Harvard University Press.

Hoffman, R.E. (1986) Verbal hallucinations and language production processes in schizophrenia. *Behavioral and Brain Sciences,* 9: 503–548.

Honig, A., Romme, M.A.J., Ensink, B.J., Escher, S.D.M.A.C., Pennings, M.H.A. and DeVries, M.W. (1998) Auditory hallucinations: A comparison between patients and nonpatients. *Journal of Nervous and Mental Disease,* 186: 646–651.

Jablensky, A. (1995) Schizophrenia: The epidemiological horizon. In S. R. Hirsch and D.R. Weinberger (eds), *Schizophrenia.* Oxford: Blackwell. pp. 206–252.

Jablensky, A. (2007) Living in a Kraepelinian world: Kraepelin's impact on modern psychiatry. *History of Psychiatry,* 18: 381–388.

Janssen, I., Hanssen, M., Bak, M., Bijl, R.V., De Graaf, R., Vollenberg, W., et al. (2003) Discrimination and delusional ideation. *British Journal of Psychiatry,* 182: 71–76.

Johns, L.C., Rossell, S., Frith, C., Ahmad, F., Hemsley, D., Kuipers, E., et al. (2001) Verbal self-monitoring and auditory hallucinations in people with schizophrenia. *Psychological Medicine,* 31: 705–715.

Johnstone, E.C., Crow, T.J., Frith, C.D., Husband, J. and Kreel, L. (1976) Cerebral ventricular size and cognitive impairment in chronic schizophrenia. *Lancet,* ii: 924–926.

Johnstone, E.C., Crow, T.J., Frith, C.D. and Owens, D.G.C. (1988) The Northwick Park 'functional' psychosis study: Diagnosis and treatment response. *Lancet,* ii: 119–125.

Jones, P.B., Rodgers, B., Murray, R.M. and Marmot, M.G. (1994) Child developmental risk factors for adult schizophrenia in the British 1946 birth cohort. *Lancet,* 344: 1398–1402.

Joseph, J. (2003) *The Gene Illusion: Genetic Research in Psychology and Psychiatry under the Microscope.* Ross-on-Wye: PCCS Books.

Kasanin, J. (1933) The acute schizoaffective psychoses. *American Journal of Psychiatry,* 90: 97–126.

Keefe, R.S.E., Bilder, R.M., Davis, S.M., Harvey, P.D., Palmer, B.W., Gold, J.M., et al. (2007) Neuro-cognitive effects of antipsychotic medication in patients with chronic schizophrenia in the CATIE trail. *Archives of General Psychiatry,* 64: 633–647.

Kendell, R.E. and Brockington, I.F. (1980) The identification of disease entities and the relationship between schizophrenic and affective psychoses. *British Journal of Psychiatry,* 137: 324–331.

Kety, S., Rosenthal, D., Wender, P.H., Schulsinger, F. and Jacobsen, B. (1975) Mental illness in the biological and adoptive families of adopted individuals who have become schizophrenic: A preliminary report based on psychiatric interviews. In R. Fieve, D. Rosenthal, and H. Brill (eds) *Genetic Research in Psychiatry.* Baltimore: Johns Hopkins University Press.

Klerman, G.L. (1978) The evolution of a scientific nosology. In J.C. Shershow (ed.) *Schizophrenia: Science and Practice.* Cambridge, Mass.: Harvard University Press. pp. 99–121.

Kraepelin, E. (1887/2005) The directions of psychiatric research. *History of Psychiatry,* 16: 350–364.

Laing, R.D. (1960) *The Divided Self.* London: Tavistock Press.

Laing, R.D. (1967) *The Politics of Experience and the Bird of Paradise.* London: Penguin Press.

Laing, R.D. and Esterson, A. (1969) *Sanity, Madness and the Family: Families of Schizophrenics,* 2nd edition. London: Tavistock.

Laroi, F., Collignon, O. and van der Linden, M. (2005) Source-monitoring for actions in hallucinations proneness. *Cognitive Neuropsychiatry,* 10: 105–123.

Leonhard, K. (1957/1979) *The Classification of Endogenous Psychoses* (R. Berman, Trans.). New York: Irvington.

Leudar, I. and Thomas, P. (2000) *Voices of Reason, Voices of Insanity: Studies of Verbal Hallucinations.* London: Routledge.

Lichtenstein, P., Yip, B.H., Bjork, C., Pawitan, Y., Cannon, T.D., Sullivan, P.F., et al. (2009) Common genetic determinants of schizophrenia and bipolar disorder in Swedish families: a population-based study. *Lancet,* 373: 234–239.

Liddle, P.F. (1987) The symptoms of chronic schizophrenia: A reexamination of the positive-negative dichotomy. *British Journal of Psychiatry,* 151: 145–151.

Lloyd, T., Kennedy, N., Fearon, P., Kirkbride, J., Mallett, R., Leff, J., et al. (2005) Incidence of bipolar affective disorder in three UK cities: Results from the AeSOP study. *British Journal of Psychiatry,* 186: 126–131.

Marangell, L.B., Bauer, M.S., Dennehy, E.B., Wisniewski, S.R., Allen, M.H., Miklowitz, D.J., et al. (2006) Prospective predictors of suicide and suicide attempts in 1,556 patients with bipolar disorders followed for up to 2 years. *Bipolar Disorders,* 8: 566–575.

Marshall, R. (1990) The genetics of schizophrenia: Axiom or hypothesis? In R.P. Bentall (ed.) *Reconstructing schizophrenia.* London: Routledge. pp. 89–117.

Marx, O. (1993) Conversation Piece: Adolf Meyer and psychiatric training at the Phipps Clinic – an interview with Theodore Lidz. *History of Psychiatry,* 4: 245–269.

McGrath, J.J. (2005) Myths and plain truths about schizophrenia epidemiology. *Acta Psychiatrica Scandinavica,* 111: 4–11.

McGuire, P.K., Shah, G.M.S. and Murray, R.M. (1993) Increased blood flow in Broca's area during auditory hallucinations. *Lancet,* 342: 703–706.

Meehl, P. (1962) Schizotaxia, schizotypia, schizophrenia. *American Psychologist,* 17: 827–838.

Melo, S., Corcoran, R. and Bentall, R.P. (2009) The Persecution and Deservedness Scale. *Psychology and Psychotherapy: Theory, Practice, research,* 82: 247–260.

Melo, S., Taylor, J. and Bentall, R.P. (2006) 'Poor me' versus 'bad me' paranoia and the instability of persecutory ideation. *Psychology and Psychotherapy – Theory, Research, Practice,* 79: 271–287.

Miller, L.J., O'Connor, E. and DePasquale, T. (1993) Patients' attitudes to hallucinations. *American Journal of Psychiatry,* 150: 584–588.

Morgan, C., Kirkbride, J., Leff, J., Craig, T., Hutchinson, G., McKenzie, K., et al. (2007) Parental separation, loss and psychosis in different ethnic groups: A case-control study. *Psychological Medicine,* 37: 495–503.

Morrison, A. P. and Haddock, G. (1997) Cognitive factors in source monitoring and auditory hallucinations. *Psychological Medicine,* 27: 669–679.

Morrison, A.P. and Wells, A. (2003) Metacognition across disorders: A comparison of patients with hallucinations, delusions, and panic disorder with non-patients. *Behaviour Research and Therapy,* 41: 251–256.

Mosher, L.R. (1999) Soteria and other alternatives to acute psychiatric hospitalization. *Journal of Nervous and Mental Disease,* 187: 142–149.

Mosher, L.R. and Menn, A.Z. (1978) Community residential treatment for schizophrenia: Two-year follow-up. *Hospital and Community Psychiatry,* 29: 715–723.

Moutoussis, M., Bentall, R.P., Williams, J. and Dayan, P. (2008) A temporal difference account of avoidance learning. *Network: Computation in Neural Systems,* 19: 137–160.

Moutoussis, M., Williams, J., Dayan, P. and Bentall, R.P. (2007) Persecutory delusions and the conditioned avoidance paradigm: Towards an integration of the psychology and biology of paranoia. *Cognitive Neuropsychiatry,* 12: 495–510.

Myhrman, A., Rantakallio, P., Isohanni, M. and Jones, P. (1996) Unwantedness of preganancy and schizophrenia in the child. *British Journal of Psychiatry,* 169: 637–640.

Nasar, S. (1998) *A Beautiful Mind.* London: Faber and Faber.

Neria, Y., Bromet, E.J., Sievers, S., Lavelle, J. and Fochtmann, L.J. (2002) Trauma exposure and posttraumatic stress disorder in psychosis: Findings from a first-admission cohort. *Journal of Consulting and Clinical Psychology,* 70: 246–251.

Norman, R.M.G. and Malla, A.K. (1991) Dysphoric mood and symptomatology in schizophrenia. *Psychological Medicine,* 21: 897–903.

Nuechterlein, K.H., Buchsbaum, M.S. and Dawson, M.E. (1994) Neuropsychological vulnerability to schizophrenia. In A.S. David and J. C. Cutting (eds) *The Neuropsychology of Schizophrenia.* Hove: Erlbaum.

Nuechterlein, K.H. and Dawson, M.E. (1984) A heuristic vulnerability-stress model of schizophrenic episodes. *Schizophrenia Bulletin,* 10: 300–312.

Nuechterlein, K.H. and Subotnik, K.L. (1998) The cognitive origins of schizophrenia and prospects for intervention. In T. Wykes, N. Tarrier and S. Lewis (eds) *Outcome and Innovation in Psychological Treatment of Schizophrenia* (Vol. 17–42). Chichester: Wiley.

Palmer, B.A., Pankratz, V.S. and Bostwick, J.M. (2005) The lifetime risk of suicide in schizophrenia: A reexamination. *Archives of General Psychiatry,* 62: 247–253.

Perala, J., Suvisaari, J., Saarni, S.I., Kuoppasalmi, K., Isometsa, E., Pirkola, S., et al. (2007) Lifetime prevalence of psychotic and bipolar I disorders in a general population. *Archives of General Psychiatry,* 64: 19–28.

Raine, A. (2006) Schizotypal personality: Neurodevelopmental and psychological trajectories. *Annual Review of Clinical Psychology,* 2: 291–326.

Read, J., Perry, B.D., Moskowitz, A. and Connolly, J. (2001) A traumagenic neurodevelopmental model of schizophrenia. *Psychiatry: Interpersonal and Biological Processes,* 64: 319–345.

Rose, S., Kamin, L.J. and Lewontin, R.C. (1985) *Not in Our Genes.* Harmondsworth: Penguin.

Rosenthal, D., Wender, P.H., Kety, S., Welner, J. and Schulsinger, F. (1971) The adopted-away offspring of schizophrenics. *American Journal of Psychiatry,* 128: 307–311.

Sanders, A.R., Duan, J., Levinson, D.F., Shi, J., He, D., Hou, C., et al. (2008) No significant association of 14 candidate genes with schizophrenia in a large European ancestry sample: Implications for psychiatric genetics. *American Journal of Psychiatry,* 165: 497–506.

Schneider, K. (1959) *Clinical psychopathology.* New York.: Grune & Stratton.

Schreier, A., Wolke, D., Thomas, K., Horwood, J., Hollis, C., Gunnell, D., et al. (2009) Prospective study of peer victimization in childhood and psychotic symptoms in a nonclinical population at age 12 years. *Archives of General Psychiatry,* 66: 527–536.

Seeman, P., Lee, T., Chau-Wong, M. and Wong, K. (1976) Antipsychotic drug dose and neuroleptic/dopamine receptors. *Nature,* 261: 717–719.

Selten, J.-P. and Cantor-Graae, E. (2005) Social defeat: Risk factor for psychosis? *British Journal of Psychiatry,* 187, 101–102.

Selten, J.-P., Veen, N., Feller, W., Blom, J.D., Schols, D., Camoenie, W., et al. (2001) Incidence of psychotic disorders in immigrant groups to The Netherlands. *British Journal of Psychiatry,* 178: 367–372.

Shevlin, M., Dorahy, M. and Adamson, G. (2007) Childhood traumas and hallucinations: An analysis of the National Comorbidity Survey. *Journal of Psychiatric Research,* 41: 222–228.

Shorter, E. (1997) *A History of Psychiatry.* New York: Wiley.

Slade, P.D. and Bentall, R.P. (1988) *Sensory Deception: A Scientific Analysis of Hallucination.* London: Croom-Helm.

Stephane, M. (2003) The internal structure and phenomenology of auditory verbal hallucinations. *Schizophrenia Research,* 61: 185–193.

Szasz, T.S. (1960) The myth of mental illness. *American Psychologist,* 15: 564–580.

Tamminga, C.A. and Davis, J.M. (2007) The neuropharmacology of psychosis. *Schizophrenia Bulletin,* 33: 937–946.

Teicher, M.H., Tomoda, A. and Andersen, S.L. (2006) Neurobiological consequences of early stress and childhood maltreatment: Are results from human and animal studies comparable? *Annals of the New York Academy of Sciences,* 1071: 313–323.

The International Schizophrenia Consortium (2009) Common polygenic variation contributes to risk of schizophrenia and bipolar disorder. *Nature,* 460(7256): 748–752.

Thewissen, V., Bentall, R.P., Lecomte, T., van Os, J. and Myin-Germeys, I. (2008) Fluctuations in self-esteem and paranoia in the context of everyday life. *Journal of Abnormal Psychology,* 117: 143–153.

Thewissen, V., Myin-Germeys, I., Bentall, R.P., de Graaf, R., Vollenberg, W. and van Os, J. (2007) Instability in self-esteem and paranoia in a general population sample. *Social Psychiatry and Psychiatric Epidemiology,* 42: 1–5.

Tien, A.Y. (1991) Distribution of hallucinations in the population. *Social Psychiatry and Psychiatric Epidemiology,* 26: 287–292.

Toomey, R., Faraone, S.V., Simpson, J.C. and Tsuang, M.T. (1998) Negative, positive and disorganized symptom dimensions in schizophrenia, major depression and bipolar disorder. *Journal of Nervous and Mental Disease,* 186: 470–476.

Torrey, E.F., Bowler, A.E., Taylor, E.H. and Gottesman, I.I. (1994) *Schizophrenia and manic-depressive disorder.* New York: Basic Books.

Trower, P. and Chadwick, P. (1995) Pathways to defense of the self: A theory of two types of paranoia. *Clinical Psychology: Science and practice,* 2: 263–278.

van Os, J., Hanssen, M., Bijl, R.V. and Ravelli, A. (2000) Strauss (1969) revisited: A psychosis continuum in the normal population? *Schizophrenia Research,* 45: 11–20.

van Os, J. and Kapur, S. (2009) Schizophrenia. *Lancet,* 374: 635–645.

Vaughn, C.E. and Leff, J. (1976) The influence of family and social factors on the course of psychiatric illness: A comparison of schizophrenic and depressed neurotic patients. *British Journal of Psychiatry,* 129: 125–137.

Veling, W., Susser, E., van Os, J., Mackenbach, J.P., Selten, J.P. and Hoek, H.W. (2008) Ethnic density of neighborhoods and incidence of psychotic disorders among immigrants. *American Journal of Psychiatry,* 165: 66–73.

Vygotsky, L.S.V. (1962) *Thought and language.* Cambidge, Mass: MIT Press.

Warner, R. (1985) *Recovery from Schizophrenia: Psychiatry and Political Economy.* New York: Routledge & Kegan Paul.

Wiersma, D., Wanderling, J., Dragomirecka, E., Ganev, K., Harrison, G., An Der Heiden, W., et al. (2000) Social disability in schizophrenia: its development and prediction over 15 years in incidence cohorts in six European centres. *Psychological Medicine,* 30: 1155–1167.

Zigler, E. and Glick, M. (1988) Is paranoid schizophrenia really camoflaged depression? *American Psychologist,* 43: 284–290.

Zubin, J. and Spring, B. (1977) Vulnerability: A new view of schizophrenia. *Journal of Abnormal Psychology,* 86: 103–126.

16

Sociological Aspects of Personality Disorder

Nick Manning

INTRODUCTION

Sociology is a discipline that focuses on human societies, and the subgroups and patterns within them, to understand human behaviour and cultural meanings. Such subgroups include families, workplaces, civic associations, governments and so on. The patterns that are of particular interest include four key clusters of behaviour and culture in relation to class, age, gender and race. Typical questions in relation to behaviour and culture might include: why and how do families reproduce or damage human beings? In what ways do people change over the life course? How and why are men and women different? How is employment distributed and where does professional power originate? What consequences do ethnic backgrounds have for health and healthcare? What are the motives and effects of government interventions?

In this chapter, we will consider how some of these sociological questions might help us to understand personality disorder. We can classify sociological approaches to personality disorder into two broad types. The first develops an analysis of personality disorder, its diagnosis and treatment and poses questions about it as an object of study. For example, what is it? How did it originate? The second takes personality disorder as a given psychiatric condition and offers supports and challenges that a sociological understanding can contribute to the diagnosis, treatment and care of personality disorder. For example, how is it distributed within the population? How effective are interventions to deal with it?

TOWARDS A SOCIOLOGY OF PERSONALITY DISORDER

The origins of personality disorder stretch back to the beginning of the nineteenth century. *Manie sans délire* was originally described in France by Pinel in 1801, but the term moral insanity was commonly used across the English speaking world until the early part of the twentieth century. European psychiatrists tend to use the term psychopathy to refer to all personality disorders, whereas in England this more often means one sub-type, the antisocial, or severe, personality disorder. The dominant classification today, however, has been imported from the US.

The process of classification is fundamental to any science. In psychiatry, it has been so difficult to arrive at an agreed approach that in the 1960s Menninger argued that diagnostic classification should be entirely abandoned (Farmer, 1997: 53). A major reason for this difficulty has been the absence of independent biological tests, or specific links between clinical features and aetiological factors. Since the nineteenth century much effort has gone into this problem. Although the US Diagnostic and Statistical Manuals of Mental Disorders (DSM) first appeared in 1952, the latest developments, starting in the 1970s, have been a wide ranging attempt to specify operational definitions for diagnoses, leading to the US series of DSMs (now up to DSM-IV) and the World Health Organization equivalent, Chapter 5 of the International Classification of Diseases, now in its tenth edition (ICD-10).

Since 1980 the DSM has assigned a special and separate axis to the personality disorders, axis II, to differentiate them from standard psychiatric syndromes covered in axis I, and there are now eleven sub-types of personality disorder. The most comprehensive definition of personality disorder is given in the DSM manual (see http://www.psychiatryonline.com/content.aspx?aID=3744). There are three clusters:

Cluster A (odd or eccentric)

- 301.0 Paranoid personality disorder
- 301.20 Schizoid personality disorder
- 301.22 Schizotypal personality disorder

Cluster B (dramatic, emotional or erratic)

- 301.7 Antisocial personality disorder
- 301.83 Borderline personality disorder
- 301.50 Histrionic personality disorder
- 301.81 Narcissistic personality disorder

Cluster C (anxious or fearful)

- 301.82 Avoidant personality disorder
- 301.6 Dependent personality disorder
- 301.4 Obsessive-compulsive personality disorder

Not otherwise specified (NOS)

- 301.9 Personality disorder NOS

Within the better known sub-types, such as borderline personality disorder, there are further sub-classifications, Higgit and Fonagy (1992), for example, identified seven different types of borderline psychopathology in the literature.

Not only has their classification proliferated, but personality disorders are also controversial since they do not include obvious psychological or organic malfunctioning, but are detected through their interpersonal effects – for example the trail of chaotic and distressing relationships in their wake, or the criminal records frequently acquired. This means that it is through behaviour rather than mental processes that personality disorder is detected and understood. A direct consequence has been difficulty and instability in their classification. This is currently under review and will be addressed in a new edition of the DSM due to be published in 2013. A draft of DSM-V appeared in February 2010 at www.dsm5.org. This suggests significant changes, including the removal of axis II, the collapse of the eleven sub-types into five and the development of a dimension of severity to each type.

A sociological approach to this diagnosis has been of two types. The most radical has been to suggest that perhaps the diagnosis is unstable because the underlying reality is itself not stable. This radical approach emerged in sociological studies of science. The process of psychiatric classification and diagnosis involves the construction of *representations* of aspects of the patient in terms of a presumed underlying reality, constructed as part of biological, medical or social science. The use of these representations in clinical situations involves the practical application of scientific knowledge to solve problems as understood by psychiatrists and others in the clinical setting. The way in which scientific representations and their technological application to clinical problems, are developed has been the subject of extensive sociological study. Where scientific knowledge and technological applications are uncertain, disputed or rapidly changing, as has been the case for personality disorder, sociological study has been able more easily to examine the way in which social factors have shaped the construction and application of knowledge. A brief review of these developments in the sociology of science and technology will help us to consider using them as explanations in the case of categorical innovation in psychiatry, particularly the rapid elaboration of the diagnosis of personality disorder.

Woolgar (1995: 159, Figure 4.1) summarizes sociological approaches to understanding science as having developed through four stages towards a state of ethnographic inversion whereby taken for granted assumptions in the 'black box' of science are exposed and examined as if they were an exotic and unfamiliar landscape. At stage one the real world was understood to be transformed into scientific representations directly, with no social influences at play, or at least with a minimum of psychological or cognitive processes, such as perception.

In stage two the observation of scientific competition, error or falsification led to a 'sociology of error' in which social influences were seen on occasion to divert or subvert true scientific representation. Following this notion, it was a relatively small step to stage three in which not only could erroneous representation be understood to have arisen out of social or cultural influences, but, equally, true representation and knowledge might also be similarly socially situated. All knowledge, both that claimed to be true and that claimed to be false, might vary with social and cultural context. It should be noted that this argument does not suggest that true knowledge, and the external reality to which it relates, is merely a cultural artefact. Such a radical stance is reserved for the fourth stage, in which the relationship between reality and observation is reversed, and the representation is taken by some sociologists of science to *constitute* reality itself. While these stages of analysis have evolved cumulatively, there is no agreement that the fourth stage is uncritically or widely accepted as correct.

From this point of view, personality disorder can be understood as a cultural category which may have little relationship to any stable underlying reality. A key focus is to bypass any judgement as to whether the underlying condition is real, or not, and to examine the circumstances under which it has appeared. Why has personality disorder, as a psychiatric category, grown rapidly in the last 40 years? In an analysis of 'transient mental illnesses' Ian Hacking (1998) suggests that a medical diagnosis, such as hysteria or chronic fatigue syndrome, emerges in a suitable 'ecological niche'. In a case study of the rapid emergence of cases of 'fugue' (compulsive travelling) in later nineteenth century France, centred particularly on Bordeaux, Hacking argues that there was a particularly conducive ecological niche composed of four key vectors: an existing medical taxonomy, cultural polarity, observability and 'release'. He means by cultural polarity an emergent popular cultural understanding in which there is both an idealized promise of new and satisfying way of life, and at the same time, a culturally demonized danger or problem. And he means by 'release' the idea that the diagnosis releases the patient from a culturally conflicted position between the two cultural poles. While he applied this very nicely to the emergence of fugue in France, it also fits the case of personality disorder remarkably well.

There is no doubt that the DSM, particularly with axis II set up in 1980, provides for the first of the four of Hacking's vectors. In particular the 'discovery' of borderline personality disorder, the most commonly diagnosed type, exhibits a distinctive pattern. Initially it was identified in 1938 by Stern, who noticed patients in his psychoanalytic office practice who disregarded the usual boundaries of therapy, and had a personality organization which differed from psychotic or neurotic types.

However this was not taken up widely until the 1960s in the USA, when a simultaneous but distinct pattern of discovery occurred. Simultaneous discovery in science, leading to the widely recognized pattern of competition and rivalry for recognition, has been used by sociologists to suggest that external social and cultural factors may be important harbingers of scientific advance (Merton,

1961). In this case the two rival worlds of private psychoanalytic therapy and academic psychiatry developed the use of the borderline type at the same time. In 1967 and 1968 Kernberg gave classic psychoanalytic definitions of the *borderline personality organization*, followed in 1972 by Masterson's extension to adolescents, using object-relations theory. The explosion of interest was remarkable. By 1975 fifty papers had been published on this theme. By 1980 there were three hundred papers, and by 1985 one thousand papers (Gunderson, 1994: 13).

At the very same time, Grinker in 1968 identified the *borderline syndrome*, describing the same type of patients, but with a tighter definition. Grinker enjoyed a particularly high status in US academic psychiatry and was, in contrast to the psychoanalysts, committed to using conventional empirical methods. This gave academic legitimacy to the syndrome and once again the development of research studies in the field took off: two in 1975, ten by 1980, one hundred by 1985 and three hundred by 1990. Between 1975 and 1980 Gunderson and others consolidated the new borderline type through literature summaries: 'The surprising attention given to those works testified to the nascent but widespread recognition of patients with this syndrome and the hunger for knowledge about them' (Gunderson, 1994: 13). Subsequent empirical research established that borderline types were not subtypes of schizophrenic or affective disorders, nor inherited, but caused by childhood trauma and neglect, and DSM status was duly conferred in 1980.

In a telling quote, Tyrer, Casey and Ferguson observe that:

> The interests of these groups at first seem opposed: one is deeply rooted in the psychodynamic tradition, with concern for the structure and development of personality and intrapsychic phenomena, and the other is preoccupied with accurate and reliable descriptions of behaviour that can be fashioned into the operational criteria of a DSM diagnosis. It says a great deal for the flexibility of personality disorder as a concept that these approaches have been married successfully, whereas for other subjects, particularly the neuroses, there has been a public and bad-tempered divorce. 'Borderline' is the common key to this success. Although it is accused of being an elusive adjective only (Akiskal et al., 1986) and unless 'used to signify a class that borders on something, has no clinical or descriptive meaning at all' (Millon, 1981: 332), it permeates the literature on personality disorder in all its contexts. Indeed, to many, 'personality disorder' is interpreted as 'borderline', illustrating the adaptability of a word that, after Lewis Carroll's *Through the Looking Glass*, could be described as a 'Humpty Dumptyism' ('when I choose a word', Humpy Dumpty said in a rather scornful tone, 'it means just what I choose it to mean – neither more nor less'). (Tyrer et al., 1991: 464)

In the psychoanalytic field there appears to have been a spontaneous response to the articulation of a new type. The key element was that it focused on instability of identity. There was alienation from stable relationships, and a mixture of grandiosity, contempt and dependency. Patients tended to polarize people between good and bad, and attacked the links between them. Feelings of rage or shame are projected onto others. Why did this strike such a chord in the late 1960s rather than pre-war? It would appear that liberalization of attitudes in the 1960s, the growth of inter-personal tolerance of varied lifestyles and values, the focus on personal fulfilment through close personal relationships, and the movement of identity issues into the heart of popular culture, meant that those who were unable to respond to these changes would have begun to differentiate themselves and appear in the offices of private psychoanalysts. The massive cultural changes of the 1960s are the key stimulus.

Turning to the world of academic psychiatry we can more easily identify Grinker as the key player. No doubt the same stranded souls, left behind by changes in the 1960s, were appearing in psychiatric clinics and hospital out-patient departments. At the same time, with the passing of the 1965 US medicare and medicaid social security amendments, there was rapidly growing concern about the control of government health spending, and the desire to contain costs. In this context Grinker was able to recruit support from academic psychiatrists, and the committee system of DSM, for his newly discovered syndrome. In both cases, the development of a new type enabled a heterogeneous group of patients that did not fit elsewhere (neither schizoid nor affective) to be *simplified* into a new category, which was *juxtaposed* with a theoretical explanation (childhood trauma), articulated with alternative theories (no evidence for heritability) and became inverted from a statement about difficult patients, to the discovery of an already pre-existing and coherent patient type: the 'borderline'.

All the elements that Hacking identifies are here. The cultural changes of the 1960s generate the cultural polarity (liberation and childhood trauma) that Hacking observed in the case of fugue. The appearance of patients in growing numbers in clinics brought them into observability, and provided 'release' through a diagnosis that explained their problems. However, this sociological explanation makes no assumption about the underlying reality of personality disorder. It merely seeks to understand it.

Turning more briefly to the other most common type, antisocial personality disorder, often termed psychopathy, we see a much longer history. In Europe the whole set of personality disorders are often grouped under the term psychopath. In the DSM system however, the psychopathic type is just one of the eleven sub-types of personality disorder. In the late 1990s in the UK the general term severe personality disorder was used by the UK Home Secretary to accentuate the dangerousness of some patients in this category to justify pre-emptive incarceration, though the legislation required that psychopaths should be treatable if they were to be compulsorily detained. In British mental health law, the category psycho-pathic disorder was very wide, covering most types of personality disorder: 'a persistent disorder or disability of mind (whether or not including subnormality of intelligence) which results in abnormally aggressive or seriously irresponsible conduct ...'. Public interest in serial killers and fictionalized characters such as Hannibal Lecter, have influenced popular views. On the other hand long standing specialist treatment units, such as Henderson Hospital in the UK, have until recently used this term to describe their patients (although it has become clear that most of them should be classified in the borderline category (Dolan et al., 1997: 275)). In fact many patients classified as dissocial would be found in prison or in severe cases in the special hospitals such as Broadmoor or Rampton.

Ramon (1986) argues that the growth of psychological models of group and organizational life after the Second World War followed by the 'open door' policies of many mental hospitals in the 1950s and the decline in mental hospital population, exposed these patients as if by a falling tide, but with a widespread concern that there was no psychiatric technology (drugs, ECT, psycho-surgery) that would work for them. They were not popular with psychiatrists who felt they were largely untreatable, and their inclusion as a special category in the 1959 Mental Health Act was controversial, and famously criticized by Baroness Wootton (1959) at the time. Here we see a clear conflict of interest between the profession and the state. Why include them under mental health law? Ramon (1986) argues that:

> The answer, I would suggest, is not to be found at the level of medical expertise but at the level of social regulation. The psychiatric concept of psychopathy makes possible a way of explaining conduct which would otherwise be socially unintelligible, regulating individuals who do not fit prevailing explanations of social need and their associated welfare systems, and confining persons who would otherwise fall outside the ambit of both the criminal justice system and the pychiatric system itself. (p. 227)

The solution to the distaste of conventional psychiatric services for the antisocial type, was to be the development of a medium secure unit service, situated on the psychiatric side of the medical–penal divide, but separate from either district services, or the special hospitals. These, recommended by the Butler Committee (Home Office/Department of Health and Social Security, 1975), were however very slow to materialize, partly because of the unwillingness of nurses to work in them. Ramon (1986) concludes that the categorization of personality disorder is a useful smokescreen for detaining difficult people, because there was no technology that commanded widespread support as effective. In recent years there has been a slow but gathering movement to make the case for therapeutic community treatment. UK research associated with the Henderson Hospital and Grendon Underwood Prison has built a sufficiently convincing case for both services to be expanded through the funding of entirely new units; and in Germany Lösel (1998) has been active in supporting the German equivalent: the social-therapeutic institution. Similar developments have been growing quickly within the US prison system (Rawlings, 1999).

In the case of the dissocial type, the key factors have been the psychiatric profession, the state and the uncertain evidence of any effective technology. The general term psychopath has been pared down to a more limited type, as other types of personality disorder have achieved separate categorization, at the hands of psychoanalytic and academic innovation. Rather than the 'discovery' of a new type of disorder, there has been the steady residualization of a rump of supposedly untreatable, and, as far as the state is concerned, intolerable people. The definition in terms of antisocial behaviour is almost identical to the definition of serious crime, and not surprisingly around 80 per cent of prison population have been shown to meet the diagnostic criteria.

SOCIOLOGY APPLIED TO PERSONALITY DISORDER

The second approach that we can take from sociology is to assume personality disorder is a given psychiatric condition, and develop a sociological analysis that can contribute to the diagnosis, treatment and care of personality disorder. For example, how is it distributed within the population? How effective are interventions to deal with it? In order to do this we need to return to some of the fundamental questions raised by sociology at the beginning of the chapter: how is personality disorder manifested in families, workplaces, civic associations, governments? What are the effects of class, age, gender and race on personality disorder?

Within clinical settings there are two definitions that are most commonly found, both from cluster B, and we will concentrate on those two: borderline and antisocial, both with treatment guidelines approved in 2009 by NICE (National Institute for Clinical Excellence) (Silk, 2010). The category of borderline, as we have seen above, emerged in the 1960s at the time of rapid cultural and social change. It is characterized by a poor sense of one's own identity, with unstable moods, fluid and changing interpersonal relationships, impulsivity and unstable affect. Fear of abandonment and self-harm are common. It appears in early adulthood, and is commonly seen to be caused by childhood trauma, particularly sexual abuse, and is three times as common amongst women as men.

Antisocial personality disorder is characterized by a casual disregard of the moral, legal and personal standards of local society. This is particularly centred on the disregard of rules, and the legal and ethical rights of others. Descriptors of this condition commonly mention lying, conning, impulsivity, recklessness, the gratification of immediate desires, often expressed as aggression or sexuality, and in general conduct likely to give rise to repeated arrest. This behaviour also appears in early adulthood, but is three times as common amongst men as women.

We see already in these short descriptions some fundamental sociological categories. The first to note is that these disorders do not manifest themselves clinically in children. While the literature often notes the contribution of family background, either genetic or psychological, to the condition, these disorders are bounded quite sharply by biographical transitions. They typically emerge in young people in their later teens and twenties, and recede markedly from middle age onwards. As far as the emergence of personality disorder is concerned, there are clear sociological processes at work. Young people are typically developing independent identities as they move away from their family context to the worlds of further education, work or early parenthood. This includes the development of new relationships, both personal and professional. Their own behaviour is less bounded by the close surveillance of family setting, and they have a wide choice of social settings in which to live and work. Later, when the conditions abate, this is typically a time of more settled life in terms of the trajectories of work, and personal life. Personality disorder emerges at times of rapid social context change and recedes when the rate of change slows. It is typically therefore a condition associated with 'biographical speed'.

Personality disorder is also segmented by gender. The literature clearly presents borderline as more often manifested by women, whereas antisocial is more often found amongst men. The difference in prevalence rates is quite marked, for example with prison populations consisting of more than 90 per cent men, and up to 75 per cent manifesting personality disorder. The reason for this is connected with the different biographical trajectories of young men and women. The cultural world of young men is externally oriented, and identity is claimed or given through the display of behaviour that celebrates independence from family control, and the testing out of physical and behavioural limits. This requires a young man to suspend or disregard typical behavioural regulators such as external approval or sensitivity to others. This suspension of cultural regulators in extreme form is at the heart of the diagnosis of anti-social personality disorder. Whether young men stay within or move beyond such cultural boundaries may result from a mixture of personal and social circumstance. We know that the rate of criminal activity self-reported by young men is relatively high. Where a young man is embedded in a strong sub-culture, in which legal, ethical and moral rule-breaking is acceptable or even celebrated, this may accentuate such behaviour. The most concentrated form and reproduction of such a sub-culture is to be found within prison itself.

By contrast as young women emerge from family relationships their struggle for identity and autonomy is a more complex process of renegotiating the way in which intimate relationships are experienced and expressed. Difficulties are less likely to be expressed outwardly, and rates of such disorders as depression and anorexia are higher for women. In addition, rates of direct damage through childhood sexual and emotional abuse are higher for women than men, and the consequent sense of betrayal and abandonment, together with the desire for secure intimacy can lead to a pattern of behaviour in which there is a poor sense of self, and the repetitive search for intimacy. The self mutilation and emotional promiscuity that can result are at the heart of the diagnosis of borderline personality disorder.

A further basic sociological category, in addition to age and gender, which has a close effect on personality disorder is social class. Rates of mental illness in general exhibit a sharp class gradient – rates are higher for lower social classes. Personality disorder is no exception. For example, prison is overwhelmingly populated by working class men. Rule-breaking, violence and personal insensitivity are typical in prison, and frequently reported as elements of working class culture. The rewards for conformity to cultural and social rules are less, as are the opportunities for personal success at school and subsequently work. Social mobility is limited and has not significantly changed in fifty years. Early teenage pregnancy can be seen as a quest for reliable emotional intimacy, and for some even a rational economic strategy for accessing independent housing, where likely employment opportunities are poor. For working class people, personality disorder diagnostic criteria seem to be an extrapolation of a cultural and social response to the limited circumstances in which working class people find themselves in the transition from childhood to adulthood.

A final and classic sociological structure is that of race. The interaction of mental disorder with race is marked, but complex. Sharply elevated rates of psychosis, especially schizophrenia, have been long noted amongst African-Caribbean young men. By contrast it is argued that Asian families are under-represented amongst the mentally ill, chiefly because families are very reluctant to seek help. Certainly the population that ends up in services for personality disorder is structured by race. Borderline personality disorder services are often populated disproportionately with Caucasian people, as are some of the most secure services for dangerous personality disorder patients. On the other hand, black men are overrepresented in the prison population, which as we have noted has high rates of personality disorder. It is difficult not to conclude that these patterns are more likely the result of family, community and social class dynamics than the distribution of psychological disturbance.

All of these sociological categories have effects during the processes of transition and emergence from childhood. These are times of tension and distress, and individual outcomes depend on networks of opportunity and rejection, support and abandonment, as they play out in the biographies of individuals with their own varying capacities for resilience. A mental disorder that is defined mainly in terms of behaviour inevitably raises the issue of how that behaviour fits with the social circumstances in which the individual finds themselves. In some circumstances it is not difficult to see why the personal distress associated with personality disorder would lead to the diagnosis of an illness. But in other circumstances personality disorder behaviour may be tolerated or even celebrated. Business or civic leaders who are ruthless may exhibit elements of antisocial personality disorder. Celebrities who self medicate with drugs and alcohol, or who repeatedly change partners may exhibit elements of borderline personality disorder. The creation and distribution of these social circumstances and the social roles they support are sociological phenomena.

A SOCIOLOGY OF TREATMENT

Personality disorder has become an illness, formally diagnosed as we detailed earlier in this chapter. The health and social care professions have developed a variety of interventions to deal with personality disorder, all of which are complex psychological or social interventions. Central to contemporary debates about health and social care interventions is the question of 'what works', and what counts as evidence. The sociology of science and technical systems can offer number of observations on this.

At the apex of the NHS hierarchy of evidence is the randomized controlled trial (RCT). The RCT evolved in the inter-war years in Britain under the leadership of the Medical Research Council. It aimed to identify the fairest and most reliable way of judging the efficacy of different medical interventions. Similar developments occurred throughout Europe and the USA at that time. The RCT has become the 'gold standard' for the experimental evaluation of medical and social interventions. The search for such evidence is a central strategy for a scientific philosophy known as positivism, typically associated with twentieth century pure science. From this point of view science progresses from the slow accumulation of evidence acquired ideally through controlled experimentation. However, it turns out that many medical and social interventions cannot be undertaken under the 'right experimental circumstances', and hence cannot draw upon the support of an RCT to demonstrate their efficacy. Treatments for personality disorder are typically of this type.

The RCT involves the experimental allocation of patients to one of several kinds of treatment, or no treatment, to determine, by comparing the results for each group, which patients do better. RCTs eliminate potential bias:

- doctors who have always been used to making decisions as to the best form of treatment for their patients might allocate patients to treatment who they think will do better – termed 'selection' bias;
- observers recording the progress of the patients might inadvertently be more likely to judge those patients getting a well known treatment as benefiting – termed 'observer bias';
- other sources of known and unknown bias, often of a random nature.

However the RCT itself is not simple:

- if the treatment is complex or multi-dimensional, and cumulative over time, such as a psychological or social intervention, then the nature of the active ingredient will be difficult to specify with any certainty;
- comparing the average response by the two groups – technically a comparison of the 'group means' – can include those patients who respond strongly, those who respond weakly, and those that have had a negative reaction;
- although practitioners are responsible for devising treatments for individual patients, we cannot generalize from the group to the individual (known as the 'ecological fallacy').

Despite the advantages that flow from the experimental comparison of treatment and control groups in RCTs, there has been a growing critical literature about the limitations of the use of RCTs in practice. First is the precision with which the treatment is developed and applied. Where an RCT is being used in a complex social situation, knowing exactly what the treatment 'mix' and 'dose' is can be difficult to specify reliably. The use of RCTs to evaluate social interventions such as crime reduction strategies (Pawson and Tilley, 1997) or active employment interventions (Stafford, 2002) have been criticized on these grounds. Second it is often difficult to disguise from patients the fact that the treatment is novel. This 'novelty', recognized many years ago in different ways as the 'Hawthorn' effect, and the placebo effect, whereby anything new tends to create a positive reaction, can generate responses that are difficult to replicate in the control group, and thereby eliminate. Third is the early drop-out of patients with a poor response from a programme, artificially concentrating those who respond well into the later stages of treatment. Fourth, many trials suffer from a surfeit of measures, such that inevitably some of them will show positive results by chance, and there is a strong temptation to report those as positive results – in fact a 'type 1' error (Campbell and Machin, 1999: 124). Fifth, there is a temptation to measure what can be measured, rather than what theory suggests we should measure, and more easily measurable outcomes might give preference to, or be more compatible with, one type of treatment than the other. Sixth, the active ingredients in the trial of a complex intervention may not themselves be independent of each other.

Treating personality disorder is therefore difficult to evidence. However government policies have nevertheless evolved steadily as the 'problem' of personality disorder has gained in significance, which we have analysed earlier in the chapter. The sociological analysis of language frequency and structure through 'corpus linguistics' shows how the language used in public policy and academic papers exhibits clear stages in the development of this public problem, moving from an eclectic distaste for an untreatable 'problem group' before the 1970s, to the adoption of a scientific and technical discourse concerning a medical disorder by the turn of the century (Parnell, 2009). These linguistic conventions are reproduced and change through the cultural life of 'policy networks' through which science, treatment and public expenditures are managed (Marsh and Rhodes, 1992). Political sociologists suggest that the British state engages with different areas of policy through policy communities with a shared culture in which the key players interact frequently, the boundaries are fairly tight and there are distinct advantages to those on the inside.

Such networks are situated within real world constraints – the substance of their concerns affects the way they work. For example, where professional interests, such as in health care, are concerned, the patterns of shared cultures and resource dependencies will be specific. Networks develop and are sustained because of mutual dependencies between individuals and networks, for example in the general relations between central and local government, or ministries and local agencies such as hospitals. The relative power between the individuals or networks will shape their interaction, and as relations develop, reproduce or change these power relations.

The outputs from networks vary between four types: economic resources, ideologies, knowledge and institutional changes (Rhodes, 1997). Much of the time there are multiple outputs of several of these factors. The government has become much more aware of the networked nature of its work, and indeed has in some respects promoted it through the differentiation between policy steering and service delivery in many parts of government (for example the purchaser-provider split in health care). This has intensified the government's own involvement in the resultant proliferation of networks, in many ways shifting its attention from 'rowing' to 'steering' (Osborne and Gaebler, 1992). The rise of 'political spin' is one consequence of this. The co-ordination of networks is based on trust and co-operation, in contrast to the price mechanism in markets, or the command structure of hierarchies. They are thus necessarily and pervasively social constructs.

Policy around personality disorder has evolved through such policy networks. A clear example has been the development of services for 'dangerous and severe personality disorder' (DSPD). The key interests in this story are, at the most general level, public perceptions of the risk of violence from personality disordered people, reflected in media attention and the activities of lobbying groups such as the Zito trust. The government feels a responsibility to respond to this perception. It could of course undertake a public education campaign to proselytize the evidence that objective levels of risk are very low and falling. However, where for example there have been attempts to relocate paedophiles in community settings there has indeed been a sharp public reaction. The government has thus adopted the alternative approach which is to bring in new legislation and to develop an expensive new service to appear to be doing something to minimize the threat that the public perceives. This is commensurate with a long term commitment of successive Home Secretaries to play tough on such issues, and vividly illustrates the ability of a key player in the network to set an agenda and a cultural tone.

This approach to the personality disorder problem has been directed by the government towards a forensic professional community which is split over its own interests and values on the issue. A core of those with special interests in this category supports the government line, and indeed has a number of potential benefits to gain. They will gain resources from active involvement in the network, and they hope to be laying the evidence base for a new branch of psychiatry. The rest, along with the large body of general psychiatrists and clinical psychologists, are distinctly cool, concerned that they might be trading in their autonomy under the new legislation. On the other hand there has been a widespread dislike of the personality disorder patient sometimes referred to as the 'heart sink' case, because of the trail of chaos and upset that they leave in their wake, both in their families and in their frequent and demanding contact with health and social services. The prospect of taking these patients out of the hair of other professional groups is a considerable external benefit outside the immediate network.

The network around personality disordered patients is not simple. One part was the academic circuit collected together in a government sponsored 'virtual institute of personality disorder'. Another has been those who deal with DSPDs in existing prisons and secure hospitals – they will also, at least a number of them, be supplying the staff for the new service under construction. Another is the central government ministry sections that deal with security issues and legal issues at the Home Office, and those more generally responsible for commissioning existing secure services in both the health and prison sectors. Another is the network of therapeutic communities that claim to have a viable treatment for personality disorders, but who are regarded by many general psychiatrists as slightly idealistic and radical (as this is the stable they came from in their early years in the 1950s and 1960s). Another is the Royal College of Psychiatrists, where support or opposition to these different networks is closely affected by the formal position that different key members of the college hold, particularly the presidency. The salience and leverage that these different networks have in relation to an issue depends both on their status, and the rules of engagement for the issue. For example, there is no doubt that evidence, preferably generated by the meta-analysis of a set of randomized controlled trials, would be the key resource for winning arguments about treatment and service development, but as we have seen this is difficult to create.

CONCLUSION

In this chapter, we have seen that sociology takes a dual role in relation to medical conditions. On the one hand it can stand outside the organization of medicine and healthcare, subjecting them to an analysis as social institutions. On the other hand it can stand shoulder to shoulder with healthcare professionals in seeking to add a sociological perspective to the diagnosis and treatment of a distressing disorder. A particular aspect is the way in which evidence is developed to try to identify effective treatments, and the way in which health policy evolves in the face of uncertain evidence.

REFERENCES

Akiskal, H.S., Chen, S.E. and Davis, G.C (1986) Borderline: an adjective in search of a noun. In M.S. Stone (ed.) *Essential Papers on Borderline Disorders: One Hundred Years at the Border.* New York: New York University Press.

Butler, R.A.B. (1975) *Report of Committee on Mentally Disordered Offenders*, cmnd 6244. London: HMSO.

Campbell, M.J. and Machin, D. (1999) *Medical Statistics: A Commonsense Approach*, 3rd edition. Chichester: John Wiley.

Dolan, B., Warren, F. and Norton, K. (1997) Change in borderline symptoms one year after therapeutic community treatment for severe personality disorder. *British Journal of Psychiatry*, 171: 274–279.

Farmer, A.E. (1997) Current approaches to classification. In R. Murray, P. Hill and P. McGuffin (eds) *The Essentials of Postgraduate Psychiatry*. Cambridge: Cambridge University Press.

Gundersen, J.G. (1994) Building structure for the borderline construct. *Acta Psychiatrica Scandinavica*, 89 (supplement 379): 12–18.

Hacking, I. (1998) *Mad Travelers: Reflections on the Reality of Transient Mental Illnesses*, Virginia: University Press of Virginia.

Higgit, A. and Fonagy, P. (1992) Psychotherapy in borderline and narcissistic personality disorder. *British Journal of Psychiatry*, 161: 23–43.

Lösel, F. (1998) The treatment and management of psychopaths. In D.J. Cooke (ed.) *Psychopathy: Theory, Research and Implications for Society*. Netherlands: Kluwer Academic Publishers.

Marsh, D. and Rhodes, R.A.W (1992) *Policy Networks in British Government*. Oxford: Oxford University Press.

Merton, R.K. (1961) Singletons and multiples in scientific discovery: a chapter in the sociology of science. *Proceedings of the American Philosophical Society*, 105(5): 470–486.

Millon, T. (1981) *Disorders of Personality, DSM-III: Axis II.* New York: Wiley and Sons.

Osborne, D. and Gaebler, T. (1992) *Reinventing Government.* Reading, MA: Addison-Wesley.

Parnell, M. (2009) *Personality Disorder and Corpus Linguistics.* PhD thesis, University of Nottingham.

Pawson, R. and Tilley, N. (1997) *Realistic Evaluation.* London: SAGE.

Ramon, S. (1986) The category of psychopathy: its professional and social context in Britain. In P. Miller and N. Rose (eds) *The Power of Psychiatry.* Cambridge: Polity Press.

Rawlings, B. (1999) Therapeutic communities in prisons. *Policy and Politics,* 27(1): 97–112.

Rhodes, R.A.W. (1997) *Understanding Governance, Policy Networks, Governance, Reflexivity and Accountability.* Buckingham: Open University Press.

Silk, K.R. (2010) Introduction: National Institute for Clinical Excellence Guidelines for the Treatment of Antisocial Personality Disorder and Borderline Personality Disorder. *Personality and Mental Health,* 4(1): 1–2 (whole issue devoted to discussion of these guidelines).

Stafford, B. (2002) Being more certain about random assignment in social policy evaluations. *Social Policy and Society,* 1(4): 275–284.

Tyrer, P., Casey, P. and Ferguson, B. (1991) Personality disorder in perspective. *British Journal of Psychiatry,* 159: 463–471.

Woolgar, S. (1995) Representation, cognition, and self: what hope for an integration of psychology and sociology? In S.L. Star (ed.) *Ecologies of Knowledge: work and politics in science and technology.* Albany: State University of New York Press.

Wootton, B. (1959) *Social Science and Social Pathology.* London: Allen and Unwin.

17

Sociological Aspects of Substance Misuse

Michael Bloor and Alison Munro

INTRODUCTION

Drug use often occurs in concert with psychiatric morbidity: psychiatric morbidity may precipitate drug use; and harmful drug use, or dependence, or intoxication, or withdrawal may lead to psychiatric morbidity, including self-harm and suicide. Such co-morbidity has a poorer prognosis: drug users with psychopathology have a poorer prognosis in the treatment of drug misuse and drug use is a predictor of poor treatment outcome for mentally ill patients (Hodges et al., 2006). This poorer prognosis for co-morbid patients/clients needs to be borne in mind in appraising the studies of treatment for drug use below. However, we begin this overview with studies of patterns of drug use.

PATTERNS OF DRUG USE AND STUDIES OF DRUG MARKETS

The illicit and hidden character of drug use has made ethnographic studies (i.e. the empathetic and immersive observation of research participants in natural settings (Atkinson et al., 2001)) a favoured method for the sociological study of drug use, although other more structured methods have also sometimes been successfully deployed in natural fieldwork settings (see, for example, Taylor et al. (2004) on the video-recording and analysis of drug users' injection techniques). The classic ethnographic study in this field is Becker's (1953) study of marijuana use among his fellow jazz musicians. Becker showed that the pleasurable effects of the drug were not experientially self-evident – a direct pharmacological consequence of ingesting the drug – but rather had to be communicated and learned just like the technique of smoking itself. MacAndrew and Edgerton (1970) subsequently made the same argument in respect of the learned and culturally diverse character of what they termed 'drunken comportment'. The cultural transmission of lay expertise in drug use has been a continuing topic in sociological studies. For example, Rhodes et al. (2005a) have documented changes over time in British injectors' propensity to inject in the groin. However, drug users also learn experimentally and incrementally, witness the account below by a steroid user, whom one might term an ethnopharmacological expert, who had gradually learned to optimize the dosages and combinations of steroids in order to maximize their 'bulking' and 'cutting' effects for success in body-building competitions:

> I pre-plan everything and I make a note of most things [...] Injections and orals, but I've tended to stay off the orals lately because they seem to suppress my appetite [...] At the moment now I'm doing a 9-week bulking cycle [...] Deca for three weeks, Heptylate for three weeks, Testoviron for three weeks. And then the last four weeks – then I'll stack them (i.e. combine them) with Pronabol ... Weeks 4 to 6 is just Deca on its own. Weeks 4 to 6 will be Hepylate. But on Week 6 I'll start the Pronabol as well [...] And then Weeks 7, 8 and 9 will be Testoviron and the Pronabol [...] With the Deca, it's about 300 mg a week, which would be three 100 mg injections. The Heptylate would be about 750 mg a week. The same with the Testoviron. And the Pronabol will be, um, week 6 will be six 5 mg tablets a day, which is 210 mg. And then Weeks 7, 8 and 9 will be 270 mg. (Bloor et al. 1998: 31)

Relatedly, ethnographic studies have emphasized the socio-cultural context – the networks of rights and obligations – in which drug use occurs. A classic pre-AIDS study of needle-sharing in San Francisco's Haight-Ashbury (Howard and Borges, 1970) emphasized how equipment-sharing was socially patterned and emblematic of relationships of intimacy and trust. In the early years of the HIV/AIDS epidemic, the relatively modest power of psychological models of risk behaviour (and particularly the then dominant Health Beliefs Model – see, for example, Joseph et al., 1987) to explain HIV-related risk behaviour encouraged sociologists to advance alternative models of risk behaviour which emphasized both the situated rationality and also the routinized nature of much HIV-related risk behaviour (Bloor, 1995).

In the developed nations, in response to concerns about HIV transmission, levels of equipment-sharing fell dramatically in the late 1980s and the early 1990s (Bloor, 1995; Stimson, 1994; van Ameijden and Coutinho, 1998), but 'residual' needle-sharing remains socially patterned (Bloor et al., 2008b). It should be noted however, that there is some division of opinion about how far equipment-sharing between sexual partners should be viewed as a sign of intimacy and trust and how far it should be seen as a sign of power relations and gender inequality, with women normally being 'second on the needle' (Bourgois and Moss, 2004). Further, although drug use and associated behaviours such as equipment-sharing are culturally transmitted, their social patterning is shaped by social structural factors, particularly population movement, population mixing and deprivation (Heimer et al., 2002; Rhodes et al., 2005b).

Studies of HIV spread among drug injectors have frequently shown a pattern of initial explosive epidemic spread in a locality followed by near-stabilization of prevalence rates. In Bangkok, for example, the prevalence of HIV infection among injectors rose from 1 per cent in late 1987 to over 40 per cent in early 1989 (Vanichseni et al., 1989) – a doubling time for the epidemic of only around 3 months. Similar explosive increases in prevalence have also been reported in localities as diverse as Edinburgh, Bari (Italy) and Manipur (India). While rapid epidemic spread in such populations is partly explicable through differential infectiousness (with newly infected persons being thought to be more infectious before they have developed antibodies to the virus), it was also due to the limited availability of injecting equipment and a consequent reliance on 'dealer's works', a form of serial anonymous sharing. Relatedly, lack of access to clean injecting equipment in prisons has also led to rapid explosions of HIV infection in the past – the HIV outbreak at Glenochil prison in Scotland being a well-documented example (Gore et al., 1995). Availability of clean injecting equipment is a necessary rather than a sufficient condition for the elimination of equipment-sharing and, as previously stated, 'residual' equipment-sharing still occurs in even the best-served drug injector populations. While these low levels of equipment-sharing may be sufficient to prevent further large-scale HIV infection among drug injectors (Bloor et al., 1994), they are insufficient to prevent further epidemic spread of hepatitis C virus ('a public health crisis' – Royal College of Physicians of Edinburgh, 2004), which is more efficiently transmitted through equipment-sharing than HIV.

Studies of drug markets tend to be either ethnographic studies of small groups of dealers (e.g. Adler, 1993) or interviews with users about their drug purchases (e.g. Best et al., 2004). As Coomber (2004) has pointed out, the information gained from such studies may be fragmentary and misleading: for example, dealers and users alike firmly believe that street-level drugs are extensively adulterated as they pass down the selling hierarchy, although forensic studies of UK police seizures show no differences in purity between seizures at national borders and seizures on the street (King, 1997). Nevertheless, the evidence that we have suggests that drug markets are highly segmented. Thus, of 189 young cannabis-using people aged 11–19 recently interviewed in the UK, the great majority rarely experimented with other drugs except ecstasy and most accessed drugs through 'social supply' (as opposed to commercial) networks, with young people 'chipping in' and sharing with friends; 22.5 per cent never bought cannabis themselves (relying on friends) and only 6 per cent bought cannabis from someone unknown to them (Duffy et al., 2008). Typically, transactions involving commercial dealers are in closed markets, where buyer and seller arrange deals in advance by mobile phone, and where exchanges take place in public spaces and involve 'runners' (generally children who were not users themselves) and look-outs (May et al., 2005).

Behaviours associated with drug use, particularly income-generating behaviours such as prostitution and criminality (e.g. McKeganey and Barnard, 1992) have also been documented ethnographically. Preble and Casey's (1969) classic paper on 'taking care of business' vividly illustrated the considerable daily effort that users must put into generating income and finding drugs. These ethnographic studies have been complemented by structured interview studies of samples of drug users recruited in treatment settings, often cohort samples followed up post-discharge. They demonstrate that post-treatment criminality, employment status and housing status all depend crucially on subsequent patterns of illicit drug use. For example, a follow-up study of more a thousand Scottish drug users starting a new treatment episode (the DORIS study – see below) showed that, after controlling for other variables, those who were abstinent 33 months later were seven times less likely to report having committed acquisitive crimes in the previous three months (McIntosh et al., 2007).

The need for quick-turnaround research to feed into new policy initiatives and rapid services-planning on HIV/AIDS epidemic spread has led to drugs researchers being among the pioneers of rapid assessment methods, using combinations of community surveys, mapping techniques, key informant interviews and brief observations to deliver reports to bodies such as the United Nations International Drug Control Programme (UNIDCP) within three-month time-periods (Rhodes et al., 1999). Another area of methodological innovation has been in studies of the prevalence of problem drug use, where sociologists have adapted the 'mark-recapture' methods that field ecologists use to estimate the size of animal, bird and fish populations to estimate local and national populations of problem drug users and to plot changes in prevalence over time (e.g. Hay et al., 2005). These studies seek to model the overlaps between different partial populations of drug users found in arrest data, drug treatment agency data and the like, to estimate the size of the 'hidden' population not in contact with any agencies (Bloor, 2005).

DRUG TREATMENT STUDIES

While drug treatment is sometimes broadly defined to encompass drug prevention, treatment for drug misuse, and harm reduction services such as needle exchange (Royal College of Psychiatrists and Royal College of Physicians, 2000), we will report separately on studies of the effectiveness of such different services here and also deal separately with drug services provided in penal institutions.

Drug prevention research

Drug prevention interventions seek to increase knowledge about drugs, to reduce the use of drugs, to delay the onset of the first use of drugs, to reduce drug abuse and/or to minimize drug-related harm (Cuijpers, 2003). The majority of initiatives and of research on drug prevention involve targeting young people of school age (Cuijpers, 2003). The results of meta analytic studies suggest that universal school-based drug prevention programmes can lead to changes in young peoples' knowledge and attitudes about drugs, and that those that utilize interactive approaches (such as role play and small group discussions), as well as those which are based on a social-influence approach, have a greater impact on reducing drug use (Tobler et al., 2000). There is currently particular interest in the potential of peer-delivered health promotion for young people both for drug prevention and for other objectives such as smoking prevention (Harden et al., 1999). However, the effects of schools-based interventions naturally tend to diminish over time (White and Pitts, 1998) and it is unclear whether interventions that have been developed in one country will be successful when introduced elsewhere (Ashton, 2003).

Mass media campaigns are another important strand of drug prevention policies, but the impacts of such initiatives are notoriously difficult to evaluate, and the few studies which have attempted to do so are hindered by methodological weaknesses (Cuijpers, 2003). It has been suggested that, while such initiatives may help to improve knowledge, their impact on behaviour is difficult to establish (ibid.). A recent review found no evidence that 'stand-alone' media interventions have any success in preventing drug use (McGrath et al., 2006).

An American programme (the Strengthening Families Program for Parents and Youth) providing guidance to parents on family management skills, communication, academic support and parent–child relations has been proven to delay initiation in both alcohol and cannabis use (Spoth et al., 2002). But it is known to be difficult to recruit and retain families in drug prevention programmes (Velleman et al., 2000). Community–based drug prevention programmes are often conducted in concert with school-based programmes. A review by Flay (2000) found no evidence that the community-based component conferred any benefits over and above the school-based programmes.

Research on harm reduction services

Syringe exchange schemes

In most of the developed world (some States in the USA were an exception), the HIV/AIDS epidemic led to the establishment of a range of services designed to reduce harm to drug users who were unable or unwilling to become abstinent. Syringe exchange schemes were the most prominent of these, but outreach services (including bleach distribution in the USA) were also developed and (in some countries) injecting rooms. The urgent need for policies to combat the epidemic meant that many of these services were introduced without prior randomized controlled trials (although in the UK the Department of Health commissioned monitoring research on pilot syringe exchange schemes (see Berridge and Strong's (1993) social history of the epidemic in the UK)). And, the near-simultaneous introduction of a range of services has made it impossible to distinguish the separate effects of different services, whose effectiveness was likely in any case to be synergistic. Evaluation efforts have therefore concentrated on longitudinal cohort studies that have compared service-users and non-users (Elliot, 1998). In respect of syringe exchange schemes, most of these studies have shown service-users reporting lower levels of equipment-sharing than non-users; where falls in sharing have occurred over time, service-users have reported larger falls than non-users (e.g. Donoghoe et al., 1989). It may be objected, of course, that syringe exchange users may be more motivated to reduce their risk behaviour than non-users.

Methadone maintenance and other substitute prescribing

One component of harm reduction services that has been comparatively well evaluated is that of substitute prescribing, particularly methadone maintenance. No randomized controlled trials have been conducted in the UK, because it is believed that drug users randomly allocated to a form of treatment that is different from that which they are seeking are likely to leave the trial prematurely and seek their preferred treatment elsewhere. However, an influential trial was conducted in (the then crown colony) Hong Kong at the time that methadone prescribing was introduced there (Newman and Whitehill, 1979). Subsequent reviews (e.g. Farrell et al., 1994), systematic reviews (e.g. Sorensen and Copeland, 2000), meta-analyses (Marsch, 1998; Semaan et al., 2002) and an overview of systematic reviews (Amato et al., 2005) have all added to an evidence base showing that methadone maintenance reduces HIV risk behaviour. Likewise, methadone maintenance has been demonstrated to be associated with reduced levels of illicit drug use and reduced criminality, with treatment effectiveness being directly associated with level of methadone dosage. Harm reduction services have proved controversial in political and policy terms and inevitably controversy has spilled over into the research field. Thus it is sometimes argued that drug misuse should be seen as a chronic condition like diabetes and therefore the research outcome measures for successful treatment should not be measures of recovery, such as abstinence, but rather should be measures of treatment retention (e.g. McClelland et al., 2005). Certainly, methadone maintenance services have generally been evaluated to perform relatively well in terms of client retention over time (e.g. Gossop et al., 2001).

Methadone is by no means the only drug used as a prescribed substitute for illicit opiates. Subutex (buprenorphine) is widely used in France for substitute prescribing and prescription heroin has also been used in some countries, particularly for clients unwilling to receive methadone. Van den Brink and colleagues (van den Brink et al., 2003) conducted two concurrent randomized control trials in the Netherlands to evaluate the effectiveness of injectable heroin and inhalable heroin for heroin users who had not fared well in traditional methadone maintenance treatments. These were multi-site trials and participants were recruited from existing methadone maintenance services in six different cities. Participants were randomly allocated to either an intervention group or a control group in one of the two RCTs in accordance with their main route of drug use, that is heroin injectors were allocated to the 'heroin injection' RCT and heroin smokers were allocated to the 'inhalable heroin' trial. The results of both trials were that drug users who received heroin (under supervised conditions) as well as methadone fared better on the study's primary outcome measures than those who received methadone alone (ibid.). However, a recent Cochrane systematic review of randomized control trials that have examined the efficacy of heroin maintenance treatment in retaining drug users in treatment claims to have found 'mixed evidence' (Ferri et al., 2006).

Research on drug treatment services

The provision of methadone is a treatment for drug use as well as a harm reduction intervention, since methadone may be used both short-term, for detoxification and longer term, on a reducing dose when maintained clients feel they wish to move towards abstinence. Other drug misuse treatments are: detoxification (non-methadone), out-patient drug free and treatment in therapeutic communities such as residential rehabilitation or twelve-step treatments (Bean and Nemitz, 2004). Psycho-social treatments such as motivational interviewing are often given in addition to such treatments.

The previously mentioned problems in setting up randomized controlled trials have had the result that the main research evidence on treatment effectiveness has come from various national, prospective, longitudinal studies. These have been conducted to assess the short and longer-term client outcomes of existing drug treatment services in the United States (DATOS: Hubbard et al., 1989) in England (NTORS: Gossop et al., 2003), in Scotland (DORIS: Neale and Robertson, 2005; McKeganey et al., 2008), in Ireland (ROSIE: Cox et al., 2006) and in Australia (ATOS: Teeson et al., 2006). All of these studies have examined treatment outcomes for drug users starting new treatment episodes contemporaneously across a number of treatment modalities including community methadone maintenance, residential rehabilitation, outpatient abstinence-based treatments and detoxification treatments for example. The ATOS study was the only one which included a control group of heroin users who were receiving no treatment.

Results from all these cohort studies were broadly similar in showing reductions in drug use and in criminality over time and improvements in physical and mental health and employment status. In the ATOS study, at one-year follow-up the improvements in recent abstinence, number of days when heroin was used in the past month and reductions in those injecting daily were all greater than in the 'no treatment' control group (ibid.). While these large scale studies provide a valuable insight into drug treatment outcomes in a 'real world' setting, these studies are limited by their non-experimental designs and the possibly limited comparability of their (non-randomly allocated) different treatment populations. It has also been pointed out (Orford, 2008) that they shed little light on questions about which elements of the treatment process, such as the quality of the therapeutic relationship, have an effect on outcome measures. And additionally it has been suggested that analyses should focus less on single treatment episodes (as is the case in much cohort study research on treatment outcomes) and more on 'treatment careers' (Hser et al., 1997) which acknowledge the often cumulative nature of treatments for drug misuse.

Detoxification treatment

With regard to withdrawal from opiates, a number of pharmacological treatments that assist the detoxification process are available. These include the administration of methadone, clonidine, lofexidine, buprenorphine and dihydrocodeine amongst others (Seivewright, 2000; Wright et al., 2007). With regard to the efficacy of these drugs in assisting the withdrawal process, a recent review of systematic reviews suggests that 'it is very difficult to draw conclusions about effective methods of managing opioid withdrawal' (Amato et al., 2005: 224). However, on the evidence available the reviewers suggested that with regard to retaining clients in treatment and in preventing relapse, methadone treatment appeared to be more effective than opioid agonists (such as clonidine and lofexidine). Recent research has made detoxification a controversial treatment because of the demonstrated greater risk of fatal overdose among relapsed clients as a consequence of their reduced tolerance of opiates (Strang et al., 2003).

Residential rehabilitation services

Residential rehabilitation facilities, like 12-step (Minnesota Model) programmes and other therapeutic communities, share the goal of seeking to achieve abstinence from drugs. While the Minnesota Model programmes can be said to focus on a disease model of addiction and therapeutic communities emphasize social learning within a highly structured programme of activities, in practice both types of facilities employ similar therapeutic techniques and principles.

A recent systematic review of randomized controlled trial evidence for the effectiveness of therapeutic communities in the treatment of substance-related disorder reviewed evidence from seven trials (included two of prison-based communities) and reported that firm conclusions on effectiveness could not be drawn because of methodological limitations (Smith et al., 2007). Referring instead to the evidence of cohort studies, the English NTORS study found that drug users who were treated in residential rehabilitation fared well on measures of drug abstinence: 50 per cent were abstinent at the 1 year follow-up point and significant reductions in drug injecting, equipment sharing and criminal activity were also found at the same follow-up point (Gossop et al., 1999).

In the Scottish DORIS study, the proportion of the study population achieving abstinence was lower than in the NTORS study, but ex-residential rehabilitation clients were significantly more likely than clients of other community-based treatments to have achieved abstinence at follow-up (McKeganey et al., 2006; McKeganey et al., 2008). The picture is a complex one since methadone maintenance clients in DORIS were significantly more likely to have reduced their use of heroin than clients of other community-based treatments (Bloor et al. 2008a;

McKeganey et al., 2008): methadone treatment is more likely to lead to reductions in illicit drug use, while residential rehabilitation is more likely to lead to abstinence.

Another cohort study of the effect of 12-step therapy on treatment outcomes for drug users was conducted by Ouimette and colleagues (Ouimette et al., 1997), comparing the outcomes between drug users in a 12-step programme and those undergoing cognitive behavioural treatment. Participants received one of three types of treatment: 12-step, cognitive behavioural, or mixed 12-step and cognitive behavioural. The study found that the three treatments were equally effective and that improvements in all of the main outcome measures were found across the three treatments.

Fiorentine and Hillhouse (2000), in a similar cohort study, compared the effects of prior and current involvement with a 12-step programme on treatment duration and outcomes for clients on a 24-week outpatient drug treatment programme. The results of the study were that weekly or more attendance at 12 step programmes prior to treatment predicted retention in treatment and treatment completion. The authors also tentatively suggest that there is evidence of an additive effect of participation in both 'types' of treatment, leading to better treatment outcomes, but caution that participation in two types of treatment may be an indicator of high motivation to change.

Therapeutic communities, like many other residential treatment settings, were also a locale for ethnographic studies in the 1960s and 1970s. Synanon, the first therapeutic community for drug users, was the subject of a widely-read book by Yablonsky (1965) and this study was followed by Sugarman's (1974) ethnography of Daytop Village. Fonkert's (1978) doctoral study of a Dutch community for drug users became one component of an eight-community comparative ethnography of the range of therapeutic community practice (Bloor et al., 1988). These ethnographic studies sought to provide a sociological description of the therapeutic community treatment process.

Therapeutic communities have as their aim the resocialization of the individual – the enduring modification of the individual's conduct, and with it his or her ways of relating to others and his or her felt identity. The techniques of achieving this resocialization or reality construction in therapeutic communities for drug users differ in some degree from those found in therapeutic communities in psychiatric hospitals or halfway houses. As described in ethnographic studies, these techniques comprised: the rigid separation of inmates from family, friends and possessions; the extensive programming of activities (including leisure activities); close supervision and exacting standards of task performance; a hierarchy of statuses with associated rights and obligations ('a boarding school run by the prefects' – Sugarman, 1974: 144); and cathartic confrontation and degradation ceremonies for poor performance and strong positive reinforcement of good performance.

To use the phrase popularized by Goffman (1968), therapeutic communities for drug users are 'total institutions' like the armed forces or religious sects, with a therapeutic objective to their resocialization techniques. Everyday therapeutic work in such communities is a cognitive act which can transform any mundane event in the community by redefining that event as an occasion for therapy in the light of some therapeutic paradigm. Just as the profane is transformed into the sacred by religious belief and ceremony, so a simple act like cleaning the toilets or mending a leaking sink is invested with new meaning and held up as relevant to the cleaner's recovery and rehabilitation (Bloor et al., 1988).

Out-patient drug free treatments

Hser and colleagues (Hser et al., 1998) compared the effectiveness of four treatment modalities (out-patient drug free, out-patient methadone, short-term in-patient and long-term residential) using data from the DATOS cohort study reported earlier. While improvements in drug use (heroin and cocaine) were found to be evident across all four treatment modalities, figures given for reductions in heroin and cocaine use for the 'average' client in treatment (ibid.) were in fact lowest for the out-patient drug free treatment group. However, this was also the group that had the lowest levels of drug use severity at intake.

Psychological treatments

In addition to the four major treatment modalities for drug misusers already discussed, psycho-social treatments are also often available to drug misusers and often in conjunction with the four major treatments. Psychological treatments include cue exposure, motivational interviewing and contingency management amongst others (Curran and Drummond, 2005).

Burke and Arkowitz (2003) conducted a meta-analysis of randomized control trials of the efficacy of motivational interviewing (MI) on changing problem behaviours, including problem drug use. Four of the thirty control trials included in this analysis involved MI with drug users, and the majority of the other studies included involved alcohol users. The authors found that MI with alcohol and drug users achieved moderate effect sizes (0.25–0.27), and concluded that MI with these groups achieved a clinically significant impact.

In an earlier study, Saunders and colleagues (Saunders et al., 1995) conducted a randomized control trial of a brief intervention using motivational interviewing with opiate users (N=122) in treatment. The authors found at 6 month follow-up that those allocated to the motivational interviewing arm of the study, as compared to those allocated to the control arm, fared better on a number of measures including commitment to abstinence, fewer drug-related problems and longer treatment compliance. However, Saunders and colleagues (Saunders et al., 1995) also found at six months follow-up that there was no difference between the groups on a measure of severity of dependence to drugs. The authors concluded though that MI could be a useful adjunct to methadone maintenance treatment.

Contingency management treatment (incentives)

Contingency management treatment programmes, which utilize positive reinforcement to help drug users to change their drug using behaviours, have evaluated well in the United States (Petry, 2006). Positive reinforcers include voucher schemes whereby drug users in treatment who submit negative urine tests receive vouchers worth a specific monetary value. The vouchers can be exchanged for goods and services but never money or any other 'inappropriate' items such as alcohol. The UK government is also seeking to assess the efficacy of such programmes as part of their new drug strategy (Home Office, 2008).

Treatment within the criminal justice system

Stallwitz and Stöver (2007) conducted a review of empirical studies which sought to evaluate the effectiveness of methadone maintenance treatment in prisons on reducing both heroin use and drug injecting. From the research evidence reviewed, the authors concluded that both the dosage level (with a preferred threshold of at least 60 mg of methadone per day) and the length of treatment (that the methadone prescription should continue for the duration of the imprisonment) may be crucial factors in the success of this type of treatment. They suggest however, that due to being under-researched, it is not possible to draw clear conclusions about the effectiveness of other substitution focused treatments in prisons.

The DORIS cohort study embraced both sample members starting a new episode of prison-based treatment and sample members starting treatment in the community. The DORIS prison treatment sub-sample received a more limited spectrum of treatments than the community sub-sample and also evaluated their experience of treatment less positively (Neale and Saville, 2004); at 33-month follow-up, those who had received prison-based treatment had significantly reduced their drug use, but this observed reduction was itself significantly less than that for those who had received community-based treatments (McKeganey et al., 2008). However, the DORIS sample was recruited in 2001/2002 which preceded the large-scale introduction of methadone prescribing in Scottish prisons, so the applicability of the DORIS findings to current treatment regimes is problematic.

Drug courts, which are criminal courts that deal exclusively with drug offenders, seek to reduce drug offending by offering drug users the opportunity of drug treatment in place of custodial sentences. Such courts which emerged initially in the United States in the late 1980s (Walker, 2001), have since been widely adopted internationally, including in Australia, Canada and the UK (Walker, 2001). A systematic review of studies of the effectiveness of drug courts on reducing criminal recidivism (Wilson et al., 2006) concluded that there is evidence that drug using offenders who participate in a drug court are less likely than similar offenders who undergo traditional criminal justice processes to re-offend. However, the authors suggest that caution has to be exercised in considering this conclusion owing to methodological weaknesses in many of the 55 studies reviewed.

Pelissier et al. (2007) conducted a systematic review of the evidence for the effectiveness of 'aftercare', defined as 'treatment provided after release from prison' (ibid.: 311) in the United States criminal justice system. A total of

15 research studies which utilized a comparison group were reviewed. The authors concluded that claims about the effectiveness of aftercare treatment are not well substantiated owing large differences in the mode, setting and intensity of the aftercare treatment being evaluated. However, in terms of outcome focused research, Pellisier et al. also concluded that in terms of reducing criminal recidivism, those people who complete both prison-based treatment and transitional treatment care after release from prison, have better outcomes than those who complete only prison-based treatment or those who receive no treatment at all.

Recovery from drug use without treatment

While it is true that for many people, drug misuse appears to be a 'chronic relapsing condition' (Hser et al., 1997; McLelland et al., 2005), which often results in numerous treatment episodes for the individuals involved, there is evidence that people can recover from drug use without any formal treatment. This is often referred to as 'natural recovery', 'maturing out' or 'spontaneous remission' (Granfield and Cloud, 2001). Since accessibility of services for drug users has improved over time and current drug users are frequently persuaded into treatment by families or propelled into treatment via the legal system, studies of natural recovery are mostly located in the pre-HIV/AIDS period where recourse to treatment was less common.

Charles Winick's (1962) pioneering study of natural recovery amongst heroin users in the United States, was an analysis of records of heroin users kept at the Federal Bureau of Narcotics. Winick (1962) found that the age of drug users correlated with 'disappearance' from the Federal records and from this it was concluded that heroin users were naturally 'maturing out' of drug use at around 35–40 years of age. However, a major criticism of this study was the assumption that because drug users disappeared from the files of the Federal Bureau, they have necessarily 'recovered' from their addiction to drugs. In other words, the possibilities that these drug users may have died, or otherwise dropped off the register, was not taken into account.

In the 1970s, Lee Robins and colleagues (Robins et al., 1974) conducted a cross-sectional study of 900 Vietnam veterans, who were interviewed at between eight and twelve months after they returned from Vietnam. The study found that while 43 per cent of the veterans reported having used opiates in Vietnam, only approximately 10 per cent reported having used any opiates since returning to the US. Robins et al. (1974) concluded from these findings that the occasional use of drugs such as heroin was possible, without a person becoming dependent or addicted. In the UK, an eight-year follow-up study of a sample of 128 heroin users recruited in 1969 found that 31 per cent were no longer addicted (with an average period of abstinence of 4.5 years) and the majority of these had given up opiate use without recourse to drug treatment services (Stimson and Oppenheimer, 1982).

CONCLUSION

Sociological studies of drug use have a chequered record. Only a very starry-eyed observer would claim that government policies on drug use in the developed world are wholly evidence-based. Fifty years of careful studies of the social world of drug users has hardly altered the public perception of drug users as vicious, amoral criminals. And study design problems and equivocal results in treatment evaluation studies have led to debates within the research community about the possible need for a change in direction in the conduct of evaluation research; from a treatment outcome focus to a change process focus (see, for example, Orford, 2008). Nevertheless, this is also a field which has been characterized by methodological innovation (e.g. in mark-recapture prevalence studies) and some of these innovations (e.g. rapid assessment techniques) have in fact been driven by a determination to provide timely, policy-relevant research evidence.

Additionally, sociological studies have played an important role in charting the HIV/AIDS epidemic and shaping the new public health services that grew up in response to that epidemic. There are surely some grounds for quiet congratulation among researchers who have demonstrated that demonized drug users, whom many (public and pundits) thought incapable of behaviour change, have made substantial reductions in risk behaviour and greatly slowed HIV epidemic spread.

REFERENCES

Adler, P. (1993) *Wheeling and Dealing: an Ethnography of an Upper-level Drug Dealing and Smuggling Community*. New York: Columbia University Press (2nd revised edition).

Amato, L., Davoli, M., Perucci, C.A., Ferri, M., Faggiano, F. and Mattick, R.P. (2005) An overview of systematic reviews of the effectiveness of opiate maintenance therapies: available evidence to inform clinical practice and research. *Journal of Substance Abuse Treatment*, 28: 321–329.

Ashton, M. (2003) The American STAR comes to England. *Drug and Alcohol Findings*, 8: 21–26.

Atkinson, P., Coffey, A., Delamont, S., Lofland, J. and Lofland, L. (2001) *Handbook of Ethnography*. London & Thousand Oaks, CA: SAGE.

Bean, P. and Nemitz, T. (2004) Introduction: drug treatment: what works? In P. Bean and T. Nemitz (eds) *Drug Treatment: What Works?* Oxford: Routledge.

Becker, H. (1953) Becoming a marijuana user. *American Journal of Sociology*, 59: 232–242.

Berridge, V. and Strong, P. (1993) *AIDS and Contemporary History*. Cambridge: Cambridge University Press.

Best, D., Beswick, T., Gossop, M., Rees, S., Coomber, R., Witton, J., et al. (2004) From the deal to the needle; drug purchasing and preparation among heroin users in drug treatment in South London. *Addiction Research and Theory*, 12: 539–548.

Bloor, M. (1995) *The Sociology of HIV Transmission*. London: SAGE.

Bloor, M. (2005) Population estimation without censuses or surveys: a discussion of mark-recapture methods illustrated by results from three studies. *Sociology*, 39: 121–138.

Bloor, M., McKeganey, N. and Fonkert, D. (1988) *One Foot in Eden, a Sociological Study of the Range of Therapeutic Community Practice*. London: Routledge.

Bloor, M., Frischer, M., Taylor, A., Covell, R., Goldberg, D., Green, S., et al. (1994) Tideline and turn? Possible reasons for the continuing low HIV prevalence among Glasgow's injecting drug users. *The Sociological Review*, 42: 738–757.

Bloor, M., Monaghan, L., Dobash, R.P. and Dobash R.E. (1998) The body as a chemistry experiment: steroid use among South Wales bodybuilders. In S. Nettleton and J. Watson (eds) *The Body in Everyday Life*. London: Routledge. pp. 27–44.

Bloor M., McIntosh, J., McKeganey, N. and Robertson, M. (2008a) Topping up methadone: an analysis of patterns of heroin use among a treatment sample of Scottish drug users. *Public Health*, doi: 10.1016/j.puhe.2008.01.007.

Bloor, M., Robertson, M., McKeganey, N. and Neale, J. (2008b) Theorising equipment-sharing in a treatment cohort of Scottish drug users. *Health, Risk and Society*, 10: 599-607, doi: 10.1080/13698570802533697.

Bourgois, P. and Moss, A. (2004) The everyday violence of hepatitis C among young women who inject drugs in San Francisco. *Human Organization*, 63: 253–264.

Burke, B. and Arkowitz, L. (2003) The efficacy of motivational interviewing: a meta-anlaysis of controlled clinical trials, *Journal of Consulting and Clinical Psychology*, 71: 843–861

Coomber, R. (2004) Editorial: Drug use and drug market intersections. *Addiction Research and Theory*, 12: 501–505.

Cox, G., Comiskey, C., Kelly, P. and Cronly, J. (2006) *Research Outcome Study in Ireland: Findings I.* Dublin: National Advisory Committee on Drugs.

Cuijpers, P. (2003) Three decades of drug prevention research. *Drugs: Education, Prevention and Policy*, 10: 7–20.

Curran, V. and Drummond, C. (2005) Psychological treatment of substance misuse and dependence. Available at:http://www.foresight.gov.uk/Brain_Science_Addiction_and_Drugs/Reports_and_Publications/ScienceReviews/Psychological%20Treatments.pdf, *Foresight Brain Science, Addiction and Drugs Project*, Office of Science and Technology, Department of Trade and Industry, UK (accessed 14 August, 2008).

Donoghoe, M., Stimson, G., Dolan, K. and Alldritt, L. (1989) Changes in HIV risk behaviour in clients of syringe exchange schemes in England and Scotland. *AIDS*, 3: 267–272.

Duffy, M., Schaefer, N., Coomber, R., O'Connell, L. and Turnbull, P. (2008) *Cannabis Supply and Young People*. York: Joseph Rowntree Foundation.

Elliot, L. (1998) Ten years of needle exchange provision, but do they work? In M. Bloor and F. Wood (eds) *Addictions and Problem Drug Use*. London: Jessica Kingsley.

Farrell, M., Ward, J. and Mattick, R. (1994) Methadone maintenance treatment in opiate dependence: a review. *British Medical Journal*, 309: 997–1001.

Ferri, M., Daviola, M. and Perruci, C.A. (2006) Heroin maintenance treatment for chronic heroin-dependent individuals: A Cochrane systematic review of effectiveness. *Journal of Substance Abuse Treatment*, 30: 63–72.

Fiorentine, R. and Hillhouse, M. (2000) Drug treatment and 12 step program participation. The additive effects of integrated recovery activities. *Journal of Substance Abuse Treatment*, 18: 65–74.

Flay, B. (2000) Approaches to substance use prevention utilising school curriculum plus social environment change. *Addictive Behaviors*, 25: 861–885.

Fonkert, D. (1978) *Reality construction in a therapeutic community for ex-drug addicts*. The Hague: doctoral dissertation.

Goffman, E. (1968) *Asylums*. Harmondsworth: Penguin.

Gore, S., Bird, G., Burns, S., Goldberg, D., Ross, A. and MacGregor, J. (1995) Drug injection and HIV prevalence in inmates of Glenochil prison. *British Medical Journal*, 310: 293–296.

Gossop, M., Marsden, J., Stewart, D. and Rolfe, A. (1999) Treatment retention and 1 year outcomes for residential programmes in England. *Drug and Alcohol Dependence*, 57: 89–98.

Gossop, M., Marsden, J., Stewart, D. and Treacy, S. (2001) Outcomes after methadone maintenance and methadone reduction treatments: two year follow-up results from the National Treatment Outcome Research Study. *Drug and Alcohol Dependence*, 62: 255–64.

Gossop, M., Marsden, J. and Stewart, D. (2003) *NTORS After Five Years*. London: National Addiction Centre.

Granfield, R. and Cloud, W. (2001) Social context and natural recovery: the role of social capital in the resolution of drug-associated problems. *Substance Use and* Misuse, 36: 1543–1570.

Harden, A., Weston, R. and Oakley, A. (1999) *A Review of the Effectiveness and Appropriateness of Peer-delivered Health Promotion Interventions for Young People*. London: EPPI-Centre.

Hay, G., Gannon, M., McKeganey, N., Hutchinson, S. and Goldberg, D. (2005) *Estimating the National and Local Prevalence of Problem Drug Misuse in Scotland*. http://www.drugmisuse. isdscotland.org (accessed 14 August, 2008).

Heimer, R., Bray, S., Burris, S., Khoshnood, K. and Blankenship, K. (2002) Structural interventions to improve opiate maintenance. *International Journal of Drug Policy*, 13: 103–111.

Hodges, C-L., Paterson, S., Taikato, M., McGarrol, S., Crome, I. and Baldacchino, A. (2006) *Co-Morbid Mental Health and Substance Misuse in Scotland*. Scottish Executive Substance Misuse Research Programme. Edinburgh: Scottish Government.

Home Office (2008) Drugs: protecting families and communities. *The 2008 Drug Strategy*. London: Home Office.

Howard, J. and Borges, P. (1970) Needle-sharing in the Haight: some social and psychological functions. *Journal of Health and Social Behavior*, 11: 220–230.

Hubbard, R., Marsden, M., Rachal, I., Harwood H., Cavanaugh, E. and Ginzburg, H. (1989) *Drug Abuse Treatment: a National Study of Effectiveness*. London: Chapel Hill.

Hser, Y.-I., Anglin, M.D. and Fletcher, B. (1998) Comparative treatment effectiveness: Effects of program modality and clinet drug dependence history on drug use reduction. *Journal of Substance Abuse Treatment*, 15: 513–523.

Hser, Y.-I., Anglin, M., Grella, C., Longshore, D. and Prendergast, M. (1997) Drug treatment careers: A conceptual framework and existing research findings. *Journal of Substance Abuse Treatment*, 14: 543–558.

Joseph J., Montgomery, S., Emmons, C. et al. (1987) Perceived risk of AIDS: assessing the behavioural and psychosocial consequences in a cohort of gay men. *Journal of Applied Social Psychology*, 17: 321–350.

King, L. (1997) Drug content of powders and other illicit drug preparations in the UK. *Forensic Science*, 85: 135–147.

MacAndrew, C. and Edgerton, R. (1970) *Drunken Comportment: a Social Explanation*. New York: Thomas Nelson & Sons.

McGrath, Y., Sumnall, H., Edmonds, K., McVeigh, J. and Bellis, M. (2006) *Review of Grey Literature on Drug Prevention Among Young People*. London: National Institute for Health and Clinical Excellence.

McIntosh, J., Bloor, M. and Robertson, M. (2007) The effect of drug treatment upon the commission of acquisitive crime. *Journal of Substance Use*, 12: 375–384.

McKeganey, N., Bloor, M., Robertson, M., Neale, J. and MacDougall, J. (2006) Abstinence and drug abuse treatment: results from the Drug Outcome Research in Scotland study. *Drugs: Education, Prevention and Policy*, 13: 537–550.

McKeganey, N., Bloor, M., McIntosh, J. and Neale J. (2008) *Key Findings from the Drug Outcome Research in Scotland (DORIS) study*. Glasgow: Centre for Drug Misuse Research Occasional Paper. www.gla.ac.uk/media/media_101969_en.pdf.

McLelland, T., McKay, J., Forman, R. et al. (2005) Reconsidering the evaluation of addiction treatment: from retrospective follow-up to concurrent recovery monitoring. *Addiction Research*, 8: 447–458.

Marsch, L. (1998) The efficacy of methadone maintenance interventions in reducing illicit opiate use, HIV risk behaviour and criminality: a meta-analysis. *Addiction*, 93: 515–532.

May, T., Duffy, M., Few, B. and Hough, M. (2005) *Understanding Drug Selling in Communities: Insider or Outsider Trading*. York: Joseph Rowntree Foundation.

McKeganey, N. and Barnard, M. (1992) *AIDS, Drugs and Sexual Risk: Lives in the Balance*. Buckingham: Open University Press.

Neale, J. and Robertson, M. (2005) Recent life problems and non-fatal overdose among heroin users entering treatment. *Addiction*, 100: 168–175.

Neale, J. and Saville, E. (2004) Comparing community and prison-based drug treatments. *Drugs: Education, Prevention and Policy*, 11: 213–228.

Newman, R. and Whitehill, W. (1979) Double blind comparison of methadone and placebo maintenance treatment of narcotic addicts in Hong Kong. *The Lancet*, ii: 485–488.

Orford, J. (2008) Asking the right questions in the right way: the need for a shift in research on psychological treatments for addiction. *Addiction*, 103: 875–885.

Ouimette, P.C., Finney, J.W. and Moos, R. H. (1997) Twelve-step and cognitive-behavioural treatment for drug abuse. A comparison of treatment effectiveness, *Journal of Consulting and Clinical Psychology*, 62: 230–240.

Pelissier, B., Jones, N. and Cadigan, T. (2007) Drug treatment aftercare in the criminal justice system: a systematic review. *Journal of Substance Abuse Treatment*, 32: 311–320.

Petry, N.M. (2006) Contingency management treatments. *The British Journal of Psychiatry*, 189: 97–98.

Preble, E. and Casey, J. (1969) Taking care of business: the heroin user's life on the street. *International Journal of the Addictions*, 4: 1–24.

Rhodes, T., Stimson, G., Fitch, C., Renton, A. and Ball, A. (1999) Rapid assessment, injecting drug use and public health. *The Lancet*, 354: 65–68.

Rhodes, T., Stoneman, A., Hope, V., Hunt, N., Martin, A. and Judd, A. (2005a) Groin injecting in the context of crack cocaine and homelessness: from 'risk boundary' to 'acceptable risk'? *International Journal of Drug Policy*, 17: 164–170.

Rhodes, T., Singer, M., Bourgois, P.,Friedmann, S. and Strathdee, S. (2005b) The social structural production of HIV risk among injecting drug users. *Social Science and Medicine*, 61: 1026–1044.

Robins, L.N., Davis, D.H. and Goodwin, D.W. (1974) Drug use by US Army enlisted men in Vietnam: A follow-up on their return home. *American Journal of Epidemiology*, 99: 235–249.

Royal College of Physicians of Edinburgh (2004) Consensus Statement on Hepatitis C. *Journal of Viral Hepatitis*, 11 (suppl.): 2–4.

Royal College of Psychiatrists and the Royal College of Physicians (2000) *Drugs: Dilemmas and Choices*. London: Gaskell.

Saunders, B., Wilkinson, C. and Phillips, M. (1995) The impact of a brief motivational intervention with opiate users attending a methadone programme. *Addiction*, 90: 415–424.

Seivewright, N. (2000) *Community Treatment of Drug Misuse: More than Methadone*. Cambridge: Cambridge University Press.

Semaan, S., Des Jarlais, D.C., Sogolow, E., Johnson, W.D. Hedges, L.V., Ramirez, G., Flores, S.A., Norman, L., Sweat, M.D. and Needle, R. (2002) A meta-analysis of the effect of HIV prevention interventions on the sex behaviors of drug users in the United States. *Journal of Acquired Immune Deficiency Syndromes*, 30: S73–S93.

Smith, L., Gates, S. and Foxcroft, D. (2007) Therapeutic communities for substance related disorder (systematic review). *Cochrane Database for Systematic Reviews*, p. 2.

Sorensen, J.L. and Copeland, A.L. (2000) Drug abuse treatment as an HIV prevention strategy. *Drug and Alcohol Dependence*, 59: 17–31.

Spoth, R., Redmond, C., Trudeau, L. and Shin, C. (2002) Longitudinal substance initiation outcomes for a universal preventive intervention combining family and school programs. *Psychology of Addictive Behaviors*, 16: 129–134.

Stallwitz, A. and Stöver, H. (2007) The impact of substitution treatment in prisons – a literature review, *International Journal of Drug Policy*, 18: 464–474.

Stimson, G. (1994) *AIDS and Drug Use – Five Years On*, Third Dorothy Black Lecture (London: Charing Cross and Westminster Medical School).

Stimson, G. and Oppenheimer, E. (1982) *Heroin Addiction: Treating and Control*. London: Tavistock.

Strang, J., McCambridge, J., Best , D., Beswick, T., Bearn, J., Rees, S. and Gossop, M. (2003) Loss of tolerance and overdose mortality after inpatient opiate detoxification: follow-up study. *British Medical Journal*, 326: 959–960.

Sugarman, B. (1974) *Daytop Village, a Therapeutic Community*. New York: Holt, Rinehart and Winston.

Taylor, A. et al. (2004) *Examining the Injecting Practices of Injecting Drug Users in Scotland*. Edinburgh: Scottish Executive.

Teeson, M., Havard, A., Ross, J. and Darke, S. (2006) Outcomes after detoxification for heroin dependence: findings from the Australian Treatment Outcome Study (ATOS). *Drug and Alcohol Review*, 25: 241–247.

Tobler, N.S., Roona, M.R., Ochshorn, P., Marshall, D.G., Streke, A.V. and Stackpole, K.M. (2000) School-based adolescent drug prevention programs: 1998 meta-analysis. *The Journal of Primary Prevention*, 20(4): 275–336.

van Ameijden, E. and Coutinho, R. (1998) Maximum impact of HIV prevention measures targeted at injecting drug users. *AIDS*, 12: 625–633.

van den Brink, W., Hendriks, V.M., Blanken, P., Koeter, M.W.J., van Zweiten, B.J. and van Ree, J.M. (2003) Medical prescription of heroin to treatment resistant heroin addicts: two randomised controlled trials. *British Medical Journal*, 327: 310–315.

Vanichseni, S., Sonchai, W., Plangringarm, K., et al. (1989) Second seroprevalence survey among Bangkok's intravenous drug addicts, Paper presented at V International Conference on AIDS, Montreal (abstract T.G.O. 23).

Velleman, R., Mistral, W. and Sanderling, L. (2000) *DPAS Paper 5: Taking the Message Home: Involving Parents in Drugs Prevention*. London: Home Office.

Walker, J. (2001) International experience of drug courts. The Scottish Executive Central Research Unit. Edinburgh: The Stationery Office Bookshop.

White, D. and Pitts, M. (1998) Educating young people about drugs: a systematic review. *Addiction*, 93: 1475–1487.

Wilson, D.B., Mitchell, O. and MacKenzie, D.L. (2006) A Systematic Review of Drug Court Effects on Recidivism. *Journal of Experimental Criminology,* 2: 459–487.

Winick, C. (1962) Maturing out of narcotic addiction. *Bulletin on Narcotics,* 14: 1–7.

Wright, N., Sheard, L., Tompkins, C., Adams, C., Allgar, V. and Oldham, N. (2007) Buprenorphine versus dihydrocodeine for opiate detoxification in primary care: a randomized controlled trial. *BMC Family Practice*, 8: 3.

Yablonsky, L. (1965) *The Tunnel Back*. New York: Macmillan.

18

Social Aspects of Psychotropic Medication

David Pilgrim, Anne Rogers
and Jonathan Gabe

INTRODUCTION

Drugs that affect mood, thinking and behaviour ('psychotropic' or 'psychoactive' substances) are peculiar for a number of reasons. They have been threaded through many social relationships, which lay beyond healing rituals. Whereas self-medication for a range of maladies has been evident throughout history and across societies, psychotropic substances have been prevalent in social interactions, outside of those concerned with the remediation of sickness. This point is evident in religious rituals and festivals (e.g. wine in Christianity and cannabis in Rastafarianism), recreational scenarios, rites of passage and celebrations of births, deaths and marriages, when alcohol and tobacco are shared habitually as part of social bonding. This recreational and social role of psychotropic drugs is only loosely connected to healing, in so far as they are used to boost happiness and at times drown sorrows.

Another peculiarity of psychotropic drugs is that, more than others, their role has been dichotomized as a result of governmental and medical strictures about the legitimacy of their use. For example, opiates are used both medicinally (legitimately) and are self-administered to induce enjoyable sedation (illegitimately). In the USA, this dichotomy has been reflected in two separate semantic forms to describe the same pharmacological agent ('analgesics' or 'narcotics').

Also, more than any other type of drug in medicine, they have been used for their generic rather than specific impact on individual functioning. Psychotropic drugs typically have a 'blunderbuss' impact on the nervous system, with a wide range of effects on cardio-vascular functioning, digestion, sexual potency, mood, cognition, perception, judgement and behavioural competence. This generic impact has created the socio-political possibility that they can be used as forms of imposed coercive social control. For example, they can be used to tranquillize and thus de-motivate deviance and nuisance in a range of settings from prisons and psychiatric hospitals to residential settings for older people or those with learning disabilities. They have even been used to suppress political dissidence and have even played a role in interrogation techniques. For example, in the old USSR, major tranquillisers were forced upon dissidents in psychiatric facilities (Bloch and Reddaway, 1977). Also in the USA the prospect of using psychiatric drugs to induce confessions in police interrogations began to be publicized after the Second World War (Gerson and Victoroff, 1948). Although the potential of 'truth drugs', such as sodium amytal was largely undemonstrated, the aspiration reflects the wide expected utility of these agents. A variant of this aspiration was inside psychiatry, in the same period, when a range of agents were experimented with in attempts at 'narco-analysis' (Houston, 1952).

Thus, whilst all forms of medication play a part in social regulation, by expediting recovery to normal functioning in voluntary patients, only psychotropic medication has a reputation for its role in coercive and non-medical state interventions. Given this common socio-political reputation of prescribed psychotropic medication, the role of the medical profession in its promotion and regulation in society has been more controversial than other medical interventions (Breggin, 1993; Fisher and Greenberg, 1997).

To illustrate the implications of the above initial arguments, the remainder of this chapter deals with the two main wings of the putative 'pharmacological revolution' of the 1950s and its wake. The first case study examines the chemical management of madness and the second turns to the treatment of misery in primary care.

MANAGING MADNESS: THE ROLE OF THE MAJOR TRANQUILLISERS

Until the 1950s most psychotic patients were warehoused semi-permanently in large mental hospitals. In many (but not all) developed countries, this pattern then began to change. More and more patients were discharged or became 'revolving door' patients. At the centre of this development was a claim that new drugs tempered or even eliminated the symptoms of psychotic patients and thus enabled them to live more of the time outside of hospital care.

Major tranquillizers (also known as 'anti-psychotics' and 'neuroleptics') were introduced in the 1950s and initially given in relatively low doses. However, during subsequent decades, average dose levels were increased by prescribing psychiatrists and adverse iatrogenic effects became more and more evident (see below).

The pharmacological revolution and decarceration

The putative 'pharmacological revolution' has remained a potent professional myth within medicine. For example, in his uncritical public relations account of the linear and unstoppable 'march' of psychiatric progress, Stone (1997) tells us this about the 1950s:

> Amazingly, in this one decade drugs became available for the relief of symptoms associated with schizophrenia, depression (especially of the 'endogenous' inherited type), mania and anxiety disorders. (Stone, 1997: 190)

Similarly, Gelder et al. argued at the turn of this century (after nearly 50 years to fairly appraise the legitimacy of the 'revolution') in a standard psychiatric textbook that:

> The introduction of chlorpromazine in 1952 made it easier to manage disturbed behaviour, and therefore easier to open wards that had been locked, to engage patients in social activities, and to discharge some of them into the community. (Gelder et al., 2001: 769)

This linking of medication with an enabling account of deinstitutionalization generates both theoretical and empirical difficulties. For example, it cannot explain why community care policies were applied to a range of care groups, such as people with learning disabilities and older people, who are not psychotic. These patients at first were not prescribed major tranquillizers, though as we noted earlier, the drugs were introduced increasingly thereafter to control disruptive, agitated or aggressive behaviour in these non-psychotic individuals.

More importantly, in some countries there was an increased pattern of discharge *prior* to the widespread use of major tranquillizers (Rogers and Pilgrim, 2005). Nor did the introduction of psychotropic drugs appear to accelerate the rate of discharge. The pattern of deinstitutionalization continued in line with that preceding the widespread use of these drugs. Moreover, in a few countries, inpatient numbers actually *increased* after the introduction of chlorpromazine in 1952, see Table 18.1. As Scull (1977) noted the data may have led to erroneous interpretations being made, since they masked '. . . earlier changes at the local level and obscure(d) the degree to which the fall in overall numbers, when it did come, represent(ed) a continuation rather than a departure from pre-existing trends'.

Other analyses of data sources indicate that organizational factors and social policy initiatives were responsible for changes in the location of psychiatric practice (Rogers and Pilgrim, 2005). Table 18.1 shows the growth in the number of psychiatric beds in a number of European countries post-Second World War, which ran counter to the run-down in the UK and the USA. While the type of increased bed use varied from one country to another (in some it was short-term beds, in others new specialist facilities) the point is that in-patient care increased during a time when the major tranquillizers were widely and increasingly utilized.

Table 18.1   Post-war growth of psychiatric beds in Europe

Country	Year	No. psychiatric beds
Belgium	1951	19,841
	1970	26,553
Austria	1950	9,868
	1975	14,314
Italy	1954	88,241
	1961	113,040
Spain	1949	25,571
	1974	42,493
Federal German Republic	1953	86,640
	1975	112,791

Source: Adapted from World Health Organization Statistics Annuals

Magic bullets for madness?

The language used by the drug companies and psychiatry about the major tranquil-lizers contributed to a scientific rhetoric of technical competence. For example, although they only helped some patients some of the time in reducing reports of auditory hallucinations and confused or confusing speech ('thought disorder'), the term 'anti-psychotic' implied some form of magic bullet that consistently targeted and eliminated symptoms. Unlike the diabetic receiving insulin, whose blood sugar could be normalized predictably by tailored amounts of a prescribed agent, this was not the case with psychiatric drugs. They were in practice 'hit and miss' interventions. Rather than concede this as a treatment failure, patients unresponsive to treatment were then further pathologized and became 'treatment resistant'.

A practical challenge facing psychiatry, when emphasizing the biological sources and implied medicinal rectification of madness, was that they only had a hammer so then everything became a nail. When symptoms persisted the hammer was made bigger and more blows applied, with serious iatrogenic consequences. For example, estimates of the prevalence of tardive dyskinesia (i.e. disfiguring movements such as facial ticks and jerking limbs) in those prescribed major tran-quillizers vary from 0.5 per cent to 50 per cent with a mean of 20 per cent (Brown and Funk, 1986). The probability of the iatrogenic effect occurring increases the longer that the drug is prescribed, the larger the dose and the more other drugs are given in a 'cocktail' (technically called 'polypharmacy') (Hemmenki, 1977; Warner, 1985). When larger doses are given ('megadosing') fatalities are also risked, warranting the invention of a new diagnosis for iatrogenic death – the 'neuroleptic malignant syndrome' (Kellam, 1987). Also, the risk of suicide increases when these drugs are initially administered, as they may cause a sudden drop of mood ('acute dysphoria') in some patients.

Brown and Funk (1986) traced how the evidence about tardive dyskinesia was available to psychiatrists in the late 1960s. However, throughout the 1970s and 1980s major tranquillizer prescription rates were undiminished (they actually increased in frequency and in dose levels). Brown and Funk note that two theories (labelling and professional dominance) have some merit in accounting for this professional resistance to change. Both acknowledge the importance of the powerless social position of patients. Labelling theory suggests that the powerless position and low social status of psychiatric patients renders them both unimportant and invisible. As a result, the patients' psychiatrists do not take their complaints about 'side effects' seriously.

The professional dominance theory focuses on the relationship between the status of psychiatry as a medical specialty and the role of physical treatment. Brown and Funk endorse a similar picture, with psychiatry tying itself to physical medicine and its attendant biological trappings to enhance its professional standing. Given this preoccupation with professional status, unfortunate consequences of biological treatment (like tardive dyskinesia) may be ignored, denied or rationalized by clinicians. According to this theory, the needs of patients are ignored in favour of the political needs of their treating psychiatrists. A study of psychiatrists' and recipient views of major tranquillizers showed that both groups concur on the risks and 'bothersomeness' of side effects. However, 'psychiatrists saw side-effects as significantly less bothersome than symptoms when considering costs to society' (Finn et al., 1990: 843). More recently, studies have established that psychiatrists are much less likely than patients to acknowledge the side effects of sedation and mental clouding caused by anti-psychotic medication and the distress caused (National Schizophrenia Fellowship, 2001; Smith and Henderson, 2000). And patients may feel they have 'not been told enough' about these side effects even where psychiatrists claim to favour a patient centred approach. This may be in part because of the asymmetrical distribution of medical expertise, which enables doctors to remain relatively free from challenges when they issue judgements about these side effects (Seale et al., 2007).

It is, perhaps, not surprising that patients who experience the adverse effects of major tranquillizers are often reluctant to comply with the regimen. In its depot form (regular injections of a slow release type of the drug) this type of medication results in an even more disempowered perception of the treatment process (Kilian et al., 2003). What is, perhaps, more surprising is that given the range and severity of adverse effects, non-adherence rates for major tranquillizers are the same as for other types of non-psychiatric medication. However, satisfaction with the drugs is also important to note. In a recent community survey of patient views about drug compliance, Moritz et al. (2009) found that only 9 per cent of patients complied *and* reported no adverse effects *and* welcomed the therapeutic value of anti-psychotic medication. This suggests that over 90 per cent of patients are not happy with these drugs.

The problems associated with traditional major tranquillizers seem to apply less to a new generation of drugs, dubbed the 'new antipsychotics'. These are more efficient at symptom reduction and are less liable to create movement disorders in patients. However, there is the risk of life-threatening blood disorders with some versions of the new anti-psychotics. In fact what seemed to be a new and better drug regime turns out to have different but equally if not more problematic unwanted side-effects than the drugs they sought to replace. Consequently, their cost-effectiveness (compared to the older agents) is now in doubt (Lieberman, et al., 2005).

The sociological significance of the prescribing of and compliance with anti-psychotics extends beyond the issue of the adverse effects and practices of the profession of psychiatry. Psychiatric patients' 'non-compliance' with medication has emerged as a significant social problem. Images of deinstitutionalization, often promoted via the mass media, have become synonymous with the occurrence of socially unacceptable behaviour by ex-psychiatric patients living in the community.

Within this oft-publicized scenario, medication has been depicted as a valid means of managing and controlling people who are viewed as a potential threat to the social order. Compliance with these drugs has come to be seen as an indicator of the success or failure of 'care in the community'. Depot medication was marketed uniquely as a means of ensuring compliance, without the need for consent to treatment or adherence to daily pill taking. Professionals, politicians and relatives' groups, who all emphasize the importance of treatment compliance for discharged patients, have simply assumed the reliable effectiveness of neuroleptics. This has even extended to legal powers to enforce medication compliance in community-based patients (community treatment orders) (Dennis and Monahan, 1996). However, this taken for granted assumption from those keen to contain madness by the singular enforcement of medication compliance has been challenged strongly by their critics. For example, Cohen (1997) points out that:

- two thirds of medicated patients eventually relapse;
- the chronic use of the drugs often diminishes social functioning;
- researchers have given relatively little attention to user experiences of the drugs.

Cohen concludes that '... the overall usefulness (of antipsychotics) in the treatment of schizophrenia . . . is far from established' (p. 195); and in the light of the conclusion of Finn et al. (1990) noted above, the question begged is 'usefulness for whom?'

Two large, non-commercial clinical trials comparing old and new ('atypical') drugs for people with a diagnosis of chronic schizophrenia, in the USA and UK, showed that both performed the same in symptom reduction (Lewis and Leiberman, 2008). Despite this outcome, professionals, politicians and the relatives of psychiatric patients remain wedded to the importance of their use with all patients at all times, with the implication that 'treatment compliance' leads to predictable behavioural outcomes for all recipients.

These drugs have been viewed as the principal means of preventing 'the revolving-door patient' phenomenon. They are a central plank of 'assertive outreach', case management, supervised discharge and the overall management of those with 'a severe and enduring mental illness'. However, given their hit and miss reputation, the drugs have been the focus of criticism from campaigning and mental health user organizations.

Policy makers are now faced with balancing the need to maintain medication adherence with the risks of clinical iatrogenesis (Rogers and Pilgrim, 1996). This dilemma has become increasingly difficult for policy makers to manage in a cultural context of high sensitivity to risk, the emergence of a consumerist philosophy within the health service, and the growing acceptance of the legitimacy of lay perceptions and assessment of medicine within modern health care systems. Major tranquillizers have been relied upon to reduce risky behaviour in all patients (and have failed in this intention). At the same time they have posed severe iatrogenic risks to the patients receiving them, even when the latter have relapsed while using them or have proved to be 'treatment resistant'. Thus these drugs satisfy neither those receiving them nor third parties, who expect them to suppress troublesome or risky conduct.

MEDICAL RESPONSES TO COMMON MISERY: ANXIOLYTICS AND ANTIDEPRESSANTS

In developed countries, the great majority of patients with mental health problems are managed in primary care (usually over 90 per cent). Most of these are never referred to specialist mental health services and even those who are, for much of their lives, are seen by primary care professionals (since deinstitutionalization). For those with so-called 'common mental disorders' the first and sometimes *only* offer of help has been a range of drugs which seek to tranquillize patients or raise their mood. At first glance, there have been two obvious groups of disorder, which have been treated by different pharmacological agents: anxiolytics and antidepressants. These have been prescribed by general practitioners (GPs) for those formally diagnosed respectively with 'anxiety disorders' or 'depression' (see Chew-Graham, this handbook).

This seemingly practical alignment between a diagnosis and its treatment is specious for two reasons. First, many patients present with mixed symptoms of anxiety and depression leading some psychiatrists to argue for a single diagnosis of common neurotic misery (Tyrer, 1990). Second, even when patients are separated diagnostically, they may still be prescribed the 'drug of choice' for another category. For example, anxiety is often treated in primary care with the use of low dose antidepressants (and occasionally even low dose major tranquillizers). This lack of treatment specificity for particular diagnosed conditions is consistent with the point made earlier about the undifferentiated 'blunderbuss' impact of psychotropic drugs on the nervous system. A lack of treatment specificity has been one of several grounds for querying the legitimacy of functional psychiatric diagnoses (Bentall, et al., 1988; Pilgrim and Bentall, 1999).

One way of analysing the use of these drugs is to focus on the societal level and consider a synergy of interests, which in turn has provoked opposition from other communities of interest. From this standpoint, certain groups of social actors are relentlessly driving the promotion and utilization of psychotropic agents for common misery. These include: the pharmaceutical industry (and its internally competing companies); the medical profession (especially psychiatrists and GPs); the advertising industry; and finally complicit patients, who submit their personal dilemmas and distress to a process of medicalization and simply assume or accept that they are ill (Koumjian, 1981). In the latter regard, people with real enough social-existential problems in life are thereby turned into patients (Dowrick, 2004). DeSwaan (1990) similarly talks of personal troubles being turned into medical problems.

At a micro level, however, we may find a more nuanced picture with both patients and doctors expressing ambivalence, at best, about the use of mood-altering drugs and patients at times self-regulating their use rather than being dominated and controlled by clinicians. Both these levels of analysis will be considered below, focusing initially on the societal level.

The rise and fall of barbiturates and amphetamines

Before the putative 'pharmacological revolution' of the 1950s, physicians had a couple of drug options for common distress, both of which were to fall into a state of disgrace. These drugs crudely sedated (barbiturates) or energized (amphetamines) the unhappy patient. Although we now associate amphetamines with recreational youth culture, they were promoted originally as a medicinal antidepressant and arguably the first of the latter category (Rasmussen, 2006). Both types of drug produced physical dependency and tolerance, which meant that dose levels had to be raised to maintain the psychotropic impact and that withdrawal provoked a distressing rebound effect of distressing symptoms. In the case of barbiturates, they were lethal in overdose, with deaths accruing accidentally, when sleepy patients took more than they needed accidentally, and if depressed patients used them deliberately for suicide. In the case of amphetamines psychotic breakdown emerged in some patients.

By 1951 concerns about these problems in the USA, prompted the Food and Drug Administration to limit their outlet to physician prescription only. Until this point, there had been a clear demarcation between those addicted to illegal 'narcotics', who were deemed to have defective personalities and decent, deserving unhappy patients, who could be treated effectively by medical paternalism.

However, these prescribed drugs and their iatrogenic toll began to introduce ambiguity about addiction. Supposing that it was not simply a matter of feckless personalities who had to be controlled by law enforcement about the use of 'narcotics'; what if medical paternalism and drug company marketing were creating addiction in innocent victims? This sort of question attended professional debates, at the very time that therapeutic optimism was being aroused and expected by the 'pharmacological revolution'. Moreover, the neat impermeable boundary between reckless users of 'narcotics' and sufferers of 'common mental disorders', prescribed 'medication' in paternalistic medical consultations, broke down completely in 1955, when the two types of drug were politically elided in the US Congress proceedings about drug abuse – *Traffic in, and Control of, Narcotics, Barbiturates and Amphetamines* (U.S. House, 1955).

The case of barbiturates also highlighted a further breakdown of common interest between the medical profession and the drug companies. The latter then, as now, funded research and development, drug marketing and educational events. All of this generated financial and other inducements to the medical profession, as well as providing packaged information and guidance about prescribing practices. However, the scale of the iatrogenic problem created by the barbiturates meant that the alliance broke down when medical researchers, previously committed to pharmaceutical advancement, inevitably had to acknowledge that the drugs were effectively as addictive as heroin. This ambivalence on the part of medical researchers and prescribers, who were financially advantaged by drug company inducements, was to become increasingly evident. However, by and large, the response of the profession was not to abandon drug solutions for medicalized distress but instead to seek out safer and more effective alternatives.

A final point of relevance to the problem of addiction to barbiturates and amphetamines was that ambiguity suddenly emerged about whether psychiatrists were experts in creating or curing substance abuse. During the 1930s a small sub-speciality of psychiatry had emerged to deal with addiction to opiates and alcohol. 'Substance abuse' was from thereon framed as a psychiatric condition; a mental disorder now appearing in the Diagnostic and Statistical Manual of the American Psychiatric Association (1994) and the International Classification of Diseases of the World Health Organization (1992). Thus a paradoxical scenario had emerged: psychiatrists were *both* experts on *and* the source of chemical addiction.

From Miltown to Prozac

The above subtitle opens Herzberg's (2009) historical examination of what he calls 'happy pills in America'. In this account interest group synergy (of doctors, advertisers, the drug companies and submissive patients) seems to be apparent at every turn. The breakdown noted above in the distinction between 'narcotics' and 'medication' reflected a number of social divisions. The first was about class and race: street heroin and marihuana were the 'narcotics' of the underclass, particularly in black ghettoes. This left white middle class patients in a legitimate and legal space under the protective wisdom of medical paternalism.

If 'narcotics' numbed the distress of oppression under capitalist relations at the bottom of the socio-economic pyramid, the stresses of surviving and conforming to the work and gender role expectations of middle class life could be ameliorated by pharmacological solutions. The latter came in the form of several generations of anxiolytics and antidepressants. This was both an enormous marketing opportunity for the pharmaceutical industry and a springboard for the psychiatric profession to extend its jurisdiction from madness to common misery and to raise its status as a true medical discipline. Profit and professionalization thus converged to promote the promise of peace of mind for the anguished white collar husband and his unhappy housewife (made famous in popular lyrics as 'mother's little helper' by the Rolling Stones in the 1960s).

During the 1950s and 1960s the drug companies altered their narrative about both 'stress' and the role expectations of husbands and wives in their marketing campaigns. The framing of 'stress' now shifted from the intra-psychic emphasis of the dynamic unconscious found in psychoanalysis to the tension between the primitive hindbrain and the developed forebrain of modern man.

Stress could now be framed as a neurochemical condition and so bio-medical authority could be claimed when physicians prescribed their psychotropic solutions to problems of living. Modern man retained his true primitive cave man brain but now had to manage the stressful challenge of expressing the finer inter-personal skills of being an office worker; this involved his developed forebrain. North American men were thus presented as red-blooded heterosexuals struggling with modern demands on their true nature. Herzberg (ibid.: 71) reproduces an advertisement for *Librium* in 1969 in the *Journal of the American Medical Association*. It shows a lion-skinned caveman looking into the jungle and alongside a be-suited office worker looking into the jungle of the modern life.

From the outset the 'minor tranquillizers' were consumed more by women than men (Ettorre and Riska, 1995). Also the masculine heterosexual ideal of the robust worker content with his lot under capitalism (but threatened by effete post-war conditions and communism, so risking a 'crisis of masculinity') posed a challenge for the drug companies and the advertising agencies they employed. In order to retain his masculinity, modern man arguably needed energizing not tranquillizing. Thus it took over a decade for this marketing challenge to be resolved by the formula just noted in the *Librium* advertisement. The danger was that if the new tranquillizers were to become a female only market, then half the population would be lost as a potential source of profit.

Women attended primary care more often than men and they adhered to (mainly male) medical ministrations. Herzberg (ibid.: 75) reproduces an advertisement for Meprospan from the *Journal of American Medical Association* in 1960. It has six captions:

1   Calm male doctor in white coat, behind his desk, listens to symptoms of housewife with a sad face and her head bowed in despair.
2   'The patient takes one' – housewife putting pill to mouth at home.
3   Housewife alert and engrossed in the label of a food can in a supermarket.
4   Housewife takes another pill at dinner table with happy family around her.
5   'Relieved, alert, attentive' – housewife sits smiling, while listening carefully to parent teacher association proposals.
6   'Peacefully asleep' – housewife in bed 'undisturbed by nervousness or tension'.

In this first phase of the 'pharmacological revolution', it therefore seems that social divisions were maintained ideologically by the promotion of drugs for common misery in two ways. The first related to class and race, by splitting off illegitimate drug use, and the trade in 'narcotics' in the ghetto, from the physician's consulting room and its 'medication' for unhappiness further up the social scale. The second, related to the role of the drugs in maintaining gendered roles. The drug companies, advertising agencies and the medical profession all gained financially and in status from this promotion of putative chemical cures for everyday distress. They shared and sustained a biomedical view about the aetiology of that misery (rooted in brain chemistry). On this view, unhappy people were turned into patients, who thereby provided both industrial profit and professional legitimacy for medicine.

The challenge to biomedical legitimacy

Two major problems emerged in relation to the above picture. The first was that medicine's own rhetoric, combined assertions about biological aetiology (a form of 'hoped-for-reductionism' common in Western psychiatry since the nineteenth century) with evidence about treatment efficacy. Uncertainty about aetiology, then as now, was tolerated by many communities of interest, including patients, *provided* that medical interventions proved to be safe and effective.

Despite repeated drug promotion campaigns, arguing that psychotropic agents were safe, effective and lacking in iatrogenic effects, medicine eventually was hoisted by its own petard; the test of research evidence. The latter began to show that these drugs were not always effective in reducing symptoms. Moreover, adverse effects (commonly and misleadingly called 'side-effects', as if they are minor and inconsequential) and tolerance were increasingly evident, as was the problem of withdrawal (Gabe and Bury, 1988). Thus, these 'non-dependency-inducing' drugs were not what they had appeared. Though safer than the barbiturates, they could still kill in overdose.

With hindsight, the advertising of these drugs involved excessive claims; that they created *selective* tranquillization for the patient, enabling him or her to sleep restfully and then discharge their gendered parental responsibilities. This was to be achieved without allegedly affecting alertness or concentration during waking hours. But the selective smartness of these drugs was logically and empirically untenable. How could drugs that depress neural activity tranquillize the person in some activities and not others? Why should culturally well-tested drugs, like alcohol, be known to sedate and impair judgements at all times, but these newly synthesized psychotropic agents be immune from the same sort of general intoxication? The new psychotropic drugs were looking just as problematic as their predecessors.

The second problem for this branch of the 'pharmacological revolution' was not about medical evidence but about political critique. Carefully avoiding an over-arching radical analysis of the divided world of underclass junkies and middle class patients (this was in the post-McCarthy era), Friedman's *Feminine Mystique* delivered a plausible attack on the drugs. By focusing on gender, rather than class, she could safely expose the dynamics of post-war heterosexual life and its nuclear family: maybe the gendered roles required for this lifestyle script made competent women capable of matching men in the labour market unhappy with their lot (Friedman, 1963). This first wave feminism suggested that medicine was playing its supportive role in the reproduction of patriarchy, a point which has been restated more recently by second wave feminists, such as Ettorre and Riska (1995).

Business as usual

Given the scientific and political disquiet about minor tranquillizers and antidepressants, expressed during the 1960s, what is striking is that the matrix of interests, involving the pharmaceutical industry, advertising agencies, medical practitioners and grateful patients proved to be highly resilient. For every doubt expressed about the iatrogenic dangers and political conservatism of psychotropic use, there came a breathless claim about a new wonder drug. The same script was written each time: the new drugs were not habit forming, were selective in their beneficial psychological impact and safe to prescribe. One after another false dawn came and went. This created a pattern or cycle of prescribing legitimacy about each drug, as it rose and fell in reputation.

Cohen et al. (2001) point to the way in which a medication life cycle evolves and mutates with social and technological change. The drug companies, the medical profession and patients themselves contribute to these changes. A study by Rogers et al. (2007) suggests that the legitimacy of psychotropic medication, despite its vulnerability to scientific and political attack in the past 50 years, is maintained through separating its legitimate, benign and sacred use from its profane and reckless misuse. Of great importance is the idea that new drugs will displace all of the problems of old drugs. In the light of the analysis of Cohen et al. and Rogers et al. just noted, we now find this sort of dualistic pattern in the discourse of prescribers:

1   New drugs good – old drugs bad;
2   Anxious and sleepless old ladies good – dysfunctional junkies bad;
3   Medically prescribed drugs good – the same drugs used recreationally bad;
4   Current medical practice good – past medical practice bad;
5   Current drug regulation good – past drug regulation bad.

While the problem of benzodiazepine dependence was first noted in the 1960s, it was a full twenty years before popular protest movements, encouraged by mass media reports, stimulated litigation against the drug companies (Lacey, 1991). This was despite the dramatic impact of the withdrawal of one tranquillizer, thalidomide, which created complex birth defects in the early 1960s. As far as the regulation of prescribed drugs was concerned, the administrative arrangements in the UK were not reviewed seriously until a GP (Harold Shipman) proved to be a mass murderer, using lethal doses of diamorphine on his elderly patients.

The role of the mass media in shifting the 'public mood' about benzodiazepines and legitimizing their status as a social problem has been discussed in a number of papers by Gabe and Bury (1988, 1991, 1996a; Bury and Gabe, 1990). These authors also analysed how the claims-making activities of medical experts and mental health pressure groups and the response of the state, together played a crucial role the development of tranquillizers as a social problem (Gabe and Bury, 1988). Subsequently, they employed this approach to explain the decision of the British Licensing Authority in 1991 to suspend the licence for the widely used sleeping tablet *Halcion* (triazolam), noting how legal challenges also played a role in this decision, alongside: claims-making by medical experts; the coverage of the media; and the interests of the state (Gabe and Bury, 1996b; Gabe, 2001).

Focusing on the same controversy about *Halcion*, Abraham and Sheppard (1998) have focused on factors within organizations like the Licensing Authority to provide an alternative explanation to that of Gabe and Bury. These factors included professional interests and the internal organizational arrangements and processes within institutions for reviewing and presenting data. Abraham and Sheppard suggested that these were more important than broader extra-institutional social influences in determining whether or not a drug remains widely available or it is withdrawn from use (cf. Gabe and Bury, 1996). It may well be that both accounts are applicable – it seems likely that social processes at both institutional and societal levels are likely to sway the extent to which drugs are viewed as acceptable by authorizing bodies, the medical profession, the public and the State.

While there has been a significant reduction in the use of benzodiazepine drugs in recent years, a question has arisen about what should replace them as a strategy for managing anxiety-based mental health problems. Moreover, despite criticisms of the drugs, they are still prescribed. They remain a quick and cheap response to complex psycho-social presenting problems in primary care settings (Groenewegen et al., 1999; Johnell et al., 2004; Pelfrene et al., 2004).

Indeed, from the outset, the proponents of psychotropic drugs for 'common mental health problems' have been ambivalent (or 'had it both ways') about their use. Psychotropics were offered as a form of mental health first aid but the existential complexity of the patient's life was still respected. Even the drug companies, with their convenient pseudo-science about neurotransmitters in the suit-wearing cave man, accepted that life was a complicated source of stress (Ross and Pam, 1995). In the US context of the 1950s, where talking treatments were the accepted aspiration for any personal difficulty, they represented a quick and simple offer of symptomatic relief in brief medical consultations (Koegler, 1965).

The working assumption, then as now, was that, in an ideal world, lengthy specialist psychotherapy would be offered, but GP prescribed drugs could bridge the gap created by prevalent need. Indeed, today the complementary rather than competing role of talking and drug treatments for 'common mental health problems' remains a dominant discourse in primary care mental health policy. Now the dilemma for the more socially-aware GP is that they can spot the particular stressors of the social context impinging on their distressed patient but the prescription pad has to be the weak response to their impotence about that context (cf. Dowrick, 2004). Doctors cannot prevent or reverse marital tensions, workplace bullying, job loss or insecurity, the stress of childrearing or the impact of living in a locality of concentrated poverty but they can offer drugs to assuage the psychological pain in their wake.

The contention about the anxiolytics has been paralleled in debates about antidepressants. The latter have been associated with a number of disabling effects, including tiredness, dry mouth, loss of libido and impotence, blurred vision, constipation, weight gain and palpitations. The tricyclic version of this type of drug was implicated in around 10 per cent of deaths from self-poisoning in Britain in the early 1980s. Tricyclics have now been superseded by the selective serotonin reuptake inhibitors (SSRIs), which are less toxic. In older people a decline in suicide has been directly attributable to prescribing this type of antidepressant (Gunnell et al., 2003) However, as these drugs have gradually superseded the tricyclics, they too are now controversial and their utilization queried. This is particularly the case when prescribing them in childhood and adolescence and warnings have been issued regarding the increased risk of suicide-related behaviour (Whittington et al., 2004).

The prescription of antidepressants for a range of psycho-social problems and their associated distress (reduced diagnostically and monolithically to 'clinical depression') (Dowrick, 2004; Pilgrim and Bentall, 1999) has implicated a number of factors. These include patient and professional characteristics, the interaction between them, the type of treatment setting and form of healthcare system. Sleath and Shih (2003) found in the USA that insurance status is influential in determining which type of antidepressant is prescribed. Patients belonging to a health management organization, which had capitated visits, were four times more likely to receive older rather than newer antidepressants.

Initially it was claimed that the SSRIs were not dependency forming and, unlike previous drugs, had a truly targeted, rather than blunderbuss, impact on the nervous system by raising serotonin levels. This good news was promoted by the drug companies and by popular psychiatric accounts. For example, Kramer (1993) argued that, unlike past products, the new wonder drug liberated rather than oppressed women and (yet again) allegedly had no major 'side effects'. By the late 1990s, these were being challenged by many, confirming the pattern of legitimation and de-legitimation of new drugs. *Prozac* and its 'me-too' versions from other companies were going the same way as *Miltown* and *Valium* (Breggin and Breggin, 1995; Healy, 1997; Metzl, 2003).

After 30 years of feminist criticism of psychotropic medication, the pharmaceutical industry modified its depiction of women. They were now 'super-mom' office workers not housewives; though the themes of alertness without sedation and a guaranteed good night's sleep connected these generations of advertisements. Herzberg (ibid.: 183) reproduces a 1998 advertisement for *Prozac* from the medical press, in which a smiling well-dressed and coiffured business woman sits by her computer, then lower down she is sleeping blissfully: women no longer in the kitchen but in the office, thanks to the very latest psychotropic medication.

At the same time, variations in gynaecological functioning became new marketing opportunities. For example, Metzl and Angel (2004) examined an increasing range of female experiences, which have been medicalized by their treatment, with the newer antidepressants, once more pointing up the synergy of interests between the pharmaceutical industry and psychiatric positivism. These reified categories of female psychopathology include 'pre-menopausal dysphoric disorder (PMDD)', 'post-partum depression' and 'peri-menopausal depression'.

It should be noted that, over the years, the pharmaceutical industry has also responded to criticism by broadening the content of drug advertisements and reduced its previous reliance on images of patients, particularly women. Now there are advertisements that employ impersonal imagery such as medical records or tablet bottles or images from nature, such as flowers or lakes (Prather, 1991). Nonetheless, it can be argued that the advertisement of the female patient as the main recipient of mood modifying drugs has informed an indelible image that continues to have consequences for prescribing behaviour.

The meaning of mood modifying drugs to patients and doctors

The argument above has demonstrated that a synergy of interests has played a central role in the promotion and use of psychotropic drugs for common distress. However, evidence at a more micro level suggests that we might need to develop a more nuanced picture that does not see these drugs simply as part of a process of medicalization and social control.

Evidence from studies of patients suggests that their relationship with the drug may be active, weighing up the risks and benefits and level of need, rather than passive, and that it is related to type of medication and pattern of use. Ambivalent attitudes were often reported. For example, a study by Gabe and Lipshitz-Phillips (1984) found that users of benzodiazepines (such as *Valium* and *Librium*) expressed mixed feelings, saying that they were fearful about the risks of dependence and of taking unnatural substances that might harm their body or mind. But they also saw them as potentially beneficial, often alongside various 'fringe' medicines and religions.

Similar ambivalence has been reported in more recent studies. For instance Stephenson (2004) has noted how interviewees in her study of people who had been offered mood modifying medicines were critical of the drugs on the grounds that they were synthetically produced and thus distanced from nature, yet still saw them as necessary. And North et al. (1995) have reported how those in their study who took their medication – mainly hypnotics – intermittently tended to emphasize the negative aspects of benzodiazepine use, such as the risks of dependence. Those who took them regularly for anxiety were more ambivalent about it and entertained trying alternatives to benzodiazepines. They also reported that users claimed that they had considerable autonomy in the use of the drugs and learned to monitor their symptoms and to self medicate.

Various typologies of users' relationship with their drug have been developed. A study by Gabe and Thorogood (1986) found that some benzodiazepine users said they used the drug as a *life-line*, as something they needed to take regularly and depended on simply to keep them going in the face of chronic unresolved problems. Others appeared to see the drug as a *standby*, to be kept in reserve and used occasionally to meet some short-lived crisis, hence keeping dependence at bay. Those who conceived the drug as a life-line were most likely to be long term users, whereas those who saw the drug as a standby were generally short-term users.

Helman (1981) noted three groups of user distinguishable in terms of per-ceived control and perceived site of action. For some benzodiazepines were a *tonic*; these users felt they had maximum control over their drug use and took their tablets episodically. Others saw it as *fuel* which enabled them to function in conformity with social expectations and reported varying degrees of control over its use, and third group saw it as a *food* which they took in order to survive and felt they had little control over its use. Both typologies are useful in drawing attention to the range of users' relationships with their drugs, the main difference being that the latter presents a more positive view, with less emphasis on risk and more on benzodiazepines as nutritional substances.

Studies of doctors have also reported an awareness of the dangers of depen-dence and expressed a range of views about their use. Gabe and Lipshitz-Phillips (1984) reported that the doctors they interviewed expressed mixed feelings about benzodiazepines and stated that prescribing ran counter to their long-term goal of promoting patient autonomy. An Australian study by Parr et al. (2006) reported a range of attitudes with some emphasizing these drugs' usefulness in assisting with acute stressful situations or as a muscle relaxant for pain, while others said they prescribed them reluctantly or not at all. And a recent British study by Rogers et al. (2007) found that the majority of GPs interviewed expressed a sense of responsibility for avoiding the risks associated with past benzodiazepine use, although a few minimized the problem of iatrogenic 'addiction'.

In contrast to the Australian study these GPs seemed to see their role to be to wean people off drugs on which they had come to depend, although they were still willing to prescribe to 'deserving' patients such as chronic users. Nonetheless, Rogers et al. suggest that, overall, the doctors in their study illustrate a cultural shift in the way in which they view the risks associated with these drugs, reflect-ing a greater consciousness of risk than in the past in the current 'risk society'. While GPs might be more forthright about accepting some moral responsibility for past actions it is clear from the above that they have been concerned about the dependence potential of benzodiazepines since the early 1980s.

In sum, at a micro level, we may find a more nuanced picture with both patients and doctors expressing ambivalence at best about the use of mood-altering drugs and patients at times regulating their use rather than being dominated and controlled by clinicians.

DISCUSSION

The above case studies of psychotropic medication have illuminated the complex matrix maintaining and extending its use in specialist mental health services and in primary care. As noted earlier, we can consider any particular aspect of mental health work by thinking about different system levels. According to Pilgrim and Rogers (1999), we can distinguish among the macro (global), meso (national and cultural) and micro (local and personal) levels.

In the case of our topic here the global context includes considerations of the pharmaceutical industry as an enduring and integral part of international capitalism. Not only is the industry constituted by multi-national companies, competing in the constant search for new international markets for new conditions to treat, it is also consequently party to the maintenance and elaboration of global claims about reified diagnostic categories, which can expand in number and so create an ever increasing market for medicinal solutions (Healy, 2006).

The synergy of interest between the drug companies and the medical profession relies upon a joint commitment to the epistemic fallacy: confusing reality with what they have preferred to call reality. Because complex unintelligibility (madness) is called 'schizophrenia' then a person who reports strange experiences becomes an embodied 'schizophrenic', suffering from an obvious disease process to be treated by doctors. Similarly, because the stress of living can lead to the experience of variations on the ordinary human experiences of sadness and fear, these become 'depression' or 'anxiety disorders' to be resolved chemically (Pilgrim, 2007).

Moreover, the constantly expanding nosologies created episodically by the American Psychiatric Association (Diagnostic and Statistical Manual) and the World Health Organization (International Classification of Disease) are then reinforced by drug company activity. Randomized controlled trials to test new drugs always have a diagnostically-related group as their target, in anticipation of marketing new agents (hence 'anti-depressant' and 'anti-psychotic').

At the meso level, national governments are faced with the challenge of controlling madness in an acceptable way for the (voting) majority who are sane by common consent, whilst conceding as much as is possible to the rhetoric of consumerism more generally applicable in health and social care systems. The narrow limits of this concession are defined by the existence of 'mental health law'; the extraordinary existence of legal means to detain some risky citizens but not others without trial, who have committed no crime (see Pilgrim and Rogers, this handbook).

The psychiatric profession in most countries has been willing to embrace this role of coercive control and medication is a useful tool because it can be imposed involuntarily. Moreover, those patients who never enter the psychiatric system can be protected from the vicissitudes of their lives inside or outside the labour market, if they can also be offered medicinal remediation for the distress experienced. In other words, psychotropic medication can oil the wheels of everyday socio-economic transactions and expectations.

At the micro-level the personal consequences for using medication are profound and not necessarily the beneficial experience offered by drug company marketing claims. All psychotropic medication because of its non-specific action alters a person's view of themselves and the world because any aspect of thoughts and feelings can be changed to some degree (for better or worse).

Let us take first major tranquillizers. Their receipt occurs in a context of the wider meaning and symbolic significance that 'psychosis' has for patients in their everyday lives and of a policy context which stresses the need to survey and control the behaviour of patients living in the community. For this reason, self-regulatory action in this group of patients has been found to be less evident, and the threat and application of external social control is greater than for other groups of patients taking medication for chronic conditions (Rogers et al. 1998).

Using data from in-depth interviews with people with a diagnosis of schizophrenia Rogers et al. explored patients' reasons for taking neuroleptics and the ways in which they self-regulate their medication on a daily basis. The data suggested that the main utility of taking neuroleptic medication was not only to control specific symptoms but in a more general way to gain personal control over managing life. However, the costs of taking medication were the 'side-effects', which at times equalled or outweighed the positive gains. Patients did not see – as mental health professionals do – 'side effects' and symptoms as separate matters. Instead, they described drugs as 'good' or 'terrible', an indication of the total impact of their treatment and its implications for subjective well-being. The latter is defined by service users as normality of function, feelings and their appearance to the outside world (Carrick et al., 2004). The same point applies when we turn now to antidepressants.

Being medicated can involve losing, as well as gaining, control. The latter tends to be emphasized selectively by health professionals and the drug companies, whilst the full experiential impact of medication may be ignored. But patients taking medication, when asked, distinguish between 'feeling better' (attributable to the benefits of say antidepressants) and 'being better' (a state of true improved emotional wellbeing in the absence of medication) (Grime and Pollock, 2004).

At the same time, studies of users and prescribers of minor tranquillizers highlight the ambivalence about taking these drugs and the variation in their use, which relates to the type of medication and pattern of use. This ambivalence can be interpreted as part of an 'anti-drug culture', in which fears about ingesting unnatural substances have been fuelled by negative mass media reporting of the side effects of a range of medications in addition to mood modifying drugs. (For patients' views about medicine taking in general, see Pound et al. (2005).) These concerns in turn resonate with a shift to a moral order based on personal responsibility, abstinence and self-reliance and also autonomy and personal freedom (Gabe and Lipshitz-Phillips, 1982; Gabe and Bury, 1996a).

The picture of patients and doctors actively choosing whether to take or prescribe mood modifying drugs in turn suggests that, at the micro level, the matter of social control is not completely obvious. It is clearly possible to prescribe and to take these medicines without creating or experiencing total dependence. At the meso and macro levels however, the generation of a series of drugs for the management of the problems of living sponsored by professional and industrial interests provide convincing support for the social control thesis.

CONCLUSION

This chapter has explored the role of psychotropic drugs in modern developed societies by focusing on their use to control madness and comfort common misery. The expectation that there are scientifically legitimate grounds and clinically efficient methods to pursue these intentions has been maintained by a matrix of interests. The latter includes: the drug companies and their need for profit in expanding global markets; the medical profession and its claims of bio-medical authority over existential matters; the advertising industry and its willingness to broker the relationship between drug producers and drug prescribers; and patients who may have accepted that their personal troubles can be eased by compliance with medical ministrations (with the relatives of patients at times at the forefront of the demand for this compliance).

This arrangement about the unquestioned legitimacy about psychotropic medication from this conservative matrix has had its fair share of critics. These include doubting professionals, feminists and disaffected service users (with the mass media spanning both conservative and critical lobbies). At the centre of these criticisms have been two major objections to the legitimacy of prescribed psychotropic medication. The first is that these drugs may endanger rather than enhance the health and wellbeing of their recipients, thus negating or undermining claims to clinical efficiency. The second is that the bio-reductionism attending the rationale of chemical responses to madness and misery obscures or mystifies social-existential complexity. While patients and doctors at the micro level may express ambivalence about these medications and look to alternative non-medicinal solutions, at the meso and macro levels the evidence that these drugs act as a means of social control is persuasive

REFERENCES

Abraham, J. and Sheppard, J. (1998) International comparative analysis and explanation in sociology: the Halcion anomaly. *Sociology*, 32(1): 141–162.

American Psychological Association (1994) *Diagnostic and Statistical Manual of Mental Disorders* (4th edition). Washington, DC: APA.

Bentall, R.P., Jackson, H. and Pilgrim, D. (1988) Abandoning the concept of schizophrenia: some implications of validity arguments for psychological research into psychotic phenomena. *British Journal of Clinical Psychology*, 27: 303–324.

Breggin, P. (1993) *Toxic Psychiatry*. London: HarperCollins.

Breggin, P. and Breggin, G.R. (1995) *Talking Back to Prozac*. New York: St. Martin's.

Brown, P. and Funk, S.C. (1986) Tardive dyskinesia: barriers to the professional recognition of iatrogenic disease. *Journal of Health and Social Behaviour*, 27: 116–132.

Bury, M. and Gabe, J. (1990) Hooked? Media responses to tranquillizer dependence. In P.Abbott and G. Payne (eds) *New Directions in the Sociology of Health*. London: Falmer Press.

Carrick R., Mitchell A., Powell R. and Lloyd K. (2004) The quest for well-being: a qualitative study of the experience of taking antipsychotic medication. *Psychology and Psychotherapy*, 77: 19–33.

Cohen, D. (1997) A critique of the use of neuroleptic drugs in psychiatry. In S. Fisher and R.P. Greenberg (eds) *From Placebo to Panacea: Putting Psychiatric Drugs to the Test*. New York: Wiley.

Cohen, D., McGubbin, B., Collin, J. and Perodeau, G. (2001) Medications as social phenomena. *Health*, 4: 441–469.

Dennis, D.L. and Monahan, J. (eds) (1996) *Coercion and Aggressive Community Treatment*. New York: Plenum Press.

DeSwaan, A. (1990) *The Management of Normality*. London: Routledge.

Dowrick, C. (2004) *Beyond Depression: A New Approach to Understanding and Management*. Oxford: Oxford University Press.

Ettorre. E. and Riska, E. (1995) *Gendered Moods. Psychotropics and Society*. London: Routledge.

Finn, S.E., Bailey, M., Schultz, R.T. and Faber, R. (1990) Subjective utility ratings of neuroleptics in treating schizophrenia. *Psychological Medicine*.

Fisher, S. and Greenberg, R.P. (eds) (1997) *From Placebo to Panacea: Putting Psychiatric Drugs to the Test*. New York: Wiley.

Friedman, B. (1963) *The Feminine Mystique*. New York: Norton.

Gabe, J. (2001) Benzodiazepines as a social problem: the case of Halcion. *Substance Use and Misuse*, 36(9&10): 1233–1259.

Gabe, J. and Lipshitz-Phillips, S. (1982) Evil necessity. The meaning of benzodiazepine use for women from one general practice. *Sociology of Health and Illness*, 4: 201–209.

Gabe, J. and Lipshitz-Phillips, S. (1984) Tranquillisers as social control? *Sociological Review*, 32(3): 524–546.

Gabe, J. and Thorogood. N. (1986) Prescribed drugs and the management of everyday life: the experiences of black and white working class women. *Sociological Review*, 34: 737–772.

Gabe, J. and Bury, M. (1988) Tranquillisers as a social problem. *Sociological Review*, 36(2): 320–352.

Gabe, J. and Bury, M. (1991) Tranquillisers and health care in crisis. *Social Science and Medicines* 32(4): 449–454.

Gabe, J. and Bury, M. (1996a) Risking tranquilliser use: cultural and lay dimensions. In S.J. Williams and M. Calnan (eds) *Modern Medicine. Lay Perspectives and Experiences*. London: UCL Press.

Gabe, J. and Bury, M. (1996b) Halcion nights: a sociological account. *Sociology*, 30(3): 447–471.

Gelder, M., Mayou, R. and Cowen, P. (2001) *Shorter Oxford Textbook of Psychiatry*. Oxford: Oxford University Press.

Gerson, M.J. and Victoroff, V. (1948) Experimental investigation into the validity of confessions obtained under sodium amytal narcosis. *Journal of Clinical and Experimental Psychopathology*, 9: 359–375.

Grime, J. and Pollock, K. (2004) Information versus experience: a comparison of an information leaflet on antidepressants with lay experience of treatment. *Patient Education and Counseling,* 54: 361–368.

Groenewegen, P.P., Leufkens, H.G., Spreeuwenberg, P. and Worm, W. (1999) Neighbourhood characteristics and use of benzodiazepines in the Netherlands. *Social Science and Medicine,* 48 (12): 1701–1711.

Gunnell, D., Middleton, N., Whitley, E. Dorling, D. and Frankel, S. (2003) Why are suicide rates rising in young men but falling in the elderly? A time series analysis of trends in England and Wales 1950–1998. *Social Science and Medicine,* 57(4): 595–611.

Healy, D. (1997). *The Antidepressant Era.* Cambridge MA: Harvard University Press.

Healy, D. (2006) *Let Them Eat Prozac: The Unhealthy Relationship Between the Pharmaceutical Industry and Depression.* New York: New York University Press.

Helman, C. (1981) `Tonic', `fuel' and `food': social and symbolic aspects of the long term use of psychotropic drugs. *Social Science and Medicine,* 15B: 521–533.

Hemmenki, E. (1977) Polypharmacy among psychiatric patients. *Acta Psychiatrica Scandinavica,* 56: 347–356.

Herzberg, D. (2009) *From Miltown to Prozac: Happy Pills in America.* Baltimore: John Hopkins University Press.

Houston, F. (1952) A preliminary investigation into abreaction comparing methedrine and sodium amytal with other methods. *Journal of Mental Science,* 98: 707–710.

Johnell, K., Merlo, J., Lynch, J. and Blennow, G. (2004) Neighbourhood participation and women's use of anxiolytic-hypnotic drugs: a multi-level analysis. *Journal of Epidemiology and Community Health* 58(1): 59–64.

Kellam, A.M.P. (1987) The neuroleptic syndrome so called: a review of the literature. *British Journal of Psychiatry,* 150: 752–759.

Kilian, R., Lindenbach, I., Lobig, U., et al. (2003) Indicators of empowerment and disempowerment in the subjective evaluation of the psychiatric treatment process by persons with severe and persistent mental illness: a qualitative and quantitative analysis. *Social Science and Medicine,* 57(6): 1127–1142.

Koegler, R. (1965) Drugs, neurosis and the family physician. *California Medicine,* 1: 5–81.

Koumjian, K. (1981) The use of valium as a form of social control. *Social Science and Medicine,* 15E(3): 245–249.

Kramer, P. (1993) *Listening to Prozac.* New York: Viking.

Lacey, R. (1991) *The Complete Guide to Psychiatric Drugs.* London: Ebury Press.

Lewis, S. and Lieberman, J. (2008) CATIE and CUtLASS: can we handle the truth? *British Journal of Psychiatry,* 192(3): 16–63.

Lieberman J., Stroup, T.S., McEvoy, J.P. Swartz, M.S., Rosenheck, R.A., Perkins, D.O., Keefe, R.S., Davis, S.M. et al. (2005) Effectiveness of antipsychotic drugs in patients with chronic schizophrenia. *New England Journal of Medicine,* 353(12): 1209–1223.

North, D., Davis, P. and Powell, A. (1995) Patient responses to benzodiazepine medicine: a typology of adaptive repertoires developed by long term users. *Sociology of Health and Illness,* 17(5): 632–650.

Metzl, J. (2003) *Prozac on the Couch: Prescribing Gender in the Era of Wonder Drugs* Durham NC: Duke University Press.

Metzl, J. and Angel, J. (2004) Assessing the impact of SSRI antidepressants on popular notions of women's depressive illness. *Social Science and Medicine,* 58(3): 577–584.

Moritz, S., Peters, M.J.V., Karow, A., Deljkovic, A., Tonn, P. and Naber, D. (2009) Cure or curse? Ambivalent attitudes towards neuroleptic medication in schizophrenia and non-schizophrenia patients. *Mental Illness* 1(1): 10–15.

National Schizophrenis Fellowship (2001) *Doesn't it Make You Sick?* London: National Schizophrenia Fellowship.

Parr, J.M., Kavanagh, D.J., Young, R. and McCafferty, K. (2006) Views of general practitioners and benzodiazepine users on benzodiazepines: a qualitative study. *Social Science and Medicine,* 62: 1237–1249.

Pelfrene, E., Vlerick, P., Moreeau, M., et al. (2004) Use of benzodiazepine drugs and perceived job stress in a cohort of working men and working women in Belgium. Results from the BELSTRESS-study. *Social Science and Medicine,* 59: 433–442.

Pilgrim, D. (2007) The survival of psychiatric diagnosis. *Social Science and Medicine,* 65(3): 536–544.

Pilgrim, D. and Bentall, R.P. (1999) The medicalisation of misery: a critical realist analysis of the concept of depression. *Journal of Mental Health,* 8(3): 261–274.

Pilgrim, D. and Rogers, A. (1999) Mental health policy and the politics of mental health: a three tier analytical framework. *Policy and Politics,* 27(1): 13–24.

Pound, P., Britten, N., Morgan, M., Yardley, L., Pope, C., Daker-White, G. and Campbell, R. (2005) Resisting medicines: a synthesis of qualitative studies of medicine taking. *Social Science and Medicine,* 61: 133–155.

Prather, J. (1991) Decoding advertising: the role of communication studies in explaining the popularity of minor tranquillisers. In J. Gabe (ed.), *Understanding Tranquilliser Use. The Role of the Social Sciences.* London: Routledge.

Rasmussen, N. (2006) Making the first anti-depressant: amphetamines in American medicine. *Journal of the History of Medicine and the Allied Sciences,* 61(3): 288–323.

Rogers, A. and Pilgrim, D. (2005) *A Sociology of Mental Health and Illness (4th edition)* Maidenhead: Open University Press.

Rogers, A., Day, J.C., Williams, B., Randall, F., Wood, P., Healy, D. and Bentall, R.P. (1998) The meaning and management of neuroleptic medicine: a study of patients with a diagnosis of schizophrenia. *Social Science and Medicine,* 47(9): 1313–1323.

Rogers, A. and Pilgrim, D. (1996) *Mental Health Policy in Britain.* London: Macmillan.

Rogers, A., Pilgrim, D., Brennan, S. et al. (2007) Prescribing benzodiazepines in general practice: a new view of an old problem. *Health,* 2: 181–198.

Ross, C.A. and Pam, A. (eds) (1995) *Pseudoscience in Biological Psychiatry: Blaming the Body.* New York: Wiley.

Scull, A. (1977) *Decarceration: Community Treatment and the Deviant – A Radical View.* Englewood Cliffs NJ: Prentice Hall.

Seale, C., Chaplin, R., Lelliott, P. and Quirk, A. (2007) Antipsychotic medication, sedation and mental clouding: An observational study of psychiatric consultations. *Social Science and Medicine,* 65: 698–711.

Sleath, B. and Shih, Y.C.T. (2003) Sociological influences on antidepressant prescribing. *Social Science and Medicine,* 56(6): 1335–1344.

Smith, S. and Henderson, M. (2000) What you don't know won't hurt you: Information given to patients about the side-effects of anti-psychotic drugs. *Psychiatric Bulletin,* 24: 172–174.

Stevenson, F. (2004) Images of nature in relation to mood modifying medicines: a user perspective. *Health,* 8(2): 241–262.

Stone, M.H. (1997) *Healing the Mind: A History of Psychiatry from Antiquity to the Present.* New York: Norton.

Tyrer, P. (1990) The division of neurosis: a failed classification. *Journal of the Royal Society of Medicine,* 83: 614–616.

U.S. House (1955) *Traffic in, and Control of, Narcotics, Barbiturates and Amphetamines.* Washington: House of Congress.

Warner, R. (1985) *Recovery from Schizophrenia: Psychiatry and Politcal Economy.* London: Routledge.

Whittington, C., Kendall, T., Fonagy, P. Cottrell, D., Cotgrove, A. and Boddington, E. (2004) Selective serotonin reuptake inhibitors in childhood depression: systematic review of published versus unpublished data. *The Lancet,* 24: 1341–1345.

World Health Organization (1992) *The ICD-10 Classification of Mental and Behavioural Disorders.* Geneva: WHO.

19

Common Mental Health Problems: Primary Care and Health Inequalities in the UK

Carolyn Chew-Graham

INTRODUCTION

According to the World Health Organization, half of all people with ill health in Western Europe have a mental illness, with the majority coming into the diagnostic categories of anxiety and depression (WHO, 2000). Mental health problems impose substantial emotional, social and economic burdens on those who experience them, their families and carers, and society as a whole (Murray and Lopez, 1996). Increased socio-economic deprivation is associated with higher prevalence of psychological distress (Eachas et al., 1996). Depression and anxiety make it much more difficult to hold down a job, while those in work are likely to have high rates of sickness absence: over 900,000 adults in England claimed sickness and disability benefits for mental health problems in 2003 (Social Exclusion Unit, 2004). Within this context, this chapter will examine the role of general practitioners (GPs) when responding to patients who consult with common mental health problems, now rarely assessed or managed by specialist mental health services in the UK.

ROLE OF PRIMARY CARE

Research and analysis on inequalities and mental health have a long tradition in epidemiology and sociology, but has tended to exclude primary care as a field from which to understand and then ameliorate inequalities in mental health. Primary Care in the UK provides the first point of contact for people and acts as a gatekeeper to other services. The National Service Framework for mental health (NSF, 1999) dictated that the majority of patients with common mental health problems should be managed in primary care. Currently 90 per cent of people with mental health problems are managed by GPs, who can refer patients to primary care mental health teams for short term psychosocial interventions, but with limited access to secondary care services (Chew-Graham et al., 2007).

In the UK, it has been estimated that an 'average' GP will undertake about 8,000 face to face clinical interactions annually (Donald, 1994) and the average consultation time is 10 minutes, although there is evidence of shorter consultations in socio-economically deprived areas (Stirling et al., 2001). The work of the GP has steadily shifted towards the management of chronic illness and incapacity in the community (DH, 2008), with an emphasis on the biomedical aspects of care. In 2004 in Britain, the new General Medical Services (GMS) contract was introduced, which aimed to shift the emphasis of general practice funding from the *volume* to the *quality* of care provided. The rationale was that financial incentives would facilitate an improvement in the quality of care. As a result, changes to the funding structure of general practice included the introduction of a *quality and outcomes framework*, in which GPs are remunerated for ensuring care for people with chronic conditions is provided according to evidence based parameters. Indicators of quality of care, based on best evidence, have been assigned to certain chronic diseases and practices are paid for achieving targets derived from these indicators.

An emphasis is placed in this contract on the management of chronic physical conditions, although screening for depression in people with some chronic conditions is now rewarded. Criticism of the contract in general, and the use of screening instruments for depression in particular, has led to the suggestion that such initiatives may encourage practitioners to take a reductionist, biomedical approach, diverting them from a broader biopsychosocial approach, particularly in the area of mental health (Dowrick, 2009).

The National Institute for Health and Clinical Excellence (NICE) produce evidence-based guidelines for the health service to support commissioning and provision of care. An updated NICE guideline for depression in adults (NICE, 2009) provides recommendations for the management of depression by healthcare professionals. The guideline shifts the emphasis from screening to identification of depression and modifies the stepped care model used in the original guideline (NICE, 2004) while recognizing the role of GPs in supporting people who have been diagnosed with depression. 'Stepped care' provides a framework in which to organize the provision of services supporting both patients and carers, and healthcare professionals in identifying and accessing the most effective interventions (NICE, 2004).

Despite the availability of such guidelines, GPs are aware of the limitations of a protocol driven approach to managing depression. For example, a survey of GPs by a leading UK charity, the *Mental Health Foundation,* found that 72 per cent of practitioners think that mindful meditation might benefit patients but most of GPs reported that they limit themselves to prescribing antidepressant medication (Mental Health Foundation, 2010).

MENTAL HEALTH AND INEQUALITIES

Tudor Hart (1971) suggested that the availability of good medical care tends to vary inversely with the need for the population served and described this as the 'inverse care law'. This is no less true for people with mental health problems. Adequate and timely support for common mental health problems within primary care is less likely to be accessed by certain groups of individuals (Borowsky et al., 2000). Many people with high levels of mental distress are disadvantaged, either because care is not available to them in the right place and time, or because when they do access care their interaction with care-givers deters help-seeking or diverts it into forms that do not address their needs.

Given that the UK's National Health Service (NHS) has an explicit equity-driven health policy framework (DH, 2008), a fundamental question is how and why inequity of access to professional help for, and inadequacy or professional response to, common mental health problems arises and is sustained.

Health Services research traditionally examines access to health care from the point of entrance to the formal system of care. Key concepts such as demand, availability, utilization and patterns of use are developed in a functionalist view of the relation between service provision and use. Access is conceptualized as an interaction between supply and demand of services mediated and codified by professionally defined needs for services (Dixon-Woods et al. 2006). Behavioural and social science traditions focus mainly on an 'out-of-service' perspective, that is, on processes that happen before the point of entrance into formal systems of care, formulating the scope of research into an umbrella term of 'help seeking'. Broadhurst's review (2003) of this literature identifies a series of a three-stage models of help-seeking, summarizing their variations in (a) problem definition, (b) deciding to seek help and (c) actively seeking help.

The concept of 'recursivity' refers to the interdependency between a user's experiences of health services and her/his future actions in regards to health and help seeking (Dowrick et al., 2009; Rogers and Pilgrim, 1997). This helps us to include user perspectives and the interaction of patients and staff in primary care when understanding the type of care given and received and its influence on future help-seeking. In other words, it is not possible to understand and predict service utilization by professional descriptions and processes alone – the view of patients, especially about their understanding of the utility of service access and the nature of their relationship with staff, needs to be taken into account, as do the organizational arrangements for delivering care.

CONTESTATION ABOUT THE UNDER-DETECTION OF DEPRESSION IN PRIMARY CARE

For over 40 years, GPs have been told that they fail to diagnose depression (Goldberg, 1992). Kessler et al., (2002) suggested that clinically significant depression (moderate to severe depressive illness) is detected by GPs at later consultations by virtue of the longitudinal patient–doctor relationship and it is milder forms, which may recover spontaneously, that go undetected and untreated. More recent studies suggest in primary care the probability of prescribing antidepressants was associated with the severity of the depression, although almost half of the patients who were prescribed antidepressants were not depressed according to standard diagnostic criteria (Kendrick et al., 2005).

Other authors draw attention to the dangers of the erroneous diagnosis of depression in patients with a slight psychological malaise and little functional repercussion, which might lead to the risk of unnecessary, and potentially dangerous, medicalization (Aragone et al., 2006). Mitchell et al. (2009) conducted a systematic search, meta-analysis and Bayesian analysis of 107 studies that examined the diagnostic accuracy of general practitioners. The focus was on their unassisted clinical ability to detect robustly-defined depression, using expert structured or semi-structured interviews as a gold standard. The analysis suggested that GPs are able to rule-out depression in most people who are not depressed with reasonable accuracy, but they have difficulty diagnosing depression in true cases. Yet given the modest prevalence of depression in most primary care settings, the number of false positive errors is larger than the number of false negatives. The authors suggested that further work is needed to examine the subsequent outcome of those false positive and false negative diagnoses and also to clarify the accuracy of GPs in diagnosing anxiety disorders, adjustment disorders and broadly defined distress.

WHY MIGHT GPS HAVE DIFFICULTY IN RECOGNIZING DEPRESSION?

According to the literature, the reasons for the lack of recognition of depression by GPs fall into three themes: the patient, the system and the general practice consultation.

The patient

Studies suggest that people may have difficulty in presenting their distress and discussing their concerns with their doctor, especially when they are uncertain that depression is a legitimate reason for seeing the doctor (Gask et al., 2003). Relationality is also important, and that GPs are, in fact, effective at identifying mental health problems in patients they know (MaGPIe Research Group, 2005) . However, for others, the GP is not considered the most appropriate person to talk to, or they believe that symptoms of distress should not be discussed at all. Other research suggests that some individuals feel that they do not deserve to take up the doctor's time, or that it is not possible for doctors to listen to them and understand how they feel (Pollock, 2002).

The oft-described barrier of stigma can be set against the arguments that depression is a social construct which is an outcome of the medicalization of chronic distress or unhappiness (Ellis, 1996; Pilgrim and Bentall, 1999). Thus, from this perspective it is suggested that chronic unhappiness or acute distress are social-existential variations on life. The challenge then is not necessarily to 'treat' an illness but to determine how the patient's needs may or may not be met within the constraints of a general medical setting. From the patient perspective, contact with primary care has been reported to be of little significance when set against the magnitude of their other experienced problems (Rogers et al., 2001).

There is increasing evidence that older people with depression are marginalized and various patient factors have been postulated. Thus, older people may complain less of depressed mood and instead somatize (Rabins, 1996). Physical co-morbidity may also make the interpretation of depressive symptoms difficult. People may have beliefs that prevent them from seeking help for depression, such as a fear of stigmatization, or that antidepressant medication is addictive or they may misattribute symptoms of major depression for 'old age', ill health or grief. This challenge about white Western older patients is similar to that of ethnic minorities (all ages) who might have different views about the body as a focus of distress, as well as a different view about individual forbearance for the sake of family duty. Some cultures have no word for 'depression' and Western medical claims that some cultures, such as those from South Asia, 'somatize' and thus disguise 'true' depression are contestable (Pilgrim and Bentall, 1999).

The system

The role of the organization within which health professionals work has been cited as a major barrier to encouraging disclosure of symptoms and a lack of resources, both personal and places to refer people with mental health problems to, added to professionals' reluctance to encourage patients to disclose their distress (Chew-Graham et al., 2008; Popay, 2007). The trend in the UK for mental health services to be 'carved out' from mainstream medical services may disadvantage depressed people, who may have difficulties in attending different sites for mental and physical disorders. The barriers described are likely to be particularly difficult for economically poor and minority populations who tend to have more ill-health and are more disabled.

The general practice consultation

The consultation has come to be identified as the cornerstone of general practice, and to be seen more than an occasion for the medical work of diagnosis and treatment (Neighbour, 1987). Beginning with the work of Balint (1957), the consultation has come to be seen as a 'meeting' of individuals in which (often undifferentiated) symptoms are expected to be understood and accommodated in relation to their social and psychological contexts. Much effort in education and research has been invested in giving the consultation this deeper meaning. Thus, whilst the importance of the doctor–patient relationship is a given in today's primary care, achieving a satisfactory doctor–patient relationship has also been elevated to be an outcome or goal of every consultation. Earlier work, using secondary analysis of qualitative data (Chew-Graham et al., 2004), suggests that doctors have over-estimated the importance of sustaining their relationships with some patients, when doing so only maintains incapacity.

It is well understood that a reductionist biomedical model of practice is unhelpful in understanding undifferentiated symptoms in primary care (May and Mead, 1999) and both doctors and patients evince a desire for humane interactions, marked by civility and an interest in the patient as a person. Recognition of the patient-as-person and the application of good communications skills play an important part in understanding the nature of symptoms and apprehending underlying pathologies, as well as securing adherence to treatment regimens (Toon, 1994). The need for GPs to reflect on their work has been recognized. For example, Fairhurst and May (2001) describe the cognitive and affective evaluations made by doctors about their patients, and how recognition of these both positive and negative evaluations is vital for GPs in reflecting upon the consultation.

GP attitudes and inequalities

Qualitative studies can illuminate the views and attitudes of health professionals and extrapolation to how this might influence the consultation and care offered by the GP. Two exemplars will be used to illustrate how GP attitudes might influence and exacerbate inequalities of care provided to people with mental health problems. The qualitative studies chosen are of semi-structured interviews with GPs (and, in the second study, other primary care professionals), exploring their views on the identification and management of depression in deprived and affluent areas, and in elderly people. There is evidence that elderly people and those deprived areas have poor access to adequate care for their mental health problems. Data from the original studies is provided to illustrate the arguments presented.

A qualitative study, in which two groups of GPs in deprived and affluent areas were interviewed (Chew-Graham et al., 2002) highlights the difficulties GPs have in applying the label of 'depression' to a patient, and how the labelling is different according to the area in which a GP works and the perceived social circumstances of the individual patient. Analysis of the two sets of interviews suggested that GPs conceptualized depression as an everyday problem of practice, rather than as an objective diagnostic category, and as a *normal* response to life events. Thus, GPs who practised in urban/inner-city areas (group one) framed their accounts of depression in relation to a variety of aetiological factors; they relied on notions of 'stress' following family breakdown, un- and under-employment, crime and poor housing as the principal causal factors of the syndrome labelled as 'depression'. These explained both the epidemiology and the phenomenology of depression:

> Here? We see loads. It's very common because of the area we work in. Because — you know — of the social factors, it's a deprived area. And that brings with it lots of stress, a lot of depression. [GP13 (group 1)]

There was nothing unexpected or surprising for doctors about the level of depression to be found in such circumstances. The kinds of social networks and resources that might sustain sufferers in other contexts were non-existent for many of their patients:

> Especially in an area like this, there is a lot of poor family support, lots of people who have very hard lives, a lot of loneliness. And yes, I think a lot of depression is circumstantial. [GP10 (1)]

If depression is conceptualized as a normal response to disadvantage, in which existential *despair* is the principal component, then the question of an appropriate diagnostic and management strategy could become as intractable as the illness itself for GPs in these environments.

Similarly, GPs described depression in older people as part of a spectrum including loneliness, lack of social network, reduction in function and very much saw depression as 'understandable' and 'justifiable':

> Our local population often have quite good reasons to be dissatisfied with life, so it's a normal response to a situation rather than a sign of pathology. (GP5)

Some GPs questioned whether depression in older people was actually a separate clinical entity:

> . . . I wonder whether actually we've got . . . patients being treated for depression . . . as a way of medicalising their discontent. (GP4)

Nurses similarly saw depression as an understandable reaction to ageing, reduction in function and disability. They seemed to normalize patients' distress or want to treat it as a separate (mental health) problem and then refer the patient onto someone else to manage the problem. There was a tension between nurses' knowledge of depression as a clinical condition and their perception as a social or existential problem:

> I think it's probably loneliness, 'cos they don't have much family around . . . and their partner's gone . . . and they don't have anywhere to go. (Practice Nurse 2)

Thus, primary care clinicians move away from the boundaries of medicalization through their recognition of the social context of depressed patients' lives. This, however, leads to problems when attempting to make a clinical diagnosis of depression and offer treatment within the biomedical model offered by the health service.

GPs practising in more deprived areas described their patients with depression as actively seeking the medicalization of their personal problems. Patients' expectations and demands were derived from their knowledge that there *is* an illness called 'depression' which is widespread and doctors are there to treat it. But there was also a sense in which some subjects construed patients as seeking a more explicit personal gain:

> What else is going on? That's the question that springs to mind. Depression is the new back pain, you know. I don't think people look hard enough at the secondary gains of illness. I think particularly now the government is willing us back towards full employment, the only way out of working for your living is to be ill. [GP17 (1)]

This kind of response is consistent with a position adopted by GPs towards other chronic problems (Chew-Graham et al., 2004). But such explicit attributions of a manipulative relationship between reported symptoms and secondary gains were rare. More common was the notion that, 'people feel conditions are being imposed upon them ... and having a mental health problem is a way out of that' [GP13, (1)]. The 'gain' that this involves is a more conventional one, conceptualized in terms strongly reminiscent of the notion of a 'sick role'. It is important to note that the notion of 'gain' does not simply apply to the patient in these accounts. GPs themselves also reported a gain in applying the diagnosis of depression:

> When we feel powerless to help the patient in any other way, or we can see that they have no other resources to turn to, then sometimes it is easy to read into the situation a diagnosis of depression. [GP6 (1)]

In this context, the 'gain' for the doctor is a diagnostic move that accommodates and acknowledges the reality of existential despair that is framed as a key component of depression by subjects. This gain also allows the GP to follow a pre-determined treatment plan:

> With the good sides of anti-depressants, it helps us to stagger the consultations, being able to prescribe and review somebody 2 to 3 weeks later, and again 2 to 3 weeks later, is a good way of breaking up those consultations we don't have time for, it makes us feel good because it feels as if we are doing something, it makes us feel good because we know that the patient will improve if we have got the diagnosis right and they take the tablets. [GP2 (2)]

Thus, applying a label of depression to the patient provides security to the GP in their work. In contrast, such feelings of security in making the diagnosis were not described by GPs reflecting on consultations with older people. Here GPs described the difficulties they had in suggesting a diagnosis of depression to an older person and perceived reluctance and resistance on the part of their elderly patients to accept depression as a diagnosis:

> you come to know the patient over a period of time . . . you're talking about things in general . . . in contrast with younger people who come in and present their depression. (GP7)

> Sometimes I will ask them how their spirits are but they think that you're saying that it's all in their head and you don't believe them. If you mention that they might be depressed they say, 'But what about my bad arm?' (GP9)

In this situation, it is the GP who is trying to impose the label on the reluctant patient, and this becomes a significant barrier, for both the GP and the patient, to progressing with management of the patient's presented problems. If there is no agreement what the problem is, the GP (and the patient) become 'stuck' with no resolution of the patient's presented problems and no satisfaction for the GP in having moved the patient forwards.

GPs in both studies reported that, having made and agreed with the patient, the diagnosis of depression, their preferred mode of treatment was unavailable:

> We don't have sufficient resources available. Psychology is something that has a long, long waiting list . . . em, counselling we have had ready access to, but because of the changes, that's going to be diluted, back to the lowest common denominator, and that's a shame. [GP9 (2)]

However, those GPs working in more affluent areas were more positive about the availability and likely success of 'talking therapies':

> It's no point stuffing people full of antidepressants, when they are still left with the problem . . . sometimes it helps to have a counsellor who puts, kind of, strategies out and enables them to move on. [GP4 (2)]

It was also apparent to GPs that some patients in these areas accessed such care privately:

> . . . it's very much a gold standard treatment, but you don't get that on the NHS. [GP5 (2)]

Similarly, when discussing alternatives to medication in consultations with older people with depression, clinicians consistently reflected on the lack of statutory agencies to refer patients to. Some GPs also admitted to managing elderly people with depression differently to younger adults, either due to simply forgetting about talking therapies or because of an assumption that they will not work in the elderly:

> We don't have a counsellor attached . . . Psychology? In the elderly I have to confess I probably . . . virtually never do'. (GP7)

Respondents described referring older patients to voluntary agencies, but perceived patient reluctance to use them:

> It's like a vicious circle once they get depressed they won't go to a lunch club. By the time they come to us they don't want to go anywhere like that. (GP2)

Primary care professionals perceived their own skills in the support and management of depression to be limited, that their time was limited and thus primary care has little to offer the patient:

> you've really got the services of the GP . . . so you've got a 10 minute appointment'. (Practice Nurse 1)

For these reasons, the majority of health care professionals described a reluctance to make the diagnosis of depression in an elderly person because of a feeling that they had nothing to offer the patient:

> I think you're probably reluctant to go looking for the diagnosis . . . if it's presented then it's a lot easier . . . but unlikely to go looking for it . . . I would feel. If there isn't a huge amount of support for following it up, and often there isn't'. (GP4)

> It's unfair to start delving and then say, 'Right fine. We've found that out [that you're depressed] but [there's] nothing we can do . . . You do have a tendency not to think about it too much'. (Practice Nurse 3)

All GPs stressed the importance of developing a therapeutic interaction in which they 'listened' to patients, and enabled them to talk. But they tempered this with the difficulties of accommodating such work within the practical exigencies of their workload. This GP notes that developing a positive personal alliance enjoyed by the patient creates time management problems given the rapid throughput expected in daily primary care:

> The more you listen, the more people come and talk to you, and the longer your surgeries run over, and the more people complain because they can't get in to see you. [GP14 (1)]

Respondents described a tension between the intractable nature of the patient and the wider demands of primary medical care. To begin with, these patients are constituted as highly demanding 'burdens' on the doctors' own psychological and professional resources:

> You have to have the emotional energy and stability to manage patients with depression. But a lot of GPs are stressed and a lot have mild depression, and when you have that combination, it's extremely difficult to look after patients who have got a depressive illness. [GP2 (2)]

In this context, GPs working with deprived populations found themselves often deeply frustrated and drained by their encounters with depressed patients:

> I suppose that people that are on long-term antidepressants are not particularly attractive people. That sounds an awful thing to say, doesn't it? But they are people that you generally find difficult to deal with anyway – people that bore you and make you tired or whatever – so it's hard to maintain an interest. [GP4 (1)]

GPs working with a less deprived population were, in contrast, more positive about the majority of people who they had diagnosed as depression as having the potential to improve:

> A lot of the GP's workload can be very mundane, matter of fact and routine, dealing with depression is always a bit more challenging and interesting. [GP3 (2)]

Thus, GPs in deprived areas viewed depression as a normal response to difficult circumstances, illnesses or life events. Depression may be under-diagnosed because of dissatisfaction with the types of treatment that can be offered, especially a lack of availability of psychological interventions. GPs practising in inner-city areas were frustrated by the intractability and time-consuming nature of depression in their practice. They emphasized structural factors and workload as inhibiting the potential for therapeutic interactions with such patients. Woven through accounts of the practical difficulties that they encountered in this work was the sense that, for these GPs, it was an unrewarding domain of clinical practice.

Similarly, primary care practitioners described a 'therapeutic nihilism' suggesting that depression is understandable and, indeed, justifiable in older people. Thus patients' feelings of distress are normalized. Respondents in all studies expressed views that suggested a move away from the biomedical view on the causation of depression to a social view. As a result, depression was regarded as the result of wider social and economic problems in the face of which primary care practitioners feel that they are powerless to intervene. This dissonance between the medical and social model of depression, does not help the clinicians identify and manage depression and leaves the patient to suffer with their symptoms. Instead of empowering practitioners within a consultation to consider psychosocial factors and describe a patient-centred model of care, this dissonance leaves the practitioner feeling impotent in the face of an older person in distress.

The doctor's capacity for empathy with the patient's presentation of symptoms is associated with the doctor's perception of a successful exit point in the consultation. Where no exit point is in sight, in elderly patients and people in deprived areas, the consultation itself becomes the focus of work to *contain* the *expression* of symptoms, rather than relieve or palliate their effects and the doctor is frustrated and the doctor-patient relationship itself has the potential to become chronic and a source of demoralization for practitioners.

IMPACT ON PROVISION OF CARE

The construction of 'depression' as a clinical condition has been shown to be contested amongst GPs (Chew-Graham et al., 2000; Pilgrim and Dowrick, 2006) and distress may be seen as intractable and not amenable to brief and easy technical solutions (May et al., 2004). The studies discussed in detail here support this proposition. These kinds of accounts have important implications for primary care and understanding the reasons for continued inequalities of care provision for people with mental health problems. Doctors working in inner cities and in consultations with elderly people may be reluctant to recognize and respond to such patients in depth because of much wider structural and social factors, as well as their own emotional responses. Elderly people living in inner city areas may be particularly poorly served (Rait et al., 1996).

Negative attributions mean that GPs exhibit a nihilistic view of the possible out-comes of individual consultations and are pessimistic about their ability to impact on patients with chronic problems, including mental health problems, presenting to them. Thus it seems that the inverse care law operates in the primary care man-agement of patients, in already disenfranchised groups, with depression. Those people more at risk of depression and anxiety, are likely to be less well understood by, and receive less appropriate and less effective care from, their GP.

AMELIORATING INEQUALITIES IN MENTAL HEALTH

So how can the effects of GP attitudes, which have the potential to increase inequalities in mental health, be ameliorated? Educational interventions alone, training GPs to identify and respond to patients' presentations of distress, based around communication skills training, are unlikely to improve patient outcome, without understanding the framework which underpins GPs' views on 'depres-sion' as a problem presented to them. A whole system approach, with intervention at the level of the patient, practice and extended primary care team, will be neces-sary to improve the provision of care for those groups currently underserved by primary care.

Thus interventions at a public health level which raise awareness of depres-sion, reduce stigma and legitimize the presentation of distress to the GP are vital to facilitate people's willingness to access primary care and disclose their feel-ings of distress. Training may enhance the health professionals' willingness to listen and bear witness to the patient's distress, and their ability and capacity to intervene within the consultation. This needs to be supported by supervision of practitioners to enable them to deal with the emotion, and frustration, generated by the fast through-put of patients with seemingly intractable problems, which adding a label of depression to may not help.

There is a need to begin to look at a recursive relationship between factors implicating inequalities at a broader population, structural level with those that operate in meso-level contexts of which general practice and primary care is a prime example.

Discussion of how much resource to support system change is needed, and will be provided, as the current organization of UK primary care with 10 minute appointments cannot realistically tackle broader psycho-social problems experi-enced by patients. Changes in national policy will be required. Thus, whilst, the National Service Framework (NSF for Older People, 2001) had as its first stan-dard the rooting out of age discrimination, little is known about the efficacy or implementation of the Framework at Primary Care Trust level. The 2009 Equality Bill will, if enacted, make age-based discrimination in the provision of health and social care illegal for the first time in the United Kingdom.

The National Service Frameworks are being superseded by the New Horizons initiative (2008), which stresses the importance of well-being and resilience, prevention and early intervention and provides a focus on the mental health of older people and recognizes the importance of socio-economic class as a determinant of mental health. Effective commissioning should take account of these policies although there is no new money for this initiative thus it's impact on primary care may be limited. The *Improving Access to Psychological Therapies* (2008) initiative aims to ensure that every patient with mental health problems who would benefit from, and agree to engage with a psychological therapy, can access such a service. Increasing awareness amongst GPs of available treatment options for their patients with mental health problems may increase the likelihood of the GP, during the consultation, being positive about making a diagnosis of depression and discussing treatment options with the patient, whatever their age or social class.

CONCLUSION

The exploration of the topic of primary care and common mental health problems in this chapter can be summarized in the following points:

- Primary Care in the UK provides the first point of contact for people and acts as a gatekeeper to other services.
- Adequate and timely support for common mental health problems within primary care is less likely to be accessed by certain groups of individuals, such as older people and people from socially deprived areas.
- 'Recursivity' refers to the interdependency between a user's experiences of health services and her/his future actions in regards to health and help seeking, emphasizing the role of the health professional and the clinical encounter in shaping care and future help-seeking.
- The primary care consultation, often seen as the 'cornerstone' of general practice, is the focus of the GP's response to the patient's distress.
- GPs practising in deprived areas view depression as a normal and understandable response to difficult circumstances, illnesses or life events.
- Depression is seen to be understandable and justifiable in older people and patients' feelings of distress are normalized.
- Negative attributions mean that GPs exhibit a nihilistic view of the possible outcomes of individual consultations and are pessimistic about their ability to be of help to patients with mental health problems presenting to them.
- Where no exit point is in sight, in elderly patients and people in deprived areas, the consultation itself becomes the focus of work to *contain* the *expression* of symptoms, rather than relieve or palliate their effects. In this scenario, the doctor may be frustrated and the doctor–patient relationship itself has the potential to become chronic and a source of demoralization for practitioners.
- The inverse care law operates in the primary care management of patients, in already disenfranchized groups, with depression.
- Interventions at the level of the general population, the individual patient, the practice and practitioners as well as NHS organizations, facilitated by policy directives, would be necessary to improve the provision of care for those groups currently under-served by primary care.

- Educational interventions alone, based around communication skills training, will not improve patient outcome without understanding the framework which underpins GPs' views on 'depression' as a problem presented to them.
- The current organisation of UK primary care with 10 minute-on-average appointments cannot realistically enable GPs to effectively manage the broader psycho-social problems experienced and presented by patients.

REFERENCES

Aragone, E., Pinol, J.L. and Labad, A. (2006) The overdiagnosis of depression in non-depressed patients in primary care. *Family Practice*, 23(3): 363–368.

Balint M. (1957) *The Doctor, His Patient and the Illness*. New York: International Universities Press.

Borowsky, S.J., Rubenstein, L.V., Meredith, L.S., Camp, P., Jackson-Triche, M. and Wells, K.B. (2000). Who is at risk of nondetection of mental health problems in primary care? *Journal of General Internal Medicine*, 15(6): 381–388.

Broadhurst, K. (2003). Engaging parents and carers with family support services: What can be learned from research on help-seeking? *Child and Family Social Work*, 8: 341–350.

Burroughs, H., Morley, M., Lovell, K., Baldwin, R. Burns, A. and Chew-Graham C.A. (2006) 'Justifiable depression': How health professionals and patients view late-life depression; a qualitative study. *Family Practice*, 23: 369–377.

Chew-Graham, C.A., May, C.R., Cole, H. and Hedley, S. (2000) The burden of depression in primary care: A qualitative investigation of general practitioners' constructs of depressed people in primary care. *Primary Care Psychiatry*, 6(4): 137–141.

Chew-Graham, C.A., Mullin, S. May, C.R., Hedley, S. and Cole, H. (2002) The management of depression in primary care: another example of the inverse care law? *Family Practice*, 19(6): 632–637.

Chew-Graham, C.A., May, C.R. and Roland, M.O. (2004) The harmful consequences of elevating the doctor-patient relationship to be a primary goal of the general practice consultation. *Family Practice*, 21: 229–231.

Chew-Graham, C., Slade, M., Montana, C., Stewart, M. and Gask, L. (2007) A qualitative study of referral to community mental health teams in the UK: exploring the rhetoric and the reality. *BMC Health Service Research*, 7:117.

Chew-Graham, C.A., Chamberlain, E., Turner, K., Folkes, L., Caulfield, L. and Sharp, D. (2008) General practitioners' and health visitors' views on the diagnosis and management of postnatal depression: a qualitative study. *BJGP*, 58: 169–176.

Department of Health (1999) *A National Service Framework for Mental Health – Modern Standards and Service Models for Mental Health*. London: HMSO.

Department of Health (2001) *National Service Framework (Older People)*. London: HMSO.

DH (2004) *Quality and Outcomes Framework*. Guidance. Department of Health.

DH (2005) *Supporting People with LTC*. London: Department of Health.

DH (2008) *Health Inequalities: Progress and Next Steps*. London: Department of Health.

Dixon-Woods, M., Cavers, D., Agarwal, S., Annandale, E., Arthur, A., Harvey, J., et al. (2006) Conducting a critical interpretive synthesis of the literature on access to healthcare by vulnerable groups. *BMC Medical Research Methodology*, p. 6.

Donald, A.G. (1994) *Doctors, Dilemmas, Decisions*. London: BMJ Publications.

Dowrick, C. (2009) *Beyond Depression* (2nd edition). Oxford: Oxford University Press.

Eachus, J., Williams, M., Chan, P. et al. (1996) Deprivation and cause-specific morbidity: evidence from the Somerset and Avon survey of health. *British Medical Journal*, 312: 287–292.

Ellis, C.G. (1996) Chronic unhappiness. Investigating the phenomenon in family practice. *Canadian Family Physician*, 42: 645–651.

Fairhurst, K. and May, C. (2001) Knowing patients and knowledge about patients: evidence of modes of reasoning in the consultation? *Family Practice*, 18(5): 501–505.

Gask, L., Rogers, A., Oliver, D., May, C. and Roland, M. (2003) Qualitative study of patients' perceptions of the quality of care for depression in general practice. *BJGP*, 53: 278–283.

Goldberg, D. et al. (1992) *Common Mental Disorders.* London: Routledge.

Government Equalities Office (2009) *A Fairer Future: the Equality Bill and Other Action to Make Equality a Reality.* www.equalities.gov.uk/pdf/NEWGEO_FairerFuture_may09_acc.pdf (accessed 3 January, 2010).

Improving Access to Psychological Therapies (2008). www.iapt.nhs.uk (accessed 3 January, 2010).

Kendrick, T. King, F. Albertella, L. and Smith, P. (2005) GP treatment decisions for patients with depression: an observational study. *British Journal of General Practice,* 55: 280–286.

Kessler, D., Bennewith, O., Lewis, G. and Sharp, D. (2002) Detection of depression and anxiety in primary care: follow-up study. *BMJ*, 325: 1016–1017.

May, C. and Mead, N. (1999) Patient-centredness: a history. In C. Dowrick and L. Frith (eds) *General Practice and Ethics: Uncertainty and Responsibility.* London: Routledge. pp. 77–89.

May, C.M., Allison, G., Chapple, A., Chew-Graham, C.A., Dixon, C., Gask, L., Graham, L., Rogers, A. and Roland, M.O. (2004) Framing the doctor–patient relationship in chronic illness: a comparative study of general practitioners' accounts. *Sociology of Health and Illness,* 26(2): 135–158.

MaGPIe Research Group (2005) The effectiveness of case-finding for mental health problems in primary care. *BJGP*, 55: 665–669.

MaGPIe Research Group (2005) Do patients want to disclose psychological problems to GPs? *Family Practice*, 22(6): 631–637.

Mental Health Foundation (2010) *Be Mindful.* London Mental Health Foundation.

Mitchell, A.J., Vaze, A. and Rao, S. (2009) Meta-analysis of unassisted recognition of depression in primary care: Importance of false positives and false negatives. *Lancet* (submitted for publication).

Murray, C.J.L. and Lopez, A.D. (1996) *The Global Burden of Disease.* Boston, Mass: World Health Organization and Harvard University Press.

National Institute for Health and Clinical Excellence (2004) *Depression: Management of Depression in Primary and Secondary Care.* Clinical Guideline 23. London: NICE.

Neighbour, R. (1987) *The Inner Consultation.* Lancaster: MTP Press.

New Horizons (2008) http://www.dh.gov.uk/en/Healthcare/Mentalhealth/NewHorizons/DH_102135 (accessed 3 January, 2010).

NICE (2009) *Depression: the Treatment and Management of Depression in Adults (update).* NICE clinical guideline 90. London: NICE.

Pilgrim, D. and Bentall, R. (1999) The medicalisation of misery: a critical realist analysis of the concept of depression. *Journal of Mental Health*, 3: 261–274.

Pilgrim, D. and Dowrick, C. (2006) From a diagnostic-therapeutic to a social-existential response to 'depression'. *Journal of Public Mental Health,* 5: 6–12.

Pollock, K. and Grime, J. (2002) Patients' perceptions of entitlement to time in general practice consultations for depression: a qualitative study. *BMJ*, 325: 687–690.

Popay, J., Kowarzik ,U., Mallinson, S., Mackian S. and Barker, J. (2007) Social problems, primary care and pathways to at the individual level. Part I: the GP perspective help and support: addressing health inequalities. *Journal of the Epidemiological Community Health,* 61: 966–971.

Rabins, P. (1996) Barriers to diagnosis and treatment of depression in elderly patients. *American Journal of Geriatric Psychiatry,* 4: 79–84.

Rait, G., Burns, A. and Chew, C.A. (1996) Old age, ethnicity and mental illness: a triple whammy [Invited Editorial]. *BMJ*, 313: 1347–1348.

Rogers, A. and Pilgrim, D. (1997) The contribution of lay knowledge to the understanding and promotion of mental health. *Journal of Mental Health,* 6(1): 23–35.

Rogers, A. May, C. and Oliver, D. (2001) Experiencing depression, experiencing the depressed: the separate worlds of patients and doctors. *Journal of Mental Health*, 10(3): 317–333.

Social Exclusion Unit (2004) *Mental Health and Social Exclusion.* London: Office of the Deputy Prime Minister.

Stirling, A.M., Wilson, P. and McConnachie, A. (2001) Deprivation, psychological distress, and consultation length in general practice. *British Journal of General Practice,* 51: 456–460.

Toon, P.D. (1994) *What is Good General Practice? A Philosophical Study of the Concept of High Quality Medical Care.* Royal College of General Practitioners Occasional Paper 65. London: Royal College of General Practitioners.

Tudor Hart, J. (1971) The inverse care law. *Lancet,* 1(7696): 405–412.

WHO International Consortium in Psychiatric Epidemiology (2000) Cross-national comparisons of the prevalences and correlates of mental disorders. *Bulletin WHO,* 78: 413–426.

WISE approach (Whole System Informing Self-Management Engagement) developed by the NPCRDC self-management programme research team. http://www.bmj.com/cgi/content/extract/335/7627/968 (accessed 3 January, 2010).

20

Promoting Mental Health

Helen Herman

INTRODUCTION

Inequities in health, avoidable health inequalities, arise because of the circumstances in which people grow, live, work and age, and the systems put in place to deal with illness. The conditions in which people live and die are, in turn, shaped by political, social and economic forces. (CSDH, 2008)

The Commission on the Social Determinants of Health (CSDH) reports that in all regions there are social gradients in health, with the poorest in any community having much worse health than those who are socioeconomically advantaged (CSDH, 2008). The CSDH was established by the World Health Organization (WHO) to marshal the evidence on effective strategies to promote health equity. As mental health is integral to health, the report directs attention to the social determinants of mental health and the needs for mental health promotion associated with these.

The recognition of mental health within public health is a recent development in many parts of the world (Herrman et al., 2005b). The significant adverse effects of wars and disasters on the mental health of those affected, especially children, women and other vulnerable groups including war veterans, are becoming apparent globally. However, until recently many governments and opinion leaders were less aware of the way that social conditions, especially poverty and disadvantage, affect the mental health and wellbeing of a population in any country. In rapidly changing social, economic and environmental conditions, governments and communities are likely to have little information about the mental health of the population and how it is affected by the policies and practices they introduce across education, employment, social development and other sectors. They may also be unaware of the evidence-based options for promoting mental health and wellbeing at a population level. This situation has much to do with how professionals and planners are trained, what they see as their role in society and, in turn, what society expects them to do (Saxena et al., 2006). There is also a limited understanding of mental health and mental illness in most communities worldwide.

Besides expanding services to those who at present receive none, preventing mental disorders and promoting mental health make critical contributions to population mental health in all parts of the world. The close connections between mental health and other aspects of health and productivity mean that promoting mental health is a necessity in low-income as well as high-income countries (Herrman and Swartz, 2007).

Reports on the global burden of disease, the release of the World Health Organization's world health report in 2001, 'Mental Health: New Understanding, New Hope' and the release of several national and international reports on mental health since 1990 have resulted in increased awareness of the need to improve the outcomes for people affected by mental illnesses or at risk of becoming ill. Even so, this attention in itself results in a restricted view of how to improve a population's mental health. Indeed the term mental health is commonly understood as referring to mental illnesses and their prevention and treatment. So it is helpful to be clear about definitions.

This chapter considers the definition of mental health and mental health promotion, the development of this field within public health and social development, and the rationale for mental health promotion as essential to improving mental health and public health in countries at all income levels. It then considers the public health framework for promoting mental health with examples from the fields of education, employment and community or social development. This includes consideration of the evidence for mental health promotion and the strategies needed for this to grow.

DEFINING MENTAL HEALTH AND MENTAL HEALTH PROMOTION

Mental health is a set of positive attributes. It is described in an extensive literature in terms of a positive emotion (affect) such as feelings of happiness, a personality trait that includes the psychological resources of self-esteem and mastery, and as resilience, or the capacity to cope with adversity. Each of these models contributes to understanding what is meant by mental health (Kovess-Masfety et al., 2005). It is defined by WHO as 'a state of well-being in which the individual realizes his or her own abilities, can cope with the normal stresses of life, can work productively and fruitfully, and is able to contribute to his or her community' (as quoted in Herrman et al., 2005: 2).

This broad definition is consistent with its wide and varied interpretation across cultures. Although the attributes defining mental health are universal, their expression differs culturally, and in relation to different contexts. Sensitivity to the factors valued by different cultures and in various political, economic and social settings will increase the relevance and success of potential interventions (Sturgeon and Orley, 2005). Understanding the effects of discrimination on the lives of women in patriarchal societies or people living with HIV/AIDS, for instance, will make a major contribution to developing intervention programmes. Most of the accessible evidence is recorded in the English language and comes from high-income countries. Progress in generating the evidence for mental health promotion depends on defining, measuring and recording mental health in all parts of the world (Kovess-Masfety et al., 2005).

Three features of mental health define the scope of mental health promotion: mental health is intrinsic to health; mental health is more than the absence of mental illness; and mental health is intimately connected with physical health and behaviour. These ideas are implicit in the well-known definition of health used by WHO: a state of complete physical, mental and social well-being and not merely the absence of disease or infirmity. The connections between mental health and other aspects of health and productivity give it importance beyond its intrinsic value.

Determinants of mental health

Mental health is determined by social, psychological and biological factors that interact with each other, just like health and illness in general. Poor mental health is associated with social disadvantage. Poverty, discrimination and violence, for instance, have a powerful influence on mental health in countries, whether they are high- or low-income (Desjarlais et al., 1995).

Consequences of mental health status

Positive mental health contributes to a person's health, wellbeing and function, and is linked with human, social and economic development. It describes a personal characteristic as well as a community characteristic. Geoffrey Rose (Rose, 1992) restated the ancient view that healthiness (including mental healthiness) is a characteristic of a whole population and not simply of its individual members. He went on to note that just as the mildest subclinical degree of depression is associated with impaired functioning of individuals, so surely the average mood of a population must influence its collective or societal functioning. Yet the measurement of population mental health and the study of its determinants are still relatively neglected.

Fundamental ideas in public health apply to the improvement of mental health (Rose, 1992; Marmot and Wilkinson, 1999; Syme, 1996). For example, health and illness are determined by multiple factors, health and illness exist on a continuum, and personal and environmental influences on health and disease may be studied and changed and the effects evaluated. Yet for many professionals and others, their views of mental health and illness are shaped by the image of long-term institutional care for people living with apparently incurable mental illnesses. Promoting population mental health is sometimes seen as diverting resources from the urgent needs for treatment and rehabilitation of people affected by mental illness. As a result, the opportunities for improving mental health in a community are not fully realized. Activities that can improve mental health include the promotion of health, the prevention of illness and disability, and the treatment and rehabilitation of those affected. As in public health overall, these are different from one another, even though the actions and outcomes overlap. They are all required, and are complementary to one another (Sartorius, 1998).

Mental health promotion

This refers to improving the mental health of everybody in the community, including those with no experience of mental illness as well as those who live with illness and disability. Evidence is available on the effectiveness of public health and social interventions for promoting the mental health of populations in locally devised and culturally appropriate ways. Evidence also links improved mental health with better health and functioning of individual people and communities (Herrman et al., 2005a; Barry and Jenkins, 2007).

Like health promotion, mental health promotion involves actions that support people to adopt and maintain healthy ways of life and create living conditions and environments that allow or foster health. Actions that promote health include advocacy, policy and project development, legislative and regulatory reform, communications, and research and evaluation. These are relevant in countries at all stages of economic development.

Often the activities are designed with vulnerable subgroups such as displaced persons or malnourished children, and in particular settings such as schools, families or in village development projects. Health promotion is concerned with the personal, social and environmental factors that support health and prevention focuses on the causes of disease. The evidence for prevention of mental disorders contributes to the evidence for the promotion of mental health, and the actions that promote mental health will often have as an important outcome the prevention of mental disorders.

The Ottawa Charter for Health Promotion provides a foundation for health promotion strategies that can be applied usefully to the promotion of mental health (Lahtinen et al., 2005). It considers the individual, social and environmental factors that influence health. It places emphasis on the control of health by people in their everyday settings in the context of healthy policy and supportive environments. The Charter's five strategies are: building healthy public policies, creating supportive environments, strengthening community action, developing personal skills and reorienting health services.

Some interventions have the primary goal of promoting mental health and others are mainly intended to achieve something else but improve mental health as a side benefit. Activities designed to promote other aspects of health, to reduce risk behaviours such as tobacco, alcohol and drug misuse and unsafe sex, to improve the relationships between teachers and students in schools, or to alleviate social and economic problems such as crime and intimate partner violence, will often promote mental health. Suicide prevention programmes in countries or districts will also typically include interventions that promote mental health.

Conversely, promoting mental health will usually have additional effects on health and on social and economic conditions. It can help, for instance, in the prevention of smoking or of unprotected sex and hence help prevent AIDS or teenage pregnancy. The evaluation of outcomes can be designed to take these wider changes into account.

Mental health promotion actions are often social and political: making changes in schools, influencing housing and working conditions, working to reduce stigma and discrimination of various types, and developing policy initiatives to reduce violence are examples. The changes are made and decisions taken by politicians, educators and members of nongovernmental organizations. Health practitioners are important as advocates and as aids to introducing the policies and programs.

HUMAN RIGHTS, MENTAL HEALTH AND DEVELOPMENT

The mental health of each person is related closely to life circumstances and experiences and also to wider contextual factors. These include a society's concern for gender, ethnicity and the human rights to education, equal social and economic participation, safety, individual autonomy and freedom from discrimination. According to the social model of health that takes all these factors into account, an individual's state of health or experience of illness is determined by personal experiences, social circumstances, culture and political environment in addition to inherited or biological factors (Fisher et al., 2010).

There are complex linkages between health and human rights (WHO, 2002a) that apply equally to mental health. First, violations or lack of attention to human rights can have serious health consequences. Examples are violence against women and children, slavery, torture, harmful traditional practices and the impact of colonialism on indigenous peoples. Second, health policies and programs can promote or violate human rights in the ways they are designed or put into practice. The rights to participation, to information, to privacy and freedom from discrimination are particularly relevant here. Third, taking steps to respect, protect and fulfill human rights can reduce vulnerability to ill health and the impact of ill health. The rights to health, education, food and nutrition and freedom from discrimination are important in policy and program development, and have a reciprocal relationship with good mental health.

Protection of human rights (civil, cultural, economic, political and social dimensions) is fundamental to mental health promotion and life with dignity (Drew et al., 2005). Every country in the world is now party to at least one United Nations human rights treaty that recognizes health-related human rights. This means that governments have committed themselves to various human rights obligations relevant to health. While the treaties neither state that good health is every person's right or that governments have a responsibility for their citizens' good health, it is the duty of every government to attempt to optimize the conditions fostering mental health and wellbeing and quality of life of all of its citizens.

Taking steps to promote and protect human rights will promote mental health and other aspects of health, given the sociopolitical and economic conditions that are prerequisites for the mental health of the population. Conversely, promoting mental health will necessarily promote and protect human rights. Effective health promotion improves fairness, dignity and participation of the local population.

The international human rights framework offers useful guidance to governments about the requirements for creating the necessary social, economic and political conditions to promote the mental health of the population. Using international human rights standards promotes accountability and the introduction of measures to end discrimination, ill treatment or violence. This provides a mechanism to consider the wide range of mental health determinants, and the need for action and involvement of a range of sectors.

Certain people and groups within society, such as women, children and refugees, are particularly vulnerable to human rights violations. Countries need to adopt specific measures to monitor, safeguard and realize their rights, including their right to mental health: that is the right to goods, services, conditions and facilities that are conducive to mental health. Discrimination and marginalization decrease the chances of good mental health and increase the propensity for mental health problems (Drew et al., 2005).

Advocating for application of human rights standards, for example, rights to healthcare, education and freedom from discrimination contributes to the creation of a protective environment and supports social protection and legal protection. Promoting population mental health particularly in settings of poverty and conflict requires the capacity to identify and monitor protection threats and failures, and respond through social protection and through legal protection (IASC, 2007).

PROMOTING MENTAL HEALTH IN LOW-INCOME COUNTRIES

Poverty, human rights abuses, conflict and emergencies associated with wars and civil unrest (conditions that are found commonly in low-income countries) are linked with poor mental health outcomes as well as poor physical health and social conditions (Baingana et al., 2005), as also noted above. Tackling important social and health concerns in these countries such as HIV prevention, maternal and child health, violence at home and in the streets, substance abuse and gender equity requires interventions that focus on self-efficacy and appropriate participation, which are in turn components of mental health. Promoting mental health and satisfying mental health needs optimally involves satisfying a range of other needs. For example, interventions to assist low-income women with breastfeeding will simultaneously address infant nutrition needs (Herrman and Swartz, 2007).

Health promotion is suited to all types of social and economic situations, and stories of health promotion success are found in all regions. An illustration of this is the World Health Organization's 'Healthy Cities' project. This is based on the principle that modern public health must tackle basic health determinants through comprehensive multi-sector policy, planning and action (Neiman and Hall, 2007).

Communities' own rituals and traditional practices can often help people affected by trauma reintegrate into normal life. Many of these rituals take the form of symbolic cleansing, of washing away the blood or the traumatic memories, of driving away bad spirits and of calling ancestors for assistance. These rituals contrast with Western and more intrusive modes of dealing with trauma, which emphasize psychotherapeutic recounting and remembering experiences. Instead, traditional rituals aim to create a rupture with the past. We await evidence about whether or not they have a positive effect on mental and psychosocial conditions, and strengthening those practices that work (Baingana et al., 2005).

For a range of reasons, including a lack of resources, far less research has been conducted in low-income than in high-income countries. It is likely, therefore, that there will be little specific evidence, in particular from randomized controlled trials (RCTs), which demonstrate the impact of social and economic development policies and programmes on the promotion of mental health. The evidence that does exist includes narrative and case study material of specific programmes and evidence from the domain of physical health promotion that may be extrapolated to mental health. These programmes focus on three major areas of action: advocacy, empowerment and social support, as described later (Patel et al., 2005).

International action would be required to generate and disseminate further evidence in low- and middle-income countries. This implies the need for international cooperation to assist low-income countries with technical support and other capacity building resources, designing dissemination strategies, publishing guidelines for effective implementation of low-cost sustainable programmes and providing training in programme planning and evaluation. Given the socio-economic conditions of poorer countries, it is unrealistic to expect that every country or district has the political will and the means to perform controlled outcome studies for each intervention they implement, however. This stresses the need to study not only the outcomes of programmes but also their working mechanisms, principles and effect moderators. Such knowledge and its translation into guidelines could support policy-makers, programme designers and practitioners in effectively adapting programmes and policies to local needs, resources and culture. This also underlines the need to use the full spectrum of research methods, including less expensive qualitative studies, to build an evidence base incrementally that has validity for the country or community in question (Saxena et al., 2005).

PLANNING AND EVALUATING MENTAL HEALTH PROMOTING INTERVENTIONS

Promoting mental health is expected to improve overall health, quality of life and social functioning. The benefits that can be measured include better mental health, lower rates of some mental illnesses, improved physical health, better educational performance, greater productivity of workers, improved relationships within families and safer communities (Wiseman et al., 2007; Zubrick and Kovess-Masfety, 2005).

The first step in any community or setting is gathering local evidence and opinion about the social and personal influences on mental health and the main problems that need to be tackled (e.g. family violence or school drop-out) and the potential gains. Local people and experts give essential advice on developing partnerships, planning interventions and their evaluation. In the case of the framework used as an example by WHO for the public health approach to promoting mental health and wellbeing (VicHealth, 2005), the three identified determinants of mental health are social inclusion, freedom from discrimination and violence, and economic participation. Local information and opinion will determine whether these or other factors are relevant to the setting, locality or country; which are the most important influences on mental health; how mental health is affected; and what interventions to introduce in which sectors, settings and population groups.

As the second step, a plan of action is agreed and partnerships established, the resources are gathered, implementation begins and monitoring of action and change processes. The third step is the evaluation and dissemination of best practices, with attention to maintaining and improving quality as dissemination unfolds (Walker et al., 2005a).

MENTAL HEALTH PROMOTION PRACTICE

Activities or interventions designed to promote health take place at several levels. Some are distant from the individual, such as policies to tax alcohol products and others are closer to the individual such as home-visiting health promotion programmes (Sartorius, 1998). The interventions may be designed to strengthen individuals (also called *micro interventions*), with an emphasis on vulnerable people such as displaced persons or malnourished children. They may be designed to strengthen communities (as in community development and neighbourhood renewal) or improve living and working conditions (e.g. adequate housing and making work conditions safer), with an emphasis on disadvantaged areas and specific sectors or settings respectively (also called *meso interventions*). Healthy policies *(macro interventions)* aim to alter the macroeconomic or cultural environment to reduce poverty and the wider adverse effects of inequality on society. These include introducing policies and regulations on legal and human rights, promoting cultural values, encouraging equal opportunities and hazard control, and 'healthier' labour laws. These policies span several sectors and work across the population as a whole.

Despite gaps in the evidence we know enough about the links between social experience and mental health to make a compelling case to apply and evaluate locally appropriate policy and practice interventions to promote mental health (Barry and Jenkins, 2007; Herrman et al., 2005b) While the published evidence on cost-effectiveness is much more limited, the evidence summarized by Friedli and Parsonage (Friedli and Parsonage, 2007) indicates that the benefits of positive mental health are likely to be considerable. Interventions targeting parents and pre-school children show a high level of effectiveness and cost-effectiveness. There is a robust case both for strengthening investment in mental health promotion in schools and for increasing educational opportunities for adults.

Support for emotional and social development is as important as help with schoolwork for young people in increasing the chances of educational success, especially for children facing difficulties at home. The effectiveness of actions to promote mental health in the employment sector and workplaces, through lifestyle messages and in the natural world and built environment are also reported.

Overall the evidence can be assembled to provide encouragement and examples for non-health and health sectors to promote mental health for mutual benefit. The UK Government Office for Science announced in 2008 the findings of the Foresight project on Mental Capital and Wellbeing (Beddington, 2008), showing that governments have tremendous opportunities to create environments in which mental capital (cognitive and emotional resources) and wellbeing (a dynamic state that refers to an individual's ability to develop their potential, work productively and creatively, build strong and positive relationships with others and contribute to their community) flourish and that failure to act could have severe consequences. Three areas of focus for the project were: childhood development, mental health and wellbeing at work and making the most of cognitive resources in older age.

This project and others demonstrate that improving mental health requires population-based policies and programmes, as well as specific activities in the health services relating to the prevention and treatment of ill-health. Population–based interventions involve health and non-health sectors in various ways. Activities in several of these sectors will now be described, aiming to illustrate in each case how mental health can be promoted in the course of other work, and how this in turn can assist the sector with its own outcomes. Mental health and public health experts can make recommendations on the scope and possibilities for mental health promotion in the work of education, employment or community sectors and provide information and resources to policymakers, leaders and practitioners. In each case this begins with broad statements of mutual benefits and extends to examples that can then be discussed with the local experts as described above.

Policymakers are now recognizing that emphasis is best placed on adding programmes that sharpen the capacity of systems, such as primary health care and school systems to be more attentive to mental health. The sustainability of mental health programmes relates more to their success as change processes within organizations or communities than to their technological aspects. Their evaluation includes analysis of factors within the programme context such as pre-existing attitudes and relationships that could predict why some programmes and not others succeed and grow (Hawe and Riley, 2005; Petersen et al., 2010; Rowling and Taylor, 2005; Swartz, 2010).

PROMOTING MENTAL HEALTH IN THE EDUCATION SECTOR

The engagement with leaders and policymakers in education to focus on improving mental health emphasizes three premises: good education, good health and good mental health are closely related in individuals and communities. Poor education and low population literacy are linked with social and economic problems, violence and ill-health and poor mental health. Educational performance for schools is typically linked to the students' mental health, physical health and behaviour.

Two areas of activity have been identified. First there is improving access to education to ensure that whole populations are literate and numerate (WorldBank, 2000). This includes support for inclusion of girls and minority groups where needed, programmes reducing truancy and school drop out and equitable access irrespective of gender, race and ability. The second activity considers the opportunities to promote mental health in schools and other education settings (considering students, teachers and the surrounding community) and through better collaboration between education, health and the community.

There is the benefit to mental health of existing policies and actions, for example, universal primary education, that are already recommended for other important reasons. The purpose of drawing these to attention is to consider how to assess the mental health outcomes and shape the policies and programmes to ensure the mental health benefits are achieved. Other programmes such as life skills training are introduced primarily for the mental health and associated benefits.

Improving access to education

A range of strategies and interventions have been shown to be effective and feasible, even in countries with limited resources. As well as programmes supporting *universal primary education*, these include *improved access to education across the lifespan*. Low levels of literacy and education are a major social problem in many countries, especially among women. Lack of education limits access to work and economic entitlements; and poor education in mothers is associated with poor health of children and families. *Adult literacy programs* can improve mental health by a number of means. For example, numeracy skills reduce the risk of being cheated; developing greater confidence allows people to assert their rights; and people who are literate and numerate gain access to social and economic opportunities. Promoting the healthy development of children *prevents school failure and dropout*. Specific programmes can also aim to engage children and reduce truancy and suspensions. Programmes can also *improve access to education for underserved populations* such as girls, immigrants and ethnic and religious minority groups. Using subsidies, improved physical access to school and culturally appropriate design can close gender gaps in education (WorldBank, 2000). Better education for women improves job prospects and child health, contributes to social equity, encourages girls and women to be more independent and lowers the risk for depression (WHO, 2000).

In September 2000, 189 member states ratified the United Nations Millennium Declaration that every woman, man and child has the right to development and freedom from want and that progress has to be measurable and demonstrable. The Declaration defines goals, targets and indicators for combating poverty, hunger, disease, illiteracy, environmental degradation and discrimination against women as central to development. UN Millenium Development Goal (MDG) 2 and its Target 3 is: Ensure that all boys and girls complete a full course of primary schooling. MDG 3 is Promote gender equality and empower women and its Target is: Eliminate gender disparity in primary and secondary education (UNDP).

Promote education settings as learning and social environments

In countries committed to universal primary education, schools are the most important institutions apart from the family for socialization and healthy development of children and adolescents. An effective school strives to help children to be healthy and successful learners to the best of their abilities. Disruptive behaviour and violence are problems in some schools. Schools can also be a safe environment for children living in dangerous places. They provide a venue for educating children about sexual abuse and protective behaviours, and an opportunity to confide in their teachers (Wild, 2007). For very disadvantaged children, schools may be the only place to find a stable and trusting relationship.

Children concentrate poorly if they are emotionally upset by conflict at home or in school. Children who become withdrawn due to depression or poor social skills are less likely to engage in classroom learning activities. Promoting the healthy development of children prevents school failure and dropout. Learning and emotional problems, including undetected learning disabilities, are important risk factors for school dropout, for example in India and South Africa (Patel et al., 2008).

Evidence from programmes promoting mental health in schools is that:

1   *Universal school mental health promotion and long-term interventions promoting the positive mental health of all pupils and involving changes to school climate* can be effective and are likely to be more successful than brief class-based mental illness prevention programmes (Wells et al., 2003).

2   *Combined programmes* including interventions to change the overall school climate and those designed to improve social competency in individual students are more effective than programmes with only one feature. Complex programmes of this type have successfully led to improved mental wellbeing and social skills as well as reduced anxiety and depressive symptoms among students. Social outcomes include reductions in aggression and bullying and increases in school achievement. Whole school mental health programmes are most effective when they include professional development training and support for teachers. Schools are a setting for promoting the health of teachers as well as students, and have an influence on family health and function. Involving parents supports some school-based programmes. WHO's health promoting schools encourage core elements of the whole school approach including: distributed leadership (or delegation) (APAPDC, 2007), inclusive policies and practices and engagement and connection (Stewart Brown, 2006).

3   *Programmes including specific interventions to improve life skills or social and emotional competence* can increase positive behaviours, reduce risk of mental health problems and increase resilience. *Life skills* include decision-making, problem-solving, creative and critical thinking, effective communication and interpersonal skills, self-awareness and coping with emotions and stress (WHO, 1997). Life skills are distinct from other important skills that young people acquire as they grow up, such as numeracy, reading and practical livelihood skills. Evidence from high-income and some low-income countries indicates that life skills education is effective in the prevention of substance abuse, adolescent pregnancy and bullying; improving academic performance and school attendance; and the promotion of mental wellbeing and healthy behaviours (Patel et al., 2008).

4   *Targeted programmes and services.* Early identification of the signs of mental illness and severe behavioural difficulties, and efficient connections to psychosocial supports and treatment where necessary can help to stop the illness developing, persisting or becoming more severe, and prevent co-occurring illnesses, substance use and disabilities. Teachers can be trained to recognize children who are likely to be distressed, offer initial interventions and refer those that require it to the appropriate sources. A psychosocial professional from the school or the community is a useful support for these school-based programmes and referral to services. (However, this early identification approach carries with it the risk of early stigmatization and remains a contested matter for professional commentators.)

5   *Partnerships across education, health and the community* can foster mentoring, family assistance and other transitional programmes, from pre-primary-secondary school and beyond, into employment. Relevant community linkages include health, social and clinical services, civic and faith based organizations, criminal justice system and youth development programmes. Out-of-school time programming (daily and seasonal) can provide enrichment and youth development, particularly for children who live in poverty.

6   *Promoting education settings as mentally healthy workplaces.* Burn out and absenteeism among teachers are big problems for teachers, students and the school climate, especially in poorly resourced schools. Where teachers are abusive or absent this needs to be detected and the situation managed actively. Teacher training and support programmes can include educational psychology, the practice of learning and teaching and how to discipline students in socially acceptable ways (Mindmatters).

PROMOTING MENTAL HEALTH IN EMPLOYMENT, LABOUR AND WORK SECTORS

Workers commonly experience brief periods of stress and anxiety at work without ill-effect, but prolonged exposure to stress is likely to harm workers' health and expose them to risk of illness. The adverse effects of job stress on mental health may be greater among lower status workers or if combined with harmful use of alcohol or other drugs, a common relation to stress. The effect of job stress on worker health and productivity is a growing concern in low-income countries, especially in countries undergoing rapid industrialization, as in Asia (Houtman et al., 2007). Work stress is already recognized as one of the most common work-related health problems in high-income countries. Job stress is rapidly emerging as the single greatest cause of work-related disease and injury and as a significant contributor to the overall burden of disease in society. Working conditions and the labour market have changed in many countries, with globalization and interdependence of the world economy, and people leaving rural areas to seek work in cities. Automation, the rapid introduction of new information technologies, and new organizational structures and processes are among the changes affecting workers (WHO and ILO, 2000).

Mental health problems at work have a negative impact on absenteeism, work performance, staff attitude and behaviour and the relationships at work. Diagnosed mental disorders are a major reason for granting disability pensions in countries with these provisions (Leka et al., 2005).

Access to meaningful employment provides an opportunity for personal development and achievement, and meaningful participation in the society. It is linked to a person's capacity to provide for themselves and their families in housing, education and health care. It is critical for people in post-conflict and refugee populations. Lack of work is associated with poor mental health and mental illness, especially in vulnerable groups such as single women with children, slum dwellers in cities and young people likely to abuse substances. This also has adverse effects on the children and families. Lack of work is a major problem in many developing countries, especially in countries affected by conflicts and with large numbers of ex-combatants and refugees (Baingana et al., 2005).

Two areas of activity are important to mental health promotion in the employment, labour and work sectors. First is *lack of employment and mental health,* and second, *working conditions and mental health* (WHO and ILO, 2000; LaMontagne et al., 2007). Policymakers attentive to these points suggest the following five interventions.

Introduce employment policies that support workers' rights, family responsibilities, role of unions and prevent discrimination

National policies are needed to provide adequate employment opportunities for the population including minority and displaced groups (employment policies, education and training); to ensure the sustenance of those who do not have or have lost work (unemployment insurance, welfare assistance); to avoid discrimination through legislation specific to employment for people with disabilities and family caregiving responsibilities; to regulate the psychosocial work environment through psychosocial risk management and legislation on safety; to define job conditions including job security, hours of work, leave entitlements (including maternity and paternity leave) and minimum wages; and to define the role of labour unions and international labour federations in improving job conditions. Employers also need to understand how these laws affect their work and planning.

Introduce policies and practices to support adequate working conditions

Certain work factors are associated with mental ill health and sickness absence among workers in a wide range of employment: long hours worked, work overload and pressure and the effects of these on personal lives; lack of control over work; little participation in decision making; poor social support; bullying and harassment; and unclear management and work role. Many of these factors can be changed. Most countries have laws and policies for safety and health in the workplace. Even when elaborated these standards focus primarily on physical health. Only some countries have special legislation concerning job stress.

Evidence in some high-income countries suggests that investment in healthy working practices and the health and wellbeing of workers improves productivity and is cost effective for business and wider society. A range of interventions in working conditions can improve mental health and lower the risk of mental disorders. These include task and technical interventions such as job enrichment with variation or incentives, as much job control as possible, reducing noise, balancing the job demand, giving appropriate reward for efforts and flexible working conditions as possible. Employers can also, for example, improve role clarity and social relationships through communication, conflict resolution and grievance processes, offer support to staff to develop roles and in case of work or personal difficulties, encourage health and fitness among employees with physical exercise and social opportunities.

Identify and support the coping capacity of vulnerable persons at work

The coping capacity of individuals at work can be improved by stress management training, stress inoculation techniques, relaxation methods and social skills and fitness training. Such methods can prevent adverse mental health outcomes.

Provide work opportunities for vulnerable groups such as refugees and ex-combatants

In countries such as Burundi, Rwanda and Sudan, socio-economic interventions contribute to the economic viability of reintegrating populations, for example vocational training, access to credit, agricultural inputs. Above all, people who have experienced mass violence and conflict need to work and earn a living. The immediate post-conflict phase is the ideal time to contribute to the reconstruction process by creating opportunities for employment. Job creation cannot wait years for factories to be built, since by then dependency has set in and economic, physical and mental damage has been done (Baingana et al., 2005).

Introduce programmes to develop personal skills for those without work

Intervention programmes to develop personal skills for those who have already lost their job or out of work can be effective. Having work is a protective factor against mental disorder. Re-employment is an effective way to promote the mental health of unemployed people. The Jobs Club or Jobs Program is used successfully in several countries (Price et al., 1992; Vuori et al., 2005)

MENTAL HEALTH PROMOTION IN COMMUNITY SECTORS (INCLUDING SOCIAL WELFARE AND ECONOMIC DEVELOPMENT SECTORS)

Throughout the world, poor mental health is associated with *poverty*. With few exceptions worldwide, the evidence shows that the lower an individual's socio-economic position the worse is his or her health (Marmot, 2007). The greater vulnerability of disadvantaged people in each community is explained by such factors as the experience of insecurity and hopelessness, rapid social change and the risks of violence and physical ill health.

Mental, social and behavioural health problems may interact so as to intensify each other's impact on behaviour and well-being. Substance abuse, violence and abuses of women and children on the one hand, and health problems such as heart disease, depression and anxiety on the other, are more prevalent and more difficult to cope with in conditions of low income, poor living conditions, gender discrimination and human rights violations (Desjarlais et al., 1995).

Conversely, decent educational opportunities, parental warmth and firm parenting and good physical health are widely recognized as conducive to good mental health, as are a sense of connection, low levels of conflict and social support (Patel et al., 2007). The right to the highest attainable level of health is enshrined in the charter of WHO and many international treaties as described above, and realizing this right requires action on the social determinants of health (Marmot, 2007).

Health has economic as well as intrinsic value (Marmot, 2007). Good mental health, just as good health overall, enables people to participate in society with potentially positive consequences for economic performance. Mental health is inextricably linked with human development and human welfare, both because the social and economic determinants of human development are strongly associated with mental health and because poor mental health will compromise longevity, general health and creativity. The factors that influence human development are those that influence mental health and it is likely that a dynamic relationship exists between human development and mental health (Patel et al., 2005).

Scope of the Interventions

In the light of the above, policymakers promoting mental health point out that communities must be consulted and actively participate in designing and implementing strategies and interventions, at all levels. These include macrolevel or national social policy to improve income security, housing and access to education and secure work and mesolevel or community action in advocacy, empowerment and social support and support for early child development (ECD) (Patel et al., 2005):

- *Advocacy* related to the mental health effects of alcohol abuse is an example, as are advocacy and public education about domestic violence, safe sex and reproductive health.
- *Empowerment* is the process by which groups in a community who have been traditionally disadvantaged in ways that compromise their health can overcome these barriers and exercise all their rights, with a view to leading a full, equal life in the best of health. Empowerment programmes and policies that have had a mental health impact include micro-credit schemes for alleviation of debt, community development programmes, violence prevention in the community and life skills education for adolescents.
- *Social support* strategies aim to strengthen community organizations and develop intersectoral alliances to allow healthy lifestyles and promote mental health. Examples of this are supporting mothers and families, promoting childhood development in the midst of adversity and befriending and income generation schemes for elderly people.

The benefits expected from promoting mental health in communities include: healthier communities, fewer disrupted families, greater productivity of workers; less crime; lower risks for mental disorder; and stronger national development as assessed by community-wide or nation-wide development indicators such as Human Development Index, Gender Related Development Index or the Gender Empowerment Index.

Examples of interventions

Having noted the scope and type of interventions possible to promote mental health, here some examples are given.

- *Macrolevel* or national policies include improved access to education and secure work (as above), and improved economic security. A formal social security net including disability insurance and social insurance supports mental health, as it reduces poverty and worries about unemployment and illness.
- *Mesolevel or community strategies that strengthen community networks.* Impoverished and socially disorganized neighbourhoods have a powerful adverse effect on mental health. For example, adverse factors in the slums of Mumbai include displacement, poor conditions, unequal distribution of amenities, demolition of housing, homelessness and communal and ethnic disharmony. Demoralization, addictions, anger, depression, hostility and violence can all be linked back to these experiences and problems (Parkar et al., 2003). Programmes are needed to reduce the clustering of these social and health problems in shantytowns and slums and at the same time help people and families cope with these circumstances (Kleinman, 1999).
- *Micro-credit schemes for alleviation of debt,* combined with organized community action in low-income countries can achieve better nutritional status, better child survival, higher educational achievement, lower rates of domestic violence and improved psychological health (Chowdhury and Bhuiya, 2005). Indebtedness is also a concern for disadvantaged groups in high-income countries. Here the problem may be lack of regulation in lending to low-income people, as well as poor access to credit for women, minority groups, unemployed people and families. Governments can consider appropriate laws and regulations.

- *Community development interventions* can focus effectively on empowering processes and building a sense of ownership and social responsibility among community members. Community development aims to develop the social, environmental and cultural wellbeing of communities with a focus on marginalized people. Community development works through the understanding of local factors relevant to a community and the empowerment of that community to solve its own problems. The subsequent improvement in the determinants of mental health (such as improved social relationships and support, including social safety nets that can be tapped during crises, improved housing, health care and education, better nutrition and cleaner environment, stronger economic development and improved health) lead to better mental health and the further benefits to health and community expected from that (Arole et al., 2005).
- *Violence prevention in the community.* The mental health of children and adults can be profoundly affected by violence at home. Child maltreatment and intimate partner violence (IPV) are prevalent public health problems in developing and developed countries. The effects on mental health often persist, and they can contribute to a generational cycle of violence and impaired wellbeing. Exposure to these types of violence and the mental health sequelae are apparently common in males as well as females in many settings (MacMillan and Wathen, 2005). Physical and sexual partner violence against women is widespread. The variation in prevalence within and between settings highlights that this violence is not inevitable, and needs to be addressed (Garcia-Moreno et al., 2006) (See Pilgrim and Rogers, this handbook.)
- *Interventions for child maltreatment and IPV* have received relatively little focus in international research (MacMillan and Wathen, 2005). Many programmes at several levels are effective in the primary outcomes of reducing violence (WHO, 2002b) and given the linkages between domestic violence and common mental disorders in women, they are likely to have a powerful impact on mental health as well. These programmes range from legal reforms to ensure the rights of abused women, community policing, training of health and law enforcement workers and politicians, improving the environments of refugee camps, and strengthening intimate relationships, one of the commonest contexts for violence, by parenting training, mentoring and marriage counselling. Some of these, such as the Stepping Stones programme, have been shown in African and Asian settings to help men communicate and give them new respect for women (WHO, 2002b). Social development programmes that emphasize competency and social skills appear to be the most effective in reducing youth violence. Systematic evaluations of the mental health impacts are needed as these programmes are introduced (MacMillan and Wathen, 2005). Violence is a pervasive experience in many developing countries through wars and civil unrest.
- *Creating safe spaces* for victims to express their feelings and providing basic relief and rehabilitation seem critical for any programme aiming to help people affected by violence, as demonstrated in the efforts to promote the psychosocial rehabilitation of the victims of riots in Gujarat, India, in 2002 (Sekar, 2002). Successful programmes aimed at promoting mental health in victims of trauma have used people's own traditions, skills and approaches to crisis (see above) and give attention to rebuilding external social worlds (Summerfield, 1999).
- *Teaching adolescents to deal effectively with the demands and challenges of everyday life.* Life skills education (see above) can teach adolescents, through improved mental health, to deal effectively with the demands and challenges of everyday life, and lead to positive changes in other aspects of health and function. This model is now being advocated, field-tested and implemented successfully in a number of developing countries (Patel et al., 2008).
- *Support for early child development (ECD).* A healthy start in life affects the child's later functioning in school, with peers, in the family and in broader connections with society. Many children younger than 5 years are exposed to multiple risks, including poverty, malnutrition, poor health and un-stimulating home environments, which detrimentally affect their cognitive, motor and social-emotional development. Worldwide over 200 million children under 5 years are not fulfilling their developmental potential. These children are likely to do poorly in school and subsequently have low incomes, high fertility and provide poor care for their children, thus

contributing to the intergenerational transmission of poverty (Grantham-McGregor et al., 2007). Child development refers to the ordered emergence of interdependent skills of sensori-motor, cognitive, language and social-emotional functioning. Brain development is modified by the quality of the environment before and after birth, and variations in the quality of maternal care can produce lasting changes in stress reactivity, anxiety and memory function in children. Despite the vulnerability of the brain to early insults, remarkable recovery is often possible with interventions and generally the earlier the interventions the greater the results. Early interventions can help prevent the loss of potential in affected children and improvements can happen rapidly (Grantham-McGregor et al., 2007).

- *Good development is promoted by several factors.* Three aspects of parenting are consistently related to young children's cognitive and social-emotional competence: cognitive stimulation, sensitivity and responsiveness to the child and emotional warmth. Early opportunities for learning in combination with improved nutrition increase the chances that a child will attend and stay in school, will learn effectively while in school and will be able to use the learning for becoming a more productive worker and caregiver of the next generation in adulthood (Fisher et al., 2010). Enabling parents to provide adequate psychosocial stimulation has been described as the single most important factor for building resilience in youth (Patel et al., 2007). The effect of these factors is sensitive to contextual factors such as level of advantage or poverty, cultural values and practices. Nonetheless these child-rearing dimensions affect children from developed and developing countries in similar ways (Walker et al., 2007).

- *Several factors adversely affect child development.* Inadequate stimulation in their first 5 years of life is identified as one of the four main causes (the others being malnutrition that leads to stunting, iodine and iron deficiency) of the millions of children failing to reach their potential in cognitive and socio-emotional development (Jolly, 2007). Several other causal factors include maternal depression and exposure to violence (as well as malaria and exposure to heavy metals). Maternal depression is a major problem in LAMICs, estimated to affect 20–30 per cent of mothers (Fisher et al., 2009). Maternal depression can disturb the attachment relationship between the mother and her young child, and has been linked to impaired cognitive development, and behavioural and emotional problems in children. Maternal mental health is apparently a critical factor in the association between social adversity and childhood failure to thrive in poor countries (Patel et al., 2004). In many LAMICs, three of the most significant risks to positive early development and later mental health commence before birth: the mother's health and nutritional status; maternal exposure to alcohol and other substances and external factors; and maternal HIV status (Richter et al., 2010).

- *Effective interventions in low- and high-income countries can promote child development and prevent or ameliorate the loss of developmental potential.* Overall, programmes that have the greatest impact on child growth and development commence prenatally and extend into infancy and early childhood in a continuous chain of support. A major series of articles on ECD in the *Lancet* concludes that despite convincing evidence, program coverage is low. To achieve the Millennium Development Goals of reducing poverty and ensuring primary school completion for girls and boys, governments and civil society should consider expanding high quality, cost-effective early child development programmes to reach all disadvantaged children (Engle et al., 2007).

Interventions for promoting ECD are optimally located within regular primary health care. There are effective and mostly low-cost actions that can be taken to prevent the damage and remedy the deficiencies (Fisher et al., 2010). The prenatal risks can all be detected, managed and referred on from the primary health care system (Richter et al., 2010). While delivery of ECD services depends on the local context, case studies illustrate that successful programmes can be implemented at all income levels. WHO in collaboration with UNICEF, the World

Bank and other partners has developed the *Care for Child Development package* that provides age-appropriate recommendations for all children up to three years of age on play, communication, nutrition and responsive feeding and includes intervention strategies when problems are identified (Engle et al., 2007). The package has a checklist for health care providers to use to identify and manage problems. It also includes recommendations for care during pregnancy and the mental health of mothers. Health workers, nutrition workers or community health workers can give these recommendations to caregivers. The feasibility of adopting the Care for Child Development programme in resource-poor settings has been demonstrated in Brazil and South Africa. In Turkey investigators found an effect on the quality of the home environment one month after a single health centre visit (Engle et al., 2007).

There is a strong argument for a range of targeted, home-based interventions including infant and child nutrition through to early stimulation and parenting (Richter et al., 2010). These may be individual level interventions in the home, directed to either parents or child, or interpersonal interventions involving both child and caregivers. In the USA where this has been studied, some forms of home-visiting programmes that target high-risk and/or low-income mothers and children, and early childhood development for low income 3- and 4-year olds (as well as some youth development programmes) are highly cost-effective. The outcomes include reduced crime, lower substance abuse, better educational outcomes, fewer teen pregnancies, fewer teen suicide attempts, lower child abuse and neglect, and reduced domestic violence (Aos et al., 2004; Olds et al., 1998).

The Prenatal and Early Childhood Nurse Home Visitation programme (Olds et al., 1998) is effective in improving parenting and attachment and reducing the risks of child maltreatment, but it is too costly for most low-income countries. A less intensive home visiting intervention for women from low-income families, designed to improve maternal sensitivity and infant–mother attachment, was tested in South Africa in a randomized control trial (Cooper et al., 2009), with promising results. Home visiting approaches need to be frequent and sustained over several years to have longer-term benefits for children (Powell and Grantham-McGregor, 1989) and have a number of other characteristics including active and engaged parental participation. Whether interventions such as these can effectively be taken to scale in low-income countries remains to be evaluated (Richter et al., 2010).

Early stimulation programmes combined with nutritional and micronutrient support reduced the effects of malnutrition and improved cognitive, educational deficits, as well as psychological functioning and long-term educational achievement and psychological functioning in at-risk children in low-income settings in Jamaica (Walker et al., 2005b). The stimulation was achieved by weekly home visits by trained community health workers to improve mother–child interaction through play (Richter et al., 2010).

Trained nurse home visitors may carry out programmes such as these, but using community resources can also be an efficient strategy. Home visiting programmes can be especially useful in low-income populations and countries because of illiteracy or constraints on access to health care or information. Developing countries have often no alternative but to train lay community family support workers and have considerable expertise in doing so. Developing the appropriate psychosocial programmes for mothers or parents requires familiarity with the local context and day-to-day tasks of parenting (Patel et al., 2008).

Group sessions and home visits by a nurse have also been found effective for mothers who are depressed or at risk of depression in a variety of settings (Small and Lumley, 2007). In rural Pakistan, integration of home-based individual cognitive behaviour therapy into the routine work of community health workers (Lady Health Workers or lay visitors) helped reduce depression among prenatally depressed women by over 50 per cent in a cluster randomized controlled trial (Rahman et al., 2008).

- *Promoting childhood development in the midst of adversity.* Parenting, nutritional and educational interventions can improve psychosocial development in disadvantaged populations in countries at all income levels. Interventions that combine psychosocial components (such as promoting mother–infant interaction) with other components such as nutritional, health, family support and educational programmes and those that are implemented as early as possible and for the longest duration have the greatest impact. That impact is evident for many years after the intervention. Providing services directly to children and including an active parenting and skill-building component is a more effective strategy than providing information alone. *The evidence base in support of these interventions is robust enough for scaling up in routine early child-care programmes.* Full-scale programmes have been implemented in some of the world's poorest countries. Despite the favourable findings, it is important to recognize that children who are nutritionally or socioeconomically disadvantaged never fully catch up with children who are well nourished or privileged. There is a need to develop and test models of combined interventions that can reach a higher proportion of children and evaluate their impact on adult mental and physical health (Engle et al., 2007; Patel et al., 2008; WHO, 2006).
- *Successful early child development interventions* have a number of characteristics (Engle et al., 2007). These include integration of health, nutrition, education, social and economic development and collaboration between governmental agencies and civil society. There is a focus on disadvantaged children. The interventions have sufficient intensity and duration, and include direct contact with children beginning early in life. Parents and families are partners with teachers or caregivers in supporting children's development. The interventions provide opportunities for children to initiate and instigate their own learning and exploration of their surroundings with age-appropriate activities, and blend traditional child-rearing practices and cultural beliefs with evidence-based approaches. The ECD staff are given systematic in-service training, supportive and continuous supervision, observational methods to monitor children's development, practice and good theoretical and learning material support.
- *Supporting migrants including refugees.* Mobile populations can be more vulnerable to mental health problems than the native population, due to their condition as migrants and their limited access to adequate services, especially if they can no longer refer to their traditional community support (IOM, 2003). Social policies and community action need to include reference to this vulnerable group.
- *Supporting mental health and psychosocial wellbeing in emergency and post-conflict settings.* Armed conflicts and natural disasters cause psychological and social suffering in the short- and long-term, threatening peace, human rights and development. One of the priorities

is therefore to protect and improve people's mental health and psychosocial wellbeing during and after emergencies and conflicts. Government and non-government humanitarian actors are increasingly active in this regard. Effective work requires coordinated action among them all (IASC, 2007). A multi-sectoral, inter-agency framework has been developed (IASC, 2007) that enables effective coordination, flags potentially harmful practices and clarifies how different approaches to mental health and psychosocial support complement one another. In the early and later phases of an emergency, social supports are essential to protect and support mental health and psychosocial wellbeing, as well as selected psychological and psychiatric interventions for specific problems. The need for cost-effectiveness studies of psychosocial interventions for populations affected by conflict is becoming increasingly apparent and some agencies including the World Bank have begun to do this work.

- *Ageing and mental health.* The elderly face a triple burden in deprived settings in all countries: a growing burden of noncommunicable and degenerative disorders associated with ageing, falling levels of family support systems and lack of adequate social welfare systems. A wide range of programmes can improve the quality of life of elders everywhere. These programmes target three risk factors for poor mental health in the elderly – financial difficulties, social isolation and poor physical health – and are all likely to have an important impact on mental health. Examples include income generation to allow a degree of independence; programmes that recruit children and youth to care for physically unwell elders; day centres, organized social events and neighbourhood visiting schemes to reduce the social isolation of elders; and aids including spectacles, and rehabilitation to minimize the effects of physical disabilities (Patel et al., 2005).

CONCLUSIONS

Just as public health and the population health approach are established in other areas such as heart health and tobacco control, so it is becoming clearer that 'Mental health is everybody's business'. The Foresight Project shows that governments and others:

> have tremendous opportunities to create environments in which mental capital and wellbeing flourish. However, failure to act could have severe consequences. A cross-governmental approach is needed to realise the full benefits. Early intervention in education could provide benefits for reducing crime, improving productivity in work, and reducing demand on health and care systems by preserving mental capital in older age. (Government departments and civil society) will need to work together more closely. And interventions may have long timescales before they see any returns. Implementing these recommendations will require significant changes in the nature of governance, placing mental capital and wellbeing at the heart of policy-making. (Beddington et al., 2008)

Particularly important for the future of mental health and economic and social development in low-income as well as high-income countries will be the scaling up and evaluation of effective participatory community-based programmes to support early child development. Required alongside these in the longer term will be effective programmes and policies for poverty alleviation and violence prevention among others. These programmes need to be expanded and their effects on mental health and its mediating variables evaluated. In this way the evidence base for mental health promotion will be expanded appropriately worldwide.

REFERENCES

Aos, S., Lieb, R., Mayfield, J., Miller, M. and Pennucci, A. (2004) Benefits and costs of prevention and early intervention programmes for youth www.wsipp.wa.gov/rptfiles/04-07-3901a.pdf. Olympia: Washington State Institute for Public Policy.

APAPDC (2007) Leading school social and emotional wellbeing: a frame for leadership for school leaders www.apapdc.edu.au. Australian Principal's Association Professional Development Council.

Arole, R., Fuller, B. and Duetschmann, P. (2005) Community development as a strategy for promoting mental health: lessons from rural India. In H. Herrman, S. Saxena and R. Moodie (eds) *Promoting Mental Health: Concepts, Emerging Evidence, Practice.* Geneva: World Health Organization.

Baingana, F., Bannon, I. and Thomas, R. (2005) Mental health and conflicts: conceptual framework and approaches *health. Nutrition and Population Discussion Paper.* Washington DC: World Bank.

Barry, M. and Jenkins, R. (2007) *Implementing Mental Health Promotion.* Churchill Livingstone: Elsevier.

Beddington, J., C.L. Cooper, et al. (2008) The mental wealth of nations. *Nature,* 455(7216): 1057–1060.

Chowdhury, A. and Bhuiya, A. (2005) Do poverty alleviation programmes reduce inequities in health? The Bangladesh experience. In D. Leon and G. Walt (eds) *Poverty, Inequality and Health.* Oxford: Oxford University Press.

Cooper, P.J., Tomlinson, M., Swartz, L., Landman, M., Molteno, C., Stein, A., McPherson, K. and Murray, L. (2009) Improving quality of mother–infant relationship and infant attachment in socioeconomically deprived community in South Africa: randomised controlled trial. *BMJ,* 338: b974.

CSDH (2008) Closing the gap in a generation: health equity through action on the social determinants of health. *Final Report of the Commission on Social Determinants of Health.* Geneva: World Health Organization.

Desjarlais, R., Eisenberg, L., Good, B. and Kleinman, A. (1995) *World Mental Health: Problems and Priorities in Low-Income Countries.* New York: Oxford University Press.

Drew, N., Funk, M., Pathare, S. and Swartz, L. (2005) Mental health and human rights. In H., Herrman, S. Saxena and R. Moodie (eds) *Promoting Mental Health: Concepts, Emerging Evidence, Practice.* Geneva: World Health Organization.

Engle, P.L., Black, M.M., Behrman, J.R., Cabral de Mello, M., Gertler, P.J., Kapiriri, L., Martorell, R. and Young, M.E. (2007) Strategies to avoid the loss of developmental potential in more than 200 million children in the developing world. *Lancet,* 369: 229–242.

Fisher, J., Cabral de Mello, M. and Izutsu, T. (2009) Pregnancy, childbirth and the postpartum year. In J.J.A. Fisher, M. Cabral de Mello and S. Saxena (eds) *Mental Health Aspects of Women's Reproductive Health. A Global Review of the Literature.* Geneva: World Health Organization and United Nations Population Fund.

Fisher, J., Rahman, A., Cabral de Mello, M., Chandra, P. and Herrman, H. (2010) How to facilitate 'good-enough parenting' in the communities of the 21st century?. In S. Tyano, M. Keren, H. Herrman and J. Cox (eds) *Parenthood and Mental Health: A Bridge Between Infant and Adult Psychiatry.* Chichester: Wiley Blackwell.

Friedli, L. and Parsonage, M. (2007) *Mental Health Promotion: Building an Economic Case.* Northern Ireland Association for Mental Health (NIAMH).

Garcia-Moreno, C., Jansen, H.A., EllsberG, M., Heise, L., and Watts, C.H. (2006) Prevalence of intimate partner violence: findings from the WHO multi-country study on women's health and domestic violence. *Lancet,* 368: 1260–1269.

Grantham-McGregor, S., Cheung, Y.B., Cueto, S., Glewwe, P., Richter, L. and Strupp, B. (2007) Developmental potential in the first 5 years for children in developing countries. *Lancet,* 369: 60–70.

Hawe, P. and Riley, T. (2005) Developing sustainable programs: theory and practice. In H. Herrman, S. Saxena and R. Moodie (eds) *Promoting Mental Health: Concepts, Emerging Evidence, Practice.* Geneva: World Health Organization.

Herrman, H., Saxena, S. and Moodie, R. (2005a) *Promoting Mental Health: Concepts, Emerging Evidence and Practice.* Geneva: World Health Organization.

Herrman, H., Saxena, S. and Moodie, R. (eds) (2005b) *Promoting Mental Health: Concepts, Emerging Evidence, Practice.* Geneva: World Health Organization.

Herrman, H. and Swartz, L. (2007) Promotion of mental health in poorly resourced countries. *Lancet,* 370: 1195–1197.

Houtman, I., Jettinghoff, K. and Cedillo, L. (2007) *Raising Awareness of Stress at Work in Developing Countries: a Modern Hazard in a Traditional Working Environment: Advice to Employers and Worker Representatives.* Geneva: World Health Organization.

IASC (2007) *IASC Guidelines on Mental Health and Psychosocial Support in Emergency Settings.* Geneva: Inter-Agency Standing Committee (IASC).

IOM (2003) *Psychocosocial and Mental Well-being of Migrants.* www.iom.int/. Geneva: International Organizarion for Migration.

Jolly, R. (2007) Early childhood development: the global challenge. *Lancet,* 369: 8–9.

Kleinman, A. (1999) Social violence: research questions on local experiences and global responses. *Archives of General Psychiatry.* 56: 978–979.

Kovess-Masfety, V., Murray, M. and Gureje, O. (2005) Evolution of our understanding of positive mental health. In H. Herrman, S. Saxena and R. Moodie (eds) *Promoting Mental Health: Concepts, Emerging Evidence, Practice.* Geneva: World Health Organization.

Lahtinen, E., Joubert, N., Raeburn, J. and Jenkins, R. (2005) Strategies for promoting the mental health of populations. In H. Herrman, S. Saxena and R. Moodie (eds) *Promoting Mental Health: Concepts, Emerging Evidence. Practice.* Geneva: WHO.

Lamontagne, A.D., Keegel, T., Louie, A.M., Ostry, A. and Landsbergis, P.A. (2007) A systematic review of the job stress intervention evaluation literature: 1990–2005. *International Journal of Occupational and Environmental Health.*

Leka, S., Griffiths, A. and Cox, T. (2005) *Work Organization and Stress: Systematic Problem Solving Approaches for Employers, Managers, and Trade Union Representatives.* Geneva: World Health Organization.

MacMillan, H.L. and Wathen, C.N. (2005) Family violence research: lessons learned and where from here? *JAMA.* 294: 618–620.

Marmot, M. (2007) Achieving health equity: from root causes to fair outcomes. *Lancet,* 370: 1153–1163.

Marmot, M. and Wilkinson, R. (eds) (1999) *The Social Determinants of Health.* Oxford: Oxford University Press.

Mindmatters www.mindmatters.edu.au.

Neiman, A. and Hall, M. (2007) Urbanization and health promotion In D., McQueen and C. M. Jones, (eds) *Global Perspectives on Health Promotion Effectiveness.* New York: Springer.

Olds, D., Henderson, C.R. Jr., Cole, R., Eckenrode, J., Kitzman, H., Luckey, D., Pettitt, L., Sidora, K., Morris, P. and Powers, J. (1998) Long-term effects of nurse home visitation on children's criminal and antisocial behavior: 15-year follow-up of a randomized controlled trial. *JAMA.* 280: 1238–1244.

Parkar, S.R., Fernandes, J. and Weiss, M.G. (2003) Contextualizing mental health: gendered experiences in a Mumbai slum. *Anthropology and Medicine.* 10: 291.

Patel, V., Flisher, A.J., Hetrick, S. and McGorry, P. (2007) Mental health of young people: a global public-health challenge. *Lancet.* 369: 1302–1313.

Patel, V., Flisher, A.J., Nikapota, A. and Malhotra, S. (2008) Promoting child and adolescent mental health in low and middle income countries. *Journal of Child Psychology and Psychiatry,* 49: 313–334.

Patel, V., Rahman, A., Jacob, K.S. and Hughes, M. (2004) Effect of maternal mental health on infant growth in low income countries: new evidence from South Asia. *BMJ,* 328: 820–823.

Patel, V., Swartz, L. and Cohen, A. (2005) The evidence for mental health promotion in developing countries. In H. Herrman, S. Saxena and R. Moodie (eds) *Promoting Mental Health: Concepts, Emerging Evidence, Practice.* Geneva: WHO.

Petersen, I., Bhana, A., Flisher, A.J., Swartz, L. and Richter, L. (eds) (2010) *Promoting Mental Health in Scarce-Resource Contexts: Emerging Evidence and Practice,* South Africa: HSRC Press.

Powell, C. and Grantham-McGregor, S. (1989) Home visiting of varying frequency and child development. *Pediatrics,* 84: 157–164.

Price, R.H., Van Ryn, M. and Vinokur, A.D. (1992) Impact of a preventive job search intervention on the likelihood of depression among the unemployed. *Journal of Health and Social Behaviour,* 33: 158–167.

Rahman, A., Malik, A., Sikander, S., Roberts, C. and Creed, F. (2008) Cognitive behaviour therapy-based intervention by community health workers for mothers with depression and their infants in rural Pakistan: a cluster-randomised controlled trial. *Lancet,* 372: 902–909.

Richter, L., Dawes, A. and de Kadt, J. (2010) Early childhood. In I. Petersen, A. Bhana, A. J. Flisher, L. Swartz and L. Richter (eds) *Promoting Mental Health in Scarce-Resource Contexts: Emerging Evidence and Practice.* South Africa: HRCS.

Rose, G. (1992) *The Strategy of Preventive Medicine.* Oxford: Oxford University Press.

Rowling, L. and Taylor, A. (2005) Intersectoral approaches to promoting mental health. In H., Herrman, S. Saxena and R. Moodie (eds) *Promoting Mental Health: Concepts, Emerging Evidence, Practice.* Geneva: World Health Organization.

Sartorius, N. (1998) Universal strategies for the prevention of mental illness and the promotion of mental health. In R. Jenkins and T.B. Ustun (eds) *Preventing Mental Illness: Mental Health Promotion in Primary Care.* Chichester: John Wiley and Sons.

Saxena, S., Herrman, H., Moodie, R. and Saraceno, B. (2005) Conclusions: the way forward. In H. Herrman, S. Saxena, R. Moodie (eds) *Promoting Mental Health: Concepts, Emerging Evidence and Practice.* Geneva: WHO.

Saxena, S., Jane-Llopis, E. and Hosman, C. (2006) Prevention of mental and behavioural disorders: implications for policy and practice. *World Psychiatry,* 5: 5–14.

Sekar, K. (2002) *Riots: Psychosocial Care by Community Level Helpers for Survivors,* Bangalore, Books for Change.

Small, R. and Lumley, J. (2007) Reduction of maternal depression: much remains to be done. *Lancet,* 370: 1593–1595.

Stewart Brown, S. (2006) What is the evidence on school health promotion in improving health or pre-venting disease and, specifically, what is the effectiveness of the healthpromoting schools approach? http://www.euro.who.int/HEN/Syntheses/healthpromotion_schools/20060224_7. Geneva: World Health Organization, Euro.

Sturgeon, S. and Orley, J. (2005) Concepts of mental health across the world. In H. Herrman, S. Saxena and R. Moodie (eds) *Promoting Mental Health: Concepts, Emerging Evidence, Practice.* Geneva: World Health Organization.

Summerfield, D. (1999) A critique of seven assumptions behind psychological trauma programmes in war-affected areas. *Soc. Sci. Med.* 48: 1449–1462.

Swartz, L. (2010) Contextual issues. In I. Petersen, A. Bhana, A. J. Flisher, L. Swartz and L. Richter (eds) *Promoting Mental Health in Scarce-Resource Contexts: Emerging Evidence and Practice.* South Africa: HRCS Press.

Syme, L. (1996) To prevent disease: the need for a new approach. In D. Blane, E. Brunner, R. Wilkinson (eds) *Health and Social Organisation.* London: Routledge.

VicHealth (2005) Mental health and wellbeing program. Victorian Health Promotion Foundation (VicHealth).

Vuori, J., Price, R.H., Mutanen, P. and Malmberg-Heimonen, I. (2005) Effective group training techniques in job-search training. *J. Occup. Health Psychol,* 10: 261–275.

Walker, L., Verins, I., Moodie, R. and Webster, K. (2005a) Responding to the social and economic deter-minants of mental health: A conceptual framework for action. In H. Herrman, S. Saxena and R., Moodie (eds) *Promoting Mental Health: Concepts, Emerging Evidence, Practice.* Geneva: World Health Organization.

Walker, S.P., Chang, S.M., Powell, C.A. and Grantham-McGregor, S.M. (2005b) Effects of early childhood psychosocial stimulation and nutritional supplementation on cognition and education in growth-stunted Jamaican children: prospective cohort study. *Lancet*, 366: 1804–1807.

Walker, S.P., Wachs, T.D., Gardner, J.M., Lozoff, B., Wasserman, G.A., Pollitt, E. and Carter, J.A. (2007) Child development: risk factors for adverse outcomes in developing countries. *Lancet*, 369: 145–157.

Wells, J., Barlow, J. and Stewart-Brown, S. (2003) A systematic review of universal approaches to mental health promotion in schools. *Health Education,* 103: 197–220.

WHO (1997) *Life Skills Education in Schools.* Geneva: Programme on Mental Health, World Health Organization.

WHO (2000) *Women's Mental Health: An Evidence Based Review.* Geneva: World Health Organization.

WHO (2002a) *25 Questions and Answers on Health and Human Rights.* Geneva: World Health Organization.

WHO (2002b) *Word Report on Violence and Health.* Geneva: World Health Organization.

WHO (2006) *Mental Health and Psychosocial Well-Being among Children in Severe Food Shortage Situations.* Geneva: World Health Organization.

WHO and ILO (2000) *Mental health and work: Impact, Issues and Good Practices.* Geneva: World Health Organization.

Wild, R. (2007) Unforseen circumstances. In J. Altman and M. Hinkinskin (eds) *Coercive Reconciliation: Stabilise, Normalise, Exit Aboriginal Australia.* Melbourne: Arena.

Wiseman, J., McLeod, J. and Zubrick, S.R. (2007) Promoting mental health and well-being: integrating individual, organisational and community-level indicators. *Health Promot. J. Austr,* 18: 198–207.

Worldbank (2000) *World Development Report: Attacking Poverty.* Oxford: Oxford Univerity Press.

Zubrick, S.R. and Kovess-Masfety, V. (2005) Indicators of mental health. In H., Herrman, S., Saxena and R., Moodie (eds) *Promoting Mental Health: Concepts, Emerging Evidence, Practice.* Geneva: WHO. pp. 148–169.

21

Institutionalization and Deinstitutionalization

Andrew Scull

For much of the twentieth century, institutional psychiatrists have shied away from the term 'asylum' (Goffman, 1961). Even a hundred years ago, the concept's associations with what Ernest Jones called the 'Chubb lock era' in psychiatry were an embarrassment for professionals desperate to escape their public image as little more than custodians of the degenerate and defective, and concerned to emphasize their ties to the more respectable sectors of the medical enterprise. Hence the eagerness with which alienists sought in those years to relabel their establishments as mental hospitals and themselves as expert practitioners of psychological medicine. In the half century since the war against Hitler and Hirohito, the reluctance to make use of the older terminology has become even more pronounced. A generation of sociological studies critical of the mental hospital's therapeutic pretensions culminated in Goffman's denunciation of such places as fundamentally and irremediably flawed. *Asylums*, his book of that title proclaimed (Goffman, 1961), stigmatized, dehumanized, and systematically disabled the inmates they purported to cure. They were 'total institutions' that, in crucial respects, resembled nothing so much as concentration camps. With institutional care for the mentally ill rapidly falling into disfavour in political circles during the same period, as policy-makers rushed to embrace the mythical vision of a community anxious to re-embrace the mentally ill, the asylum's fate seemed sealed on still another front. Its paymasters increasingly dismissed it as a well-meaning experiment gone wrong, an expensive irrelevance now thankfully to be relegated to the dustbin of history. In the words of the inimitable

Enoch Powell (1961), mental hospitals were 'doomed institutions', and governments contemplating their fate ought to be 'erring on the side of ruthlessness'.
Confronting the ramshackle and decaying empire of asylumdom bequeathed us
by our Victorian forebears, the way forward was simply to set 'the torch to the
funeral pyre' (Powell, 1961).

In view of its ignominious end, it is difficult to recall how differently the found-
ers of the asylum era in Britain and North America expected asylumdom to turn
out. The lunacy reform movement of the early nineteenth century was driven
forward, in substantial measure, by a utopian vision of the possibilities of asylum
life. So far from being 'a moral lazar house' (Combe, 1850) wherein the deranged
were hidden and hope and humanity abandoned, the asylum in their imagination
was transmuted into the 'moral machinery' through which the mind was to be
strengthened and reason restored.

To be sure, on the far side of the Atlantic, the moral outrage that gave
energy and urgency to the reformers' efforts was periodically refuelled by
new revelations about the deficiencies of the traditional trade in lunacy, the prof-
it-making madhouses which had become a visible and notorious element in
English responses to insanity over the course of the eighteenth century. A series
of early nineteenth century parliamentary inquiries appeared to provide compelling confirmation of the public's worst gothic nightmares about what transpired
behind the high walls and barred windows of the madhouse. The reports of the
Select Committees themselves, and the books and pamphlets produced by
those agitating for lunacy reform, contained a compelling amalgam of sex, madness, maltreatment and murder, mixed together in a fashion guaranteed at once to
titillate and repel: patients bled and drugged into insensibility; their public display, 'like animals in a menagerie'; unregarded deaths from botched force-feed-
ing and the brutality of uncaring attendants; the corrupt confinement of the sane,
amidst the shrieks and ravings of the mad; the placing of even those madwomen
who retained some semblance of 'innate' female purity and modesty at the
disposal of the lascivious ruffians who served as madhouse attendants; and
the ingenious array of 'bolts, bars, chains, muffs, collars, and strait-jackets'
madhouse proprietors had devised to coerce a measure of order from recalcitrant
raw materials.

At least as vital to the achievement of lunacy reform, however, was the construction of a positive image for the reformed asylum. Here, if its proponents
were to be believed, were 'miniature worlds, whence all the disagreeable alloys
of modern life are as much as possible excluded, and the more pleasing portions
carefully cultivated' (Anon, 1836). Most famously realized by Tuke (1813)
and Jepson at a Quaker institution, the York Retreat, this novel version of a haven
for the mentally ill, presented a very different scene to those with occasion
to view it.

The asylum was now to be a home, where the patient was to be known and
treated as an individual, where his mind was to be constantly stimulated and
encouraged to return to its natural state. Mental patients required dedicated

and unremitting care, which could not be administered on a mass basis, but rather must be flexible and adapted to the needs and progress of each case. Such a regime demanded kindness and an unusual degree of forbearance on the part of the staff. If the ideal were to be successfully realized, the attendants would have to be taught to keep constantly in mind the idea that 'the patient is really under the influence of a disease, which deprives him of responsibility, and frequently leads him into expressions and conduct the most opposite to his character and natural dispositions' (Tuke, 1813). Crucial, too, was the moral influence of the asylum's governor. By paying 'minute attention' to all aspects of the day-to-day conduct of the institution, by always setting, through his own example, a high standard for subordinates to emulate in their dealings with the inmates, by observing the patients daily, sometimes hourly, he could foster the kind of intimate and benevolent familial environment in which acts of violence would become rare. Indeed, as the autocratic guiding spirit of the whole curative apparatus, the superior moral and intellectual character of the medical superintendent was an essential precondition for success.

Classification, separation, and employment, all central features of Tuke's version of moral treatment, were to be combined with careful attention to the architecture and physical setting of the asylum. Since it was recognized that the insane were very sensitive to their surroundings, buildings ought to emphasize as little as possible the idea of imprisonment or confinement. Indeed, spacious and attractive accommodations could make their own contributions to the inmates' 'moral training', and to replacing 'their morbid feelings ... [with] healthy trains of thought' (Browne, 1837). Treatment could thus be individualized and adapted to the peculiarities of the particular case, and interaction managed and controlled within carefully constructed communities of the mad.

Similar ideas were soon equally prevalent in 'enlightened' circles in North America, a development that should occasion little surprise given the close intellectual, religious, and often personal ties that bound together activists on both sides of the Atlantic (Gollaher, 1989). Isaac Ray (1863), for instance, who was among the most prominent of the early American alienists, acknowledged that 'to sever a man's domestic ties, to take him out of the circle of friends and relatives most deeply interested in his welfare ... and place him ... in the hands of strangers, and in the company of persons as disordered as himself – at first sight would seem ... little likely to exert a restorative effect'. But such sentiments were the very contrary of the truth: 'While at large, the patient is every moment exposed to circumstances that maintain the morbid activity of his mind ... In the hospital, on the other hand, he is beyond the reach of all these causes of excitement' (Ray, 1863). American discussions of the asylum, like their British counterparts, employed transparently Utopian imagery, and insisted that, given early treatment within a well-ordered institution, 'this deplorable malady [insanity] is equally with other diseases of the human system under the control of proper medical treatment, the proportion of cures being as great' (*Friend's Asylum*, 1835). Expenditures on asylums could thus be justified, not just by appeals to humanity, but by cold calculation. There existed, that is, what Ellen Dwyer (1987) has termed 'an economics of compassion' whereby the higher initial costs of a properly constituted asylum system would be rapidly offset by the high proportion of cures that would result, and the subsequent return of the dependent to the ranks of the productive citizenry (cf. Pennsylvania Prison Discipline Society, 1845).

Here was an ideological vision of extraordinary resonance and surpassing attractiveness, of the asylum as a social universe constituting an organic, harmonious whole wherein even the rage of madness could be reigned in without whips, chains, or corporal punishment, amidst the comforts of domesticity and the invisible yet infinitely potent fetters of 'the desire for esteem' (Tuke, 1813). Men like William Tuke, William Alexander Francis Browne, and John Conolly in Britain, and Eli Todd, Amariah Brigham, and Luther Bell in the United States, insisted, moreover, that theirs was a 'description ... not ... of a theorist, or of an enthusiast, but of ... practical [men] long accustomed to the management of lunatics' (Conolly, 1835). It was, said Browne, 'a faithful picture of what may been seen in many institutions, and of what might been seen in all, were asylums conducted as they ought to be' (Browne, 1837). Within the controlled confines of the institution, even the irrational and the raving could be reduced to docility and cured of their madness, and by moral persuasion and self-sacrifice, rather than by force. With all the fervour of a new convert (for he had earlier been a stern critic of the idea of confining the mad in institutions), John Conolly (1847) delivered a panegyric to the new asylum:

> the place where calmness will come; hope will revive; satisfaction will prevail. Some unmanageable tempers, some violent or sullen patients, there must always be; but much of the violence, much of the ill-humour, almost all the disposition to meditate mischievous or fatal revenge, or self-destruction will disappear ... Cleanliness and decency will be maintained or restored; and despair itself will sometimes be found to give place to cheerfulness or secure tranquility.[The asylum is the place] where humanity, if anywhere on earth, shall reign supreme. (p. 143)

Crusading across the American continent in behalf of a network of state asylums, the indefatigable Dorothea Dix (1845) drew repeatedly upon claims of this sort, coupling them with her own vivid (and sometimes imaginary) recital of the abuses to which the insane were exposed in the community in order to loosen politicians' purse-strings. If those afflicted were treated by 'a combination of medical and moral treatment' in an asylum, she insisted, 'all experience shows that insanity ... is as certainly curable as a cold or a fever' (Dix, 1845: 13–15, 57).

The small, intimate institution which allowed even a remote approximation to this idyll did not survive for long. The influx of a horde of pauper lunatics into the new public establishments brought the swift demise of the notion that the asylum should be a substitute household. Instead, local magistrates in England and state legislators in America insisted on taking advantage of presumed economies of scale, and until well into the twentieth century, the average size of county asylums and state hospitals grew almost yearly. The degree of regimentation needed to administer institutions of five hundred, a thousand, and more ensured that such asylums would be the virtual antithesis of their supposed inspiration, the York Retreat. To Tuke, moral treatment had meant the creation of a stimulating environment where routine could be sacrificed to the needs of the individual. Here the same term disguised a monotonous reality in which the needs of the patients were necessarily subordinated to those of the institution; indeed, where a patient's needs were unlikely even to find expression. Hence John Arlidge's trenchant conclusion that 'a gigantic asylum is a gigantic evil' (1859: 102).

At the margin, among those newly admitted to an asylum, turnover remained reasonably rapid, with between a quarter and two fifths being discharged within a year or so of their arrival. Each year, however, a very substantial fraction remained behind to swell the population of chronic, long-stay patients, and as the size of county asylums and state hospitals grew remorselessly, annual admissions formed a smaller and smaller fraction of the whole. An overwhelming and growing proportion of the asylum population thus came to be composed of patients who lingered year after year; and it was this spectre of chronicity, this horde of the hopeless, which was to haunt the popular imagination, to constitute the public identity of the asylums, and to dominate Victorian and Edwardian psychiatric theorizing and practice.

At Utica State Hospital in New York, for instance, recoveries calculated on total numbers resident never rose above 16 per cent after 1856, and by 1890, had fallen below 11 per cent (Dwyer, 1987: 150). On the other side of the Atlantic, at the Lancaster County Asylum, 'After 1850, the figure [for cures] never again reached 10 per cent , and the death rate was almost always higher than the cures' (Walton, 1840: 150). These outcomes were replicated throughout the still expanding empire of asylumdom. For the remainder of the nineteenth century, and beyond, the proportion of their patients alienists claimed to cure was to fall still further, till ultimately more of their charges left the asylum in coffins each year than were restored to society in the possession of their senses.

Mired in such depressing surroundings, W.A.F. Browne (1857) despairingly viewed the collapse of the vision he had once propagated of the asylum as a curative establishment under the weight of 'a vast assemblage of incurable cases'. Their numbers ensured, he said, that:

> The community becomes unwieldy; the cares are beyond the capacity of the medical officers; personal intimacy is impossible; recent cases are lost, and overlooked in the mass; and patients are treated in groups and classes. An unhealthy moral atmosphere is created; a mental epidemic arises, where delusion, and debility, and extravagance are propagated from individual to individual, and the intellect is dwarfed and enfeebled by monotony, routine, and subjection. (p. 8)

This sense that mental hospitals could prove actively harmful to those they purported to cure, already spreading in the 1860s, grew still more pronounced in the following decade. Henry Maudsley (1871), for instance, widely regarded as the leading English alienist of the age, confessed that 'I cannot help feeling, from my experience, that one effect of asylums is to make permanent lunatics'. Spitzka, Hammond, and Weir Mitchell, among the most prominent American neurologists of the Gilded Age, were equally emphatic, complaining of the pernicious effects of incarceration, and of 'the sadness ... of the wards ... [in which] the insane, who have lost even the memory of hope, sit in rows, too dull to know despair, watched by attendants, silent, grewsome [sic.] machines which eat and sleep, sleep and eat' (Hammond, 1879; Mitchell, 1894; Spitzka, 1878). Lay critics were even less inhibited, denouncing mental hospitals' failings, calling into question the superintendents' claims to expertise, and claiming that mistreatment and abuse were routine (Eaton, 1881; Packard, 1873; Lowe, 1883).

As asylums silted up with the chronically crazy, those Browne dubbed 'the waifs and strays, the weak and wayward of our race', (*Journal of Mental Science*, 1857) so Victorian psychiatry on both sides of the Atlantic moved steadily towards a grim determinism, a view of madness as the irreversible product of a process of mental degeneration and decay. The madman, as Maudsley (1879) put it, 'is the necessary organic consequent of certain organic antecedents: and it is impossible he should escape the tyranny of his organization'. Insanity constituted nothing less than a form of phylogenetic regression – which accounted, of course, for its social location and for the lunatic's loss of civilized standards of behaviour and regression to the status of a brute. 'Whence', Maudsley (1870) rhetorically asked, 'came the savage snarl, the destructive disposition, the obscene language, the wild howl, the offensive habits displayed by some of the sane? Why should a human being deprived of his reason ever become so brutal in character as some do, unless he has the brute nature within him?' Employing ever harsher language which combined a physiological account of madness with 'the look and tone of moral condemnation' (Turner, 1988). Psychiatric discourse now exhibited a barely disguised contempt for those 'tainted persons' (Strahan, 1890) whom it sequestered on society's behalf. And within such a world-view, given that the notion of mass sterilization never acquired the status of a serious option in Britain and was employed on a sizeable but still limited scale in the United States (Grob, 1983). The asylum was naturally accorded a wholly new significance in the battle to contain social pathology and to defend the social order.

Certainly, whatever the institutions' therapeutic deficiencies, the community beyond the asylum's walls evinced no enthusiasm for the prospect of lunatics at large. In his Presidential Address to the assembled British alienists, John Charles (1860) Bucknill (whose efforts to mitigate the isolation of his patients at the Devon County Asylum) had provoked widespread public outrage and opposition, bitterly complained of the public's hypocrisy:

> The feeling and conduct of the British public towards the insane remind one of nothing so much as that the enlightened citizens of the free States of America. Noble and just sentiments towards the negro race are in every one's mouth, but personal antipathy is in every man's heart. (p. 6)

Though 'the idea which the public now have of an asylum is, that it is a place where madmen are consigned until they die ... ', (Burdett, 1891) the prospect appeared to disturb most of them not one whit, for it safely removed from their midst 'the branded bondmen of disease', and spared them the polluting presence of these products 'of morbid passions, of ignorant and wicked habits, of the physical accidents and the tainted descent which cause their disease' – to quote Bucknill (1860) once more.

States and local authorities were always reluctant to spend 'extravagant' sums of money on the poor, and the funds for a predominantly custodial operation were predictably scarce, rarely more than what was needed to supply a bare minimum of care. Occasionally, indeed, the cheeseparing went too far, as in Buckinghamshire between 1916 and 1918, when the official dietary tables for St. John's Hospital suggest that a male patient's daily food allowance provided only 40 grams of protein and 750 calories a day (which may be compared with what is now estimated to be a minimum requirement for a sedentary man of 60 grams of protein and 2100 calories). Female patients received even less. With a deliberate policy of semi-starvation carried to this extreme, the result (as J.L. Crammer (1991) has noted) was a very sharp increase in asylum mortality rates, till in 1918, a third of the asylum population died in the space of twelve months, a denouement which finally shamed the authorities into action.

Recent work has shown that even in small, richly endowed private facilities – the Crichton Royal Asylum in Dumfries, the Ticehurst Asylum (the favourite resort for deranged English aristocrats), the Pennsylvania Hospital in Philadelphia, and the York Retreat itself (Digby, 1985; MacKenzie, 1992; Scull, 1991; Tomes, 1984) – the quality of care provided by an essentially custodial operation tended to diminish steadily over time. Although, as Anne Digby (1985) summarizes her findings for the York Retreat, 'individuality was not crushed into helpless anonymity' (as in the county asylums), still by the last third of the nineteenth century, control and discipline were the paramount goals of the institution, and 'patients were no longer subjects to be treated but objects to be managed' all of which serves, I think, to re-emphasize just how difficult it is to sustain staff and patient morale and to maintain the quality of care in the absence of some prospect of therapeutic success.

Not surprisingly under the circumstances, for the overwhelming majority of a profession that had begun with such elevated, even utopian hopes for the future, the nineteenth century thus ended on a note of quiet desperation and despair, as psychiatrists (as they now called themselves) confronted what they themselves recognized as the Sisyphean task of wrestling with 'the most repulsive features of man's weakness, an atmosphere of moral miasma, an almost hopeless struggle, day by day, to retrieve or reset the broken fragments of reason' (Hawkes, 1875). The central mission of institutional psychiatry had been reduced to quarantining the incurable, rather than restoring the temporarily distracted to sanity. And by and large, asylum superintendents seem to have accepted the somewhat ambiguous professional status this brought them, working uncomplainingly within the limits of the authority granted by their employers.

Living as we now do in the twilight of the empire of asylumdom, we are aware that this isolation and somnolence were not to last forever. As early as the 1860s, in fact, we can observe some members of the psychiatric elite seeking to escape the institution's stultifying grasp, and to carve out alternative career paths outside the walls of the asylum. To lavish consultation fees from cases they recommended for asylum treatment, they increasingly added income from a whole new class of 'nervous' patients, the denizens of those shadowy regions Mortimer Granville labelled 'Mazeland, Dazeland and Driftland, perilous territories others preferred to call 'the borderlands of insanity' (Wynter, 1877). Such 'incipient lunatics', the carriers of 'latent brain disease', included a whole array of neurotics, hysterics, anorexics and sufferers from the newly fashionable 'neurasthenia', or weakness of the nerves. Disproportionately female, and desperate to avoid the stigma and hopelessness associated with certification and confinement in an asylum, they provided a promising basis for an office-based practice (Oppenheim, 1991; Shorter, 1992; Showalter, 1985), a financially lucrative if therapeutically frustrating clientele which was to be thoroughly exploited only in our own century.

Even as the vanguard of the psychiatric profession began to abandon the chronically crazy (Grob, 1983; 1991), the institutional response remained the dominant approach to the problems posed by the mentally ill till past the middle of our own century. The pattern of consistent year-by-year increases in the number of inmates confined in mental hospitals, so noticeable a feature of the nineteenth-century asylum system, persisted almost unchanged until 1954 in Britain, and 1955 in the United States. And for most of the time since then, mental hospital admissions have continued to rise quite sharply, keeping the now decrepit nineteenth-century structures in constant use. Nevertheless, this latter period has witnessed a major departure from historical precedent, a reversal of the remorseless secular increase in the size of the mental hospital population. In the face of a century-and-a-half-old trend in precisely the opposite direction, the number of patients resident in English mental hospitals fell sharply, from 148,000 in 1954 to fewer than 60,000 three and a half decades later. In the United States, in the quarter century between 1955 and 1980, the in-patient census fell from 560,000 to just over 130,000, and the decline has continued uninterruptedly since then. Still more abrupt has been the mental hospitals' decline from official favour. Under mounting attack because of their negative effects on those they treat, segregative techniques in their traditional form are now steadily losing ground to newer 'community-based' alternatives.

Madness seems to attract more than its share of myths. In the nineteenth century, the myth of the Noble Savage – free from the stress, the artificiality, the vices of modern life (and thus free from the insanity which was part of the price of civilization) – was given a widespread currency. The propagation of such a notion had obvious value for those bent on reforming the treatment of lunatics and bringing them the benefits of modern science; for only the adoption of their programme of a network of specially designed, medically run asylums could hope to stem the rising tide of madness with which the advance of civilization threatened the social order. The contemporary equivalent of the Noble Savage (in some intellectual circles at least) seems to be a mythical pre-institutional Golden Age, when the population at large enjoyed the blessings of living in 'communities' – an innocent rustic society, uncorrupted by the evils of bureaucracy, where neighbour helped neighbour and families gladly ministered to the needs of their own troublesome members, while a benevolent squirearchy looked on, always ready to lend a helping hand. Once again, a myth has had its uses for those bent on changing social policy, this time providing a counterpoint to a mass of social scientific research on the mental hospital which amounts to a full-blown assault on its therapeutic failings (Caudil, 1958; Belknap, 1956; Goffman, 1961; Perrucci, 1974). For such people, lunacy reform is seen as simply one colossal mistake.

Certainly, there is much in what I have said about the nineteenth-century asylum which can but serve as grist for their mill. But realism about the awfulness of asylum existence ought not to prompt us to opt for a blind faith in the virtues of its presumed antithesis. One can – indeed, I think must – be deeply sceptical about claims made on the mental hospital's behalf: yet one must not fall prey to equally groundless fantasies and illusions about the available alternatives. If one were to believe the devotees of the contemporary cult of the community, if we would only bring the mentally disturbed back into our midst, not only would we avoid the isolating and labelling effects of commitment to an institution, but 'by enlisting the good will and the desire to serve, the ability to understand which is found in every neighbourhood, we shall meet the challenge which such groups of persons present ...' Apparently, what is needed is a return to:

> a simpler time not so very long ago ... when the problems of the mentally retarded and disturbed, the aged and the troubled young, were dealt with in the communities where each of these people lived. A greater continuity or integration of the entire age spectrum seems to have prevailed in those days: ... and those who were deficient in intelligence or emotional balance were not only tolerated but accommodated. (Alper, 1972: vii-viii)

We may reasonably doubt whether such idylls existed in seventeenth- or eighteenth-century England or in colonial America, the Paradise presumably Lost when the insane were consigned to the asylum. The available evidence on the treatment accorded the insane in the community in this period is sketchy and inadequate, a situation complicated by the then prevalent failure to distinguish at all carefully between the mad and other deviant and dependent groups. Nevertheless, what we do know of the treatment either of the clearly frenzied or of problematic people in general lends little support to such romantic speculations. Nor should this come as a surprise, given what we know of the general tenor of eighteenth-century English social life, particularly, though not exclusively, among the lower orders. Even among their 'betters' the widespread credence given to the idea of the continuity of all forms of creation, including man, in the imperceptible gradations of a single great chain of being brought with it a ready acceptance of the notion that some men were indistinguishable from brutes – an easy equation between apes and savages, and between apes and men lacking in 'reason' (Bynum, 1974; Lovejoy, 1960). And what we know of the treatment of brutes in this period scarcely inspires confidence about the treatment of human beings equated with them (cf. Thomas, 1983: Chapters 3 and 4).

More recent experiences with 'community treatment' have certainly not proved to be much of an advertisement for its virtues either. Cutting through the clouds of rhetoric and wishful thinking with which the subject abounds, it is apparent that the whole policy was undertaken with little prior investigation of its likely effects, and that even now we lack 'substantiation that community care [as it has actually been implemented] is advantageous for clients' (Wolpert, 1976; 1984). As one of the most perspicacious English psychiatrists has indicated, under the new dispensation, while the acutely disturbed continue to receive some attention, frequently being dealt with through short-term hospitalization, this contrasts 'with a second class service, or no service at all, for the chronic patient' (Wing, 1971).

In the midst of all the excitement about the replacement of the mental hospital and the breathless proclamations about the virtues of the community, it seems that few people noticed the degree to which the new programmes remained castles in the air, figments of their planners' imaginations. Nor did many appear to realize, for some considerable time, that despite all the rhetoric on both sides of the Atlantic about 'better services for the mentally handicapped' (the title of an official statement of British policy) (Department of Health and Society Security, 1971). The reality was the much darker one of retrenchment or even elimination of state supported programmes for victims of severe and chronic forms of mental disorder. As Peter Sedgwick (1981) put it, with pardonable sarcasm, 'the reduction in the register of patients ... has been achieved through the creation of rhetoric of "community care facilities" whose influence over policy in hospital admission and discharge has been particularly remarkable when one considers that they do not, in the actual world, exist'.

Sooner or later, however, any audience becomes disenchanted with a shell game in which there is no pea. For almost a quarter century, there was a remarkable dearth of 'major research projects of academic respectability that [showed] either the extent of the need or the extent of the failure' of mental health policy (Jone, 1979). But more recently, the implementation of community care has finally begun to attract more critical attention, much of it journalistic, but some of it (belatedly) from scholarly sources (Arnhoff, 1973; Bassuk and Gerson, 1978; Kirk and Thierren, 1976, 1981; Reich and Siegal, 1973; Rose, 1979; Wolpert and Wolpert, 1976). In consequence, it is now generally conceded that on both sides of the Atlantic, a policy of de-institutionalization was implemented with little or no prior consideration of such basic issues as where the patients who were released would end up; who would provide the services they needed;

and who would pay for those services (General Accounting Office, 1977). What is perhaps more surprising, the massive reassignment of patients has continued in the face of continuing lack of attention to these matters, with the predictable consequences I shall discuss below.

Ex-patients, and those who would formerly have been sent to mental hospitals (for many jurisdictions have sharply cut back the criteria justifying commitment), are to be found, of course, in a wide variety of settings, and attempting to generalize about their situations is necessarily a hazardous business. The problem is intensified by 'the paucity of follow-up studies whose data can be generalized and compared, and that trace the movement of discharged patients through the labyrinth of psychiatric facilities and living conditions after their release' (Bassuk and Gerson, 1978). And it is, of course, still more acute when one is discussing more than one country. Among state mental health bureaucrats, ignorance about the fate of their former charges is often so great that they may not even know where the discharged patients are to be found. The American General Accounting Office, for example, commented on the disconcerting regularity that 'information on what happened to former mental hospital patients and residents in institutions for the retarded was generally not available. Follow-up of released patients was generally haphazard, fragmented, or non-existent' (General Accounting Office, 1977).

We do know, however, that the overwhelming majority of them are not being serviced by the community mental health centres that the Federal Government began to subsidize in the United States during the Johnson years. The existence of several hundred of these centres in the United States has fostered the comforting notion, particularly among overseas observers (Jones, 1979). That those discharged from state hospitals have simply been transferred to a setting that provides a more modern and effective way of delivering treatment. Such assumptions are quite natural. (After all, the patients are allegedly being discharged to receive 'community treatment' and the community mental health centres are one of the few places where community treatment is conceivably being dispensed.) Nevertheless, they are also quite mistaken. Even if one disregards the centres' uneven geographical distribution and their current fiscal problems, it remains the case that 'both their ideology and their most common services are not directed at the needs of those who have traditionally resided in state psychiatric institutions' (Kirk and Thierren, 1974). From the outset, those running the new centres have displayed a pronounced preference for treating "good patients" [rather] than chronic schizophrenics, alcoholics or senile psychotics ...' (Rieder, 1974) – in other words, precisely a desire not to treat the patients being discharged from state institutions. Unsurprisingly, therefore, studies show 'no large consistent relationship between the opening of centres and changes in state hospitals resident rates' (Windle and Scully, 1976). Indeed, National Institute of Mental Health data demonstrate that 'public mental hospitals accounted for fewer referrals to community mental health centres [less than 4 per cent] than any other referral source reported, except for the clergy' (General Accounting Office, 1977).

Partly as a consequence, community health centres 'have no direct bearing on the bulk of publicly funded mental health care in the public sector' (Okin, 19878; Rose, 1979; Sharfstein, 1978).

Nevertheless, one must acknowledge that some of those discharged from mental hospitals have unambiguously benefited from the shift in social policy. Victims of an earlier tendency toward what the Wolperts (1978) have called 'overhospitalization', they have experienced few problems obtaining employment and housing, maintaining social ties and so forth, blending all but imperceptibly into the general population. Such benign outcomes are, however, far from constituting the norm.

Among those with more noticeable continuing impairment, it comes as no surprise that ex-patients placed with their families seem on the whole to have fared best. It would be a serious mistake, though, to suppose that even here deinstitutionalization has proceeded smoothly and has proved unambiguously beneficial. John Wing has recently expressed 'surprise' that, in view of the greatly increased likelihood of someone with schizophrenia living at home instead of in a hospital, so little research is being done on the problems experienced by their relatives (Wing, 1978). His own work, and that of his associates, has provided us with much of what little data we do possess on this subject, and demonstrates that 'the burden on relatives and the community was rarely negligible, and in some cases it was intolerable' (Alcaron and Sainsbury, 1963; Creer and Wing, 1974; Wing and Brown, 1970). A good deal of the distress and misery has remained hidden because of families' reticence about complaining, a natural tendency, but one which has helped to sustain a false optimism about the effects of the shifts to community treatment. As George Brown puts it, 'relatives are not in a strong position to complain – they are not experts, they may be ashamed to talk about their problems and they have come to the conclusion that no help can be offered which will substantially reduce their difficulties' (Brown et al. 1966). (Such conclusions may have a strong factual basis, in view of the widespread inadequacies or even absence of after-care facilities, and the reluctance, often refusal, of the authorities to countenance re-hospitalization.) The new policy has thus unquestionably seen 'a considerable burden being placed on the health, leisure and finances of the families [involved]' (Wing, 1971). The evidence may not be sufficient yet to warrant Arnhoff's claim that 'the consequences of indiscriminate community treatment may often have profound iatrogenic effects ... we may be producing more psychological and social disturbance than we correct' (Arnhoff, 1975). But at the very least, we must recognize that 'if ... state policy is to shift more responsibility on to "the family" then the physical and psychological burdens on individuals will increase disproportionately' (Gough, 1979; Lamb, 1982).

Yet whatever the difficulties encountered by these ex-patients and their families, they pale by comparison with the experiences of the greater number of ex-patients who have no families, or whose families simply refuse to accept responsibility for them. Particularly in the United States the precipitous decline in mental hospital populations from the mid-1960s onwards has been matched by an equally dramatic upsurge in the numbers of psychiatrically impaired residents of nursing homes. This trend is particularly marked among, but not confined to, the aged mentally ill. That the majority of these elderly people have simply been transferred from one institutional setting to another is suggested by the fact that between 1963 and 1969 the number of nursing home inmates with mental disorders virtually doubled, and evidence from the National Center for Health Statistics that shows a further 48 per cent increase through mid-1974, from 607,400 to 899,500 (General Accounting Office, 1977). NIMH data show that by the mid-1970s, nursing homes had become the 'largest single place of care for the mentally ill', absorbing 29.3 per cent of the direct costs associated with coping with them (General Accounting Office, 1977). More than 50 per cent of these nursing home residents were placed in facilities with more than a hundred beds and more than 15 per cent in 'homes' with more than 200 beds (General Accounting Office, 1977).

These numbers alone might cause one to suspect that 'the return of patients to the community has, in many ways, extended the philosophy of custodialism to the community rather than ending it at the gates of the hospital' (Kirk and Thierren, 1975). But there is a growing volume of more direct evidence which demonstrates the 'ghettoization of the returning ex-patients along with other dependent groups in the population; the growing succession of inner city land use to institutions providing services to the dependent and needy ... the forced immobility of the chronically disabled within deteriorated urban neighbourhoods ... areas where land use deterioration has proceeded to such a point that the land market is substantially unaffected by the introduction of community services and their clients' (Senate Committee on Aging, 1971). The 1977 General Accounting Office study of the institutionalization reported 'a general tendency to place formerly institutionalized persons in those nursing homes where the quality of care was poorer and safety standards not complied with as rigidly as in other nursing homes ... generally speaking, the more mental patients there were in a facility, the worse the conditions'. Despite their titles, these places frequently provided neither nursing nor a home. In the words of an Oregon Task Force, 'a typical day for a mentally ill person in a nursing home was sleeping, eating, watching television, smoking cigarettes, sitting in groups in the largest room, or looking out the window [sic.]; there was no evidence of an organized plan to meet their needs' (General Accounting Office, 1977). To make matters worse, state agencies typically provide few or no follow-up services, and little in the way of effective supervision or inspection. In the absence of such controls and lacking the bureaucratic encrustations of state enterprises, nursing home operators have found ways to pare down on even the miserable subsistence existence characteristic of state institutions.

Of course, many discharged mental patients of all ages end up in other, perhaps still less salubrious settings – board and care homes and so-called welfare hotels, or among the ranks of the sidewalk psychotics who have in recent decades become a taken-for-granted aspect of urban existence. In Philadelphia, for example, a Temple University study revealed that some 15,000 ex-patients were living in approximately 1,500 boarding homes in the city. In New Jersey, a whole new industry has sprung up, utilizing the huge, cheap, run-down Victorian hotels in formerly fashionable beach resorts as accommodation for several thousand more discharged mental patients. In New York, there have been repeated media exposes of the massive concentrations of ex-inmates in the squalid single room occupancy welfare hotels of the upper west side of Manhattan, and in the Long Island communities surrounding Pilgrim and Central Islip State Hospitals. Many of the boarding homes in the latter area, in a pattern which is becoming all too familiar, were opened by those formerly employed by the state hospitals (see Mesnikoff, 1978). In Michigan, the pattern is depressingly similar: 'many of the foster care homes serving the mentally disabled were in inner-city areas with high crime rates, abandoned buildings, sub-standard housing, poor economic conditions and little or no recreational opportunities. Of a total of 378 community placement residences in Detroit serving the mentally disabled, 165 were located in the inner-city with 101 on one street. State officials attributed this to the availability of large homes at relatively low prices ... and to restrictive zoning which limits after-care homes to the older, run-down sections of the city. Although the number of mentally disabled in these facilities was not known, it has been estimated to be several thousand. The only service being provided many released mentally ill patients was medication' (General Accounting Office, 1977).

Such developments have not occurred without implicit and explicit state sponsorship and encouragement. In New York State, the scandals associated with the connections between the board and care industry and the political establishment eventually forced a full scale inquiry and subsequent prosecutions (see *New York Times*, 1975). Pennsylvania, with remarkable foresight, repealed its provisions for inspecting boarding homes the same year (1967) it began 'a massive deinstitutionalization program aimed at moving patients out of mental hospitals into community programs' (*Philadelphia Inquirer*, 1975). Hawaii faced a massive shortage of beds in licensed boarding homes when it adopted a policy of accelerated discharge. The problem was resolved, with unusual bureaucratic flexibility, through 'the proliferation, with the explicit encouragement of the state mental health division, of unlicensed boarding homes for the placement of ex-hospitalized patients' (Kirk and Thierran, 1975: 211). Nebraska at first shied away from such a laissez-faire approach, deciding apparently that some form of state oversight was called for. Accordingly, in a splendidly original variant on the ancient practice of treating the mad like cattle, the state placed licensing and inspection of the board and care homes in the hands of its State Department of Agriculture. Subsequent citizen complaints about the conditions which resulted led to the withdrawal of licenses, but not the patients, 'from an estimated 320 of these homes, leaving them without state supervision or regulation' (Kirk and Thierren, 1975: 19). Missouri simply noted the existence of some '755 unlicensed facilities in [the] State housing more than 10,000 patients' (Senate Committee on Aging, 1976: 724) and continued to dispense the state funds on which their operators depended. And still other states, like Maryland and Oregon, opted for perhaps the safest course of all – no follow-up of those they released and hence a blissful official ignorance about their subsequent fate (General Accounting Office, 1977: 95).

Such systematic academic research as has been done on conditions in board and care facilities (and again the research is noticeable mainly by its absence) confirms the picture. Lamb and Goertzel (1971: 29–34) concluded that: 'it is only an illusion that patients who were placed in board and care homes are "in the community" ... These facilities are for the most part like small long-term state hospital wards isolated from the community. One is overcome by the depressing atmosphere, not because of the physical appearance of the boarding home, but because of the passivity, isolation, and inactivity of the residents'. Kirk and Thierren (1975: 212) use remarkably similar language to describe their findings in Hawaii: 'many ex-patients are placed in "ward-like" environments where they are supervised by ex-state hospital staff, and they participate in a state hospital routine, albeit now "in the community". But many of these former patients do not even have the limited involvement provided by a day hospital. They spend the majority of their time in a boarding home which promotes dependency, passivity, isolation and inactivity'.

In the United States over the past quarter century, with the wholesale assistance of federal funds – Supplemental Security Income (SSI), Medicaid, Medicare and so forth – mental patients have been transformed into a commodity from which various professionals and entrepreneurs extract a profit. The consequence has been the emergence of a new 'trade in lunacy' (Jones, 1972). which in many ways bears a remarkable resemblance to the private madhouses which were employed to deal with the mentally disordered and distracted in eighteenth century England. In that earlier period, any one could enter this business, and there was no regulation of conduct, with the result that gross exploitation and maltreatment of patients were commonplace. As critics at the time pointed out, in such 'trading speculations [operated] with a view to pecuniary profit ... the extent of the profit must depend on the amount that can be saved out of the sum paid for the board of each individual' (Commissioners in Lunacy, 1847). Proprietors must therefore 'have a strong tendency to consider the interests of the patients and their own at direct variance' (Nicoll, 1828). Given free entry into the business and the difficulties associated with the inspection and supervision of a multitude of operations, the least scrupulous were likely to be the most successful, and appalling results were all but structurally guaranteed. So it proved: it was precisely the abuses to which this system was prone that led to a campaign for reform and to the establishment of England's state mental hospitals (cf. Scull, 1993).

Again the cycle is repeating itself. We now live in a period, also hailed as an era of reform, when anyone can open a boarding home for mentally ill patients discharged from the state system. Once more the mentally disturbed are at the mercy of speculators who have every incentive to warehouse their charges as cheaply as possible, since the volume of profit is inversely proportional to the amount expended on the inmates (Senate Committee on Aging, 1971; 1976). We possess a handful of studies which systematically compare the social functioning and clinical condition of hospitalized chronic patients with those of their counterparts in quasi-institutional community settings. 'From both American and Canadian studies we have reports that fewer of the [hospitalized] patients were incontinent, fewer took no part in bathing, more were able to bathe without help, fewer took no responsibility for their own grooming, more dressed without assistance, fewer failed to dress and remain in hospital gowns and more had money available and were capable of making occasional purchases' (Epstein and Simon, 1968; Swan, 1973). More dramatically, a number of studies appear to demonstrate a close correlation between the relocation of chronic patients and sharp increases in their mortality rates (cf. Marlowe, 1976; Aldrich and Mendkoff, 1963; Jasman, 1969; Markus et al., 1971).

Intended as a cheap alternative to the state hospital, the ramshackle network of board and care homes and welfare hotels and the swelling presence of the seriously mentally disabled among the ranks of the homeless stand as an indictment of contemporary American mental 'health' policy. They constitute perhaps the most extreme example of what has become the new orthodoxy, an 'almost unanimous abdication from the task of proposing and securing any provision for a humane and continuous form of care for those mental patients who need something rather more than short-term therapy for an acute phase of their illness' (Sedgwick,1982). Here, ecologically separated and isolated from the rest of us, the most useless and unwanted segments of our society can be left to decompose, quietly and, save for the occasional media expose, all but invisibly.

In view of the depths of the misery and maltreatment associated with recent American mental health policy, Kathleen Jones (1979: 567) claim that 'so far the United States has made a much better job of the business of deinstitutionalization' would, if accurate, constitute an even more damning indictment of British practice than she perhaps intended. Apparently, what led her to make this unfortunate assertion was the combination of a relatively intimate knowledge of the failures of British policies with a rather naive acceptance at face value of the claims made by American advocates of deinstitutionalization. And certainly at the level of rhetoric, Americans have by and large been the more active and shameless. Practically, however, the British experience has not (yet?) been quite as awful.

In part this is because de-institutionalization has simply not been as rapid or far-reaching in Britain. In general, the shift away from the mental hospital in both societies has been powerfully influenced by fiscal considerations, the savings realizable by substituting neglect for even minimal custodial care (Murphy and Datel, 1976; Rose, 1979; Scull, 1977; Sheehan and Atkinson, 1974). In the United States, however, these pressures have been magnified by the fragmentation of the political structure. Care of the mentally ill has traditionally been a responsibility of the states, but de-institutionalization has allowed and has been promoted by the states' ability to transfer most of the costs of community support to the federal level. (The causal linkage is particularly plain in the case of the mass discharges of the elderly beginning in the late 1960s) (Lerman, 1982). In the absence of this additional incentive, the rush to empty mental hospitals has been somewhat less headlong in Britain.

Ex-patients there have also for the most part been spared the excesses associated with the new trade in lunacy (Scull, 1981). The chains of private board and care homes and the dilapidated welfare hotels, now so large a part of American mental health 'services', have few precise British equivalents (Edward et al., 1978; Tidmarsh, 1974). In part, this probably reflects the somewhat lower numbers of chronic patients discharged. Undoubtedly too, it also mirrors the more entrepreneurial character of American capitalism, and the greater legitimacy accorded to the process of the privatization of state and welfare services (Spitzer and Scull, 1977). in a society still wedded to the myth of 'free enterprise'.

All these qualifications notwithstanding, the British experience with community care remains dismal and depressing in its own right. As Peter Sedgwick (1982) points out:

> in Britain no less than in the United States, 'community care' and 'the replacement of the mental hospital' were slogans which masked the growing depletion of real services for mental patients; the accumulating numbers of impaired, retarded and demented males in the prisons and common lodging houses; the scarcity not only of local authority residential provisions for the mentally disabled but of day care centers and skilled social work resources; the jettisoning of mental patients in their thousands into the isolated helpless environment of their families of origin, who appealed in vain for hospital admission (even for a temporary period of respite), for counselling or support, and even for basic information and advice .... (pp. 193–194)

Britain, like the United States, has sharply curtailed its reliance on the traditional mental hospital while systematically neglecting to build up the infrastructure of services and financial supports essential for any workable system of community care. During 1973–1974, for example, while 300 million pounds was spent on the mentally ill still receiving institutional treatment, a mere 6.5 million pounds was spent on residential and day care services for those 'in the community'. Local authority spending on residential facilities for the mentally ill was a derisory 0.04 per cent of their total expenditure (Sedwick, 1982). Three years later, 116 out of 170 local authorities did not provide a single residential place for the elderly mentally infirm (*The Guardian*, 1976; cited in Sedgwick, 1982). And more recently still, the intensifying fiscal crisis of the Thatcher–Reaganite years has simply reinforced the existing conservative hostility to social welfare services, and made the prospect of providing even minimal levels of supportive services still more remote (see Clare).

It should be starkly apparent, from the history I have reviewed here, that our collective reluctance to make a serious and sustained effort to provide a humane and caring environment for those manifesting grave and persistent mental disturbance has far deeper roots than the callousness of our contemporary political leadership. Still, recent changes in our political culture – in Britain just as clearly as in the United States – have scarcely improved the prospects for a satisfactory resolution of what one recent Maudsley lecturer, speaking to the Royal College of Psychiatrists, has called 'Scull's dilemma' (Jones, 1982). The idea that we bear a collective moral responsibility to provide for the unfortunate – indeed, that one of the marks of a civilized society is its determination to provide as of right certain minimum standards of living for all its citizens – has been steadily eroding over the past two decades. In its place, we have seen the resurgence of an ideology far more congenial and comforting to the privileged: the myth of the benevolent 'Invisible Hand' of the marketplace, and its corollary, an unabashed moral individualism. There is little place (and less sympathy) within such a worldview for those who are excluded from the race for material well-being by chronic disabilities and handicaps – whether physical or mental disease, or the more diffuse but cumulatively devastating penalties accruing to those belonging to racial minorities or living in dire poverty.

The punitive sentiments directed against those who must feed from the public trough extend only too easily to embrace those who suffer from the most severe forms of psychiatric misery. Those who seek to protect the long-term mental patient from the opprobrium visited upon the welfare recipient may do so by arguing that the patient is both dependent and *sick*. But I fear this approach has only a limited chance of success. After all, despite two centuries of propaganda, the public still resists the straightforward equation of mental and physical illness. Moreover, the long-term mental patient in most instances will not get better, and often fails to collaborate with his or her therapist to seek recovery. Such blatant violations of the norms governing access to the sick role in our societies (see Parsons, 1951) make it unlikely that chronic schizophrenics will be extended the courtesies and exemptions accorded to the conventionally sick. Instead, even those incapacitated by psychiatric disability all too often find themselves the targets of those who would abolish social programs because they consider any social dependency immoral.

Few of us, I suspect, would welcome the reincarnation of an unreconstructed psychiatric Victorianism, and there seems in any event little prospect of its rebirth, if only on grounds of cost. And yet we can feel no more confident than our Victorian forebears that we have devised a satisfactory system of humane and continuous care for those grossly disabled by what we call psychosis. Clearly, for some substantial sub-set of this population, one vital component of the needed array of services is a form of sheltered care – asylum, if you please – that will satisfy the basic human need for shelter, for occupation, for the embrace of a community that cares. How we are to reach such a Utopia, when the alternatives history presents us with are inadequate, often inhumane, and always underfunded mental hospitals or a grossly underdeveloped and frequently non-existent system of community care, is, dare I say it, not Scull's dilemma at all – but that of the psychiatric profession which claims to govern this territory; and of the all-too-indifferent larger society in which we collectively reside.

REFERENCES

Alcaron, J.G. and Sainsbury, P. (1963) 'Mental Illness and the Family', *The Lancet* i, pp. 544–547.

Alper, B. (1972) Foreword to Y. Bakal (ed.), *Closing Correctional Institutions*. Lexington, Massachusetts: Lexington Books, pp. vii–viii.

Aldrich, C. and Mendkoff, E. (1963) 'Relocation of the Aged and Disabled: A Mortality Study', *Journal of the American Geriatrics Society*, 11: 105–194.

Anon, (1837) Review of *What Asylums Were, Are, and Ought to Be*, *Phrenological Journal* (1836–1837), 10(53): 697.

Arlidge, J.T. (1859) *On the State of Lunacy and the Legal Provision for the Insane*. London: Churchill, p. 102.

Arnhoff, F. (1975) 'Social Consequences of Policy Toward Mental Illness', *Science*, 188: 1277–1281.

Bassuk, E. and Gerson, S. (1978) 'Deinstitutionalization and Mental Health Services', *Scientific American*, 238: 46–53.

Brown, G.W., Bone, M., Dalison, B. and Wing, J. (1966) *Schizophrenia and Social Care*, London: Oxford University Press, p. 59.

Browne, W.A.F. (1837) *What Asylums Were, Are, and Ought to Be*. Edinburgh: Black, p. 191, 231.

Bucknill, J.C. (1860) 'President's Address', *Journal of Mental Science*, 7: 6.

Burdett, H.C. (1891) *Hospitals and Asylums of the World*, London: Churchill, 2: viii.

Bynum, W.F. (1974) 'Time's Noblest Offspring: The Problem of Man in the British Natural Historical Sciences', unpublished Ph.D. dissertation, Cambridge University.

Caudill, W. (1958) *The Psychiatric Hospital as a Small Society*. Cambridge, Massachusetts: Harvard University Press. Belknap, I. (1956) *Human Problems of a State Mental Hospital*. New York: McGraw Hill.

Charles Hynes (1977), *Proprietary Homes for Adults: Their Administration, Management, Control, Operation, Supervision, Funding, and Quality*. New York: Deputy Attorney General's Office.

Chu, F. and Trotter, S. (1974) *The Madness Establishment*, New York: Grossman.

Clare, A. (1976) *Psychiatry in Dissent*, London: Travistock Publications. pp. 434–435.

Combe, G. (1850) *The Life and Correspondence of Andrew Combe, M.D.* Edinburgh: Maclachlan and Stewart, p. 376.

Commissioners in Lunacy (1847) *Further Report Relative to the Haydock Lodge Lunatic Asylum*. London: Spottiswoode and Shaw.

Conolly, J. (1835) 'Review of *What Asylums Were, Are, and Ought to Be*', *British and Foreign Medical Review*, 5(4): 74.

Conolly, J. (1847) *On the Construction and Government of Lunatic Asylums*. London: Churchill, p. 143.

Crammer, J.L. (1991) *Asylum History: Buckinghamshire County Pauper Lunatic Asylum – St. John's*. London: Gaskell, pp. 76–77, 113, 126–127.

Creer, C. and Wing, J.K. (1974) *Schizophrenia at Home*. London: Institute of Psychiatry.

Crichton Royal Asylum, (1857) *18th Annual Report*, p. 8.

Department of Health and Social Security [England] (1971) *Better Services for the Mentally Handicapped*, Cmnd 4683. London: HMSO.

Digby, A. (1985) *Madness, Morality and Medicine: A Study of the York Retreat 1796–1914*. Cambridge: Cambridge University Press. pp. 56, 199.

Dix, D. (1845) *Memorial Soliciting an Appropriation for the State [of Kentucky]*. Lexington: Hodge, p. 10.

Dix, D. (1845) *Memorial to the Senate and House of Representatives of the State of Illinois*. Springfield, Illinois: State Printer, p. 19.

Dix, D. (1849) *Memorial Soliciting a State Hospital for … Alabama*. Montgomery, Alabama: Office of the Advertizer, pp. 13–15.

Dwyer, E. (1987) *Homes for the Mad: Life in Two Nineteenth Century Asylums*. New Brunswick, New Jersey: Rutgers University Press, p. 150.

Eaton, D.B. (1881) 'Despotism in Lunatic Asylums', *North American Review,* 132: 263–275.

Edwards, G. Williamson, V., Hawker, A., Hensman, C. and Postoyan, S. 'Census of a Reception Centre', *British Journal of Psychiatry*, 114: 1031–1039.

Epstein, L. and Simon, A. (1968) 'Alternatives to State Hospitalization for the Geriatric Mentally Ill', *American Journal of Psychiatry* 124, pp. 955–961.

Friends' Asylum, (1835) *11th Annual Report,* Frankford, Pennsylvania, p. 8.

General Accounting Office (1977), *The Mentally Ill in the Community* : Government Needs to Do More. Washington, D.C.: Government Printing Office. pp. 11, 13–18, 39, 95.

Goffman, E. (1961) *Asylums: Essays on the Social Situation of Mental Patients and Other Inmates* Garden City, New York: Doubleday.

Gollaher D. (1989) *Social Order/Mental Disorder: Anglo-American Psychiatry in Historical Perspective.* Berkeley: University of California Press/London: Routledge.

Gough, I. (1979) *The Welfare State,* London: Macmillan p. 92. Lamb, H.R. (1982) *Treating the Long-Term Mentally Ill.* San Francisco: Jossey Bass.

Grob, G. (1983) 'Between 1907 and 1940, a total of 18,552 mentally ill persons in state hospitals were surgically sterilized'. *Mental Illness and American Society, 1875–1940.* Princeton, New Jersey: Princeton University Press, p. 173.

Hammond, W. (1879) 'The Non-Asylum Treatment of the Insane', *Transactions of the Medical Society of New York,* pp. 280–297.

Hawkes, J.M. (1875) *On the General Management of Public Lunatic Asylums in England and Wales.* London: Churchill, p. 32.

Jasman, K. (1969) 'Individualized Versus Mass Transfer of Nonpsychotic Geriatric Patients from the Mental Hospital to the Nursing Home', *Journal of American Geriatrics Society,* 15: 280–284.

Jones, K. (1979) 'Deinstitutionalization in Context'. *Milbank Memorial Fund Quarterly,* 57(4): 552–569.

Jones, K. (1982) 'Scull's Dilemma', *British Journal of Psychiatry,* 141: 221–226.

Kirk, S. and Thierren, M. (1975) 'Community Mental Health Myths and the Fate of Formerly Hospitalized Mental Patients', *Psychiatry*, p. 210.

Lamb, R. and Goertzel, V. (1971) 'Discharged Mental Patients: Are They Really in the Community?' *Archives of General Psychiatry,* 24: 29–34.

Laycock, T. (1869) 'The Objects and Organization of the Medico-Psychological Association', *Journal of Mental Science,* 15: 332.

Lerman, P. (1982) *Deinstitutionalization and the Welfare State.* New Brunswick, New Jersey: Rutgers University Press.

Lovejoy, A.O. (1960) *The Great Chain of Being.* New York: Harper.

Lowe, L. (1883) *The Bastilles of England; or, The Lunacy Laws at Work.* London: Crookenden.

MacKenzie, C. (1992) *Psychiatry for the Rich: A History of Ticehurst Private Asylum.* London: Routledge.

Markus, E., Blenker, M. and Downs, T. (1971) 'The Impact of Relocation Upon Mortality Rates of Institutionalized Aged Persons', *Journal of Gerontology,* 26: 537–541.

Marlowe, R. (1976) 'When They Closed the Doors at Modesto'. In P. Ahmed and S. Plog (eds), *State Mental Hospitals: What Happens When They Close?* New York: Plenum.

Maudsley, H. (1867) *The Physiology and Pathology of Mind.* London: Macmillan, pp. 494–495.

Maudsley, H. (1870) *Body and Mind.* London: Macmillan, p. 53.

Mesnikoff, A. (1978) 'Barriers to the Delivery of Mental Health Services: The New York City Experience', *Hospital and Community Psychiatry,* 29: 373–378.

Mitchell, S.W. (1894) *Address Before the American Medico-Psychological Association.* Philadelphia, p. 19.

Murphy, J. and Datel, W. (1976) 'A Cost-Benefit Analysis of Community Versus Institutional Living', *Health and Community Psychiatry,* 25: 165–170.

Nicoll, S.W. (1828) *An Enquiry into the Present State of Visitation in Asylums for the Reception of the Insane.* London: Harvey and Darnton, pp. 2–3.

Okin, R.L. (1978) 'The Future of State Mental Health Programs for the Chronic Psychiatric Patient in the Community', *American Journal of Psychiatry,* 135: 1355–1358.

Oppenheim, J. (1991) *'Shattered Nerves': Doctors, Patients, and Depression in Victorian England.* New York: Oxford University Press.

Packard, E. (1873) *Modern Persecution, or Insane Asylums Unveiled,* 2 vols, Hartford, Connecticut: Case, Lockw and Brainard.

Parry-Jones, W. (1972) *The Trade In Lunacy.* London: Routledge and Kegan Paul.

Parsons, T. (1951) *The Social System.* New York: Free Press.

Pennsylvania Prison Discipline Society (1845) 'The expense incurred in making a proper provision for this class of paupers is a very profitable investment'. *Pennsylvania Journal of Prison Discipline and Philanthropy,* p. 60.

Perrucci, R. (1974) *Circle of Madness .* Englewood Cliffs, New Jersey: Prentice-Hall.

Reich, R. and Siegal, L. (1973) 'Psychiatry Under Seige: The Mentally Ill Shuffle to Oblivion', *Psychiatric Annals,* 3: 37–50. F.

Rieder, R.O. (1974) 'Hospital, Patients and Politics', *Schizophrenia Bulletin,* 11: 11.

Rose, S. 'Deciphering Deinstitutionalization'. *Milbank Memorial Fund Quarterly,* 57(4): 552–569. p. 44.

Rose, S. (1979) 'Deciphering Deinstitutionalization', *Milbank Memories Fund Quarterly,* 57: 429–460.

Rothman, D. (1971) *The Discovery of the Asylum.* Boston: Little, Brown, p. 177.

Scull, A. (1976) 'The Decarceration of the Mentally Ill: A Critical View', *Politics and Society,* 6: 173–212.

Scull, A. (1977) *Decarceration .* Englewood Cliffs, New Jersey: Prentice Hall Inc.

Scull, A. (1981) 'A New Trade in Lunacy: The Recommodification of the Mental Patient', *American Behavioral Scientist,* 24: 741–754.

Scull, A. (1981) 'Deinstitutionalization and the Rights of the Deviant', *Journal of Social Issues,* pp. 6–20.

Scull, A. (1991)*The Asylum as Utopia: W.A.F. Browne and the Mid-Nineteenth Century Consolidation of Psychiatry.* London: Routledge.

Scull, A. (1993) *The Most Solitary of Afflictions: Madness and Society in Britain, 1700–1900.* London and New Haven: Yale University Press.

Sedgwick, P. (1981) 'Psychiatry and Liberation', unpublished paper (Leeds University, 1981), p. 9.

Sedgwick, P. (1982) *Psychopolitics,* London: Pluto Press, pp. 193–194.

Senate Committee on Aging, (1971) *Trends in Long Term Care, Hearings Parts 12 and 13, Chicago, Illinois.* Washington, D.C.: Government Printing Office, pp. 1239, 1256.

Senate Committee on Aging, (1976) *The Role of Nursing Homes in Caring for Discharged Mental Patients.* Washington, D.C.: Government Printing Office, p. 753.

Sharfstein, S. (1978) 'Will Community Mental Health Survive in the 1980s?' *American Journal of Psychiatry,* 135: 1363–1365.

Sheehan, D.N. and Atkinson, J. (1974) 'Comparative Cost of State Hospitals and Community Based In-Patient Care in Texas', *Hospital and Community Psychiatry,* 25: 242–244.

Shorter, E. (1992) *From Paralysis to Fatigue: A History of Psychosomatic Medicine in the Modern Era.* New York: Free Press.

Showalter, E. (1985) *The Female Malady: Madness and English Culture, 1830–1980.* New York: Pantheon.

Spitzer, S. and Scull, A. (1977) 'Privatization and State Control: The Case of the Private Police', *Social Problems,* p. 25.

Spitzka, E. (1878) 'Reform in the Scientific Study of Psychiatry', *Journal of Nervous and Mental Diseases,* 5: 200–229.

Strahan, S.A.K. (1890) 'The Propagation of Insanity and Other Neuroses', *Journal of Mental Science,* 36: 337.

Swan, R. (1973) 'A Survey of a Boarding Home Program for Former Mental Patients', *Hospital and Community Psychiatry,* 24: 485–486.

Thomas, K. (1983) *Man and the Natural World: Changing Attitudes in England 1500–1800.* London: Allen Lane.

Tidmarsh, D. (1974) 'Secure Hospital Units', *British Medical Journal,* p. 216.

Tomes, N. (1984) *A Generous Confidence: Thomas Story Kirkbride and the Art of Asylum Keeping.* Cambridge: Cambridge University Press.

Tuke, S. (1813) *Description of the Retreat.* York: Alexander, p. 147, 175.

Turner, T. (1988) 'Henry Maudsley: Psychiatrist, Philosopher, Entrepreneur'. In W.F. Bynum, R. Porter and M. Shepherd (eds) *The Anatomy of Madness,* London: Routledge, 3: 179.

Walton, J. (1985) 'Casting Out and Bringing Back in Victorian England: Pauper Lunatics, 1840–70'. In W.F. Bynum, R. Porter and M. Shepherd (eds), *The Anatomy of Madness,* London: Tavistock, 2: 142.

Windle, C. and Scully, D. (1976) 'Community Mental Health Centers and the Decreasing Use of State Mental Hospitals', *Community Mental Health Journal,* 12: 11.

Wing, J.K. (1971) 'How Many Psychiatric Beds?' *Psychological Medicine,* 1: 190.

Wing, J.K. and Brown, G.W. (1970) *Institutionalism and Schizophrenia,* Cambridge: Cambridge University Press, p. 192.

Wolpert, E. and Wolpert, J. (1976) 'The Relocation of Released Mental Hospital Patients into Residential Communities', *Policy Science:* Spring.

Wolpert, E. and Wolpert, J. (1976) 'The Relocation of Released Mental Patients into Residential Communities,' *Policy Sciences,* 7: 31–51.

Wolpert, E. and Wolpert, J. (1984) *Decarceration: Community Treatment and the Deviant–A Radical View,* 2nd edition. Oxford: Polity Press/New Brunswick: Rutgers University Press.

Wynter, A. (1877) *The Borderlands of Insanity,* 2nd edition. London: Renshaw.

22

Action for Change in the UK: Thirty Years of the User/ Survivor Movement

Peter Campbell and Diana Rose

INTRODUCTION

Any observer of mental health services in the United Kingdom over the last thirty years would have to acknowledge the important changes that have taken place in the role of service users. Service users are now extensively involved: as individuals in their own care and treatment and collectively in the development of mental health services. It is now scarcely possible to undertake major initiatives in the mental health sphere without involving service users. Service users have moved from being a notable absence to a significant presence in all important mental health matters. Listening to service users has become absolutely necessary.

Nevertheless, there is some danger in celebrating too enthusiastically the pervasive nature of service user involvement. Evidence, not least that of service users themselves, suggests that involvement in care and treatment does not go as far as all that. Recent findings from the Healthcare Commission and elsewhere suggest that as few as 50 per cent of mental health service users are being involved in significant aspects of their care (HCC, 2005). At the same time activists continue to complain at the tokenistic approach to collective involvement and cite examples of organizations where involvement is badly carried out. Some activists go as far as to question whether involvement really delivers the goods in terms of meaningful positive change. While recognizing the important advances that have occurred, the history of service user action in the last 30 years is one of gains and failures, acceptance, resistance and struggle. It is by no means a story of unrelieved triumphs (Campbell, 2008).

The reader will find this chapter different to the others particularly with respect to referencing. We are relatively light on the 'peer reviewed' literature and strong on user literature and government reports. We have also relied on our own individual archives and experiences in service user activism over the last 30 years. In this respect, a word should be said about the authors. We worked together closely in the 1980s but took different turns. Much of the historical material in this chapter comes from Peter Campbell's personal archive. Diana Rose took a different turn, into user research, so her contribution is more mainstream academic than the grounded historical approach of Peter Campbell.

LANGUAGE

Mental health is a controversial field. Some concepts and language remain fiercely contested. It has been customary to see service user activists as having an 'anti-medical' bias and there could be good justification for this although the picture may be more complicated now than it was in the 1980s and there is a danger in overemphasizing the radical nature of current action. Nevertheless, the increasing involvement of service users has seen the rise of non-medical/non-psychiatric language. There is a tendency to talk about mental distress rather than mental illness. Hallucinations are now seen as hearing voices. Anorexia nervosa and builimia are replaced by eating distress. Hypochondria becomes health anxiety. While it is probably wrong to see these shifts as a the result of a full-scale assault on the medical model (such an assault may not been the intention of the majority of service user activists nowadays) they are clear evidence that the demedicalization of mental health is seen as advantageous for a number of reasons including the difficulties of stigmatization and mystification that attend traditional concepts and language.

The issue of identity is central to the lives of people with a mental illness diagnosis, not least because they have been shunted by that diagnosis into a negative category of citizen and human being and have to live with the prejudice that results from this. Having the opportunity to self-identify both as an individual and as a collective has often been seen as one way to challenge negative preconceptions. Self identification, as the term suggests, has not led to a 100 per cent agreement at a collective level. While it is clear that many service users (whether activists or not) no longer wish to be called 'the mentally ill' or schizophrenics, manic depressives or similar diagnosis-based descriptions, what is seen as positive alternatives, is not so clear. In the 1980s, talk was often of consumers rather than mental patients but this was often challenged by activists who denied the usefulness of the term 'consumer' to describe their powerlessness within the system or to recognize that substantial numbers were using services against their will. Some activists identified themselves as recipients rather than consumers to emphasize this powerlessness.

Service user has largely replaced consumer in the UK (though not in the United States where the shortened form 'user' is linked strongly to the use of illegal drugs). But service user is an essentially neutral term and many activists have preferred to use the term 'survivor' which implies a degree of criticism – people are not just using services but are surviving the obstacle course they present. It should not be assumed that everyone who identifies as a survivor sees themselves as surviving the same problems. There may for instance be differences of emphasis or substance between someone who calls themselves a psychiatric survivor and someone who calls themselves a mental health system survivor. At the same time, there has always been a temptation to see the self-identifying survivor as more radical than the self-identifying service user. Although there is some truth in this, it is a simplification of a more complex reality. Debates about collective self-identification break out regularly. This can be seen as a healthy thing. The terms which have endured longest so far are 'service user' and 'survivor'. It is probably pointless to argue which is best.

EARLY DAYS AND INFLUENCES

Although individual mad people have for centuries protested at the way society responds to them, it is not until the 1970s that we had real evidence of collective action for change by service users in the United Kingdom (Crossley, 2006). The Mental Patients' Union (MPU), established in 1972 and slightly predated by the short-lived Scottish Union of Mental Patients (SUMP), has a strong claim to be the original group from which the current service user movement sprang. Originating in a meeting of 150 individuals, the MPU grew rapidly with a number of cells in London and throughout the United Kingdom, including some groups within psychiatric hospitals. While it did not survive into the 1980s, there are clear links between its activities and those of the early 1980s and some members of the MPU were to play significant roles in the local and national service user groups that developed in the mid-1980s. It is now clear that, while there was a marked upsurge in action by service users in the second half of the 1980s, we need to look to the 1970s for the true origins of the movement. This is exceptionally well documented on the Survivor History Group website: www.studymore.org.uk.

Nevertheless, the growth of activity in the 1980s is remarkable and worthy of attention. In the early years of the decade, service user action groups were few and far between. Service users, whether in their own action groups or not, were on the margins, more likely to be excluded from discussions about mental health services than included, substantially lacking a credible voice in key areas that concerned them. The 1983 Mental Health Act seems to have been formulated without meaningful input from those to whom it was to be applied. Yet by the end of the 1980s, there were more than 50 independent, service user action groups in England and Wales and service users were being invited into meetings about the development and monitoring of services or were involved in the education and training of certain professional groups. The establishment's desire to involve service users that was to become overwhelming in the 1990s was already intensifying. Listening to service users, whether it resulted in positive change or not, was happening in a way it had never done before.

The reasons for service users becoming a presence where hitherto they had been an absence are complex. One important factor, some might say the predominant factor, was the Conservative government's intention to open up all health services to market economics (NHS and Community Care Act, 1990). This necessitated an increased attention to the service 'consumer' as a means of securing services that were as efficient and as cost-effective as possible. It can well be argued that service user activists first rode into the corridors of power in the United Kingdom on the back of health service consumerism. While their intentions, certainly in the 1980s, were not the same as the government's, they were not battering at a door that was totally closed against them but at one that was being opened ever wider from within.

Of course, activists of the time were not looking to the government for their influences. These came from elsewhere, from the movements of oppressed groups in previous decades: black people and women, gays and lesbians, the disability movement. Contacts with service user movements in other countries, which had sometimes achieved much more, were extremely important. Visits from activists in the USA and the Netherlands were influential. By the 1980s there was a generation of service users in the United Kingdom who had been receiving services for decades but for whom the community rather than the asylum was home. They had absorbed a civil-rights culture, they could see how it applied to them and, unlike previous generations of mad people, were in a position to do something about it. The growth of service user action in the 1980s may owe a great deal to the policies of the Conservative government but it may also be an example of an idea whose time had finally come.

Some commentators (Crossley, 2006; Pilgrim, 2005) emphasize the influence of 'anti-psychiatry' on the service user movement in the 1980s and since. It is certainly true that British Network for Alternatives to Psychiatry (BNAP), an important group in the early 1980s where a number of service user activists first came together, contained mental health professionals who had been close to R.D. Laing and David Cooper. It is also true that much of the discourse for criticizing psychiatry at that time depended on language and concepts traceable to 'anti-psychiatry'. On the other hand, there were strands in service user action that owed little or nothing to 'anti-psychiatry'. Self-advocacy, an important concept in the service user movement in the 1980s came from the learning disability field. Anti-psychiatry said little or nothing about independent mental health advocacy that became one of the enduring demands of service user activists. It can also be questioned whether service user involvement in consultation about service development was close to the heart of most 'anti-psychiatrists'. While more research needs to be done on the linkages, it is notable that many activists of the time now play down connections with 'anti-psychiatry' and emphasize what they learned from other sources, including fellow activists.

It is possible to regard the five or six years from 1985 onwards as a pioneering time for the service user movement. Organizations like Survivors Speak Out and Nottingham Advocacy Group were spending considerable time spreading the word about service user action, persuading mental health professionals and service users of its possibilities. There was much scepticism and some obstruction. Although it was clear that involving service users was coming into fashion, most of their action groups were small and underfunded, without office premises or paid workers. User Development Workers, employed to set up service user groups in local areas, were at this stage comparatively rare.

The growth of service user groups accelerated after the NHS and Community Care Act 1991. More resources were made available and a number of new networking groups emerged: United Kingdom Advocacy Network (UKAN), Hearing Voices Network (HVN) (http://www.hearing-voices.org/), National Self-Harm Network (NSHN) (http://www.nshn.co.uk/) for example. The NSHN published a handbook with a radical new take on self harm calling it 'harm minimization' (http://www.kreativeinterventions.com/resources_7.html). When a Government Task Force was set up between 1992 and 1994 to stimulate good community health services, it included a User Group which produced a prototype charter and other publications and held an England-wide conference in Derby. As the 1997 election approached, it seemed this group might become a fixture at the Department of Health representing the concerns of English service users at a high level.

THE USER MOVEMENT UNDER NEW LABOUR

The impetus to user involvement started under the last conservative government of the 1980s–1990s (the 'Major years') promised to continue when New Labour came to power in 1997. There were forward looking MPs who were prepared to listen to service user activists but it soon became clear that they tended to act as individuals. Relatively early on, an ominous note was struck when Frank Dobson, then Secretary of State for Health, called service users 'a nuisance and a danger' in the foreword to the National Service Framework for Mental Health (DH, 1999).

However, the New Labour government did seem to wish to continue the emphasis on public involvement which it had inherited. Most initiatives were generic but in mental health there was the specific National Service Framework for Mental Health (DH 1999). The process leading up to this involved an intense national exercise bringing together psychiatrists, other practitioners, policy makers and commissioners. These made up what was known as the 'Internal Reference Group (IRG)'.

The IRG included six service users. One of the authors of this chapter (DR) interviewed five of the six (Wallcraft et al., 2002). All found it a very negative experience. Three resigned before the process was complete. There were issues around 'cherry-picking' users to sit on the IRG, insufficient attention to people's expertise and very difficult issues for users from Black and Minority Ethnic Users. When asked whether they would participate in such a process again, four immediately said 'no'. The fifth said it would depend on the circumstances.

As time progressed, it became clear that New Labour's impact on service user activism was mixed. As Survivors Speak Out waned and UKAN lost much of its impact, the development of the National Service Framework was perhaps the last time there was a strong user presence in a national initiative until very recently. Thereafter it seemed that the user movement devolved into a large but disparate series of local groups. Wallcraft et al. (2002) counted 383 groups by 2002 with very varying memberships and resources.

The devolution into local groups can be argued to have been at least partially a result of subsequent involvement policies in the last decade of the last century. Involvement policy was targeted at Trusts and Local Authorities who eventually had a duty laid upon them to consult with and involve patients and the public (PPI). Thus, the Wallcraft survey found that one of the commonest activities groups engaged in was 'consultation with planners and policy makers'. Some had contracts where consultation was a condition of funding.

As the first decade of the twenty-first century wore on, the structure and nature of PPI changed at a dizzying pace. Different fora were opened up and then closed or replaced by new ones. Local activists often found themselves bemused about meetings they were being invited to. The involvement agenda was generic and covered all health care groups or all social care groups. There is a lack of a place for people who participate in these kinds of activities to come together and decide collectively which, if any, is helpful. And mental health has a specific issue when it comes to compulsion and coercion. Negotiating about services with people who could detain you is not a comfortable thing to do.

The main point, however, is that it can be argued that the demise of national organizations and the rise of local groups as a result of initiatives at national and local levels undermined the earlier radicalism of the user movement. The pressure from government for local involvement coupled with the strain that this put on small groups meant that networking diminished and service users had to concentrate on their own patch. Not least, this was their only route to funding and resources.

The nature of the involvement that authorities want in mental health is worth noting. According to Gummer and Furney (1998) providers want to hear the 'authentic voice of experience'. However, they do not want that voice to be *too* authentic. Outbursts of emotion such as anger are readily pathologized as a return of mental illness. As we write, a new initiative for a national network of service user groups is underway. Named NSUN (www.nsun.org.uk), it is to be a 'network or networks' and attempts to counter criticisms of elitism having been initiated by well-known users/survivors. Thus far its approach is managerial, for example, advising groups on how to attain charitable status. It is well-funded. Whether in the future it can revive some of the ideas of the user movement of two and a half decades ago remains to be seen.

INTRODUCTION TO SERVICE USER ACTIONS

The service user movement is notable for its diversity of action. It is impossible to do full justice to this aspect in this chapter. Government and mental health service providers are probably most interested in the service user movement as a partner in consultations about the monitoring of existing services and the development of new ones. But the movement has gone beyond such functions, although they still make up a large proportion of the activities of many local groups. In the following paragraphs, some of the other areas of service user action are examined and an assessment made of positive impacts and problematic issues.

ADVOCACY

In many respects, independent mental health advocacy can be viewed as an area of positive achievement for the service user movement. Whereas many of the more radical demands of activists, for less compulsion, less medication, for 24 hour non-medical crisis houses for example, have produced little or no positive change, the demand for advocacy has achieved results. In the early 1980s, there was little or no advocacy support available to service users. The need for advocacy was not widely discussed. Now, in 2009, we have advocacy services, albeit of varying quality, in most areas of the country and a right to advocacy for detained patients in England and Wales and Scotland. It can be argued that the main reason we have gone as far as we have done in terms of advocacy, is very largely due to the efforts of service user action groups.

Activists have always made advocacy provision a basic demand in their work for better community mental health services. They took a lead in promoting advocacy in the 1980s when government was not much interested and major voluntary organizations like Mind and the National Schizophrenia Fellowship (now Rethink) were cautious or sceptical. Advocacy was on the service user movement's list of priorities before those of most agencies and has remained a key requirement. Service users were also much involved in the establishment of early advocacy projects and in the development of advocacy skills. The United Kingdom Advocacy Network, a service user-controlled organization, played a key role in the development of advocacy during the 1990s and early years of the new century, including providing vital support to local projects and developing codes of good practice and training manuals (UKAN, 2001, 2004; Wood, 2003).

But the success of service user action in relation to advocacy is by no means unalloyed. Many action groups, including UKAN, have been committed to the ideal of service user-led advocacy, where service users, if not acting as advocates themselves, are certainly in control of the organizations providing advocacy. This ideal has not been realized. As advocacy has been increasingly recognized as a vital element in good services and, in particular, as it has been given a definite role in the new Mental Health Act 2007, so the service user element in advocacy provision has become more marginal. Although we are currently at the very earliest stages of introducing advocacy for detained patients across England and Wales, it seems clear that there is no real commitment to service users having an active role in advocacy provision. The provision of advocacy, perhaps inevitably, is undergoing a process of professionalization in which it appears service user input has a quite limited part to play. Having taken advocacy forward as part of a grassroots initiative, service users appear to have no choice but to place it in the hands of more credible operators.

UNDERSTANDINGS

Service user activists have not confined their activities to the improvement of mental health services, to working for more choice, more information, greater individual control over care and treatment. A significant number have also explored new understandings about the true nature of madness/mental illness itself. It is sometimes said that the service user movement is opposed to the 'medical model'. While there is a good deal of truth in such a generalization, the reality is rather more complex.

There are certainly activists who fundamentally challenge medical understandings, who question whether the idea of mental illness stands up scientifically and doubt the validity and usefulness of diagnostic categories. But they may be a minority within the movement. A greater number take their criticisms less far and focus on improving the consequences of medical understandings of madness rather than trying to be rid of them entirely. Although the situation has never been properly researched, it is quite possible that a substantial portion of the service user movement would be happy if the medical model could be made to work better and still believe that it can be.

One drawback for those activists who see a full-blooded attack on the medical model as being essential, is the lack of a convincing model to replace it with. The service user movement has nothing equivalent to the social model of disability that has been so central to the work and effectiveness of the disability movement. Service user activists have not been enthusiastic in taking up this model for themselves, partly through ignorance of it and partly because many of them do not feel their mental distress as being an impairment. In recent years, there has been an attempt by a small group of activists to develop a social model of madness and distress but this is very much a work in progress and may not be seen as a real priority by the majority of the movement.

Nevertheless, the lack of a coherent model to replace the medical model has not prevented groups of activists from putting forward alternative understandings of their problems. This has occurred in relation to a diversity of experiences. One of the most notable has been the reconfiguration of ideas and practices around hallucinations, a key indicator for a diagnosis of schizophrenia. The Hearing Voices Network, founded in 1990, has become an important vehicle for alternative understandings of aural and visual hallucinations and a source of novel coping strategies and mutual support. However, once again such ideas can be taken up and then radically diluted by mainstream professionals. Psychologists run what they call 'hearing voices groups' but these may contain a significant element of medication compliance.

Another example of alternative understandings starting to challenge traditional practice is the National Self Harm Network which has enabled people with direct experience to come out of the shadows and present their own view of their predicament for the first time. It is perhaps significant that the first ever conference in the UK where people who self harm came together with professionals in the field was organized not by professionals but by people with direct experience. The National Self Harm Network has gone on to challenge some of the deep-rooted prejudices attached to self harm, to promote the idea of self-harm as a vital coping strategy and to introduce the idea of practical harm minimization. A group of people who self harm and their allies have just produced a DVD which will be available shortly (http://www.selfharm-mindvd.co.uk/).

There is no doubt that both mental health services and wider society are now much more willing to listen to people with a mental illness talking about their personal experience. Personal testimony of this kind does not just occur in training sessions for mental health professionals but increasingly in the media, in books, journals and magazines directed at the general public. What is not yet clear is precisely what value or credibility is attached to such material. Mainstream psychiatry is certainly starting to listen to the voice of direct experience. It may be slower in accepting the new understandings and analysis service users are deriving from that experience. The challenge coming from the service user movement, or at least significant elements within it, is twofold. First, accept our understandings of our own experiences as equally valid as professional understandings. Second, acknowledge that our ability and expertise in self-help and mutual support is commensurate to that of professional expertise. In short that service users are not merely consumers of mental health care and treatment but are primarily 'experts by experience'.

RESEARCH

User/survivor research can be dated from the mid-1990s. Two publications mark this beginning and both were user-controlled projects carried out in NGOs. User-focused monitoring detailed a method for user evaluation of services illustrating this with data from over 500 service users across seven sites in England.

Strategies for Living (Faulkner and Layzell, 2001) described a project where peer interviewers investigated how people dealt with mental distress particularly outside formal services or complementarily to them. There had been small local projects before this. A prominent local group, Camden Mental Health Consortium, did a piece of research on the views of service users about the move of inpatient wards from the local large asylum to provision in a community hospital (Good Practices in Mental Health/Camden Mental Health Consortium, 1998). However, UFM and S4L were large, well funded user-led research projects.

It is important to note that the co-ordinators of these projects were active in the wider user movement. They sought to bring their research skills to bear on the agenda for research and developed research methods that would be commensurate with the aims of the movement. Strategies for Living went on to fund a network of small projects throughout England (Nicholls et al., 2003) but no longer exists. User-Focused Monitoring has been rolled out in approximately 20 projects in England (Kotecha et al., 2007). Its aim of effecting change in services is often achieved but not always. There exists a UFM network, no longer based in the original NGO. There are face-to-face meetings and there is a co-ordinator but most activity is web-based. Currently, UFM projects may be experiencing difficulties as local authorities try to bring user involvement 'in-house'.

A development in the early 2000s was that user/survivor research moved into the universities. Examples are SURESearch in Birmingham which now works closely with the Centre of Excellence in Interdisciplinary Mental Health Research and the Service User Research Enterprise (SURE) at the Institute of Psychiatry, King's College, London. These endeavours were no longer user-controlled but collaborative as between service user researchers and mainstream researchers. As such, there were issues of power and hierarchies of evidence that needed to be addressed (Rose, 2009). The process was helped by the Department of Health setting up a dedicated unit to promote user involvement in research, known first as Consumers in NHS Research and then INVOLVE (www.invo.org. uk). INVOLVE is generic and its membership is diverse. It is interesting that amongst the consumer members the majority are mental health service user researchers. This speaks to the greater conflict in terms of agendas for research and research methodologies in mental health as opposed to other conditions and client groups. This itself seems to be a consequence of the greater critiques of psychiatry by the mental health service user movement.

User/survivor research in universities does not commend itself to everyone (Sweeney et al., 2009). Mainstream researchers are often suspicious, even denigrating. However, user involvement in research is now a condition of funding for DH research and so mainstream researchers approach user teams in their universities. The concern is that this is a 'tick box' exercise. At the same time, this move into the universities is sometimes criticized by other user researchers on the grounds that the entry into the mainstream is a form of co-option and that user researchers have lost their independence. The opposite point of view is that user research has indeed made inroads into health and social care research.

There exists one research organization that is user-controlled – Shaping Our Lives (Beresford). It concentrates on social care and covers all social care client groups. It is resolute that it will remain user-controlled thus avoiding the pitfalls of collaborative research.

User research has begun to develop its own methodologies and epistemologies. SURE has developed a model of 'Patient Centred Systematic Reviews'. This was first applied to users' experiences of Electro-Convulsive Therapy (ECT) (Rose et al., 2003, 2005). The review showed marked differences in what patients said about the benefit of ECT according to whether they were asked by a professional or a peer. People who had had ECT tended to say it helped if the interviewer was a psychiatrist but not if the question came from a fellow user. The study also showed that long-term memory loss was a serious problem for many, something denied by most clinicians. Two of the researchers on this review had received ECT themselves. When this was published, it drew a very hostile response from the Royal College of Psychiatrists. Nevertheless, the review was influential on the National Institute for Clinical Excellence (NICE) when it drew up new guidelines for ECT and the Royal College itself did become more accepting.

User/survivor research critiques the way in which certain methods are prized in providing an 'evidence base' for mental health services. This particularly applies to Randomized Controlled Trials (RCT). Claimed as neutral, they nevertheless always use outcome measures devised by clinicians and academics. A 'good outcome' is defined by clinicians but they never reflect on this. So we can argue that they leave implicit their philosophical assumptions. Mainstream psychiatry believes its research is 'obviously' objective. It sees no need to question its philosophical underpinnings. User researchers are teasing out the philosophical underpinnings of mainstream research as a form of critique and developing new models to serve as the basis for a user-focused research methodology (Beresford, 2003; Rose, 2009).

MENTAL HEALTH ACTS

The 1959 Mental Health Act marked a watershed in hospital care for people with a mental illness diagnosis. It ushered in an era where psychiatric care was allegedly aligned with physical care and where people who would previously been under an 'order' could be treated as voluntary patients. The 1983 Act continued this focus on restricting compulsion although it was procedurally much more complex. Now we have the 2007 Amendments to the 1983 Act, of which more below.

But have these changes led to a reduction in coercion? In fact, it seems that the proportion of patients admitted compulsorily has steadily increased since 1983 and particularly in the period between 1996 and 2006 (Keown et al., 2008). These facts are, today, well-known to users of mental health services. However, there was little or no consultation or involvement in the development of either the 1959 or 1983 Acts. The NAMH (now MIND) was responsible for intense lobbying to bring more rights for patients into the 1983 Act but they did not consult meaningfully with service users. The period of development leading up to the 1983 Act did coincide with the formation of an embryonic user movement, such as the Mental Patients' Union, but this voice was not yet strong enough, or maybe was disinclined, to be much involved with debates about the Act.

Things were very different in the decade 1997 to 2007. When New Labour was elected, they proposed a new Act 'fit for the twenty-first century'. This saw the establishment of a committee chaired by the lawyer Genevra Richardson. The Richardson Committee proposed that a new Mental Health Act be based on the principle of 'capacity'. That is, a patient should only be subject to compulsory powers if they cannot make treatment decisions. It has been made explicit that the capacity principle also applies in general medicine and so it is argued that the very existence of a separate Mental Health act constitutes discrimination against those with mental health problems (Szmukler et al., in press).

The government almost immediately rejected the recommendations of the Richardson Committee and replaced it with a focus on protection of the public. A 'new' category of mental disorder was introduced – Severe and Dangerous Personality Disorder (SDPD). Those so designated could be subject to compulsory powers even if they had not offended. Treatment was to be 'appropriate' but need not confer benefit. This provision, it was argued by opponents, stemmed from media reporting of high-profile tragedies.

A further new provision was to treat patients not only in hospital but under compulsory powers in the community. This was proposed to offer the 'least restrictive environment' for 'revolving doors' patients. Patients were to comply with treatment in the community. This basically meant medication as it is impossible to be compelled to receive psychological treatments. In addition, those subject to Compulsory Treatment Orders (now called Supervised Treatment Orders) could be forced to live or spend their days in situations specified by the Orders. These, and other provisions, were too much for service users and many other organizations. A coalition called the 'Mental Health Alliance' was formed with user groups, including those from BME communities well-represented. Some of these were national user groups – such as the United Kingdom Advocacy Network (UKAN) and the Voices Forum. Some, however, were local user groups. The Mental Health Alliance was far from user-controlled. It was formed also of professional bodies including the Royal College of Psychiatrists. The Royal College had a slightly different agenda arguing that the new powers could not work as there were insufficient psychiatrists to staff various new bodies, such as tribunals. The slogan of the Mental Health Alliance is 'Rights not Compulsion'. The situation regarding user involvement seemed to represent a dramatic change from that leading up to the 1983 Act.

The progression of the Act through Parliament was tortuous taking ten years from the establishment of the Richardson Committee to the final Act in 2007.

Two Bills were introduced – in 2002 and 2004 – and both fell under public scrutiny in a campaign led by the Alliance including user groups and individual service users. Finally, the government used parliamentary procedure to pass the amendments. The Alliance claimed some achievements such as the right to independent advocacy and the provision that treatments be not just 'appropriate' but known to confer benefit. From the point of view many service users and user groups, however, the right to independent advocacy was disappointing as the tradition in the user movement of peer advocacy was replaced by professional advocacy.

Finally, user involvement in Mental Health Legislation was gradually adopted by the Mental Health Act Commission which oversees the rights of detained patients. The Commission introduced a Service User Reference Panel made up of people who had been detained and were still currently detained. It also appointed some commissioners who were service users (Mental Health Act Commission, 2009). However, the Commission has now been merged into the Care Quality Commission which oversees health and social care generally. It is an open question as to how far the old MHAC initiatives to adopt service user involvement will develop or fall by the wayside.

The Mental Health Alliance has been called an 'unholy alliance' embracing as it does everything from the Royal College of Psychiatrists to very radical user groups. But it seems that user involvement in this complicated process leading up to the implementation of the Act (it was not actually implemented until the end of 2008) had a real effect not only on the Act itself but on the status of user involvement as such.

On the other hand, service user involvement in the process has not been without problems. Two service users were initially invited onto the Richardson Committee but rapidly disinvited when they declared in public that they opposed the introduction of Community Treatment Orders. There is anecdotal evidence that some activists involved in the Mental Health Alliance felt their voice was not being listened to. It is possible, once again, that the more radical voices were not easily heard or accommodated.

What is clear is that, overall, the Mental Health Act 2007 has taken services in a direction contrary to that desired by most of the service user movement. They have campaigned continuously since the 1980s for no extension of compulsory powers, and have opposed successive attempts to introduce community treatment orders. Although, it is true that service users have been more involved in the debate and that their contribution may have heightened awareness of the negative implications of compulsion, in the end more compulsion is what has become enshrined in law. In the final analysis, the Mental Health Act 2007 can only be seen as a defeat for service user action. This is illustrated by the Care Quality Commission having to 'apologise' for delays in processing Community Treatment Orders because the expected number of cases of 200 patients in the first phase turned out to be 2,868 instead.

STIGMA AND DISCRIMINATION

The issue of stigma in mental health has a long history. Goffman (1986) described persons with a 'spoiled identity' who were 'discredited' by society and in this he included people with mental health problems. Falk (2001) describes people with mental health problems as carrying the 'ultimate stigma' eliciting more disapprobation from society than any other group.

From the point of view of service users the work of the sociologist Scheff is notable (1966). He proposed that many instances of 'mental illness' were in fact the *effects* of being labelled as such, due to an individual behaving in a way that did not adhere to societal rules and that these effects could be the source of stigma and discrimination. The influence of Scheff's work was subject to much critique but lately it has been reinstated (Corrigan, et al., 2003; Hayward and Bright, 1997). Link and Phelan (2001) also argue that concepts of stigma must include the effect of power and structural discrimination.

A further development in the literature is that of the concept of 'self-stigma' (Link and Phelan, 2001). This approach argues that those with a diagnosis of mental illness internalize stigma and that this leads to hopelessness, low self-esteem and low self-worth. This idea has shortcomings. It portrays people with a mental illness diagnosis as helpless and as objects of pity. The argument that people with a diagnosis do not disclose their condition because they feel ashamed further intensifies this portrayal.

An alternative perspective is provided by the idea of 'anticipated discrimination' (Rose and Thornicroft, 2010). This concept suggests that those with a diagnosis of mental illness stop themselves from participating in social life because they anticipate discrimination. This is the reason why many do not disclose. Whilst avoiding some of the negative overtones of the concept of 'self-stigma' this argument retains the idea of passivity. It might rather be argued that non-disclosure is for some a positive choice made in clear conscience in order to avoid unpleasant situations and to preserve integrity.

Although service users have long been aware of discrimination as an important barrier in their lives, activists have until fairly recently focused more on issues within services than in society as a whole. It is notable that the service user movement played only a small part in the Rights Now campaign leading up to the Disability Discrimination Act, focusing instead on the Mental Health Act as the piece of legislation that had a prime influence on their lives. But the situation is changing now. Whereas in the 1980s, activists could be heard saying the response of services to their distress was the biggest problem they faced, in the last decade, discrimination has come to be identified in such a way.

Service users have identified the media as a potent carrier of stigma and discrimination. Representations of service users as violent and unpredictable are argued to contribute to negative public views of those with a mental illness diagnosis. The English Department of Health has a unit called Shift which was set up to try to reduce stigma and discrimination against those with a mental illness diagnosis and they conduct an analysis of the written press every year. Positive representations are virtually absent (Callard et al., 2008).

Service users have worked with the organization Mental Health Media. One of the activities of this group was to set up a 'Speakers Bureau' whereby the press and broadcast media could have direct access to the experience of those with a mental illness diagnosis. This initiative has not been formally evaluated but those involved see it positively. Mental Health Media extended their activities with a project called 'Open Up' which trained service users in anti-discrimination tactics, at the same time continuing the focus on media interventions. Open Up is due to be evaluated as part of the Time to Change campaign (see below).

It is not just the public who hold stigmatizing attitudes. More subtly, psychiatrists and mental health services can themselves contribute to stigma. The process of diagnosis can itself be seen as discriminatory. Although some people, on receiving a diagnostic label feel relieved, many others reject or deny it and see it as pernicious (Rose and Thornicroft, 2010). Diagnosis is critical as it marks the point when a service user formally enters the psychiatric system. Other ways that psychiatry may contribute to stigma and discrimination include secrecy concerning people's condition and treatment and straightforward advice that a person should avoid normal activities in case it leads to a relapse.

There has been an exponential rise in literature on stigma and discrimination recently and also a burgeoning of campaigns across the world. As we write, Time to Change has been launched in England funded for nearly £20 million by the Big Lottery Fund and Comic Relief. It includes a Lived Experience Advisory Panel (LEAP) but there have been resignations particularly around issues for people from Black and Minority Ethnic Groups. Time to Change contains a 'social marketing' strand, using posters, films and the like. This has not commended itself to all service users. One part of this campaign was the installation of 'padded cells' in a transport system in a Northern city apparently designed to show that 'we can all go to work together'. As one service user pointed out, this is deeply offensive when it is noted that 11,500 service users a year are locked in police cells waiting for a Mental Health Act assessment and that seclusion is routinely used in many psychiatric hospitals. It remains to be seen how effective the LEAP will be in this campaign.

RECOVERY

During the last decade there has been increasing enthusiasm among many service providers and service users for Recovery. Recovery comes in a number of guises and this can affect analysis of how positive a development it really is. Recovery can be a unique personal journey that 'involves the development of new meaning and purpose in one's life as one grows beyond the catastrophic effects of mental illness …' (Anthony, 1993). It can be a vision or mission statement. It can be a series of principles or a new approach to the delivery of care, treatment and support. In this later guise, it can be moulded into a number of competencies for good recovery practice.

Much has been made of the fact that Recovery seems to have emerged from the grassroots of the service user/survivor movement in North America and in New Zealand. This has been cited as evidence that it is a particularly 'user-friendly' development. It is much harder to see the development of Recovery in the United Kingdom as an example of a grassroots initiative, so swiftly has it been taken up by the mental health establishment (Slade, 2009). Yet, in its ideal form, it does encapsulate some of the important beliefs and desires expressed by the service user movement in this country over the last quarter of a century.

A recovery approach is a hopeful one that believes people with a mental illness diagnosis can come to terms with their difficulties and live a meaningful life. It puts the service user at the centre of action and pays proper attention to the resources and expertise of the individual. It recognizes that mental health professionals do not hold all the answers and that service users can obtain assistance from non-professionals, including fellow service users. Recovery puts a high value on collaboration as equals and on openness. In all these ways, Recovery can be seen as making a constructive response to some of the key demands of service user activists in the United Kingdom and elsewhere.

Despite this, it is becoming clear that support for Recovery among service user activists is by no means unanimous (Mind, 2008). This is partly due to the perception that service users do not have ownership of Recovery and that the way it is being developed, particularly in England, shows signs of a top-down approach. But there are other objections being raised. A recovery approach places higher expectations on service users. While this is frequently welcomed, a substantial number of service users feel they are being pushed forward too quickly and are having vital supports taken away from them. In some areas, adoption of Recovery has been accompanied by cuts to services and seen as problematic for that reason. It is not clear what will happen to those who cannot live up to the blossoming number of recovery outcomes. The fact that each person should be allowed and encouraged to set out their own goals and outcomes is respected in principle but endangered by the ongoing search for key stages of recovery and lists of desired outcomes.

One particular difficulty is the apparent linking of recovery to the ability to hold down a paid job and the fear both that more service users will be cajoled into unfulfilling employment and that those who do not or cannot follow them will be seen as 'unrecovered' and inferior. At the same time a recovery approach often seems to overlook the very real structural disadvantages service users face in their lives. Emphasizing the capacity and self-responsibility of service users to recover can misread exactly what service users are recovering from. The 'catastrophic effects of mental illness' mentioned above, perhaps. But also the damage inflicted by mental health services obsessed by treatment compliance and adept at manipulating service users in the name of collaboration. While Recovery certainly places services users at the centre of things, they continue to face multiple disempowerments and may not have yet won significantly greater control of their destinies. In this respect, Recovery may fall a good dealt short of the 'paradigm shift' some have claimed for it.

CONCLUSION

Assessing the success or failure of service user action is not an easy task. Much action has taken place at a local level and has resulted in small scale changes that have not been well documented. At the same time, there have been different ideas about just what service user action is trying to change. What is desirable and what is realistically possible? While some activists have been looking for quite radical changes to services or the creation of alternatives to them, others seem to be happy with incremental improvements. It is possible that the latter have more to feel pleased about than the former.

After 30 years, it now appears unlikely that government and service providers will easily turn their backs on service users and renege on their commitment to service user involvement. Involvement is here to stay, though whether it requires a service user movement of independent action groups to provide it is a somewhat different matter. It is by no means clear that the mental health establishment is much concerned about exactly how the service user involvement they desire is actually delivered. As time goes on, involvement provided by voluntary organizations that are not service user-led may appear just as fit for purpose as involvement provided by local service user-led groups. Although the service user movement has been successful enough in delivering involvement to suggest that it has now achieved a degree of permanence, its exact shape could evolve significantly in the future.

A more urgent question relates to just what service user involvement has actually achieved in changing services or in empowering service users. This chapter has shown a story of mixed success. Many of the more radical demands of service user activists have clearly not been met. In England we have services that are still heavily dependent on medication, where choice is limited and the percentage of involuntary admissions is rising. Widespread demands for non-medical crisis services have had poor results. Black and minority ethnic groups continue to receive a raw deal. In all these respects, mental health services seem to be evolving in ways that are directly opposite to the direction of progress many service user activists are fighting for. When services do start to change, it happens at a slow pace and always according to agendas other than those of service users. It has taken 30 years for the grassroots demand for more talking and listening to lead to coherent action and then it is met by the wholesale provision of Cognitive Behavioural Therapy in the form of the initiative Increasing Access to Psychological Therapy which has the explicit goal of getting people back to work and reducing the welfare benefits bill. A more sensitive and differentiated response is absent. Overall, it is probably accurate to conclude that the views and opinions of the service user activists are rarely in themselves enough to achieve change. If partnerships exist, service users remain very much the junior partner.

Casual use of the term 'empowerment' has been a bugbear of the mental health scene in recent years. Nevertheless, if empowerment is taken to mean having control over the significant aspects of your life, it seems fair to conclude that the majority of service users are not empowered. Involvement in services may have increased influence. It has not, generally speaking, enabled power to be grasped. Beyond services, most service users are disempowered, living lives encumbered by poverty and significant social exclusion. The service user movement has by and large not chosen to, or not been able to, address this wider dimension and has focused on the inadequacies of mental health services. The great challenge for the movement is how to take on the task of combating social exclusion while at the same time continuing to address the problematic predicaments of service users within services. In both these areas, a key concern will remain how to make involvement a truly effective agent of change.

REFERENCES

Anthony, W. A. (1993) Recovery from mental illness: the guiding vision of the mental health system in the 1990s. *Innovations and Research*, 2: 17–24.

Beresford, P. (2003) *It's Our Lives: A Short Theory of Knowledge, Distance and Experience.* London: Citizen Press in association with Shaping Our Lives.

Campbell, P. (2008) The service user/survivor movement. In J. Reynolds, R. Muston, T. Heller, J. Leach, M. McCormick, J. Wallcraft and M. Walsh (eds) *Mental Health Still Matters.* Basingstoke: Palgrave Macmillan. pp 46–52.

Corrigan, P. W., Markowitz, F. E., Watson, A., Rowan, D. and Kubiak, M. A. (2003) An attribution model of public discrimination towards persons with mental illness. *Journal of Health Social Behaviour*, 44: 162–179.

Callard, F. Thornicroft, G. and Rose, D. (2008) *Mind over Matter 2.* London: Shift.

Crossley, N. (2006) *Contesting Psychiatry: Social Movements in Mental Health.* Abingdon: Routledge.

Department of Health (1990) *NHS and Community Care Act.* London: The Stationery Office.

Department of Health (1999) *A National Service Framework for Mental Health.* London: The Stationery Office.

Faulkner, A. and Layzell (2001) *A Strategies for Living.* London: Mental Health Foundation.

Good Practices in Mental Health/Camden Consortium (1988) *Treated Well: A Code of Practice for Psychiatric Hospitals.* London: GPMH.

Health care commission performance ratings (2005) http://ratings2005.healthcarecommission.org.uk/Search/SearchResults.asp?TrustType=MH (accessed 1 December, 2009).

Falk, G. (2001) *Stigma: How We Treat Outsiders.* New York: Prometheus Books.

Goffman, E. (1986) *Stigma: Notes on the Management of Spoiled Identity.* Touchstone.

Gummer, T. and Furney, S. (1998) The business of listening. *Health Management*, 2(3): 12–13.

Hayward, P. and Bright, J. A. (1997) Stigma and mental illness: a review and critique. *Journal of Mental Health*, 6(4): 345–354.

Keown, P., Mercer, G. and Scott, J. (2008) Retrospective analysis of hospital episode statistics, involuntary admissions under the Mental Health Act 1983, and number of psychiatric beds in England 1996–2006. *BMJ*, 337: a1837.

Kotecha, N., Fowler, C., Donskoy, A-L., Johnson, P., Shaw, T. and Doherty, K. (2007). *A Guide to User Focused Monitoring: Setting Up and Running a Project.* London: The Sainsbury Centre for Mental Health.

Link, B. G. and Phelan, J. C. (2001) Conceptualizing stigma. *Annual Review of Sociology,* 27: 363–385.

MindThink Report 3 (2008) *Life and Times of a Supermodel: The Recovery Paradigm for Mental Health.* London: Mind.

Nicholls, V., Wright, S., Waters, R. and Wells, S. (2003) *Surviving User-led Research: Reflections on Supporting User-led Research Projects.* London: Mental Health Foundation.

Pilgrim, D. (2005) *Key Concepts in Mental Health.* London: SAGE.

Rose, D. (2009) Survivor produced knowledge. In A., Sweeney, P., Beresford, A., Faulkner, M., Nettle and D. Rose (eds) *This is Survivor Research.* Ross-on-Wye: PPCS Books.

Rose, D., Wykes, T., Leese, M., Bindman, J. and Fleischmann, P. (2003) Patients' perspectives on electroconvulsive therapy: systematic review. *BMJ,* 326: 1363–136.

Rose, D., Wykes, T., Bindman, J. and Fleischmann, P. (2005) Information, consent and perceived coercion: Consumers' views on ECT. *British Journal of Psychiatry,* 186: 54–59.

Rose, D and Thornicroft, G. (2010) Service users perspectives on the impact of mental illness diagnosis. *Epidemiologica Psychiatrica Sociale* 19(2): 140–147.

Scheff, T. J. (1966) *Being Mentally Ill: A Sociological Theory.* Chicago, Illinois: Aldine.

Slade, M. (2009) *Personal Recovery and Mental Illness: a Guide for Mental Health Professionals.* Cambridge: Cambridge University Press.

Sweeney, A., Beresford, P., Faulkner, A., Nettle, M. and Rose, D. (2009) *This is Survivor Research.* Ross-on-Wye: PPCS Books.

Szmukler, G., Daw, R. and Dawson, J. (in press) A model law fusing incapacity and mental health legislation. *Special Issue of Journal of Mental Health Law.*

UKAN (2001) *A Clear Voice, a Clear Vision: an Advocacy Reader.* Sheffield: UKAN.

UKAN (2004) *Advocacy Today and Tomorrow – UKAN Training Tool.* Sheffield: UKAN.

Wallcraft, J., Read, J. and Sweeney, S. (2002) *On Our Own Terms.* London: The Sainsbury Centre for Mental Health.

Wood, P. (2003) *Advocacy Standards: Standards for Advocacy in Mental Health.* Sheffield: UKAN.

23

Recovery in Mental Illness: The Roots, Meanings, and Implementations of a "New" Services Movement

Ann McCranie

The history of the care and treatment of the mentally ill in America for almost four centuries offers a sobering example of a cyclical pattern that has alternated between enthusiastic optimism and fatalistic pessimism. (Gerald Grob, 1997, *The Mad Among Us*, pp. 309)

INTRODUCTION

Moral treatment, moral hygiene, asylums, psycho-pharmaceuticals, community mental health, and community support: all have been heralded as positive new directions for the treatment of severe and chronic mental illness. But the reality of all of these models has fallen short of providing a permanent solution or even the ideal support for treatment. Some have come to be seen in the long run as actually harmful with people with serious mental illness. It was against this backdrop of unsatisfactory, incremental, and unintentional consequences – what Frank and Glied (2006) called "better but not well" in the US context – that the movement of "recovery" has taken root modern mental health services.

"Recovery" for in the field of mental health services is actually a complex of ideas – but I propose it can be understood most simply as *hope* that someone, particularly someone in the throes of suffering acutely from a serious and persistent mental health problem, can reclaim their life or create a newly meaningful one. "Recovery-oriented" systems of care, then, are those that help rather than hinder that individual in their "recovery." But admittedly, that broad brush fails to captures what the range of meanings that "recovery" in the context of mental illness means and has meant to different actors – individuals with mental illness, family members, service providers, and policy makers – over time. Hopper offers another start: "If a provisional consensus may be hazarded, it would read something like this: recovery is difficult, idiosyncratic, and requires *faith* – but it is possible" (2007: 870, emphasis added).

But how do concepts such as "hope" and "faith" fare in a mental health service system? How do these concepts become embodied in the interaction between provider and individual? How do those concepts become institutionalized and embedded in a system of care marked with disappointment, lack of resources, disorganization, and invisibility? What happens if these terms and movements are co-opted or fail to take root? And what if Grob's historical view of the pendulum swings from enthusiastic optimism to fatalistic pessimism proves prophetic – and this is just the moment before the plunge?

The impact of major reform movements in mental health services, such as deinstitutionalization (Brown, 1985; Jones, 1993), community care in Britain (Rogers and Pilgrim, 2001) and the even the serendipitous origins of psychopharmacology (Healy, 2002) reveal that shifts in treatment can have profound effects at individual, family, institutional, and state levels. The movement toward "recovery" and "recovery-oriented services" has already had some impact on the direction of recent mental health policy in the United States (Department of Health and Human Services, 2003) and England (Department of Health, 2001, 2004) and research (Lieberman et al., 2008). The challenge this concept "recovery" presents to individuals to understand serious mental illness differently is one important matter, but so too is the challenge the idea's promotion has had on individual and organizational practices and structures of care in a changing fiscal, policy, and scientific environment.

The focus of this chapter is on the organizational field of mental health services. The purpose is not to define "recovery" – as many have attempted this already and the definition continues to change and be debated (Bellack, 2006; Davidson and Roe, 2007; Hopper, 2007; Jacobson and Greenley, 2001; National Consensus Conference on Mental Health Recovery and Mental Health Systems Transformation, 2004; Noordsy et al., 2002; Onken et al., 2007). Instead, it is to argue that recovery is a concept and movement in modern mental health services. To that end, this chapter will present a brief history of the concept in the mental health services field, including a set of key (but not uncontested) definitions for recovery. It will also highlight the critiques, largely from within the movement and offer a brief description of the diffusion of recovery-oriented services and some of the most relevant social science research on recovery.

Whether recovery is truly the "guiding vision" (Anthony, 1993), the "heart and soul of treatment" (Townsend and Glasser, 2003), "old wine in new bottles" (Davidson et al., 2005; Pilgrim, 2008), or it is just another pendulum swing up to the "enthusiastic optimism" that Grob (1997) warned about, the concept's diffusion throughout the field marks an important moment in modern mental health services. This movement has different implications for the different cultural and material environments it enters. While this chapter focuses on the US context, it will also briefly discuss how the concept of recovery has been received in several other contexts, such as the United Kingdom and Australia.

A BRIEF HISTORY OF "RECOVERY" IN THE MENTAL HEALTH SERVICES FIELD

There is nothing new about the term "recovery" for people with mental illness. The term has been used for many years to refer to a remission or reduction of symptoms. In 1937, Abraham Low, a psychiatrist working in state mental hospitals in Illinois founded a group called "Recovery, Inc." devoted to structured self-help groups to provide "after-care" for recently discharged hospital patients. Recovery, Inc. focused on reducing "relapses," through social coping skills, goal-setting, and increasing self-confidence. While Low's original organization failed to gain acceptance in the larger research and treatment community and was dissolved, it was reborn as a peer-led group model (Low, [1991] 1943) that still exists today.

However, the roots of a concept of recovery – if not the term – have been traced back to over 200 years ago to Philippe Pinel and his *traitement moral* in Paris asylums (Davidson et al., 2010). And certainly the concept of recovery is familiar from the field of addictions treatment (Davidson and White, 2007). Yet, at some points in recent history, recovery was, for some seen as impossible. In the case of schizophrenia, even the clinical definition asserted a declining course and a permanent state of illness – such as in Emil Kraepelin criteria for "dementia praecox." Remission or recovery was seen as *prima fascia* evidence that the illness had not been dementia praecox. Eugen Bleuler, who challenged this diagnosis and renamed this condition "schizophrenia" in part to remove the connotation with dementia, also challenged the chronicity of the problems, recognizing that people diagnosed with it could get better.

This early dispute is often cited in the literature about recovery (Bellack, 2006; Corrigan et al., 1999; Jacobson, 2004; Lieberman et al., 2008). In addition, several longitudinal studies of the outcomes of individuals who had been institutionalized or diagnosed with schizophrenia suggested that a large percentage, perhaps a large majority, of individuals were improved after a period of time, particularly in the area of remission of symptoms (Bleuler, 1974; Harding et al., 1987;

Jacobson, 2004; Lieberman et al., 2008; Tsuang et al., 1979). The concept of recovery in mental health services is often less concrete and posits a more expansive view of the possibilities for individuals than the outcomes investigated in these studies (e.g., symptom reduction, decreased medication usage, living independently, working, etc.). However, as studies showed evidence that improved quality of life in some key life domains was possible, they provided an "evidence base" of recovery and had a particular meaning to researchers who sought to promote the ideological concept (Jacobson, 2004).

In one of the first and most cited articles about recovery, clinical psychologist, and advocate Patricia Deegan (1988) wrote a first person account of her illness and recovery experience and argued that recovery is different from psychosocial (or psychiatric) rehabilitation. Rehabilitation, she argued, is about services and technologies, but "recovery refers to the lived or real experiences of persons as they accept and overcome the challenge of the disability" (1988: 7). Early first person accounts had a strong influence on the direction researchers went with their recovery writing and pushed beyond the traditional concepts of symptom reduction, independent living, treatment utilization, and employment that were hallmarks of psychiatric outcomes work.

Themes that emerge from Deegan's work, and that three other notable first person accounts of recovery from mental illness – Marcia Lovejoy (1982), Esso Leete (1989), and Rae Unzicker (1989) – include hope, acceptance, engagement in social life, active coping, and reclaiming a positive sense of self (Ridgway, 2001). First person accounts such as these became the basis for establishing a definition of recovery, and even now comprise a large basis of research for recovery researchers and for seeing recovery as a unique "journey" into finding purpose in one's life (Davidson, 2003; Deegan, 2003; Mead and Copeland, 2000; Ridgway, 2001; Roe and Lachman, 2005; Wisdom et al., 2008).

It would not be long before researchers and providers were also promoting the concept of recovery. After publishing a short piece addressing the topic in 1991, William Anthony, a psychologist and director of the Boston University Center for Psychiatric Rehabilitation, returned to the topic wrote the recovery "call to arms" in the mental health services literature (1993). In this he outlined both the "vision" of recovery that would guide services in the years to come and what a recovery-oriented system would look like. Recovery is:

> a deeply personal, unique process of changing one's attitudes, values, feelings, goals, skills, and/or roles. It is a way of living a satisfying, hopeful, and contributing life even with limitations caused by illness. Recovery involves the development of new meaning and purpose in one's life as one grows beyond the catastrophic effects of mental illness. (1993: 527)

Anthony asserts that "(r)ecovery is what people with disabilities do … Recovery is a truly unifying human experience" (1993: 527–528). Recovery, according to Anthony, is multi-dimensional, defying simplistic measurement. However, he laid out a set of assumptions to which providers in a recovery-oriented system of care should adhere: recovery happens with or without treatment; it requires social support; it is independent of etiological beliefs about illness; and it can continue even if symptoms re-occur (i.e., recovery being a "non-linear process"). For Anthony, recovery is unique to each person, requires that the person have choices about their situation, and must also take place in a social context in which recovery from the consequences of the illness (such as stigma) can be harder to overcome than the mental health problem. Recovery-oriented services would not just rely on more traditional activities such as treatment, crisis intervention, case management, and rehabilitation, but would also seek to enrich lives, protect rights, and enable basic support and self-help.

Anthony's work is still highly cited, even though the effort to find a commonly accepted definition of recovery has so far been elusive, even by those quite motivated to promote and carry it out in services (e.g., Clay et al., 2005; Davidson et al., 2005). Several comprehensive reviews and proposed reformulations have been attempted (Bellack, 2006; Corrigan and Ralph, 2005; Jacobson, 2001; Jacobson and Greenley, 2001; Lunt, 2002; Noordsy et al., 2002; Onken et al., 2007; Ralph, 2000; Roe et al., 2007). But there is broad agreement among those who study recovery is that the notion is subject to much "confusion, dialogue, and debate" (Davidson et al., 2006: 6) and that "(l)ike mental illness itself, the notion of recovery represents a multidimensional set of phenomena which may share nothing more than a Wittgensteinian sense of 'family resemblance'" (Davidson and Roe, 2007: 460).

Two often cited distinctions that appear in the literature are "recovery in" vs. "recovery from" (Davidson and Roe, 2007) or to internal vs. external processes in recovery (Jacobson and Greenley, 2001). Davidson and Roe distinguish between the meaning of recovery "from" mental illness as a more symptom-based remission type of return to function, whereas recovery "in" mental illness can refer to moving ahead with life even as symptoms persist and functions are not returned. Jacobson and Greenley (2001) refer to the "internal" components of recovery, such as hope, attitudes, experiences and processes of individual change, whereas "external" conditions – such as material circumstances, services, policies, practices, can aid or hinder the process. These themes are echoed again and again as researchers attempt to clarify the meaning of recovery.

Recovery in the United States

In the United States, the banner of recovery was seen as an opportunity for common ground for individuals with mental illness and providers (Frese, 1998). It was lauded as a goal for individuals and for systems in the 1999 Surgeon General's Report (Department of Health and Human Services, 1999). Two of the more influential recent definitions came from high profile public reports on the "transformation" of the mental health systems, one from President George W. Bush's New Freedom Commission on Mental Health (New Freedom Commission on Mental Health, 2003) and the other from the Substance Abuse and Mental Health Services Administration (SAMHSA)'s National Consensus

Statement (2004). In the New Freedom Commission report, recovery was a central organizing concept:

> Recovery refers to the process in which people are able to live, work, learn, and participate fully in their communities. For some individuals, recovery is the ability to live a fulfilling and productive life despite a disability. For others, recovery implies the reduction or complete remission of symptoms. Science has shown that having hope plays an integral role in an individual's recovery. (2003: 5)

Shortly after, the US Substance Abuse and Mental Health Services Administration (SAMHSA) produced a "consensus statement" that defined recovery as "a journey of healing and transformation enabling a person with a mental health problem to live a meaningful life in a community of his or her choice while striving to achieve his or her full potential." The consensus was reached after a series of reports and paper on topics surrounding recovery was commissioned and over 100 stakeholders in mental health service providers – individuals with mental illness, family members, academic researchers, providers, government officials, etc. – worked to find agreement on the meaning. The consensus statement also identifies ten "dimensions" of recovery: self-direction, individualized and person-centred, empowerment, holism, non-linearity, strengths-based, peer support, respect, responsibility, and finally, hope (National Consensus Conference on Mental Health Recovery and Mental Health Systems Transformation, 2004).

Critiquing the concept of recovery

Even among supporters for the concept of "recovery" in the mental health services field, some have pointed out that studying recovery is a problem for scientists because it can become overly broad and meaningless (Roe et al., 2007). While arguing for understanding that would draw from economist and philosopher Amartya Sen's capabilities approach, Hopper described the current state of affairs of the concept of recovery a "co-opted, near-toothless gospel of hope" (2007: 877). He noted the lack of contentiousness about the varied meanings reflect "working misunderstandings" of the meanings and values attached to the concept (2008: 307). Pilgrim (2008, 2009) makes a similar argument about the "polyvalent concept" of recovery and argues that ethnographic study of the concept is needed to untangle meanings and enactments lest these misunderstandings continue. Others have argued recovery could be in some instances a veiled attempt to further cut services or to leave behind those in most need in the name of reaching an elusive goal (Dickerson, 2006; Johnson, 2005). Peyser (2001) warned that it could actually harm individuals by interfering with treatment goals of symptom reduction. As the call for recovery-oriented services was (and still is) happening alongside managed care reforms and calls for the "transformation" of US mental health services, Jacobson and Curtis (2000) note that recovery could be co-opted as a concept and left without content.

The moving target of the definition, coupled with the difficulty of pinning down concepts as "hope" and "unique processes," have led to frustration and scepticism and some suggestion that recovery ought to be rooted in "objectively measureable" functional criteria focused on symptom reduction and remission (Bellack, 2006; Liberman et al., 2002; Roe et al., 2007). This is a direct challenge to the view that recovery is not about symptoms or functional improvement. However, the focus on functional remission may serve as a *de facto* answer for researchers frustrated with concepts too difficult to operationalize. Liberman and Kopelowicz (2005), for instance distinguishes between the "process" and "outcome" of recovery. A recent special issue of *Schizophrenia Bulletin* (see Essock and Sederer, 2009) published a series of seven reports on measurement of "functional recovery." The focus of this "functional recovery" that it is focused more on an individual's ability to be able to perform daily activities (such as self-care and work) and be integrated into social life.

Leiberman et al. (2008) suggests that in order for it to be a useful heuristic, recovery should be qualified with the domain of life in which it is achieved – such as "recovery of vocational function" or "recovery of cognitive function." This account of a way to pull together neuroscience and psychiatry with the recovery movement allows the focus to stay on more traditional issues of symptomatology and "acknowledges" but does not address the other issues of living so close to the recovery movement: "civil rights, stigma, housing, vocational opportunities, and other community issues" (Leiberman et al., 2008: 488). Some within the movement have also argued that recovery as a term suggests going or looking back to a previous, perhaps mythical "state of health," whereas the true goal should be moving forward. Advocate Kathleen Crowley has termed this idea "Procovery" (Crowley, 2000) and has developed a set of trainings for providers and individuals and "Procovery Circles" that function like peer-led support groups.

But the component parts of recovery remain difficult to measure. An effort by European researchers to review the literature for the use of the concept of "hope" found 49 different definitions and 32 different measurement tools (Schrank et al., 2008). In an era of increased interest and demand for evidence-based practices in mental health services, some have questioned (Browne, 2006) whether recovery can be even be appropriately tied to outcomes, while others have said that it can and should be done (Anthony et al., 2003; Frese et al., 2001). Tanenbaum (2006) identifies the tensions between the tenets of evidence-base practice (EBP), so heavily dependent on randomized control trials and experimental methods and aggregate results, and the tenets of recovery, so focused on individualized and self-determining recovery goals. In short, she argues that recovery demands a new standard for EBP studies, one that involves individuals with mental illness in the meaning making of research framing and interpretation.

It is important to note *where* in the mental health services literature rigorous discussion has been taking place. Discussion and disagreements about the meaning of recovery in the psychiatric/psychosocial rehabilitation and community mental health journals have been answered with a more muted critique – even silence – from the larger clinical psychiatric and psychological community. For instance, a recent working group of prominent psychiatrists and neuroscientists considered criteria for remission of schizophrenia and came up with some significant changes, but explicitly avoided engaging the criteria for recovery, as the concept is underspecified and reflects "ongoing multidisciplinary efforts seeking to incorporate the viewpoints of patients, caregivers, and clinicians, as well as an evolving appreciation for the relationship between improvements in symptoms, cognition, and functionality" (Andreasen et al., 2005: 442). The relatively supportive language about the potential for recovery as a concept – if only it can be more clearly specified – belies a larger silence by some of the most prominent journals in the fields of clinical psychiatry (such as the *Archives of General Psychiatry*, *Journal of Clinical Psychiatry*, and the *American Journal of Psychiatry*) or clinical psychology (such as *Psychological Medicine*, or the influential *Annual Review of Psychology* or *Annual Review of Clinical Psychology*) about anything other than a functional recovery outcome measure (far more akin to a remission paradigm). One exception to this is the *British Journal of Psychiatry*, which has published a number of pieces taking the issue head-on (Dickens, 2009; Dinniss, 2006; Lester and Gask, 2006), perhaps reflecting a different national response to the concept (discussed more below). In the United States, academic discussion has been largely relegated to journals that are focused on services research (*Psychiatric Services, Journal of Psychiatric Rehabilitation,* and *Community Mental Health Journal*) and the more narrowly focused journal, *Schizophrenia Bulletin* (which, not coincidentally, published some of those early first-person accounts (Leete, 1989; Lovejoy, 1982) that came to influence the concept's development.

As George Bernard Shaw wrote, "Silence is the most perfect expression of scorn" and this quiet could portend a larger battle for this community of service researchers to have the idea of recovery, with its messy multiple constituencies, recognized in larger academic circles. This silence in the broader community, after a 20-year history of writing high profile policy involvement, and the emergence of new treatment models, speaks volumes of the "fractiousness that has yet to face the fact" (Hopper, 2007: 307). Sociologists would do well to pay attention to these cleavages – as they reflect long-standing divisions in the treatment and research of mental illness within psychology and psychiatry – between medical and social understandings of illness.

MARCHING AHEAD: "RECOVERY-ORIENTED SERVICES" IN AN AGE OF "EVIDENCE-BASED PRACTICES"

As recovery has gained currency, so have efforts to tie specific models of treatment to it. Davidson defined recovery-oriented services as those that emphasize the shared decision making of individual and provider (Davidson et al., 2009). Psychosocial, or psychiatric, rehabilitation models, which emphasize goal setting, skill-building and community integration were a welcome home for recovery principles (Lamb, 1994; Stromwall and Hurdle, 2003; Taylor and

Yuen, 2008). One the field's leading journals, *Psychiatric Rehabilitation Journal*, (founded and edited by Anthony), has become central for publications on recovery. The connection between the field of rehabilitation and recovery is an early one with Anthony's involvement and Deegan's warning in 1988 that rehabilitation was not synonymous with a recovery-oriented approach. The United States Psychiatric Rehabilitation Association, the field's professional certification organization, has adopted recovery language in its mission statement and recovery-oriented services as a center point in its training efforts.

The concept of recovery has focused on new individual service models, practices, types of actors, and the interaction between care providers and those they work with. Simultaneously, there has been an interest in developing and implementing evidence-based practices (analogous to the evidence-based medicine movement in general health research). How to square the goals of evidence-based practices with the more subjective terms of recovery has been the subject of much discussion (Anthony et al., 2003; Bellack, 2006; Farkas et al., 2005; Fisher and Ahern, 2002; O'Connor and Delaney, 2007; Tanenbaum, 2006). Frese et al. (2001) suggests that recovery-based models of treatment (those that emphasize more choice, empowerment, and regaining control of one's life) would be more appropriate when the individual is experiencing less severe symptoms of illness and is not as highly impaired in their decision-making ability. A more evidence-based medical model approach could be appropriate when individuals are more impaired. Frese et al. points out that among activists, support for "recovery-oriented services" vs. "evidence-based practices" varies along a continuum of severity of illness for which the activists advocate. This illustrates a tension between functional remission (recovery "from") and personal journeys of recovery (recovery "in").

One identified evidence-based practice that is explicitly tied to recovery movement and stresses empowerment of individuals is "Illness Management and Recovery" (Mueser et al., 2002; Roe et al., 2009). Illness Management and Recovery is a structured program for providers that encourages them to work in concert with individual consumers/users to plan for and pursue individual goals. It stresses educating individuals about mental illness, about the "stress vulnerability model" and how to reduce their chances of stressful circumstances that could lead to relapse. Individuals are also walked through steps to build their own social support networks, counselled about their medication use, and to navigate the mental health system.

Deegan, in attempting to address some of the problems that individuals face when they talk to their providers about their medication use, has introduced "CommonGround" (Deegan et al., 2008). This model offers a web-based software package to help individuals talk more openly about their psychotropic (and other) medication usage with their doctors. An individual would use CommonGround, which asks questions about usage, side effects, and other issues involving medication, before seeing their provider. They would also be prompted to share information with their doctor about their "personal medicine,"

(Deegan, 2005) or non-pharmaceutical techniques, like walking or gardening, they use to gain relief from their problems. This intervention, still in the pilot stage, is one of many efforts to foster collaboration between individuals and their providers and to provide a more "recovery-oriented" approach to care.

But the recovery movement has also advanced the creation of a new category of professional caregivers – that offered by peers who also have mental illness who then are trained to work with others (Clay et al., 2005; Corrigan et al., 2005). Peer support is nothing particularly new – recall Low's reliance on peers in the late 1930s for his Recovery, Inc. and the emphasis on peer-run support programs such as clubhouses and advocacy organizations (Clay et al., 2005). But, the new emphasis on training and certifying peers ("Peer Recovery Support Specialists") to provide mental health services to other individuals, has added a new professional category for individuals with mental illness (or their family members). Special certification programs (at the Institute for Recovery and Community Integration, for instance), special billing codes for services, and a national professional organization (the National Association of Peer Specialists, Inc.) have developed. Certification as a peer specialist depends on an individual's identity as someone diagnosed with a mental illness, but other identity-based professional statuses are available. In Florida, for instance, certification is available as a "peer," as a "family peer" and as both.

One of the motivations behind peer support as recovery-oriented services hearkens back to advocate demands for more involvement in the treatment system by individuals affected with mental illness. But there is also Deegan's concept of the contagiousness of hope (1988) – that by modeling recovery, peers can provide inspiration to others to pursue their own goals.

CONCORDANCE AND CONTRASTS: RECOVERY IN NON-US CONTEXTS

The discussion above is not to suggest that recovery is a conceptual product or discovery of the United States (indeed, international scholars are engaged in discussions with US scholars cited above). The concept of recovery has a much longer history, crossing many eras and national borders (Davidson et al., 2010). It is perhaps more appropriate to talk about the "rediscovery" of recovery (Ramon et al., 2007). But as others have noted (Allott and Loganathan 2002; Ramon et al., 2007), the influence of some US (and New Zealand) researchers and policy makers has been felt in the United Kingdom, particularly through policy documents, such as those from the Ohio Department of Mental Health, and through specific recovery approaches, such as the Wellness Action Recovery Plan (Copeland, 1997[2002]).

However, the modern recovery movement met a somewhat different set of circumstances when it began to be recognized and written about in the UK. It meshed with the political agenda of "social inclusion" in welfare policies since

New Labour came to power in 1997 (Ramon et al., 2007) and with a more general focus on lay-lead self-management of chronic physical and mental conditions (Davidson et al., 2005). The meaning of that social inclusion rhetoric has been questioned by some (Pilgrim, 2008; Rogers and Pilgrim, 2001), as they note the concurrent fascination with "risk management" of individuals with mental illness. While social inclusion is a clearly stated goal of many US policy documents, it is clearly not a central focus of most recovery work – which is far more focused on individuals. Appealing to Amartya Sen, some US researchers (Hopper, 2007; Ware et al., 2008) have called for a reconceptualization of recovery from a capabilities approach and social model of disabilities approach – yet another example of the border-crossing of ideas.

Similar to the "transformation" effort of the United States, mental health services in the UK have also been the subject of a decade of concerted transformation efforts begun in 1999 called the National Services Framework. This framework, while ambitious and underfunded, has been focused largely on deinstitutionalization and a community support model (Department of Health, 2001; Sainsbury Center for Mental Health, 2003). Ramon et al. (2007) declare it a largely unimplemented process, with few clear guidelines for seeing it through. Throughout Britain and Ireland there are varying degrees of implementation. Ireland, for instance, has only recently begun to address recovery in policy documents (Kartalova-O'Doherty and Doherty, 2010), whereas Scotland has already developed and begun implementing its own recovery indicator tool – based on one developed in New York State – and has made a concerted effort to train peer recovery specialists (Scottish Recovery Network, 2005; Slade, 2009).

Australia, as Ramon et al. (2007) points out, might not have been using the term "recovery" in policy documents until 2003, when it was addressed as a core concept in the National Mental Health Service Plan. But as early as 1989, language that echoed central tenets in most recovery definitions – optimism for improvement and the importance of involving people with mental illness in their own treatment planning process – were central to Australian national policy. There, recovery oriented work is being pushed largely by consumer/service user groups, and is largely housed in a somewhat separate psychosocial rehabilitation system heavily influenced by consumers/service users. This stands outside the more "clinical" approach of most public mental health clinics (Ramon et al., 2007).

While Anglophone researchers and writers of recovery often refer and even import work from other national contexts, the conceptual flexibility can mean important differences are lost. This international diffusion of ideas and practices deserves attention.

CONSIDERING RECOVERY IN THE SOCIAL SCIENCES

Some sociologists have already begun addressing recovery and recovery-oriented services and the impact they could have on individuals and mental health systems.

Nora Jacobson's articles (Jacobson, 2001, 2003; Jacobson and Greenley, 2001) and book length treatment on recovery efforts in the state of Wisconsin (2004) is expansive in its scope and places recovery in the US federalist context. In an effort to understand the definition, process, and consequences of recovery in mental health services, she (2004) deconstructs the various usages of the term recovery and identifies five key meanings: evidence, experience, ideology, policy, and politics. These "recovery-as" meanings each operate at different levels and convey different meanings about what recovery is.

Jacobson parses the various definitions of recovery that mental health stakeholder draw upon. "Recovery-as-evidence" refers particularly to the growing understanding by mental health service researchers that individuals with serious mental illness could, and did, in fact get better over time and see a remission of symptoms. "Recovery-as-experience" drew meaning from the lived experiences and narratives of those with mental illness, and drew more from a political and social-disabilities based understanding of the individual embedded within a social context. "Recovery-as-ideology" drew from the two previous wells of meaning and crafted a new stream of research and writing about how providers and services ought to be organized to support recovery. "Recovery-as-policy" developed as policy-setting bodies (like state governments) tried to make sense of this new emphasis to translate it into policy and practice. "Recovery-as-politics" is the ongoing process of how to deal with the consequences of the movement in light of other realities, such as constricted finances, more calls for evidence-based practices, and peer involvement in the provision of treatment.

Jacobson (2004) poses seminal questions about the consequences of recovery: what will a recovery-oriented system looks like, who benefits, how it will be compatible with other system changes, and how its success or failure will be evaluated? Further, who will have the right to evaluate success? As she noted earlier (Jacobson and Curtis, 2000), the questions start as questions of epistemology and end with questions of policies and values.

Others find different sets of meanings and interest groups. Pilgrim (2008, 2009) cautions that recovery is a "polyvalent concept," and using Britain as a case study, finds it to have at least three distinct and sometimes contradictory meanings. In one, it refers to a notion that biomedical psychiatric biological recovery from illness is possible – a direct contradiction to the Kraepelin pessimism of a declining course. A second meaning, held by those providers offering a social skills or rehabilitation approach, takes another optimistic view of the course of illness from a different philosophy of treatment. A third, what Pilgrim refers to as the "dissenting service user" approach is a more social model of recovery, focused on empowerment and autonomy, sometimes in opposition to the oppressiveness of treatment regimes. These three meanings, all operating under the same banner of recovery, can be used simultaneously or individually, but can mask critical ontological positions and make meaningful policy consensus precarious or impossible.

Other sociologists have taken interest in recovery – particularly as an outcome. For instance, one groups of researchers (Link et al., 2001) have taken a sociological approach to understanding how stigma can impede recovery and found that experienced stigma impacts later self-esteem measures. Relatedly, Markovitz (2001) has approached recovery from the outcomes perspective, and has proposed a recovery model that incorporates symptoms, self-concept, and life satisfaction as all reciprocally related to one another in the lives of individuals with mental illness. Finding support in his work for both a social stress/social support argument that social circumstances contribute to illness and to medical/psychiatric view of symptoms causing social distress, Markovitz concludes that that treatment that incorporates both symptom management and social and vocation skills training are key to being "recovery-oriented."

Echoing (but not drawing from) Jacobson and Greenley's (2001) distinctions of "internal" vs. "external" conditions for recovery, Yanos et al. (2007) argue that sociologists understanding of both structure and agency can be enhanced by paying attention to the ways in which individual choices and constraints and collective action can reconfigure social structures and enhance or inhibit recovery for individuals. Individual actions, such as coping and goal-setting coupled with structural transformation through collective political action, can increase individuals' abilities to recover. Both social structure and individual agency become critical considerations when considering recovery, a task made no easier when outcomes for individuals are often considered outside a structure/agency framework, and rather a function of biology and of symptomatology.

With an explicitly political economic take on recovery, Warner (1994) argues provocatively that recovery from schizophrenia is tied to socioeconomic conditions. Oppressive economic conditions create stressors for people who then suffer disproportionately when economic conditions keep them from resuming meaningful adult social roles (such as employment) or from enjoying basic necessities (such as secure housing and food). Furthermore, systems of care that do not ameliorate stress on caregivers and families leave individuals adrift and socially isolated, stressed further.

All of these arguments about the nature of recovery, particularly as they impact the individual are important. However, there is a further set of questions about what recovery suggests for the future of the mental health service system, and how it is organized that are only now beginning to be answerable. What, for instance, does it mean when the meaningful and unique personal journey of recovery is a valued concept by researchers and providers, but remains so illusive in definition and measurement? What does this portend for policy choices? What happens when "recovery" meets a policy environment interested in enacting performance-based standards and "transformation" (in the United States). The literature on engaging recovery and evidence-based practices begins to suggest that there is no simple answer.

CONCLUSION: AGENDA FOR THE SOCIOLOGICAL STUDY OF RECOVERY

Brand new technologies and revolutionary ideas can rapidly displace old ways. But the history of mental health treatments reveals that many elements of care for people with serious mental illness – such as moral treatment, moral hygiene, asylums, psycho-pharmaceuticals, community mental health, and community support – do not simply appear or disappear, but rather wax and wane in importance, and get reinvented and rediscovered over time. Perhaps the concept of recovery will be something similar. While it has increased in prominence in rhetoric, policy, and services over the last two decades, the concept has a long history.

While it is clear that the rhetoric of recovery has permeated at least one corner of the modern mental health services field, that of rehabilitation, this material impact of this "guiding vision" is still unfolding. Certainly services have been challenged, efforts to change attitudes and outlooks are underway, and the diffusion of this idea and language has crossed many borders.

For a field that has been so active and fruitful in discussing the social construction of mental illness, few sociologists of mental health have taken on the flip: the social construction of recovery. It is time and we are well-equipped. For instance, sociology can and should explore further the provocative political economic research of Warner (1994) and the questions it raised. Sociologists of mental health have done excellent work in understanding how mental illness and stress is stratified, but paid less attention to how recovery from that same problem is also stratified. If we are to believe Warner, understanding this could point us to clear ways in which systems can be strengthened for the most vulnerable.

In addition, drawing the concept of recovery from the stories of the successful can draw on a rich history of the sociology of mental illness of identity research. In addition to the obvious contributions we can offer to understanding the lived experiences of people with serious mental illness who are recovering or are recovered, sociologists of mental health should attend to this social movement both inside and outside of research circles as it develops or withers. Who will win in this nascent dispute over whether outcome or process should come to represent recovery in the academic literature? Will recovery become another fad of the mental health services literature and fade away, or will it have staying power as it is ingratiated into treatment models and policy statements? What impact does this recovery have on traditional social pressures such as stigma? And finally, who "recovers," and who does not?

REFERENCES

Allott, P. and Linda L. (2002) *Discovering Hope For Recovery From A British Perspective – A Review of a Sample of Recovery Literature, Implications for Practice and Systems Change.* Birmingham: West Midlands Partnerships for Mental Health.

Andreasen, Nancy C., William T. Carpenter, Jr., John M. Kane, Robert A. Lasser, Stephen R. Marder, and Daniel R. Weinberger (2005) Remission in schizophrenia: proposed criteria and rationale for consensus. *American Journal of Psychiatry*, 162: 441–449.

Anthony, William A. (1991) Recovery from mental illness: the new vision of service researchers. *Innovations and Research*, 1: 13–14.

Anthony, William A. (1993) Recovery from mental illness: the guiding vision of the mental heath service sustem in the 1990s. *Psychosocial Rehabilitation Journal*, 16: 11–23.

Anthony, William A., Sally Rogers, E. and Marianne Farkas (2003) Research on evidence-based practices: future directions in an era of recovery. *Community Mental Health Journal*, 39: 101–14.

Bellack, Alan S. (2006) Scientific and consumer models of recovery in schizophrenia: concordance, contrasts, and implications. *Schizophrenia Bulletin*, 32: 432–442.

Bleuler, M. (1974) The long-term course of the schizophrenic psychoses. *Psychological Medicine*, 4: 244–254.

Brown, P. (1985) *The Transfer of Care*. Boston: Routledge and Kegan Paul.

Browne, G. (2006) Outcome measures: do they fit with a recovery model? *International Journal of Mental Health Nursing*, 15: 153–4.

Clay, Sally, Bonnie Schell, Patrick W. Corrigan, and Ruth O. Ralph (2005) *On Our Own, Together.* Nashville: Vanderbilt University Press.

Copeland, Mary Ellen (1997[2002]) *Wellness Action Recovery Plan*. West Dummerston, VT: Peach Press.

Corrigan, Patrick W., Daniel Giffort, Fadwa Rashid, Matthew Leary, and Iheoma Okeke (1999) Recovery as a psychological construct. *Community Mental Health Journal*, 35: 231–239.

Corrigan, Patrick W. and Ruth O. Ralph (2005) Introduction: recovery as consumer vision. In R.O. Ralph and P.W. Corrigan (eds). *Recovery in Mental Illness: Broadening Our Understanding of Wellness.* Washington, DC: American Psychological Association, pp. 3–18.

Corrigan, Patrick W., Natalie Slopen, Gabriela Gracia, Sean Phelan, Cornelius B. Keogh, and Lorraine Keck. (2005) Some recovery processes in mutual-help groups for persons with mental illness; II: qualitative analysis of participant interviews. *Community Mental Health Journal*, 41: 721–735.

Crowley, Kathleen (2000) *The Power of Procovery in Healing Mental Illness: Just Start Anywhere.* Los Angeles: Kennedy Carlisle Publishing.

Davidson, Larry (2003) *Living Outside Mental Illness: Qualitative Studies of Recovery in Schizophrenia.* New York: New York University Press.

Davidson, Larry and David Roe (2007) Recovery from versus recovery in serious mental illness: One strategy for lessening confusion plaguing recovery. *Journal of Mental Health*, 16: 459–470.

Davidson, Larry and William White (2007) The concept of recovery as an organizing principle for integrating mental health and addiction services. *Journal of Behavioral Health Services and Research*, 34: 109–120.

Davidson, Larry, Martha S. Lawless, and Fiona Leary (2005) Concepts of recovery: competing or complementary? *Current Opinion in Psychiatry*, 18: 664–667.

Davidson, Larry, Maria J. O'Connell, Janis Tondora, Martha Lawless, and Arthur C. Evans (2005) Recovery in serious mental illness: a new wine or just an old bottle? *Professional Psychology Research and Practice*, 36: 480–487.

Davidson, Larry, Maria O'Connell, Janis Todora, M. Staeheli, and Arthur C. Evans (2005) Recovery in serious mental illness: paradigm shift or Shibboleth? In L. Davidson, C.M. Harding, and L. Spaniol (eds). *Recovery from Serious Mental Illness: Research Evidence and Implications for Practice*. Boston: Center for Psychiatric Rehabilitation, pp. 5–24.

Davidson, Larry, Maria O'Connell, Janis Tondora, Thomas Styron, and Karen Kangas (2006) The top ten concerns about recovery encountered in mental health system transformation. *Psychiatric Services*, 57: 640–645.

Davidson, Larry, Robert E. Drake, Timothy Schmutte, Thomas Dinzeo, and Raquel Andres-Hyman (2009) Oil and water or oil and vinegar? Evidence-based medicine meets recovery. *Community Mental Health Journal*, 45: 323–332.

Davidson, Larry, Jaak Rakfeldt, and John S. Strauss (2010) *The Roots of the Recovery Movement in Psychiatry: Lessons Learned*. Hoboken, NJ: Wiley-Blackwell.

Davidson, Laurie (2005) Recovery, self management and the expert patient – Changing the culture of mental health from a UK perspective. *Journal of Mental Health*, 14: 25–35.

Deegan, Gene (2003) Discovering recovery. *Psychiatric Rehabilitation Journal*, 26: 368–76.

Deegan, Patricia E. (1988) Recovery: the lived experience of rehabiliation. *Psychosocial Rehabilitation Journal*, 11: 11–19.

Deegan, Patricia E. (2005) The importance of personal medicine: a qualitative study of resilience in people with psychiatric disabilities. *Scandinavian Journal of Public Health. Supplement*, 66: 29–35.

Deegan, Patricia E., Charlie Rapp, Mark Holter, and Melody Riefer (2008) Best practices: a program to support shared decision making in an outpatient psychiatric medication clinic. *Psychiatric Services*, 59: 603–605.

Department of Health and Human Services (1999) *Mental Health: A Report of the Surgeon General*. Department of Health and Human Services, Rockville, MD.

Department of Health and Human Services (2003) *Achieving the Promise: Transforming Mental Health Care in America*. Department of Health and Human Services, President's New Freedom Commission on Mental Health, Rockville, MD.

Department of Health (2001) *The Journey to Recovery – The Government's Vision for Mental Health Care*. Department of Health London.

Department of Health (2004) *The Ten Essential Shared Capabilities – A Framework for the Whole of the Mental Health Workforce*. Department of Health, London.

Dickens, Geoff (2009) Mental health outcome measures in the age of recovery-based services. *British Journal of Nursing*, 18: 940–943.

Dickerson, Faith B. (2006) Commentary: disquieting aspects of the recovery paradigm. *Psychiatric Services*, 57: 647.

Dinniss, Stephen (2006) Recovery-oriented mental healthcare. *The British Journal of Psychiatry*, 189: 384.

Essock, Susan and Lloyd Sederer (2009) Editorial: understanding and measuring recovery. *Schizophrenia Bulletin*, 35: 279–281.

Farkas, Marianne, Cheryl Gagne, William Anthony, and Judi Chamberlin (2005) Implementing recovery oriented evidence based programs: identifying the critical dimensions. *Community Mental Health Journal*, 41: 141–158.

Fisher, Daniel B. and Laurie Ahern (2002) Evidence-based practices and recovery. *Psychiatric Services* 53: 632–633.

Frank, Richard G. and Glied, Sherry A. (2006) *Better But Not Well: Mental Health Policy in the USA Since 1950*. Baltimore: Johns Hopkins University Press.

Frese, Frederick J. (1998) Advocacy, recovery, and the challenges of consumerism for schizophrenia. *Psychiatric Clinics of North America*, 21: 233–249.

Frese, Frederick J., Jonathan Stanley, Ken Kress, and Suzanne Vogel-Scibilia (2001) Integrating evidence-based practices and the recovery model. *Psychiatric Services*, 52: 1462–1468.

Grob, Gerald N. (1997) *The Mad Among Us*. New York: Free Press.

Harding, Courtenay M., George W. Brooks, Takamaru Ashikaga, John S. Strauss, and Alan Breier (1987) The Vermont longitudinal study of persons with severe mental illness, I: Methodology, study sample, and overall status 32 years later. *American Journal of Psychiatry*, 144: 718–726.

Healy, David (2002) *The Creation of Psychopharmacology*. Boston, MA: Harvard University Press.

Hopper, Kim (2007) Rethinking social recovery in schizophrenia: What a capabilities approach might offer. *Social Science and Medicine*, 65: 868–879.

Hopper, Kim (2008) A confusion of tongues, a reform on hold. *Chronic Illness*, 4: 307–308.

Jacobson, Nora (2001) Experiencing recovery: a dimensional analysis of recovery narratives. *Psychiatric Rehabilitation Journal*, 24: 248–256.

Jacobson, Nora (2003) Defining recovery: an interactionist analysis of mental health policy development, Wisconsin 1996–1999. *Qualitative Health Research*, 13: 378–393.

Jacobson, Nora (2004) *In Recovery: The Making of Mental Health Policy.* Nashville: Vanderbilt University Press.

Jacobson, Nora and Laurie Curtis (2000) Recovery as policy in mental services: strategies emerging from the states. *Psychosocial Rehabilitation Journal*, 23: 333–341.

Jacobson, Nora and Dianne Greenley (2001) What is recovery? A conceptual model and explication. *Psychiatric Services*, 52: 482–485.

Johnson, Shaun (2005) Misuse and abuse of 'recovery' by the psychiatric system. *Mental Health Today.* 37.

Jones, Kathleen (1993) *Asylums and After: A Revised History of the Mental Health Services, from the Early Eighteenth Century to the 1990s.* London: Athalone Press.

Kartalova-O'Doherty Yulia and Donna Tedstone Doherty (2010) *Reconnecting with Life: Personal Experiences of Recovering from Mental Health Problems in Ireland.* HRB Research Series 8. Dublin: Health Research Board.

Lamb, H. and Richard (1994) A century and a half of psychiatric rehabilitation in the United States. *Hospital and Community Psychiatry*, 45: 1015–1020.

Leete, Esso (1989) How I perceive and manage my illness. *Schizophrenia Bulletin*, 15: 197–200.

Lester, Helen and Linda Gask (2006) Delivering medical care for patients with serious mental illness or promoting a collaborative model of recovery? *The British Journal of Psychiatry*, 188: 401–402.

Liberman, Robert P., Alex Kopelowicz, Joseph Venture, and Daniel Gutkind (2002) Operational criteria and factors related to recovery from schizophrenia. *International Review of Psychiatry*, 14: 256–272.

Liberman, Robert Paul and Alex Kopelowicz (2005) Recovery from schizophrenia: a concept in search of Research. *Psychiatric Services,* 56: 735–742.

Lieberman, Jeffrey A., Robert E. Drake, Lloyd I. Sederer, Aysenil Belger, Richard Keefe, Diana Perkins, and Scott Stroup (2008) Science and recovery in schizophrenia. *Psychiatric Services*, 59: 487–496.

Link, Bruce G., Elmer L. Struening, Sheree Neese-Todd, Sara Asmussen, and Jo Phelan (2001) The consequences of stigma for the self-esteem of people with mental illnesses. *Psychiatric Services*, 52: 1621–1627.

Lovejoy, Marcia (1982) Expectations and the recovery process. *Schizophrenia Bulletin*, 9: 604–609.

Low, Abraham A. ([1991] 1943) *Mental Illness, Stigma and Self-Help.* Glencoe, IL: Willett Publishing.

Lunt, Alan (2002) A theory of recovery. *Journal of Psychosocial Nursing and Mental Health Services* 40: 32–39.

Markowitz, Fred E. (2001) Modeling processes in recovery from mental illness: relationships between symptoms, life satisfaction, and self-concept. *Journal of Health and Social Behavior*, 42: 64–79.

Mead, Sheryl and Mary Ellen Copeland (2000) What recovery means to us: consumers' perspectives. *Community Mental Health Journal*, 36: 315–328.

Mueser, Kim T., Patrick W. Corrigan, David W. Hilton, Beth Tanzman, Annette Schaub, Susan Gingerich, Susan M. Essock, Nick Tarrier, Bodie Morey, Suzanne Vogel-Scibilia, and Marvin I. Herz (2002) Illness management and recovery: a review of the research. *Psychiatric Services*, 53: 1272–1284.

National Consensus Conference on Mental Health Recovery and Mental Health Systems Transformation (2004) *National Consensus Statement on Mental Health Recovery.* Rockville, MD: Substance Abuse and Mental Health Services Administration, U.S. Department of Health and Human Services.

New Freedom Commission on Mental Health (2003) *Achieving the Promise: Transforming Mental Health Care in America. Final Report.* Rockville, MD: U.S. Department of Health and Human Services, DHHS Pub. No. SMA-03-3832.

Noordsy, Douglas, William Torrey, Kim Mueser, Shery Mead, Chris O'Keefe, and Lindy Fox (2002) Recovery from severe mental illness: an intrapersonal and functional outcome definition. *International Review of Psychiatry*, 14: 318–326.

O'Connor, Frederica W. and Kathleen R. Delaney (2007) The recovery movement: defining evidence-based processes. *Archives of Psychiatric Nursing*, 21: 172–175.

Onken, Steven J., Catherine M. Craig, Priscilla Ridgway, Ruth O. Ralph, and Judith, A. Cook (2007) An analysis of the defintions and elements of recovery: a review of the literature. *Psychiatric Rehabilitation Journal*, 31: 9–22.

Peyser, Herbert (2001) What is recovery? A commentary. *Psychiatric Services*, 52: 486–487.

Pilgrim, David (2008) 'Recovery' and current mental health policy. *Chronic Illness*, 4: 295–304.

Pilgrim, David (2009) Recovery from mental health problems: scratching the surface without ethnography. *Journal of Social Work Practice*, 23: 475–487.

Ralph, Ruth O. (2000) Review of recovery literature: A synthesis of a sample of literature. National Technical Assistance Center for State Mental Health Planning (NTAC), National Association for State Mental Health Program Directors (NASMHPD), Alexandria, VA.

Ramon, Shulamit, Bill Heay and Noel Renouf (2007) Recovery from mental illness as an emergent concept and practice in Australia and the UK. *International Journal of Social Psychiatry*, 53: 108–122.

Ridgway, Priscilla (2001) Restorying psychiatric disability: learning from first person recovery narratives. *Psychiatric Rehabilitation Journal*, 24: 335–343.

Roberts, Glenn and Paul Wolfson (2004) The rediscovery of recovery: open to all. *Advances in Psychiatric Treatment*, 10: 37–48.

Roe, David and Max Lachman (2005) The subjective experience of people with severe mental illness: A potentially crucial piece of the puzzle. *Israel Journal of Psychiatry and Related Sciences*, 42: 223–230.

Roe, David, Abraham Rudnick, and Kenneth J. Gill (2007) Commentary: the concept of 'being in recovery'. *Psychiatric Rehabilitation Journal*, 3: 171–173.

Roe, David, Ilanit Hasson-Ohayon, Michelle P. Salyers, and Shlomo Kravetz (2009) A one year follow-up of illness management and recovery: participants' accounts of its impact and uniqueness. *Psychiatric Rehabilitation Journal*, 32: 285–291.

Rogers, Anne and David Pilgrim (2001) *Mental Health Policy in Britain*. London: Palgrave.

Sainsbury Centre for Mental Health (2003) *Money for Mental Health: A Review of Public Spending on Mental Health*. London: Sainsbury Centre for Mental Health.

Schrank, Beate, Giovanni Stanghellini, and Mike Slade (2008) Hope in psychiatry: A review of the literature. *Acta Psychiatrica Scandinavica*, 118: 421–433.

Scottish Recovery Network (2005) *The Role and Potential Development of Peer Support Services*. Glasgow: Scottish Recovery Network.

Slade, Mike (2009) *Personal Recovery and Mental Illness: A Guide for Mental Health Professionals*. Cambridge: Cambridge University Press.

Stromwall, Layne K. and Donna Hurdle (2003) Psychiatric rehabilitation: An empowerment-based approach to mental health services. *Health and Social Work*, 28: 206–213.

Tanenbaum, Sandra J. (2006) The role of 'evidence' in recovery from mental illness. *Health Care Analysis*, 14: 195–201.

Taylor, Susan and Francis Yuen (2008) Psychiatric rehabilitation and recovery: a journey in reframing disability. *Journal of Social Work in Disability and Rehabilitation*, 7: 131–135.

Townsend, Wilma and Nicole Glasser (2003) Recovery: the heart and soul of treatment. *Psychiatric Rehabilitation Journal*, 27: 83–86.

Tsuang, Ming T., Robert Woolson, and Jerome A. Fleming (1979) Long-term outcome of major psychoses. I. Schizophrenia and affective disorders compared with psychiatrically symptom-free surgical conditions. *Archives of General Psychiatry*, 36: 1295–1301.

Unzicker, Rae (1989) On my own: A personal journey through madness and re-emergence. *Psychosocial Rehabilitation Journal*, 13: 71–77.

Ware, Norma C., Kim Hopper, Toni Tugenberg, Barbara Dickey, and Daniel Fisher (2008) A theory of social integration as quality of life. *Psychiatric Services*, 59: 27–32.

Warner, Richard (1994) *Recovery from Schizophrenia: Psychiatry and Political Economy.* New York: Routledge.

Wisdom, Jennifer P, Kevin Bruce, Goal Auzeen Saedi, Teresa Weis, and Carla A Green (2008) 'Stealing me from myself': Identity and recovery in personal accounts of mental illness. *The Australian and New Zealand Journal of Psychiatry*, 42: 489–495.

Yanos, Philip T., Edward L. Knight, and David Roe (2007) Recognizing a role for structure and agency: integrating sociological perspectives into the study of recovery from severe mental illness. In W.R. Avison, J.D. McLeod, and B.A. Pescosolido (eds). *Mental Health, Social Mirror.* New York: Springer Publishing, pp. 407–433.

24

Mental Health Problems, Social Exclusion and Social Inclusion: A UK Perspective

Jenny Secker

INTRODUCTION

The concept of social exclusion has been influential in European social policy for around 20 years and was given momentum by the European Union's establishment in 1991 of an Observatory to monitor national policies to combat exclusion. However, the term was not widely used in the UK until 1997, when the newly elected Labour government established a cross-departmental body, the Social Exclusion Unit (SEU), to coordinate national policy initiatives aimed at tackling the disadvantages faced by people seen as unable to participate in social, economic, political and cultural life. Since 1997, the use of the term 'social exclusion' has proliferated to the extent that it has passed into everyday use and is adopted by interest groups ranging from disability rights groups to the Rail Passenger Council, who wish to highlight perceived injustices (Schneider and Bramley, 2008).

Within mental health policy development, the publication of an SEU report (Office of the Deputy Prime Minister, 2004a) has been influential. This highlighted the impact of stigma and discrimination on unemployment and restricted opportunities to participate in mainstream education and community activities. It was followed by an action plan and guide to promoting social inclusion (Office of the Deputy Prime Minister, 2004b) together with the establishment of a National Social Inclusion Programme to coordinate cross-departmental delivery of the recommendations. The shift in terminology from 'social exclusion' to 'social inclusion' evident here is not insignificant and will be considered in subsequent sections of this chapter.

Given the widespread use of the terms 'social exclusion' and 'social inclusion', and the development of related initiatives within UK mental health policy, it is easy to assume that the concepts are straightforward and that we instinctively know what they mean. However, the definition of 'social exclusion' has been a topic of considerable debate, not least because it is similar to, and overlaps with, other social concepts. The assumption that 'social inclusion' is its opposite is also open to question. The first two sections of this chapter therefore look at the ways in which 'social exclusion' has been defined, at its relationship to other key concepts and at the relationship between 'social exclusion' and 'inclusion'. The following two sections then consider 'social exclusion' and 'inclusion' in the context of mental health. In the fifth section the particular position of people from Black and minority ethnic groups is considered. Thus far, and in much of the mental health literature, 'social inclusion' is taken uncritically to be self-evidently desirable. However, mental health service users do not necessarily see it that way, and from a political perspective too the assumption is open to question. The final section of the chapter therefore critiques the concept of 'social inclusion' from political and service user perspectives. Hereon in the text, the terms 'social inclusion' and 'social exclusion' will no longer be placed in speech marks for convenience but the above cautions about terminology will still obtain and are explored further now.

DEFINING SOCIAL EXCLUSION

As Schneider and Bramley (2008) point out, in most everyday use 'disadvantage' or 'poverty' could be substituted for social exclusion without any loss of meaning. However, researchers in the poverty tradition in Europe see exclusion as more comprehensive than poverty alone and a considerable amount of analysis aimed at clarifying and mapping out the scope of the concept has been undertaken. The ways of thinking about social exclusion, which emerge, can be described as relating to social systems, rights and opportunities and dimensions of exclusion. This section presents an overview of each approach.

Social systems and exclusion

Researchers in the poverty tradition in Europe have made a distinction between poverty and social exclusion. Whereas poverty is defined succinctly as a lack of resources, social exclusion is seen as a more comprehensive concept encompassing processes that involve the failure of one or more of four systems on which our sense of belonging in society depends. The four systems are described by Commins (1993) as:

- The democratic and legal system, which promotes civic integration, that is being an equal citizen in a democratic system.
- The labour market, which promotes economic integration in terms of having a valued economic function.
- The welfare state system which promotes social integration so that we are able to avail ourselves of the social services provided by the state.
- The family and community system, which promotes interpersonal integration, in terms of having family and friends, neighbours and social networks to provide care and companionship and moral support when these are needed.

All four systems are seen as important and as complementing one another; when one or two are weak the others need to be strong, and the worst off are those for whom all four systems have failed (Commins, 1993).

Rights and opportunities

A literature review around mental health and social exclusion carried out by Burchardt et al. (2002) identified two broad schools of thought about social exclusion. The first is a rights-based approach strongly associated with the international literature (e.g. Rodgers et al., 1995) within which social exclusion is seen as reflecting the deprivation of rights as a member or a citizen of a particular group, community, society or country. The second approach revolves around the opportunity to participate in key functions or activities of the society in question. This approach is a development of the traditional concerns of social science and especially social policy, with measuring poverty and deprivation (Townsend, 1979; Pantazis et al., 2006).

A not dissimilar distinction has been drawn by Huxley and Thornicroft (2003) between two types of social exclusion – that which corresponds to the Greek idea of demos – the political community, which grants (or withholds) rights; and that which corresponds to ethnos – the cultural community, which is about belonging. A person's membership of demos means that he or she may participate in political life and has the status of citizen in legal terms, but this does not necessarily imply acceptance by the cultural community as a member of that group (ethnos).

Dimensions of social exclusion

In their analysis of the literature, Schneider and Bramley (2008) identify four dimensions of social exclusion within which exclusion is seen as relative, multifactorial, dynamic and transactional. The first and second of these dimensions appear to overlap considerably with ideas of disadvantage, inequality and multiple deprivation. Like disadvantage, social exclusion is seen as relative because it describes the position of an individual or group in relation to other people or groups and thus encompasses ideas of inequality. In turn, this relative disadvantage is seen as due to multiple factors (Burchardt et al., 2002) such as poverty, poor housing, poor education and poor health, which may be inter-related, an idea also encompassed by the term multiple deprivation.

However, the third dimension takes the concept beyond disadvantage and multiple deprivation. Social exclusion is described as dynamic because it may be a long-term experience, but it may also be transient, episodic or recurrent. Thus an analysis of data from 1991 to 1995 carried out by Burchardt et al. (1999) found no distinct group of socially excluded individuals; few were excluded on all dimensions in any one year and even fewer experienced multiple exclusion for the whole period investigated.

People may move in and out of the conditions which lead to exclusion, such as poverty, unemployment or ill health. Thus, the mechanisms that bring about movement into and out of social exclusion are of interest to those concerned with social change.

Finally, and most distinctively, social exclusion has a transactional dimension because it locates individuals or groups in relation to wider structures of society. From this perspective, exclusion limits the interactions that are possible between individuals, families and communities. Since these interactions are reciprocal, not only the excluded are affected; the rest of society is also affected, for better or worse.

This transactional aspect of social exclusion indicates that remedies cannot be found solely from the perspective of the excluded. Exclusion cannot exist unless someone or something brings it about, be it through inadvertence, the operation of systems such as those described by Commins (1993) or active discrimination by individuals.

THE RELATIONSHIP BETWEEN EXCLUSION AND INCLUSION

As has been noted, in the course of the translation of concerns with social exclusion into UK mental health policy a second term, social inclusion, has come into widespread use and now dominates the policy discourse. Although the Social Exclusion Unit report on mental health and social exclusion focused on the causes of exclusion (Office of the Deputy Prime Minister, 2004a), its recommendations and subsequent developments have seamlessly moved towards endorsing inclusion as the way forward, as illustrated by the action plan and guide to promoting social inclusion that followed the SEU report (Office of the Deputy Prime Minister, 2004b).

Within the mental health policy discourse there appears to an unquestioned assumption that social exclusion and inclusion can be understood as the end-points of a single continuum, with inclusion seen as the polar opposite of exclusion. It is arguably more helpful, however, to separate out the two and to think of exclusion as operating on a structural level through barriers that work to exclude individuals and groups from full participation in society. By contrast, inclusion operates on an individual or group level and relates to the extent to which people are accepted and feel they belong within different social contexts.

The analyses outlined in the previous section offer some support for this approach. Taking Commins' systems of integration for example (Commins, 1993), while the first three systems – democratic and legal, labour market and welfare state – can be seen to involve political, economic and social structures, the fourth system – family and community – implies social relationships based on mutual acceptance. Similarly, the rights and participation approaches identified by Burchardt et al. (2002) and the demos/ethnos distinction drawn by Huxley and Thornicroft (2003) can be seen to involve social structures that can work for or against exclusion on the one hand, and on the other individual attitudinal factors, such as prejudice and discrimination, that influence opportunities for participation and belonging.

If they are separated out and treated as distinct concepts, social exclusion and inclusion can be depicted not on a single continuum but in terms of two intersecting continua depicting high and low levels of exclusion and inclusion as shown in Figure 24.1. This then allows us to think of conditions of exclusion and inclusion in terms of movement between the four quadrants created by the intersecting axes. Quadrant A can be seen to depict the worst case condition of high levels of exclusion coupled with low levels of inclusion, while quadrant C depicts the ideal condition, combining low levels of exclusion with high levels of inclusion. Quadrants B and D depict more complex conditions. In quadrant B, low levels of inclusion are combined with low levels of exclusion. For example, someone with mental health needs might have a job and to that extent not be excluded from the labour market, but if they are ostracized or bullied at work on account of their mental health needs they can hardly be said to be included. Quadrant D depicts high levels of inclusion

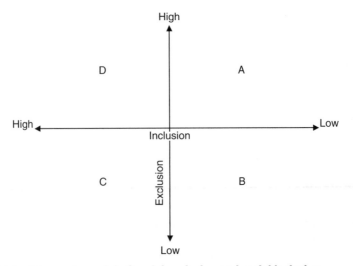

Figure 24.1   A two-axis model of social exclusion and social inclusion

despite low levels of exclusion. For example, people with mental health needs may be excluded from work and other mainstream activities, but be accepted, and therefore feel included, in other social milieus, such as those affording peer support from people with whom they share similar experiences and concerns.

SOCIAL EXCLUSION AND MENTAL HEALTH

The SEU's report on mental health and social exclusion (Office of the Deputy Prime Minister, 2004a) described adults with mental health needs as 'one of the most excluded groups in society'. In this section the four social systems described by Commins (1993) are used as framework within which to examine the evidence for that statement.

Democracy and the law

The Disability Discrimination Act of 2005 provides protection for people with 'a physical or mental impairment' against discrimination on the part of employers and service providers. The Act includes a duty to make reasonable adjustments to enable people defined as disabled to work and to access services. It also creates a positive duty on public sector organizations to promote disability equality. Although the current Act and its predecessor in 1995 marked an important milestone in protecting people with mental health problems from discrimination and upholding their rights, there is some evidence that they and their current or prospective employers lack awareness of the implications of the Act (Office of the Deputy Prime Minister, 2004a). People with mental health problems may not see themselves, or wish to be described as 'disabled'. In addition, to claim protection under the Act requires disclosure of a mental health problem and in some contexts, for example when applying for a job, people may be reluctant to disclose for fear that this will prejudice their chances of success.

There are also limitations to the protection afforded under the Act, particularly in relation to people compulsorily detained under the Mental Health Act. It is beyond the scope of this chapter to consider the complex and contentious issues that stem from legislation relating to mental health. However, it is important to note that the powers of compulsory detention and treatment enshrined in successive Mental Health Acts and the recent extension in the Mental Health Act 1983 as amended by the Mental Health Act 2007 of compulsory treatment to people living in the community raise questions of human rights that are of grave concern to service users, mental health organisations and the Disability Rights Commission, now part of the Equality and Human Rights Commission (Disability Rights Commission, 2007; Mental Health Alliance, 2007; Wallcraft et al., 2003).

As the Disability Rights Commission (2007) noted in its briefing on the second reading of the Mental Health Bill in the British parliament, the use of compulsory powers has wide-ranging and damaging consequences for the individual and society, in particular by bringing about discrimination in other areas of civic life. Examples include disqualification from civic roles, such as school governorship, parliamentary membership and jury service.

Where school governorship is concerned, the most contentious issue has now been addressed. Whereas the original regulations specified that an individual *liable* to be detained under mental health legislation was disqualified from serving, this has now been amended to encompass only those who are actually detained (Department for Education and Skills, 2004). Nonetheless, the inclusion of anyone liable to be detained in the original wording is a clear illustration of the potential for widespread exclusion from civic roles related to compulsory detention.

The position regarding parliamentary membership remains unchanged. The Mental Health Act 1983 specified that Members of Parliament (MPs) could be removed from their seat if detained, on the grounds that they would no longer be able to fulfil their duties, and this has been retained in the 2007 Act. Despite the fact that an MP admitted to hospital due to physical illness might be equally unable to fulfil her or his duties, the same provision does not apply.

The position regarding jury service also remains unchanged and, in this case, the exclusionary impact goes beyond compulsory detention to the treatment of mental health problems in the community, whether compulsory or not. Current regulations state that individuals are disqualified from jury service if they have a mental health problem that has led to hospital admission, or regular attendance for medical treatment. The jury summoning form requires any such experience to be declared, and declaration results in automatic disqualification (Schedule 1, Juries Act 1974). Given that one in six adults in the UK are estimated to experience mental health problems at any one point in time (with a one in four life prevalence) (Singleton et al., 2001), the exclusionary potential is far reaching. However, attempts to address the issue so far appear to have failed to make progress (National Social Inclusion Programme, 2006).

Beyond the exclusionary impact of mental health legislation, people with mental health problems can experience difficulty in accessing the same legal protection as other citizens because they may be seen as unreliable witnesses or unable to cope with the pressure of legal proceedings (Office of the Deputy Prime Minister, 2004a). In addition, the prevalence of mental health problems amongst people in prison is over four times higher than in the general population (Singleton et al., 1998) and the quality of mental health care available in prisons is often poor (Sainsbury Centre for Mental Health, 2007). Lack of access to appropriate care while in prison clearly has the potential to compound the exclusionary effects of high levels of unemployment and homelessness experienced on release (Niven and Stewart, 2005; Williamson, 2006).

The labour market

Across the literature on social exclusion, unemployment is seen as a major exclusionary factor and the remedy for exclusion is sometimes portrayed as residing solely in increasing employment rates amongst excluded groups. In the UK, people with mental health problems have the lowest employment rate of any of the main groups of disabled people, with only 21 per cent currently in work in England (Office of National Statistics, 2006). Estimates for people with severe and enduring problems are estimated at 8 per cent and for people with a diagnosis of schizophrenia at only 4 per cent (Perkins and Rinaldi, 2002; and see Bentall, this handbook). In addition to the negative impact on confidence, self esteem and mental health itself, unemployment can result in restricted income, fewer opportunities to meet with other people or develop skills, and loss of a productive identity that for many people is central to a sense of belonging within society.

Contrary to previous assumptions, the majority of unemployed people with mental problems want to work, even when they have been out of the labour market for many years (Bates, 1996; Secker et al., 2001; South Essex Service User Research Group et al., 2006). Research in the United States indicates that these aspirations are by no means unrealistic in that far higher proportions of people with mental health problems than are currently in work have been shown to be capable of holding down a job (Ecdawi and Conning, 1994). Studies aimed at identifying the characteristics of those most likely to get back to work have been unable to find any clear association with clinical factors such as diagnosis, symptoms or hospitalization history, or with measures of social functioning (Grove and Membrey, 2005). Indeed there is evidence that getting back to work can have long-term beneficial effects on clinical outcomes (Anthony et al., 1995, Arns and Linney, 1993, Bell et al., 1993, Lehman 1995) and social functioning (Lysaker and Bell, 1995).

While some psychological factors, particularly self efficacy and motivation to work, have been shown to be associated with gaining employment, access to effective employment support using the Individual Placement and Support (IPS) approach has emerged from the research as a significant factor. Fifteen randomised controlled trials, mainly in the United States but also in Australia, Canada and Hong Kong, have demonstrated significantly better work outcomes for IPS compared with more traditional approaches or standard care (Drake and Bond, 2008). Although doubts have been expressed as to whether the benefits of IPS would translate to the European context, a trial covering seven European locations, including England, has recently produced results similar to those obtained elsewhere (Burns et al., 2007).

Despite the proven effectiveness of the approach, access to IPS-based services is currently very limited in the UK (Schneider, 2005). For this reason commissioning guidance published by the Department of Health (2006a) promotes the development of IPS services alongside other initiatives such as social enterprises.

The welfare state

For people with mental health needs in the UK, social exclusion issues relating to the welfare state revolve mainly around the supply, quality and flexibility of provision. Housing and welfare benefits emerge from the literature as key areas of concern.

Housing

The SEU's report on mental health and social exclusion (Office of the Deputy Prime Minister, 2004) highlights housing as one of the basics which needs to be 'got right', as stable, appropriate housing is critical for people to work and take part in community life. However, people with mental health problems are particularly vulnerable to housing problems, including uncertainty about length of tenure in rented accommodation, dissatisfaction with housing and its state of repair (Meltzer et al., 2002) and a high risk of rent arrears (Shelter, 2003).

People with mental health needs may be considered to have a priority need for accommodation under homelessness legislation, but placement in temporary housing due to shortages of settled accommodation is common and is particularly problematic for people who need stability. A lack of suitable mainstream accommodation can also delay discharge from hospital, or result in inappropriate placement in segregated housing or residential care (Tarpey and Watson, 1997). Although the great majority of people do live in mainstream housing, over half live alone, a factor that can have its own implications for social exclusion.

While recognizing that some people will need specialist supported housing or residential care, the National Institute for Mental Health in England (2003) identified four characteristics of housing practices aimed at supporting people to obtain ordinary housing with ordinary landlords:

1   Full tenancies, with the full rights and responsibilities of a tenant, including for example the right to refuse admission to visitors except on the terms agreed in the tenancy.
2   The housing broadly reflects the aspirations of tenants – the housing stock is of averagely decent quality, and service users can be offered a range of appropriate housing options without loss of support service.
3   The arrangements meet the landlord's requirements – the landlord (whether local authority, Registered Social Landlord or private sector) has access to sufficient support, information and training, and any other resources to enable them to carry out their normal role, though with sufficient sensitivity.
4   There is just enough help to ensure success. The support can be flexible in intensity over time and between individuals; and also flexible in the range of support tasks, from relatively simple practical help such as arranging benefits and bill payments, through the teaching of lifeskills and dealing with neighbour disputes, to active attempts to help the individual engage constructively within their local community and achieve a sense of belonging.

A review of ten studies of the outcomes of supported housing in the United States provides evidence for a focus on mainstream housing with flexible support (Rog, 2004). There was strong evidence that supported housing tenants experienced decreased homelessness and hospital admission and some evidence, limited by methodological weaknesses in the studies reviewed, that these outcomes were better than for people living in other forms of housing provision.

Welfare benefits

High rates of unemployment amongst people with mental health needs mean that large numbers of people are dependent on welfare benefits for their financial security. In recent years, mental health problems have overtaken musculo-skeletal problems as the single biggest reason for incapacity benefit claims (Department for Work and Pensions, 2006). Additional means tested benefits to which many claimants of incapacity benefit (IB) and its successor, Employment Support Allowance (ESA), are entitled include Housing Benefit and Council Tax Benefit. Although therefore clearly an important welfare provision, aspects of the welfare benefit system can also be a disincentive to work. Although most people who claim incapacity benefit expect to return to work, after six months they have only a 50 per cent chance of returning (British Association of Rehabilitation Medicine, 2003). After 12 months their chances of returning to work within five years are only one in five (Department for Work and Pensions, 2002).

The disincentive to work stems from what is widely perceived to be a 'benefits trap', whereby returning to paid work can result in loss of secure income. In surveys of mental health service users, fear of losing benefits has consistently emerged as one of the main perceived barriers to work, cited by around 70 per cent of respondents (Secker et al., 2001; South Essex Service User Research Group, 2006). As well as concerns about loss of income, people fear that if their job does not work out they may not be entitled to reclaim benefits, or will have to go through a lengthy claim process in order to regain financial security (Seebohm and Scott, 2004).

In line with the UK government's commitment to 'make work pay', a range of changes to the system have been introduced to address the disincentives. These include:

- introduction of a national minimum wage;
- introduction of a working tax credit for people in low paid work working 16 hours a week or more (30 hours or more if not previously in receipt of incapacity-based benefits);
- permitted work arrangements under which people can retain their incapacity benefit within certain limits relating to hours of work and earnings levels;
- linking rules that entitle people who leave incapacity benefit to return to work to automatically re-qualify for the same level of benefit if they reclaim within two years with the same health condition or disability;
- extension of housing benefit for the first four weeks in work and a shortened claim process for people reclaiming housing benefit within 12 weeks of leaving it;
- a £40 per week return to work credit payable for one year to customers of the Department for Work and Pension's Pathways to Work programme;
- an Access to Work fund for people with a disability or mental health problem who need practical assistance to get and keep a job.

A further change being introduced for claimants doing permitted work from April 2010 (DWP, 2009) is an increase from £20 to £92 per week in the earnings disregard to which means tested benefits are subject. As opposed to being able to work fewer than four hours a week at minimum wage without losing means tested benefits for every pound earned thereafter, eligible claimants will be able to work up to 16 hours per week (at the time of writing the national minimum wage was set at £5.73 for people aged 22 and over).

This is a significant change with the potential to shift the perceived 'benefits trap' that deters people with mental health needs from seeking work. A persistent disincentive, however, is the sheer complexity of the welfare benefits system itself. Many people are not aware of all their entitlements and the decisions that have to be made about hours of work and earnings are daunting. With ESA now in place for new claimants the complexity is arguably increasing due to the introduction of four new benefits and different conditions for permitted work.

Family and community

This fourth social system identified by Commins (1993) highlights the importance of engagement with social networks. As well as being valuable in its own right, participation in social networks widens access to other opportunities and some types of engagement, such as volunteering and undertaking courses of education and training, increase the chances of paid employment for those who want to get back to work.

In comparison with the general population, people with mental health needs report lower levels of social engagement. They are more likely to be dissatisfied with levels of participation in family, social and leisure activities (Office of the Deputy Prime Minister, 2004a) and four times more likely to report feeling isolated (Mind, 2004).

One survey of 200 people using local mental health services found that 43 per cent had no regular daytime activities (South Essex Service User Research Group et al., 2006) and research with a larger sample of over 3,000 people found that even amongst those in contact with support organizations a quarter had no or very limited involvement with community activities.

Although the vast majority of people with mental health needs now live within their local communities, a significant proportion are reported to experience continued segregation, in that their social networks are restricted to other people within mental health services (Repper and Perkins, 2003). It is suggested that mental health day service provision has played a part in maintaining this segregation by focusing on providing specialized support only for people with mental health needs. Services tend to be buildings-based, with activities taking place within a centre. Contact with local communities is often limited to inviting local organizations such as colleges to provide sessions within the centre, or to group outings to community facilities such as the cinema or sports centre. Although highly valued by some, such provision is rejected by people who do not want to be constrained to a service user identity, particularly younger people and people recently experiencing mental health problems (Office of the Deputy Prime Minister, 2004a).

Commissioning guidance for day services issued by the Department of Health (2006b) is intended to encourage a shift away from buildings-based services towards greater provision of community bridge building services that support

individuals to engage with mainstream organizations and work with those organizations to widen opportunities for people with mental health needs. Other initiatives include regional partnerships between the National Social Inclusion
Programme, the National Institute of Adult Continuing Education (NIACE) and
the Learning Skills Council to encourage and assist adult and further education
providers to promote learning opportunities for adults with mental health needs.

In addition, under legislation passed in 1996 and strengthened in 2003, local
authorities now have a duty to make direct payments to people with disabilities,
including people with mental health needs, who are eligible and want them. The
payments are intended to enable people to purchase their own care, based on an
agreed needs assessment, thus enabling them to look beyond 'off-the-peg' provision as well as funding personal assistance or support. Examples of their use by
people with mental health needs include employment of trained artists to motivate exploration of creativity and assist in turning creative ideas into reality
(Spandler and Vick, 2006), gym membership and financing college courses
(National Social Inclusion Programme, 2005).

The take up rate of direct payments by people with mental health needs has
increased steadily over the last three years, but is still the lowest compared to the
other main adult service groups, and is less than a third of the rate for people with
learning difficulties. The latest figures available, from March 2007, show that
whilst just 6 local authorities in England were not making any direct payments in
lieu of mental health services, over a third (61) were making five or fewer. The
low uptake has been identified as stemming from inadequate leadership, a lack of
awareness and promotion of direct payments, and staff concerns about people's
ability to manage payments (Spandler and Vick, 2006). Guidance issued by the
Department of Health (2006d) is intended to help health services and local
authorities to address these problems.

SOCIAL INCLUSION AND MENTAL HEALTH

It was argued earlier that whereas social exclusion relates to structural barriers
that work to exclude individuals and groups from full participation in society,
inclusion works at an individual level and is concerned with the extent to which
people are accepted and feel they belong within different social contexts. No
matter whether people with mental health problems have a job, decent housing
and access to activities in their community, and to that extent are not socially
excluded, if they do not *feel* accepted in their workplace, neighbourhood and
community they can hardly be said to be socially included.

The evidence suggests that many people with mental health problems do not
feel included in society. Over 80 per cent of respondents to a consultation carried
out by the SEU identified the stigmatization of mental health problems and associated discrimination as the main barrier to inclusion, 55 per cent identified
stigma as a barrier to employment and 52 per cent reported negative attitudes to

people with mental health needs in the community (Office of the Deputy Prime Minister, 2004a). Similarly, an inquiry carried out by Mind, the national mental health association for England, received strong and consistent evidence of the discrimination people experience as a direct result of their mental health needs (Dunn, 1999). Around three-quarters of respondents to a more recent Mind survey felt a lack of understanding about mental health issues was a key cause of social isolation (Mind, 2004).

The discrimination reported by people with mental health needs is reflected in the results of research into public attitudes. In a survey of attitudes amongst the adult general public in Britain, around 70 per cent of respondents rated people with a diagnosis of schizophrenia as dangerous to others (Crisp et al., 2000), despite evidence that very few people actually display violent behaviour and are far more likely to be victims of violence (Department of Health, 2001; Pilgrim and Rogers, this handbook, Walsh et al., 2003;). Within specific groups, a survey of employers found that fewer than four in ten would consider employing someone with a history of mental health problems, compared to more than six in ten for a physical disability (Manning and White, 1995). Also, research into the views of Metropolitan police officers found that many had very negative attitudes towards mental health issues (Fahy and Dunn, 1987).

It is important to note that the attitudes expressed in response to these surveys may reflect prejudice that is not translated into discriminatory actions or inaction. However, for people with mental health problems themselves, fear of stigma and discrimination, whether actually experienced or not, can lead to severe loss of confidence and reluctance to engage with social networks, beyond those involving others in the mental health system, a process described by some authors as 'self-stigmatization' (Green et al., 2003; Knight et al., 2003).

Stigma is understood as a relationship between characteristics that are perceived to mark an individual or group out as somehow 'different' and socially constructed negative attitudes (National Institute for Mental Health in England, 2004; Scambler, this handbook). It is not possible within the scope of this chapter to explore the processes of stigmatization in detail, but where people with mental health needs are concerned, these may be rooted in fears that are deeply embedded within societies. For example, a four-year participant observation study in rural France revealed how the hygiene practices of families with whom people with mental health problems were lodged, in the expectation of their integration within the communities concerned, stemmed from ancient magical thinking about the powers of itinerants and contributed to the segregation of the very people for whom integration was the aim (Jodelet, 1989). In the UK, a study of audience response to negative media portrayals of those with a psychiatric diagnosis found that, contrary to the results of studies of negative portrayals of other groups such as striking miners, such portrayals could overwhelm even more positive direct personal experience of people with patients (Philo et al., 1994). The researchers concluded that the power of negative portrayals to overwhelm personal experience may stem from deep rooted fears of madness and distress.

Philo and colleagues (1994) also analyzed coverage of mental health matters over one month in a range of British print and visual media. They found that items linking mental distress with violence to others comprised two thirds of the coverage and tended to receive headline treatment. In contrast, more sympathetic items comprised only 18 per cent of the coverage and tended to be found in health columns or problem pages. Whether negative media coverage influences public attitudes or simply reflects public opinion is open to question. However, in a further Mind survey around a third of people with mental health problems reported that such coverage made them reluctant to apply for a job or to volunteer and that their friends and family reacted differently to them following negative media coverage (Mind, 2000).

A review of international literature on work to tackle stigma and discrimination around mental health (National Institute for Mental Health in England, 2004) found few rigorous studies but the evidence that was available indicated that approaches were more effective when:

- people with experience of mental distress were involved throughout;
- a combination of approaches and methods is used at a range of levels;
- behaviour change rather than changes in attitudes and awareness is the focus;
- clear consistent messages are delivered in targeted ways to specific audiences;
- long term planning and funding supports sustainable programmes of work.

Little previous work in the UK had encompassed these indicators of effectiveness and a five year campaign, *Shift*, was established in 2004 to tackle stigma and discrimination more comprehensively in England (www.shift.org.uk). In Scotland the *See Me* campaign was launched in 2002 by an alliance of five mental health organizations with funding from the Scottish Executive (www.seemescotland. org). A review of the first four years of the Scottish campaign reports significant achievements including a 57 per cent reduction in the use of derogatory terms in the Scottish media.

SOCIAL EXCLUSION, SOCIAL INCLUSION AND ETHNICITY

There is reason to believe that people with mental health problems from Black and minority ethnic groups face particular exclusionary barriers and difficulties in relation to social inclusion.

The evidence is particularly strong in relation to democracy and the law. People from Black and minority ethnic groups are six times more likely than white people to be detained under the Mental Health Act (Audini and Lelliott, 2003), with implications for access to civic roles from which people detained under the legislation are excluded. They are also overrepresented in prisons (Sandamas and Hogman, 2000), particularly in the male prison population (Home Office, 2003), and can therefore be disproportionately affected by a lack of mental health care in the criminal justice system. In terms of access to justice, Black people are eight times more likely to be stopped and searched than white people, and five times more likely to be arrested.

Where the labour market is concerned, reliable data on employment rates amongst people with mental health problems from Black and minority ethnic communities are not available. However, it is likely that these are lower than for white people since in the general working age population only 58 per cent of people from Black and minority ethnic groups are in work, compared to 75 per cent of the white population (Department for Work and Pensions, 2003). There is some evidence that people with mental health needs from Black and minority ethnic groups are under-represented in specialist employment services (Pozner et al., 1996). This may well relate to a widespread fear of mental health services within Black and minority ethnic communities (Sainsbury Centre for Mental Health, 2002). In addition, employment support workers may lack the knowledge and skills to provide appropriate support, for example in enterprise development which is of particular interest to some people from Black and minority ethnic groups (Office of the Deputy Prime Minister, 2004a).

Likely higher rates of unemployment mean that people with mental health needs from Black and minority ethnic groups may be particularly vulnerable to disincentives to work within the welfare benefits system. In relation to housing, amongst heads of household people from Black and minority ethnic groups are three times more likely to have experienced homelessness than white people (Harrison and Phillips, 2003). Although data are not separately available for people with mental health problems, it is not unlikely that they experience particular difficulty in obtaining the secure, stable housing required to work and take part in community life.

Turning to community engagement itself, in the Mind survey cited earlier, people with mental health needs from Black and minority ethnic groups were amongst the groups most likely to report isolation (Mind, 2004). They may also be less able to access education and training due to low expectations within mental health services or language barriers arising from a lack of confidence in speaking English coupled with inflexibility in the provision of English language courses (Office of the Deputy Prime Minister, 2004a).

What evidence there is, then, indicates that people with mental health needs from Black and minority ethnic groups face exclusionary barriers that are heightened by their position in relation to the legal, labour market, welfare state and community systems. In the light of increasing recognition of the ways in which society's institutions promulgate racism through processes, attitudes and behaviour that amount to discrimination (Macpherson, 1999), it is clear that underpinning those heightened exclusionary barriers are deep rooted barriers to the acceptance within society that arguably defines social inclusion.

A CRITIQUE OF THE INCLUSION IMPERATIVE IN MENTAL HEALTH

As has been seen, although originally informed by European social policy concerns with social exclusion, the UK mental health policy discourse is now dominated by the concept of social inclusion. Whereas the concept of social exclusion has attracted much interest and debate, the notion of social inclusion is presented as self evidently desirable and has received less critical attention (Ratcliffe, 2000). A recent exception is a critique put forward by Spandler (2007). This section draws on her critique to question the assumptions underpinning the shift to a discourse of social inclusion, in the sense of 'bringing people with mental illness into mainstream society, enabling access to ordinary opportunities for employment, leisure, family and community life' (Rankin, 2005).

A first set of assumptions identified by Spandler (2007) concerns the society from which people with mental health needs are seen to be excluded, namely that the quality of mainstream society is not only desirable, but unproblematic and legitimate. As Spandler argues, this fails to take account of the difficulties, conflicts and inequalities apparent in the wider society, which actually generate and sustain *both* exclusion *and* mental health problems (Burden and Hamm, 2000; Kleinman, 1998). A pertinent example, in view of the emphasis placed on paid employment as a route to inclusion, is the impact of modern employment conditions on mental health. A recent review concluded that the 'evidence is clear that, for working people, the design and management of work can be a major threat to their mental health' (Cox et al., 2004). Modern employment is increasingly poorly paid, un-unionized, insecure and characterized by longer working hours, short term contracts, increasing workloads, stress and uncertainty (Stewart, 2004). In addition, focusing on employment as *the* route to inclusion ignores the necessity, value and gendered nature of unpaid work and also undermines the legitimacy of non-employment (Kleinman, 1998; Levitas, 2004).

Spandler (2007) goes on to point out that the broader view of inclusion as involving not simply paid employment but also involvement in a wide range of community settings also makes assumptions about mainstream society, in that the 'normal' population are themselves assumed to be 'socially included' in a variety of aspects and social and community life. Yet it is well known that people in full time work spend little time on non-work related activities and full time work can negatively affect people's ability to socialize, volunteer or help others (Lader et al., 2005; Ruston, 2000). Similarly, research has noted how the inhabitants of middle class suburbs (the core of 'mainstream society') are often socially isolated and rarely mix with others outside their own socio-cultural group (Baumgartner 1998; Kleinman 1998).

In assuming that the 'mainstream' is ideal and desirable, Spandler (2007) notes, discourses around mental health are deficit-focused. This constructs the 'socially excluded' as lacking in the skills and dispositions required for paid work and other 'mainstream activities'. In this way, the problems which need to be addressed are not the structural barriers that work to exclude people, but cultures of low aspiration and fatalism (Fairclough, 2000). The moral imperative for service users to engage in a way which is defined as appropriate by government, policy makers and services can lead to those who do not cooperate being viewed as dysfunctional. Moreover, this limits discussions of social inequalities to ones about *aspirations and opportunities* for individuals and excludes any consideration of structural inequalities which are about group power, wealth and ownership.

A related set of assumptions identified by Spandler (2007) concern people with mental health problems themselves and the desirability or undesirability of the kinds of relationships they form, especially with mental health services, the state and other mental health service users. Increasingly, service users are constructed as being 'dependent' on welfare services if they use services in particular ways. The notion of dependency is almost invariably construed in negative terms and is opposed to the ideal of 'independence' (usually through employment). In this way, service users' reliance on benefit payments, services and other people with mental health difficulties becomes a 'moral hazard' (Levitas, 2004) which encourages dependency, rather than a social good which prevents destitution or provides support, solidarity and care (Burden and Hamm, 2000).

The assumptions underpinning the discourse of social inclusion have a number of potential consequences. If service users are constructed as 'lacking' or 'dependent', the problem then becomes how to 'help, cajole or coerce' those perceived as outsiders back into mainstream society (Levitas, 2004). Although the mantra of 'individual choice' and 'person centeredness' often accompanies social inclusion initiatives, in effect the inclusion imperative inadvertently imposes certain choices as more desirable than others. In other words some choices are privileged and encouraged while others are problematized or pathologized.

If inclusion shifts attention to changing individuals' behaviours and choices, then a final consequence of the inclusion imperative is that the conditions of possibility for collectivist demands and solutions are undermined (Stewart, 2000). In this way, initiatives such as direct payments may actually encourage a minority of social care users to find individual solutions to the effects of social exclusion rather than address the fundamental divisions which cause exclusionary practices (Lyons, 2005; Spandler, 2004).

In summary, despite good intentions, there is a risk that a narrow social inclusion agenda may foster a disproportionate focus on 'slotting in, rather than transforming society' (Bates and Davis, 2004). Such concerns have led to some disquiet amongst service users/survivors about the social inclusion agenda:

> Survivors don't necessarily want to be part of a mainstream society which has rejected them and in which they will never easily fit until society itself redresses its prejudiced attitudes and tunnel vision. Where is the problem located, in the individual who has dropped out or been excluded, or in society, which tries to force people to fit its stereotypes? 'Social inclusion', if we are not careful, can sound rather like 'normalisation', which appeared to mean making people more normal so they would fit in (Wallcraft, 2001).

CONCLUSION

This chapter has examined the various approaches taken to defining social exclusion and has argued that it is more helpful to separate out the concepts of social exclusion and inclusion than to unquestioningly assume that they are opposites at each end of a single continuum. Instead it was proposed that social inclusion operates at an individual or group level and is concerned with the extent to which people are accepted and feel they belong within different social contexts. Social exclusion, on the other hand, can be seen as relating to structural barriers that work to exclude individuals and groups from full participation in society. The evidence that people with mental health needs are socially excluded in the terms of this definition was then examined in relation to four social systems: democracy and the law, the labour market, the welfare state and family and community.

On the basis of the available evidence there are grounds for concluding that this group, and particularly people with mental health needs from Black and minority ethnic communities, are amongst the most excluded in society. There are also grounds for concluding that structural barriers play a part in that exclusion, for example the regulations around jury service, disincentives to work within the welfare benefit system and mental health services that inhibit return to work and community engagement.

However, the evidence relating to social inclusion highlights the difficulties people with mental health needs face in feeling accepted within mainstream society. Even if the structural barriers to their participation were removed, stigmatization, prejudice and discrimination are deeply embedded within mainstream society, underpinning and reinforcing exclusionary mechanisms within the four social systems. Examples include the prejudiced attitudes found amongst the police and amongst employers, and the negative stereotypes prevalent in media representations and in the attitudes of the general public.

It follows from the evidence examined that mental health and wider social policy initiatives need to focus both on tackling the structural barriers that work to exclude people with mental health needs, and on challenging the deep rooted prejudice and stigmatization that reinforce those barriers. As has been seen, efforts are being made on both fronts. However, the critique of the shift from a discourse of social exclusion to a discourse of inclusion put forward by Spandler (2007) goes further in highlighting the questionable assumptions about mainstream society and social relations on which the inclusion discourse is based. As she notes:

> To ensure that social inclusion does not become a 'new tyranny' we need to be mindful of the context in which inclusion policies are implemented, the assumptions that become implicit within these policies, and the possible consequences of their adoption as a moral imperative.

From this perspective, without radical intervention to bring about change in social relations within mainstream society, some people with mental health problems will prefer to remain within social milieus in which they are accepted and supported, as depicted in quadrant D of Figure 24.1. That choice needs to be recognized as equally legitimate to the aspirations of others to move beyond a service user identity and to reengage with mainstream society. Otherwise, 'social inclusion' will become co-opted as a modern form of moral and social governance which reproduces and legitimises the prevailing socio-economic order.

ACKNOWLEDGEMENT

I am especially grateful to Helen Spandler, Research Fellow in the Department of Social Work, University of Central Lancashire, for allowing me to draw so extensively on her critique of social inclusion and for keeping me thinking.

REFERENCES

Anthony, W.A., Rogers, E.S. Cohen, M. and Davies, R.R. (1995) Relationships between psychiatric symptomatology, work skills and future vocational performance. *Psychiatric Services,* 46(4): 353–358.

Arns, P.G. and Linney, J.A. (1993) Work, self and life satisfaction for persons with severe and persistent mental disorders. *Psychosocial Rehabilitation Journal,* 17(2): 63–80.

Audini, B. and Lelliott, P. (2003) Age, gender and ethnicity of those detained under Part II of the Mental Health Act 1983. *British Journal of Psychiatry,* 180: 222–226.

Bates, P. (1996) Stuff as dreams are made on. *Health Service Journal,* 4(33): 1.

Bates, P. and Davis, F.A. (2004) Social capital, social inclusion and services for people with learning disabilities. *Disability and Society,* 19(3): 195–207.

Baumgartner, M. (1988) *The Moral Order of the Suburb.* New York: Oxford University Press.

Bell, M.D., Milstein, R.M. and Lysaker, P. (1993) Pay and participation in work activity: clinical benefits for clients with schizophrenia. *Psychosocial Rehabilitation Journal,* 17(2): 173–177.

Burchardt, T., Le Grand, J. and Piachaud, D. (1999) Social exclusion in Britain, 1991–1995. *Social Policy and Administration,* 33(3): 227–244.

Burchardt, T., Le Grand, J. and Piachaud, D. (2002) Degrees of exclusion: Developing a dynamic, multi-dimensional measure. In J. Hills, J. Le Grand and D. Piachaud (eds) *Understanding Social Exclusion,* Oxford: Oxford University Press. pp. 30–43.

Burden, T. and Hamm, T. (2000). In J. Perry-Smith (ed.) *Policy Responses to Social Inclusion.* Buckingham: Open University Press. pp. 184–200.

Burns, T., Catty, J., Becker, T., Drake, R.E., Fioritti, A., Knapp, M., Lauber, C., Rössler, W., Tomov, T., van Busschbach, White, S. and Wiersma, D. (2007) The effectiveness of supported employment for people with severe mental illness: a randomised controlled trial. *Lancet,* 370: 1146–1152.

Care Services Improvement Partnership/National Institute for Mental Health in England (2007) *Valuing Involvement: Making a Real Difference – Strengthening Service User and Carer Involvement in NIMHE and CSIP – Benefit Conditions and Systems Relating to Paid and Voluntary Service User and Carer Involvement Activity.* London: CSIP/NIMHE.

Commins, P. (1993) *Combating Exclusion in Ireland 1990–1994, A Midway Report.* Brussels: European Commission.

Cox, T., Leka, S., Ivanov, I. and Kortum, E. (2004) Work, employment and mental health in Europe. *Work and Stress,* 18(2):179–185.

Crisp, A.H., Gelder, M.G., Rix, S., Meltzer, H. and Rowlands, O.J. (2000) Stigmatisation of people with mental illnesses. *British Journal of Psychiatry,* 177: 4–7.

Department for Education and Skills (2004) *School Governance (Constitution, Procedures and New Schools) (England) (Amendment) Regulations.* Norwich: The Stationery Office.

Department of Health (2001) *Safety First: Five year report of the national confidential inquiry into suicide and homicide by people with mental illness.* London: Department of Health.

Department of Health (2006a) *Vocational Services for People with Severe Mental Health Problems: Commissioning Guidance.* London: Department of Health.

Department of Health (2006b) *From Segregation to Inclusion: Commissioning Guidance on Day Services for People with Mental Health Problems.* London: Department of Health.

Department of Health (2006c) *Reward and Recognition: the Principles and Practice of Service User Payment and Reimbursement in Health and Social Care.* London: Department of Health.

Department of Health (2006d) *Direct Payments for People with Mental Health Problems: a Guide to Action.* London: Department of Health.

Department for Work and Pensions (2003) *Opportunity For All: 5th Annual Report.* London, Department for Work and Pensions.

Department for Work and Pensions (2006) *A New Deal for Welfare: Empowering People to Work.* Norwich: The Stationery Office.

Department for Work and Pensions (2009) *Permitted Work and Incapacity Benefits.* London: Department for Work and Pensions.

Disability Rights Commission (2007) *Parliamentary Briefing. Mental Health Bill, Second Reading, House of Commons, Monday 16th April 2007.* London: Disability Rights Commission.

Drake, B. and Bond, G (2008) The future of supported employment for people with severe mental illness. *Psychiatric Rehabilitation Journal,* 31: 367–376.

Dunn, S. (1999) *Creating Accepting Communities. Report of the Mind Inquiry into Social Exclusion and Mental Health Problems.* London: Mind.

Ecdawi, M. and Conning, A. (1994) *Psychiatric Rehabilitation: A Practical Guide.* London: Chapman Hall.

Fahy, T.A. and Dunn, J. (1987) Where Section 136 fails. *Police Review,* 95:1580–1581.

Fairclough, N. (2000) *New Labour, New Language?* London: Routledge.

Green, G., Hayes, C., Dickenson, D., Gilheany, B. and Whittaker, A. (2003) A mental health service users' perspective to stigmatisation. *Journal of Mental Health,* 12(3): 223–234.

Grove, B. and Membrey, H. (2005) Sheep and goats: new thinking on employability. In B, Grove, J, Secker and P, Seebohm (eds) *New Thinking about Employment and Mental Health.* Abingdon: Radcliffe Medical Publishing, pp. 3–9.

Harrison, M. and Phillips, D. (2003) *Housing Black and Minority Ethnic Communities: review of the Evidence Base.* London: Office of the Deputy Prime Minister.

Home Office (2003) *Statistics on Race and the Criminal Justice System, 2002.* London: Home Office.

Huxley, P. and Thornicroft, G. (2003) Social inclusion, social quality and mental illness. *British Journal of Psychiatry,* 182: 289–290.

Jodelet, D. (1989) *Madness and Social Representations.* Hemel Hempstead: Harvest Wheatsheaf.

Kleinman, M. (1998) *Include Me Out? The New Politics of Place and Poverty.* CASE paper No. 11. London: Centre for Analysis of Social Exclusion, London School of Economics, http://sticerd.lse.ac.uk/dps/case/cp/paper11.pdf

Knight, M., Wykes, T. and Hayward, P. (2003) 'People don't understand': An investigation of stigma in schizophrenia using Interpretative Phenomenological Analysis (IPA). *Journal of Mental Health,* 12(3): 209–222.

Lader, D., Short, S. and Gershuny, J. (2005) *The Time Use Survey.* London, Office for National Statistics.

Lehman, A.F. (1995) Vocational rehabilitation in schizophrenia. *Schizophrenia Bulletin,* 21: 645–656.

Levitas, R. (2004) Let's hear it for Humpty: social exclusion, the third way and cultural capital. *Cultural Trends,* 13(2): 1–15.

Lyons, J. (2005) A systems approach to direct payments: a response to 'friend or foe'? Towards a critical assessment of direct payments. *Critical Social Policy,* 25(2): 240–252.

Lysaker, P. and Bell, M.D. (1995) Work performance over time for people with schizophrenia. *Psychiatric Rehabilitation Journal,* 18(3): 141–145.

Macpherson, W. (1999) *The Stephen Lawrence Inquiry.* Norwich: The Stationery Office.

Manning, C. and White, P.D. (1995) Attitudes of employers to the mentally ill. *Psychiatric Bulletin,* 19: 541–543.

Meltzer, H., Singleton, N., Lee, A., Bebbington, P., Brugha, T. and Jenkins, R. (2002) *The Social and Economic Circumstances of Adults with Mental Disorders*. Norwich: The Stationery Office.

Mental Health Alliance (2007) *The Mental Health Act 2007: the Final Report*. London: Mental Health Alliance.

Mind (2000) *Counting the Cost: Mental Health in the Media*. London, Mind.

Mind (2004) *Not alone? Isolation and mental distress*. London, Mind.

National Institute for Mental Health in England (2003) *Making Inclusion Work*. Leeds: National Institute for Mental Health in England.

National Institute for Mental Health in England (2004) *From Here to equality: a Strategic Plan to Tackle Stigma and Discrimination on Mental Health Grounds*. Leeds: National Institute for Mental Health in England.

National Social Inclusion Programme (2005) *Direct Payments in Mental Health: What Are They Being Used For?* London: National Social Inclusion Programme.

National Social Inclusion Programme (2006) *Second Annual Report*. London: National Social Inclusion Programme.

NHS Information Centre (2009) *Adult Psychiatric Morbidity in England, 2007*. Leeds, NHS Information Centre for Health and Social Care.

Niven, S. and Stewart, D. (2005) *Resettlement Outcomes on Release from Prison in 2003. Findings 248*. London, Home Office.

Office of the Deputy Prime Minister (2004a) *Mental Health and Social Exclusion*. London, Office of the Deputy Prime Minister.

Office of the Deputy Prime Minister (2004b) *Action on Mental Health: A Guide to Promoting Social Inclusion*. London, Office of the Deputy Prime Minister.

Office for National Statistics (2006) *Labour Force Survey* 2006. Available at www.statistics.gov.uk

Pantazis, C., Gordon, D. and Levitas, R. (eds) (2006) *Poverty and Social Exclusion in Britain*. Bristol, The Policy Press.

Perkins, R. and Rinaldi, M. (2002) Unemployment rates among patients with long-term mental health problems: a decade of rising unemployment. *Psychiatric Bulletin,* 26: 295–298.

Philo, G., Secker, J., Platt, S., Henderson, L., McLaughlin, G. and Burnside, J. (1994) The impact of the mass media on public images of mental illness: media content and audience belief. *Health Education Journal,* 53: 271–281.

Pozner, A., Hammond, M.L. and Shepherd, G. (1996) *Working it out: Creating Work Opportunities for People with Mental. Health Problems*. Brighton: Pavilion Publishing.

Rankin, J. (2005) *Mental Health in the Mainstream: Mental Health and Social Inclusion*. London, Institute for Public Policy Research.

Ratcliffe, P. (2000) Is the assertion of minority identity compatible with the idea of a socially inclusive society? In P. Askonas and A. Stewart (eds) *Social Inclusion: Possibilities and Tensions*. Basingstoke: McMillan Press Ltd.

Repper, J. and Perkins, R. (2003) *Social Inclusion and Recovery: a Model for Mental Health Practice*. Edinburgh: Balliere Tindall.

Rodgers, G., Gore, C. and Figueiredo, J. (eds) (1995) *Social Exclusion: Rhetoric, Reality, Responses*. Geneva, International Institute for Labour Studies.

Rog, D. (2004) The evidence on supported housing. *Psychiatric Rehabilitation Journal,* 27(4): 334–344.

Ruston, D. (2000) *Volunteer, Helpers and Socialisers: Social Capital and Time Use*. London: Office for National Statistics

Sainsbury Centre for Mental Health (2002) *Breaking the Circles of Fear. A Review of the Relationship between Mental Health Services and African and Caribbean Communities*. London: Sainsbury Centre for Mental Health.

Sainsbury Centre for Mental Health (2007) *Mental Health Care in Prisons. Briefing 32*. London: Sainsbury Centre for Mental Health.

Sandamas, G. and Hogman, G. (2000) *No Change?* London: National Schizophrenia Fellowship (now Rethink).

Schneider, J. (2005) Employment support in the UK: where are we now? In Grove, B., Secker, J. and Seebohm, P. (eds) *New Thinking about Employment and Mental Health*. Abingdon, Radcliffe Medical Publishing, pp. 51–59.

Schneider, J. and Bramley, C. (2008) Towards social inclusion in mental health? *Advances in Psychiatric Treatment*, 14: 131–138.

Secker, J., Grove, B. and Seebohm, P. (2001) Challenging barriers to employment, training and education for mental health service users: the service user's perspective. *Journal of Mental Health*, 10(4): 395–404.

Seebohm, P. and Scott, J. (2004) *Benefits and Work for People with Mental Health Problems. Briefing 27*. London: Sainsbury Centre for Mental Health.

Shelter (2003) *House Keeping: Preventing Homelessness through Tackling Rent Arrears in Social Housing*. London: Shelter.

Singleton, N., Bumpstead, R., O'Brien, M., Lee, A. and Meltzer, H. (2001) *Psychiatric morbidity among adults living in private households, 2000*. Norwich: The Stationery Office.

Singleton, N., Meltzer, H., Gatward, R., Coid, J. and Deasy, D. (1998) *Psychiatric Morbidity Among Prisoners in England and Wales*. Norwich, The Stationery Office.

Spandler, H. (2004) Friend or foe: towards a critical assessment of direct payments. *Critical Social Policy* 24(2): 187–209.

Spandler, H. (2007) From social exclusion to inclusion? A critique of the social inclusion imperative in mental health. *Medical Sociology Online*, 2(2): 3–16.

Spandler, H. and Vick, N. (2006) Opportunities for independent living using direct payments in mental health. *Health and Social Care in the Community*, 14(2): 107–115.

South Essex Service User Research Group, Secker, J. and Gelling, L. (2006) Still dreaming: service users' employment, education and training goals. *Journal of Mental Health*, 15(1): 103–111.

Stewart, A. (2000) Social inclusion: a radical agenda. In P. Askonas and A. Stewart (eds) *Social Inclusion: Possibilities and Tensions*. Basingstoke: McMillan Press Ltd.

Stewart, P. (ed) (2004) *Employment, Trade Union Renewal and Future of Work*. Basingstoke: Palgrave.

Tarpey, M. and Watson, L. (1997) *Housing Need in Merton: People with Severe Mental Illness Living in Households*. London: London Borough of Merton.

Townsend, P. (1979) *Poverty in the United Kingdom*. Harmondsworth: Penguin.

Wallcraft, J. (2001) *Social Inclusion, Strategies for Living and Recovery*. Sainsbury Centre for Mental Health threaded discussion 20/06/2001 http://www.scmh.org.uk/website/threaded_discussion.nsf/0/17dbdfb0f19eb63c80256a71002c59c4?OpenDocument. Accessed March 2007.

Wallcraft, J., Read, J. and Sweeney, A. (2003) *On Our Own Terms*. London: Sainsbury Centre for Mental Health.

Walsh, E., Moran, P., Scott C., McKenzie, K., Burns, T., Creed, F., Tyrer P., Murray, R. M. and Fahy, T., (2003) Prevalence of violent victimisation in severe mental illness. *British Journal of Psychiatry*, 183(3): 233–238.

Williamson, M. (2006) *Improving the Health and Social Outcomes of People Recently Released from Prisons in the UK: A Perspective from Primary Care*. London, Sainsbury Centre for Mental Health.

25

Social Network Influence in Mental Health and Illness, Service Use and Settings, and Treatment Outcomes

Bernice A. Pescosolido

INTRODUCTION

Social networks, the ties or connections that exist among individuals in the community, in treatment systems, and in other institutions, have increasingly come to the fore in explaining a wide range of illness and disease prevalence, health behaviors, and health outcomes. We have been told that social networks are critical in understanding physical health problems like obesity and heart disease (Berkman and Syme, 1979; Christakis and Fowler, 2007), mental health problems such as suicide and substance abuse (Bearman, 1989; Pescosolido and Georgianna, 1989; Pescosolido et al., 2008), and negative behavioral health choices like smoking (Christakis and Fowler, 2008). Networks are even operant in the protein messaging system that influences key genetic processes implicated in disease (Barabasi, 2003).

Most of this is no surprise to sociologists, in general, or sociologists of mental health and illness, in particular, where the role of social networks has been implicated and studied in issues of onset (Pearlin and Aneshensel, 1986), treatment pathways (Clausen and Yarrow, 1955), treatment environments (Coser, 1958; Pescosolido et al., 1995), and outcomes like stigma (Goffman, 1963) since the beginnings of the discipline (Freeman, 2004; Pescosolido, 2000b, 2006b; Pescosolido and Levy, 2002). However, the recent resurgence of interest and activity surrounding social networks has brought about "new" claims. For example, Castells (2000) sees contemporary society as the "Network Society" and researchers from a wide variety of disciplines talk about the advent of "Network Science." For those who have drawn from and developed the social network perspective over the last hundred years of sociology, this may seem like either a welcome "rediscovery" of the central salience of a social network perspective or a sign of the lack of integration of social science into medical and mental health research. As Simmel (1955) originally noted and Castells (2000) recently reminded us, social networks are a very old form of social organization.

The purpose of this chapter is to review the nature, meaning and impact of social networks on all phases of the illness career for persons facing mental health problems. While a seemingly simple task, there are a number of confounding issues that prohibit a straightforward accounting of a cumulated body of findings. Despite the pervasive role of "others" in understanding mental health and mental illness, there have been different theoretical traditions, diverse methodological approaches, and even debates, about the proper focus of research. As a result, the chapter begins with some definitions and clarifications that allow a discussion of what the sociology of mental health has learned from the network perspective, and then ends with a conceptual map to facilitate the yet-to-be done research.

THE MEANING OF A SOCIAL NETWORK PERSPECTIVE

Social networks are basic building blocks of human experience. In a U.S. Institute of Medicine report, *From Neurons to Neighborhoods* (Shonkoff and Phillips, 2000), social network relationships are viewed as the "fundamental mediators of human adaptations" and the "active ingredients of environmental influence." Networks map the connections that individual or collective social actors have to one another. The generalized terms of "individual or collective social actors" is critical, and not jargon *per se*, because, in the mental health, social networks are often thought of as characteristics attached only to individuals (e.g., social support). However, networks also map relationships among organizations, for example, helping to describe the "cultural climate" in treatment units and its impact on care (Wright, 1997), or locating the "cracks" in social service systems (McKinney, 2002; Morrissey et al., 1994).

In a network perspective, individual actors are neither puppets of the social structure nor purely rational, calculating individuals. Individuals are "sociosyncratic," both acting and reacting to the social networks in their environment (Pescosolido, 1992). Individual actors are, however, always seen as interdependent rather than independent (Wasserman and Faust, 1994). Some theorists, like the 2009 Nobel Laureate Elinor Ostrom see networks as purposive action

(Ostrom, 1990; see also Coleman, 1990); however, networks may also be seen in a broader framework which includes habits and norms where the rational cost-benefit activation of network ties represents only one type of action (Pescosolido, 1992). In any case, the underlying engine of action in a social network approach is real human contact. As such, social network ties link levels of the environment and influences across time as social interactions influence what others do as individuals and as groups (Coleman, 1990; Giddens, 1990; Pescosolido, 1992; Stryker, 1980; Tilly, 1984).

This is the key: social networks provide the structural element of the mechanism of social interaction. Social networks build individuals' personal social support systems, they are the foundation of the therapeutic alliance, and they determine whether health care systems are integrated or fragmented. However, social networks are more than impartial or sterile connecting structures. They are neither randomly distributed nor egalitarian. They can be flat or hierarchical, facilitating or restricting access to resources, including treatment. Further, they hold important content. Interaction in social networks creates cultures of information (e.g., where can one get help for mental health problems), beliefs (e.g., what others, providers or friends, say causes mental illness), and action scripts (e.g., whether or not to seek formal care, what treatment regimes are suggested, and whether or not one should follow provider's recommendations). Network cultures can be parochial or cosmopolitan (Suchman, 1964); that is, they may support modern medicine views or reject them in favor of other systems of healing (e.g., traditional medicine, religion; Freidson, 1970).

Traditions, terms, and dimensions

One of the most vexing problems for mental health researchers and providers is trying to make sense of the different languages used in research on social ties and social interaction. Different strands of research have different theoretical starting points, data requirements and measures, methods of data collection, and analytic techniques. They continue to use different terms and draw only sporadically from one another (Pescosolido, 2006b; Thoits, 1995).

Perhaps the most "pure" network approach is represented by the *complete or full* network approach, which attempts to describe and analyze whole network system. This approach is seen in the recent findings on health behaviors and health status from the famous Framingham Heart Study in the U.S. Using the contact information that was collected to ensure finding respondents for later waves of the multi-decade study, Christakis and his colleagues (e.g., 2007) used this information to define the universe of ties for a specific and single geographical area (i.e., a small city in Massachusetts). With this creative use of what is usually practical information for study continuity, they have been able to show, for example, that individuals over time tended to form clusters of obese and normal weight individuals. This suggests that social interaction processes may underlie weight problems.

The *local or ego-centred approach* targets the ties surrounding particular individual actors. Here, the focus is on examining whether and how the structure of ties surrounding individuals who are selected for some reason (e.g., they have been diagnosed with mental illness) have been influential in shaping their entry into care or treatment outcomes. For example, early research (Hammer, 1983) documented that individuals who experience institutional care are likely to have small social networks to support them in their return to the community.

The *social support* perspective is more general and theory oriented, often using network imagery but tending to focus on the perceived overall state of an individual's social relationships and summary measures of the availability and effectiveness of ties. Here, in the classic Alameda County Study in the state of California, Berkman and Syme (1979) reported that individuals with more social support had lower rates of cardiac disease.

The *social capital* perspective is the most recent (and perhaps the most popularly persuasive) approach, focusing on the "good" things that flow along network ties (i.e., trust, solidarity) which are complementary to more economically focused human capital (e.g., education; Lin, 2000). For example, in one of many studies, Australian researchers found that three types of social capital (having trust in others, feeling safe and reporting reciprocity in social ties) were associated with lower risk for mental distress (Phongsavan et al., 2006). This approach is also represented in the mental health arena by the work of Nan Lin and his colleagues (e.g., Song and Lin, 2009).

The central "units" that have networks are referred to as nodes or actors. "Ties" are network connections between and among actors. They can be directed (e.g., advice about mental health problems sent or received from social ties) or not directed (e.g., the existence of contractual arrangements between two organizations in the mental health care system). Ties can simply map the existence of a relationship (e.g., a person is named or not named as a confidant) or be "valued" (e.g., a "closeness" value of the friendship or the monetary value of existing contracts). Given network ties, we can measure their number, strength (intensity or potency) and multiplexity (more than one type of connection underlying social interaction) which can tap into the potential impact and durability of connections and influence. The content or functions of networks include practical resources such as assistance (instrumental support); love, caring, and nurturing (emotional support); evaluations (appraisal); and guidance (monitoring). Ties can be latent (potential or dormant) or activated (used).

In sum, networks can have many possible features, forms, and functions. This complexity both belies the way most network research, especially mental health research, is conducted at this point, but speaks to the incredible potential to understand when, why and how individuals experience the onset of mental illness, how they respond, and whether treatment systems can help (see Pescosolido, 2006b for more substantive and technical detail on each tradition as well as graphical and terminologically description of network characteristics).

What networks are not

First, social networks are often cast as good; however, social interactions can be positive or negative, helpful or harmful. Networks can integrate individuals into a community and, just as powerfully, isolate individuals and regulate their behavior. They hold the potential to be rich sources of support, care and information, as well as monitoring, control and hassle (Pescosolido, 2000b). In fact, while sparse, research exploring the influence of negative ties in people's lives has found them to have powerful effects (Berkman, 1986; Pagel et al., 1987). Further, "more" is not necessarily better with regard to social ties. Too much oversight (regulation) or support (integration) can be stifling and repressive (Durkheim, 1951; Falci and McNeely, 2009; Pescosolido, 1994). While "strong" ties are often assumed to be better, "weak" ties can act as a bridge to different information and resources (Granovetter, 1982). The focus on social support, and now social capital, which tends to emphasize the positive, somewhat obfuscates the power of the "dark" aspects of social networks in research.

Second, while social networks create structures, they are not static. Ties are dynamic, and the ability to form and maintain social ties may be just as important as their state at one point in time. There may be changes in the total structure of networks or internal changes in membership. In fact, research suggests that while turnover rates in individuals' personal networks may hover around 50 percent, looking from the outside, there often appears to be little change in overall structure (Moody et al., 2005; Perry, 2005). Even when institutions change, what may matter is how network ties change. For example, health care reform inevitably involves shifts in social networks of power, changes in social networks within and between medical and social systems, and alterations in possible ties between patients and providers.

Third, while network theory focuses on the power of social interactions, it does not ignore other influences. While a network approach may reject the central focus on individuals, mental events, cognitive maps, or technological determinism (White, 1992), many of these factors come into play in shaping, modifying or mediating networks and their effects. Understanding how identity, cognition, technology, and biology shape the nature and influence of social ties becomes a critical part of unraveling complex health and health care outcomes (Pescosolido et al., 2008).

Fourth, despite the most visible social networks research on health at present (e.g., Christakis and Fowler, 2009), network research does not take a quantitative approach exclusively. In fact, a network perspective allows for, and even calls for, multimethod approaches. As, Jinnett et al. (2002) conclude, quantitative research is powerful in documenting the effects of social networks but only when accompanied by qualitative research that describes why they operate and look the way they do. There is no standard way to chart network relationships – they may be derived from a list on a survey where individuals are asked to name the people they ask for help or with whom they share health information (Pescosolido et al., 1998a). Alternatively, network data may come from observing the behavior of individuals (e.g., who they talk to as they solve health problems; Janzen, 1978) or from archival sources such as contact information in the Framingham Heart Study described above.

THE NETWORK PERSPECTIVE AND MENTAL HEALTH

Since the basic premise of network theory is that what individuals, organizations, and nations do is shaped, at least in part if not mainly, through consultation, resource sharing, suggestion, support, and nagging, it offers a dynamic approach, rooted in the community and its institutions, to understand (1) persons' risk of illness, disease, or disability; (2) their experiences in health care systems; and (3) their outcomes confronting these problems back in the receiving community. Because interaction in networks is conceptualized as the underlying *mechanism*, rather than one more "contingency" or "utility," they contextualize the response to health and health problems in everyday life.

Thus, social network theory and research "offer a way to think about community-based care or the health care system by looking to the set of social interactions that occur within them" (Pescosolido and Levy, 2002). Networks set a context in formal organizations and institutions for those who work in, or are served by them, which, in turn, affect what people do, how they feel, and what happens to them (Wright, 1997). Importantly, then, for issues of health and health care, social networks exist not only in the "lay" community, as is most commonly conceived, but also in the formal health care system since all health care is provided through human communication, with or without human touch, aided or devoid of human compassion, and in concert or opposition to community cultures (Hohmann, 1999; Pescosolido et al., 1995).

Social network approaches may have come to the fore in health and mental health research because of a basic frustration with research using socio-demographics. Variables such as age, race, education and gender are increasingly poor predictors of mental health and mental health/illness behavior and do not allow us to get underneath what is happening by offering a realistic mechanism to change mental health profiles or treatment systems. That is, networks provide a point of intervention that more stable or diffuse concepts do not. To change the risk of mental health or the efficacy of treatment, researchers and providers cannot alter individuals age, gender, ethnicity or income; however, they can try to change the social networks surrounding the delivery of care or that integrate providers and community ties, for example, through peer support efforts. As suggested earlier, what policy change often does is to affect the contacts that certain categories of people can or cannot have in the health care system and what kinds of ties can be sustained after treatment.

What do we know about networks and mental health?

All of the research that can be embraced under the umbrella of social networks cannot be summarized as an orderly set of findings. However, looking across these studies begins to produce some reliable conclusions. Below, I suggest six findings from contemporary research.

Finding #1. Social networks are implicated in mental health status and mental health care but their effects depend on the nature of the tie, and often the social context in which the network processes are operating

Networks can influence mental health, including severe mental illness like major depression as well as suicide, and substance abuse. The most expected findings suggest that individuals who report better family and friendship ties or who engage in more community participation have better mental health (Berry, 2008), while those who do not are likely to experience mental health problems from distress to disorder. For example, in the European KIDSCREEN study, families' poorer social support systems was associated with poorer mental health in children (Berry, 2008). Inadequate social support has been reported in the lives of individuals diagnosed with severe psychiatric problems (Okoro et al., 2009) and among users of a free clinic diagnosed with anxiety and depression (Cadzow and Servoss, 2009). Pearlin and Aneshensel (1986), using the stress process model, summarize the two ways that social networks can result in positive mental health outcomes. First, individuals who have better support systems tend to have fewer life events, experience less stress, and as a result, report fewer mental health problems. Second, social supports can buffer stress and interfere in the negative effect of life events on mental health.

However, social network ties do not always work the same for different groups of people or operate in expected, protective ways. In the National Latino and Asian-American Study (NLAAS) in the U.S., for women, the critical network ties that increased distress targeted the lack of family support, while for men distress was increased in the presence of family conflict (Masood et al., 2009). In Shanghai, China, male migrant workers reported negative mental health when confronted with difficulties in interpersonal or social companion ties, while women reported a lack of "esteem support" to be problematic (Wong and Leung, 2008).

Even more importantly perhaps, social networks can have complicated and simultaneous effects. Within the same social support systems, problematic social relationships result in more involuntary entrance to care while supportive ones in the same individuals" network bring individuals voluntarily into the mental health system. McLaughlin et al. (2002) show that the effects of positive and negative networks are not zero sums. In a study of individuals with dual diagnoses, they reported that family ties were both "good news and bad news" with regard to their mental health problems (Padgett et al., 2008), providing supports and producing hassles. Among school age populations, suicidal ideation was increased among those students who reported "too many" friends (Falci and McNeely, 2009).

On a larger scale, research on suicide suggests that even the same kinds of ties can operate differently. Religious ties can produce contexts of either too little or too much integration and regulation or offer a moderate level of both to create a social safety net in times of trouble. As Figure 25.1 indicates, county suicide rates are lowest where there are greater proportions of Catholics. However, in contemporary

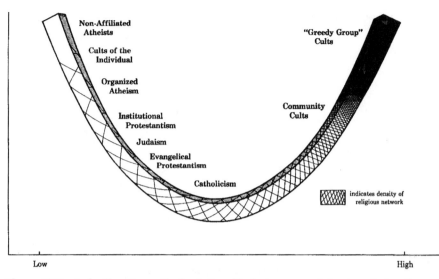

Non-Affiliated Atheists

Cults of the Individual

Organized Atheism

Institutional Protestantism

Judaism

Evangelical Protestantism

Catholicism

"Greedy Group" Cults

Community Cults

indicates density of religious network

Low   High

Figure 25.1   Inductive theoretical relationship between social network density and U.S. aggregate potential suicide rate, Pescosolido and Georgianna (1989). Reprinted with permission

U.S. populations, the negative effect of Protestantism that Durkheim (1951) predicted really depends on whether areas have more evangelical protestant groups like Seventh Day Adventists, or liberal/institutional protestant groups, such as Episcopalians. Individuals in the U.S. who belong to the evangelical protestant groups tend to report social networks made up of more coreligionists than those who belong to the liberal institutional protestant groups. In extreme cases where individuals have no ties into religious networks (e.g., atheists) or belong to cults, the propensity to suicide is heightened (Pescosolido and Georgianna, 1989).

Finding #2. Social networks and biological processes are both in operation in mental health status and mental health care. More central to the arguments here, networks can work with biology or genetics to interfere with or trigger genetic predispositions to mental health problems
Using data from one of the premier medical studies of alcoholism, a multidisciplinary team of researchers replicated findings on the importance of the GABRA2 gene in predisposing individuals to alcoholism. However, as Figure 25.2 illustrates, as individuals report greater amounts of social support from their families, the role of genetics may be virtually eliminated (Pescosolido et al., 2008). Research suggests that the parasympathetic system is involved when affect is regulated by social engagement (Willemen et al., 2008).

With regard to health care utilization for mental health problems, data from the Indianapolis Network Mental Health Study documented the joint operation of biological and social network influences in shaping pathways to care. Specifically, the interaction of networks (i.e., large networks) and one type of symptom profile

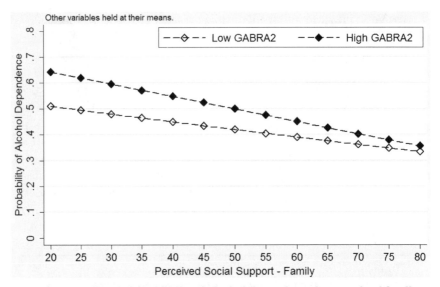

Figure 25.2 Predicted probabilities of alcohol dependence by perceived family support and GABRA 2 interaction, Collaborative Study of the Genetics of Alcoholism (COGA, N = 2,516), from Pescosolido et al. (2008). Reprinted with permission

(i.e., bipolar disorder) together shaped the coercive or involuntary pathways to treatment (Pescosolido et al., 1998; see also Carpentier and White, 2002).

Finding #3. Network contacts activated during an illness episode create a pathway to care; and these pathways, in tone as well as type, are shaped by the structure and content of individuals' network support system
Social interactions in the face of the onset of mental health problems not only influence what individuals do but, under a network perspective, are reconceptualized as network links that create a "treatment" pathway. In the U.K. Pathways to Care Study, Rogers et al. (1999) document that about 2/3 of people said that, during the episode of illness reported in their diaries, friends or relatives offered advice about self-care or suggested some form of treatment.

Individuals can combine different "advisors" to confront medical health problems. Even using a conservative accounting, the National Survey of American Life, which targeted American blacks, documented that almost half (41 percent) of individuals who indicated lifetime mood, anxiety or substance abuse disorders used both formal and informal sources of care and advice while 14 percent reported only formal care, 23 percent sought out only informal care and 22 percent reported no help-seeking. Those with greater social support used more informal sources which the authors see as an indication of the strong, preventive role that informal networks play in the lives of ethnic groups (Woodward et al., 2008). Other research suggests that this may be a more general response to mental illness, not limited to ethnic groups. For example, among older adults with serious mental illness, both formal and informal support reduced psychological distress; however the former also provided information while the latter provided no information on self-care (Cummings and Kropf, 2009).

Not only do the network lay and formal ties which are activated in response to mental illness create a pathway that ends up or does not end up in formal care, but they (1) set a tone for the pathways, (2) are shaped by the larger structure and content of the whole social network system in which individuals are embedded; and (3) help to explain inconsistencies in the mental health services literature that frustrated researchers for almost four decades. In a study of "first timers" of individuals using mental health services, fewer than half of individuals reported that their social interactions shaped pathways in which they made a decision, at some point, to use mental health care (45.9 percent, choice pathway). However, despite social pressure to the contrary, almost one-quarter of respondents (22.9 percent) reported that they actively resisted suggestions to seek formal care and continued to oppose treatment even as they received care (coercive pathways). They came into the mental health system against their will, forced into care by family, employers, and even the police. The remainder of this cohort were passive, entering care with neither choice nor resistance, through the actions of others (i.e., "muddling through"; 31.2 percent). And, as described above, those who reported coercive pathways to care had a unique combination of large social networks and bipolar disorder (Pescosolido et al., 1998).

However, the role of social networks in health care utilization research has been chequered, at best. For the most part, early research posited and documented, in both qualitative and quantitative studies, that social networks were essential to get into formal services (e.g., Lee, 1969). Horwitz's (1977) study of entry into the psychiatric emergency room found that social networks were critical, and in one of the most influential studies, Kadushin (1966) also documented that networks facilitated entry into treatment.

Yet, almost a decade of research followed that produced a series of inconsistent findings, leading researchers to abandon study of the role of social networks (McKinlay, 1972). More recently, using Puerto Rico as a case where social networks harbored negative beliefs and attitudes about the mental health system, we argued that the larger context in which networks are embedded matter. In a traditional, family-oriented society (unlike the upper west side of Manhattan which was the site of Kadushin's study), we found that large social networks in more traditional communities keep people out of formal treatment (Pescosolido et al., 1998b).

Theoretically, these findings help to unravel how social networks work in health care utilization. The structure of networks calibrated the "push" or amount of social influence, but only cultural context determined the direction of the trajectory, i.e. either toward or away from the formal medical system. When the push is great (i.e. in extended social networks) and beliefs held are in concert with modern scientific medical methods, the "lay referral system," as Freidson (1970) called it, pushes individuals into care. A similar network structure with beliefs in opposition to modern medical care would exert the same amount of influence but would likely do so in the opposite direction.

Finding #4. Networks in mental health treatment systems shape care and individuals'
recovery possibilities

Social networks among providers and between providers and clients exist inside
of treatment programs, shaping how health care services are provided; whether
they are accepted or rejected by individuals and the community; and what effect
they may have in the longer run (Coser, 1958; Wright, 1997). In treatment organizations characterized by supportive social ties among providers, families were
more likely to be brought into the treatment process (Wright, 1997) and these ties
were the major determinant of successful outcomes in treatment teams serving
children with mental health problems (Glisson and Hemmelgarn, 1998). Among
veterans, individuals with chronic psychological disorders who participated in
peer support activities longer and more often reported a greater recovery orientation (Barber et al., 2008). Further, individuals with serious mental illness who
received care in supportive (i.e., therapeutic community orientation) as opposed
to transitional (i.e., emphasis on practical skill development) sheltered care housing programs were more likely to develop emotional and instrumental networks
in the community (Segal and Holschuh, 1995). However, those who had been
treated in institutional settings had fewer multiplex ties (Holschuh and Segal,
2002). This was crucial since community-based social networks, in turn, resulted
in symptom reduction, prevented relapse and have been shown to be critical to
recovery (see also Cummings and Kropf, 2009).

Finding #5. Social networks not only affect the mental health status and behaviors of
individuals with mental illness, but they can reverberate through the community and
boomerang on the mental health of those who provide care

Outcomes are dependent not only on the social networks of the person with serious mental illness but also on the supports of the supporters. In the Finnish Health
2000 Study, the treatment team climate was associated with depression and antidepressant use among mental health *workers* (Sinokki et al., 2009). Outside of
the treatment staff, Suitor and Pillemer (2002) examined over 4,000 ties for over
400 caregivers of individuals with serious dementia, finding that women's social
ties influenced caregiver stress. Because women have more often taken on the
role of caregiver, their experience provided them with greater support resources
to face the stress of caregiving. Further, those who received support often mentioned the value of these experientially-based insights in and suggestions from
those who have been in similar situations. In other studies, family support mediated the intensity of the mental health distress experienced by daughters in their
role of caregivers of aging parents (Ron, 2009).

Findings #6: Networks exist within the mental health system organizations and between
the larger set of organizations that are critical for the housing, work and fiscal support
required for individuals with serious mental illness to recover in the community

A perennial complaint for both clients and providers is the lack of integrated
care among the organizations that compose the broader "mental health system"

including those that provide financial, housing and employment support. In the Robert Wood Johnson Program on Chronic Mental Illness, the establishment of a central mental health authority was able to reengineer the social network in this system, providing a more integrated set of network ties among them (Morrissey et al., 1994). Yet, it is in this aspect of illness careers and network systems that the research is most thin. In fact, despite the path breaking network approach in the RWJ-PCMI, the research that was designed to determine whether changes at the system level would "trickle down" to improve client outcomes simply used a parallel rather than integrated approach. That is, the researchers monitored client outcomes across the study period, but did not address whether and how clients' connections into the changing treatment and community systems may have been altered. Using this approach, researchers were unable to document positive changes in outcomes for clients (Shern et al., 1994). This conclusion and the lack of network research connecting these levels highlight the need for new designs, discussed in the conclusion, and for the centrality of integrated theoretical frameworks, which is discussed next. As Hawe et al. (2009) note, interventions are events in larger treatment and social service systems in which social networks connect people to the setting.

Providing a multi-level, dynamic frame for epidemiological, services, and outcomes research: The Network Episode Model

Elsewhere, I have argued that to address critical problems in understanding mental health, mental health service utilization and the outcomes of both, we need to have an organizing framework that can integrate our critical understandings about network influences and how they operate with other factors to affect the onset, recognition, response and outcomes of mental health problems. Such a framework or model to be used in integration must: (1) consider and articulate the full set of contextual levels documented in past empirical research to have impact; (2) offer an underlying mechanism or "engine of action" that connects levels, is dynamic, and allows for a way to narrow down focal research questions; (3) employ a metaphor and analytic language familiar to both social and natural science, so as to facilitate synergy; and (4) understand the need for and use the full range of methodological tools proven useful in the social and natural sciences (Pescosolido, 2006a). While many multilevel frameworks exist, they have not been widely adopted because they do not meet these requirements. As Mechanic (1990) notes, no widely shared and convincing view is available to replace the dominant individually focused theories of health and health care.

The Network-Episode Model (Pescosolido, 1991, 2006a, 2010; Pescosolido and Boyer, 1999) was developed to fill this gap. It holds the potential to answer the two critical problems facing the integration of biomedical science and social science conceptions of context. First, how do we pare down the innumerable possible hypotheses about the environment? Second, given the abstract nature of these influences, how can findings be translated into effective social and medical interventions?

The network perspective both simplifies and enriches theorizing, selection of research questions, and data collection in the complicated designs required to answer complex questions about the society–individual–biology interface. It starts with two basic ideas. First, the onset of mental health problems is fundamentally tied to the social network contexts in which individuals live their lives. Even in the presence of genetic predispositions, uncontrollable life events, or damaged organ systems, the social network ties that individuals have can play a role in shaping their effects on mental health or mental illness. While geneticists may find how networks among DNA clusters and messaging systems linked to RNA shape the predisposition to mental illness, social networks in personal network systems, organizations and communities likely shape and are shaped by these individual and biological systems. Social networks, whether lay or professional, may work to buffer or trigger that translation of predispositions into "treatable diagnoses." Second, dealing with mental health problems is a social process managed through the contacts that individuals have in the community, the treatment system and social service agencies. Interaction in social networks is the underlying mechanism at work in the recognition, diagnosis and treatment of mental health problems, thereby contextualizing the response to mental illness in everyday life.

In line with the general tenets of the network perspective described earlier, individuals are seen as pragmatic, having common-sense knowledge and cultural routines that they draw from past experience. People face mental illness by interacting with other people who may recognize (or deny) a mental health problem; send them to (or provide) treatment; and support, cajole or nag them about appointments, medications or lifestyle. Those who provide mental health or medical services as well as those who provide social services (including the all-too-often contact with the criminal justice system) have their own social networks and ties in a work culture that also sets norms and values regarding persons with mental illness; what could and should be done for them; and whether they, themselves, may confront psychological stressors in the face of the challenges of mental illness. These day-to-day encounters for lay and professional caregivers provide meaning to issues surrounding mental health and shape outcomes for persons with mental illness.

The naming of the NEM, in its early development, targeted the two most critical aspects of an approach which veered away from the dominant approaches to health services utilization (Pescosolido, 1991). First, as depicted in its original version, Figure 25.3 highlights the entire illness career, rather than any decision to seek assistance. Most research on mental health utilization focused on whether or not individuals received formal care. The typical dichotomy, as a dependent variable, de-contextualized the response to mental illness, even ignoring foundational sociological work which located the "sick role" in lay community networks (Parsons, 1951). The fundamental idea of the NEM-Phase I lay in the notion that the use of general or specialty providers was likely one in a series of ties that individuals activated to understand and respond to changes. In addition,

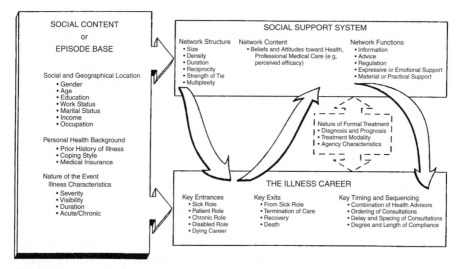

Figure 25.3   The Network-Episode Model – phase I. Pescosolido (1991). Reprinted with permission

individuals may end up in the same place (e.g., hospitalized), but, via different pathways which may be shaped by social network access and the resources (e.g., information, stigma) that they hold. To even understand how individuals with mental health problem get to formal care, their use (voluntary, involuntary or even by happenstance) of the wide range of available "medical advisors" is critical. Thus, the NEM Phase I shifted attention from a yes–no use of formal care or a count of the volume of visits/hospitalizations, etc. to the timing and sequencing of key role exits and entrances across an entire *episode*. Rather than "use," patterns and pathways to care, as part of a larger illness career, became the central focus. The initial version, as pictured, attempted to convey an emphasis on fluidity, time, and the co-construction of the problem and solutions to changes in mental health.

The NEM conceptualized response to illness as a social-influences process that works through the mechanism of networks. As described earlier, the NEM took from Freidson (1970) the idea that the content and structure of social networks in the community work together to determine the strength of social influence and the trajectory of addressing the mental health problem. Thus, the NEM begins with a focus on the illness career, with networks between and among individuals as an integrating mechanism. Primacy is given to studying interaction directly, and seeing networks as determining how individuals evaluate need, gather data, and perceive the sociocultural fit of available options. Similarly, because social networks can be harsh and controlling as well as supportive, the NEM-Phase I opened the question of the tone of the different pathways and gateways to care, bringing together research strands on utilization and forensics that had previously existed apart. In this initial phase, the nature of the illness, social location, or the effect of treatment were conceptualized as static, starting or potential intervention points affecting network and illness career trajectories.

Thus, the NEM-Phase I elaborated the central context and processes that distinguished it from other health and mental health utilization models (Pescosolido, 1991, 1992). A second version NEM (NEM Phase II, not pictured; see Pescosolido and Boyer, 1999, 2010) recognized the power of social networks in and between treatment and social service organizations and acknowledged the dynamic aspects of networks in these organizations. Social networks within large and sometimes daunting institutions such as the health care system were conceptualized as the organizing vector of environmental influences on treatment and outcomes. This conceptualization elaborated the effect of the dynamics of organizing and financing treatment systems on network ties in treatment sites, among providers, and between providers and patients, which reverberated on outcomes. It stipulated that if and how networks, whether lay or in other service systems, reinforced or clashed with treatment network recommendations was critical to individual and contextual outcomes. Thus, the NEM–Phase II moved from the notion that social networks are everywhere and can be anything to a more sophisticated view of real organizational structures, distinct levels of analysis, and the changing dynamics of health care systems.

Until recently, the NEM has focused primarily on the *consequences* of illnesses – it was a health services research model. However, the line between the community and treatment systems is both an artificial one from the client's perspective and an unnecessary one from the point of view of the NEM which targeted individuals' illness careers – *in situ* from the community to wherever individuals "travelled." The NEM-Phase III recalibrated its starting point to the *causes* of disease, which bridges the artificial divide between epidemiology, services and outcomes research to consider the totality of people's lives. This not only opened the way to think about the interaction between biology and society in the causes and responses to illness but also to the potential ways that illness careers can change individuals biologically.

Figure 25.4 presents the Network Episode Model (NEM-Phase III). While space and goals for this chapter do not permit a full elaboration of the propositions and hypotheses under the this version, (see Pescosolido, 2010) Figure 25.4 provides a visual elaboration of contexts or network systems that are in operation three levels above the individual's illness career and two levels below it. The complexities of the illness career remain as the central set of phenomena to be examined and explained. Networks remain as the mechanism connecting different levels and marking changing processes and dynamics. While the NEM-Phase III allows for research by geneticists and other biomedical scientists who are moving to network models within their areas of research (e.g., Antonov et al., 2006; Brazhnik, 2005), the NEM's goals at this point are limited only to understanding social network influences at contextual levels "at" or "above" the illness career and interactions with levels "below" it that shape illness careers and outcomes.

Depicted in the top level of Figure 25.4, and reflecting the recent resurgence on intent on "space" or "place," geographic areas have been shown to influence

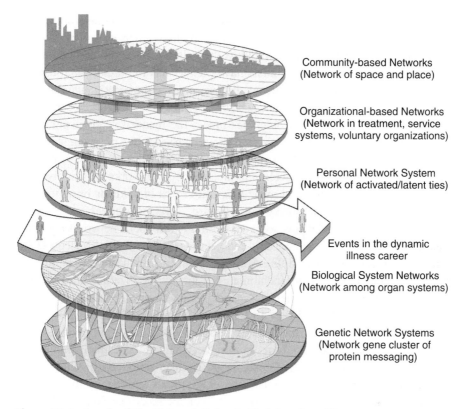

Community-based Networks
(Network of space and place)

Organizational-based Networks
(Network in treatment, service
systems, voluntary organizations)

Personal Network System
(Network of activated/latent ties)

Events in the dynamic
illness career

Biological System Networks
(Network among organ systems)

Genetic Network Systems
(Network gene cluster of
protein messaging)

Figure 25.4   Levels of the Network-Episode Model – phase III

health, illness, preventive care, treatment rates and types, and outcomes. More to the point, "place-based contacts' have been shown to shape important mental health phenomena (e.g., PTSD, Kadushin, 1983; suicide, Pescosolido and Georgianna, 1989). Even in the era of the internet, social networks in communities can facilitate or hinder the formation and activation of social networks, the access to and use of different networks of "advisors," and outcomes.

Similarly, a second contextual level shaping the dynamics of the illness career lies in the social networks within and among organizations, whether they are designed to provide care or not. Certainly, workplaces and worker networks are crucial to service use since Employee Assistance Programs (EAPs) in the U.S. can recommend or even require use of mental health services, and events as simple as health exams for insurance benefits, can begin illness careers not yet even acknowledged by individuals or their personal social network support system. With regard to treatment organizations, a network approach opens up the "black box" of formal care by seeing services, at least in part, as the human provision of care (Pescosolido, 2000a). While internal networks are not "treatment," any diagnostic, treatment or rehabilitation instrument, medication or manipulation is delivered by human providers in human service organizations. Interventions determine "what" is offered. Internal networks shape "how" it is implemented, whether potential challenges are reconciled with the community network or not, and ultimately, what outcomes are experienced by individuals with mental health problems. This separation of community, writ large, from the community of organizations with which individuals have contact has important ramifications for potential policy and system change. For example, setting up a standard mental health facility in a community that does or does not have networks of trust can produce less than satisfactory outcomes unless the medical needs, community context, and critical community partners are addressed in the planning stages.

Finally, the NEM-Phase III acknowledges the importance of two systems that exist "below" the individual level. Individuals' social networks are not divorced from the body and the physical/mental capacities that individuals bring to them (Leventhal et al., 1997; Orlinsky and Howard, 1987; Rosenfeld and Wenzel, 1997). For example, social psychologists examine how social networks and their influences vary with personality, age, and gender (Gadalla, 2008; Hurlbert et al., 2000; Suitor and Pillemer, 2002). Self and identity provide the filter through which the social environment, including community, organization, and personal networks, come to have personal meaning and encounter biology (Crocker and Quinn, 2001; McLeod and Lively, 2003; Stryker, 1980). The onset of symptoms of mental illness, for example, causes profound disruptions and shapes basic cognitive processes that have, in turn, been linked to treatment and health outcomes (Breier et al., 1991; Green, 1996; Lysaker et al., 2000). Further, no matter what social networks are available, individuals' abilities to use them or even acknowledge them may be hindered by genetic inheritance and predispositions, as well as by the symptoms. As depicted in Figure 25.2, even relatively poor measures of social network supports reveal a powerful dampening effect on a widely accepted deleterious candidate gene for the probability of alcohol dependence (Pescosolido et al., 2008). The NEM-Phase III emphasizes that the network approach requires a systematic accounting of whether the number, duration, valence, and strength of social ties make phenotypic expression from genotypic predisposition either more likely or less likely, or whether social ties are even implicated in adaptations of genetic profiles (see Pescosolido, 2010).

FUTURE CHALLENGES FOR THEORY, RESEARCH, AND POLICY

What we know about the role of social networks in the onset, treatment, and outcomes of mental illness is noteworthy and promising. Taking this approach allows us to take a new, but perhaps more complex, look at how human interconnections matter for mental health, for mental health research and for directions in social policy. However, caution is warranted. The broad-based findings which seem to lead us to this point have been carved out more with a machete than a scalpel. At this point in time, we know much more about the basic empirical finding that having social networks matter, than how or why they operate, where they come from, how they are activated or how they are meshed with psychological, biological or clinical factors. Though it is scientifically comforting that different traditions, different methods and different data all seem to coincide to reach the six major findings that are reported here, much more work needs to be done before particular programs are enacted.

Current research is useful in changing the awareness of researchers, providers and policymakers to the potential of changing systems through reengineering social contacts. But the question arises as to what kinds of contacts and how to intervene within the bounds of ethics. Certainly, it is easier to suggest a different medication than it is to suggest different friends. And, which friends? Researchers have documented that significant others played, in their words, "a variable role" in medication adherence among individuals with schizophrenia (McCann et al., 2008). Other research found "intentional friends" to be a potent and cost-effective way to help integrate individuals with serious mental illness into the wider receiving community (McCorkle et al., 2009).

Nevertheless, existing network research provides a critical sensitizing function: perhaps the human networks around individuals in the community and the treatment center need to be considered and studied along with the introduction of technological, programmatic or pharmacological intervention. Detailed social network data on form, content and function should be included in randomized clinical trials, and in epidemiological survey-based and institutional data collection. This will not be easily accomplished since these data require revamping of our measurement tools and require more time than the typical social support battery.

If networks matter, do we need to know *which* networks are potent vectors of disorder or protection? Researchers call for understanding how perceived need for mental health treatment is shaped by social networks (Garrido et al., 2009); but, again, *which* networks? The most commonly used "network generator" in ego-centric research is the "important matters" question in the U.S. General Social Survey (i.e., "From time to time, most people discuss important matters with other people. Looking back over the last six months – who are the people with whom you discussed matters important to you? Just tell me their first names or initials'; Marsden, 1987). However, in recent analyses, we have found that it is the specific "health matters" network, rather than the "important matters" network that seems to be associated with better outcomes for "first timers" in the Indianapolis Network Mental Health Study of respondents with serious mental illness (Perry and Pescosolido, 2010).

In addition, we need to take general ideas about networks and tailor them to particular populations or problems. To some extent, this has been done as the NEM has been adapted for children (Costello et al., 1998), and for understanding the implications of different "portals" into the social service system for children with mental health problems (Stiffman et al., 2004), and for understanding how the interface between community and treatment systems shapes health disparities (Alegria et al., 2010). Further, we are past the point where researchers can choose between the social support and a social traditions approach, for instance. Both hold a piece of the network and have to be considered together in more sophisticated ways in future research. As an interdisciplinary and international workgroup has done, and continues to do for the problems surrounding sustainability in socio-ecological systems, we need to detail the primary and secondary levels of factors at work and the measures that capture them reliably (Ostrom, 2009). In sum, deciding which kinds of social networks are of interest, how to elicit the ties, and how to track their dynamics remain as critical issues (Berkman, 1986; House et al., 1982; Leik and Chalkey, 1996; O'Reilly, 1998; Suitor et al., 1996; Wellman et al., 1996).

Relevant networks can be measured reliably and accurately, at least to accepted standards (Pescosolido and Wright, 2004; Wright and Pescosolido, 2002). This is important because data from individuals who may have been seen as too impaired by some to provide accurate information (i.e., persons with serious mental health problems), reinforce notions of empowerment and align with consumer perspectives (Jivanjee et al., 2008). But some studies echo concerns of families and advocates, finding that clinical staff had much less regard for informal support in treatment than did potential clients (Jorm et al., 2008). As pharmacological solutions and insurance reimbursement continue to both help and hinder the range of treatment that can be offered by mental health providers, the social network perspective reminds us that the therapeutic community, both inside and outside the formal walls of clinics and hospitals, present an enormous opportunity for improving the lives of people with mental illness.

ACKNOWLEDGEMENTS

Parts of this paper were presented at the U.S. National Institute of Drug Abuse (NIDA), *Exploring Interconnections: A Network Dynamics Workshop for Understanding and Preventing Adolescent and Young Adults Substance Abuse*, January, 2010. Support is acknowledged from the National Institute of Mental Health; the Indiana Consortium for Mental Health Services Research (ISMHSR), Indiana University; and the College of Arts and Sciences (COAS), Indiana University.

REFERENCES

Alegria, Margarita, and Bernice A. Pescosolido (2010) Taking health disparities to task: the socio-cultural framework. In Bernice A. Pescosolido, Jane D. McLeod, Jack K. Martin, and Anne Rogers (eds) *The Handbook of the Sociology of Health, Illness, and Healing: Blueprint for the 21st Century*. New York, NY: Springer.

Antonov, Alexey V., Igor V. Tetko, and Hans-Werner Mewes (2006) A systematic approach to infer biological relevance and biases of gene network structures. *Nucleic Acids, Research*, 34: e6.

Barabasi, Albert-Laszlo (2003) *Linked: How Everything is Connected to Everything Else and What It Means*. New York: Plume.

Barber, Jessica A., Robert A. Rosenheck, Moe Armstrong, and Sandra G. Resnick (2008) Monitoring the dissemination of peer support in the VA healthcare system. *Community Mental Health Journal*, 44: 433–441.

Bearman, Peter (1989) Social structures: a network approach. *American Journal of Sociology*, 94(6): 1512–1514.

Berkman, Lisa (1986) Social networks, support, and health: taking the next step forward. *American Journal of Epidemiology*, 123: 559–562.

Berkman, Lisa F. and S. Leonard Syme (1979) Social networks, host resistance, and mortality: a nine-year follow-up study of Alameda County residents. *American Journal of Epidemiology*, 109: 186–204.

Berry, Helen Louise (2008) Social capital elite, excluded participators, busy working parents and aging, participating less: Types of community participators and their mental health. *Social Psychiatry and Psychiatric Epidemiology*, 43: 527–537.

Brazhnik, Paul (2005) Inferring gene networks from steady-state response to single-gene perturbations. *Journal of Theoretical Biology*, 237: 427–440.

Breier, Alan, Judith L. Schreiber, Janyce Dyer, and David Pickar (1991) National Institute of Mental Health longitudinal study of chronic schizophrenia: prognosis and predictors of outcome. *Archives of General Psychiatry*, 48: 239–246.

Cadzow, R.B. and T.J. Servoss (2009) The association between perceived social support and health among patients at a free urban clinic. *Journal of the National Medical Association*, 101: 243–250.

Carpentier, Normand and Deena White (2002) Cohesion of the primary social network and sustained service use before the first psychiatric hospitalization. *Journal of Behavioral Health Services and Research*, 29: 404–418.

Castells, M. (2000) Toward a sociology of the network society. *Contemporary Sociology*, 29: 693–699.

Christakis, Nicholas A. and J.H. Fowler (2007) The spread of obesity in a large social network over 32 years. *New England Journal of Medicine*, 357: 370–379.

Christakis, Nicholas A. and J.H. Fowler (2008) Dynamics of smoking behavior in a large social network. *New England Journal of Medicine*, 358: 2249–2258.

Christakis, Nicholas A. and J.H. Fowler (2009) *Connected: The Surprising Power of Our Social Networks and How They Shape Our Lives*. New York: Little Brown.

Clausen, John A. and Marian Radke Yarrow (1955) Pathways to the mental hospital. *Journal of Social Issues*, 11: 25–32.

Coleman, James S. (1990) *Foundations of Social Theory*. Cambridge, MA: The Belknap Press of Harvard University.

Coser, Rose Laub (1958) Authority and decision-making in a hospital: a comparative analysis. *American Sociological Review*, 23: 56–63.

Costello, E. Jane, Bernice A. Pescosolido, Adrian Angold, and Barbara J. Burns (1998) A family network-based model of access to child mental health services. In J.P. Morissey (ed.) *Social Networks and Mental Illness*. Stamford, CT: JAI Press. pp. 165–190.

Crocker, Jennifer and Diane M. Quinn (2001) Psychological consequences of devalued identities. In R. Brown and S. Gaertner (eds) *Blackwell Handbook in Social Psychology*. Malden, MA: Blackwell. pp. 238–257.

Cummings, Sherry M. and Nancy P. Kropf (2009) Formal and informal support for older adults with severe mental illness. *Aging and Mental Health*, 13: 619–627.

Durkheim, Emile (1951) *Suicide*. New York: Free Press.

Falci, Christina, and Clea McNeely (2009) Too many friends: social integration, network cohesion and adolescent depressive symptoms. *Social Forces*, 87: 2031–2062.

Freeman, Linton C. (2004) *The Development of Social Network Analysis: A Study in the Sociology of Science*. Vancouver, BC: Empirical Press.

Freidson, Eliot (1970) *Profession of Medicine: A Study of the Sociology of Applied Knowledge*. New York: Dodd, Mead, and Co.

Gadalla, Tahany M. (2008) Comparison of users and non-users of mental health services among depressed women: A national study. *Women and Health*, 47: 1–19.

Garrido, Melissa M., Robert L. Kane, Merrie Kaas, and Rosalie Kane (2009) Perceived need for mental health care among community-dwelling older adults. *Journals of Gerontology: Series B – Psychological Sciences and Social Sciences*, 64: 704–712.

Giddens, Anthony (1990) *The Consequences of Modernity*. Stanford, CA: Stanford University Press.

Glisson, Charles and Anthony Hemmelgarn (1998) The effects of organizational climate and interorganizational coordination on the quality and outcomes of children's service systems. *Child Abuse and Neglect*, 22: 401–421.

Goffman, Erving (1963) *Stigma: Notes on the Management of Spoiled Identity*. Englewood Cliffs, NJ: Prentice-Hall.

Granovetter, Mark (1982) The strength of weak ties: A network theory revisited. In P. Marsden and N. Lin (eds) *Social Structure and Network Analysis*. Thousand Oaks, CA: SAGE. pp. 105–130.

Green, Michael F. (1996) What are the functional consequences of neurocognitive deficits in schizophrenia? *American Journal of Psychiatry*, 153: 321–330.

Hammer, Muriel (1983) 'Core' and 'extended' social networks in relation to health and illness. *Social Science and Medicine*, 17: 405–411.

Hawe, Penelope, Alan Shiell, and Therese Riley (2009) Theorising interventions as events in systems. *American Journal of Community Psychology*, 43: 267–276.

Hohmann, Ann A. (1999) A contextual model for clinical mental health effectiveness research. *Mental Health Services Research*, 1: 83–91.

Holschuh, Jane and Steven P. Segal (2002) Factors related to multiplexity in support networks of persons with severe mental illness. In Judith A. Levy and Bernice A. Pescosolido (eds) *Social Networks and Health*. New York: JAI/Elsevier Science. pp 293–322.

Horwitz, Allan V. (1977) The pathways into psychiatric treatment: Some differences between men and women. *Journal of Health and Social Behavior*, 18: 169–178.

House, J.S., Robbins, C. and Metzner H.L. (1982) The association of social relationships and activities with mortality: Prospective evidence from the Tecumseh Community Health Study. *American Journal of Epidemiology*, 116: 123–140.

Hurlbert, Jeanne S., Valerie A. Haines, and John J. Beggs (2000) Core networks and tie activation: what kinds of routine networks allocate resources in nonroutine situations. *Amercian Sociological Review*, 65: 598–618.

Janzen, John M. (1978) *The Quest for Therapy in Lower Zaire*. Berkeley, CA: University of California Press.

Jinnett, K., Coulter, I. and Koegel P. (2002) Cases, context and care: The need for grounded network analysis. In Judith A. Levy and Bernice A. Pescosolido (eds) *Advences in Medical Sociology: Social Networks and Health*. Oxford, U.K.: Elsevier Science.

Jivanjee, Pauline, Jean Kruzich, and Lynwood J. Gordon (2008) Community integration of transition-age individuals: Views of young with mental health disorders. *Journal of Behavioral Health Services and Research*, 35: 402–418.

Jorm, Anthony F., Amy J. Morgan, and Annemarie Wright (2008) Interventions that are helpful for depression and anxiety in young people: A comparison of clinicians' beliefs with those of youth and their parents. *Journal of Affective Disorders*, 111: 227–234.

Kadushin, Charles (1966) The friends and supporters of psychotherapy: On social circles in urban life. *American Sociological Review*, 31: 786.

Kadushin, Charles (1983) Mental health and the interpersonal environment: Reexamination of some effects of social structure on mental health. *American Sociological Review*, 48: 188–198.

Lee, Nancy Howell (1969) *The Search for an Abortionist*. Chicago, IL: University of Chicago Press.

Leik, R.K. and M.A. Chalkey (1996) On the stability of network relations under stress. *Social Networks*, 19: 63–74.

Leventhal, Howard, Elaine A. Leventhal, and Richard J. Contrada (1997) Self-regulation, health and behavior: A perceptual-cognitive approach. *Psychology and Health*, 12: 1–17.

Lin, Nan (2000) Inequality in social capital. *Contemporary Sociology*, 29: 785–795.

Lysaker, Paul H., Gary Bryson, Tamasine Greig, and Morris D. Bell (2000) Emotional discomfort and impairments in verbal memory in schizophrenia. *Psychiatry Research*, 97: 51–59.

Marsden, Peter (1987) Core discussion networks of Americans. *American Sociological Review*, 52: 122–131.

Masood, Nausheen, Sumie Okazaki, and David T. Takeuchi (2009) Gender, family, and community correlates of mental health in South Asian Americans. *Cultural Diversity and Ethnic Minority Psychology*, 15: 265–274.

McCann, T.V., G. Boardman, E. Clark, and S. Lu (2008) Risk profiles for non-adherence to antipsychotic medications. *Journal of Psychiatric and Mental Health Nursing*, 15: 622–629.

McCorkle, Brian H., Erin C. Dunn, Mui Wan Yu, and Cheryl Gagne (2009) Compeer friends: A qualitative study of a volunteer friendship programme for people with serious mental illness. *International Journal of Social Psychiatry*, 55: 291–305.

McKinlay, John (1972) Some approaches and problems in the study of the use of services: An overview. *Journal of Health and Social Behavior*, 13: 115–152.

McKinney, Martha M. (2002) Variations in rural AIDS epidemiology and service delivery models in the united states. *Journal of Rural Health*, 18: 455–466.

McLaughlin, Julie, Allan Horwitz, and Helene Raskin White (2002) The differential importance of friend, relative and partner relationships for the mental health of young adults. In Judith A. Levy and Bernice A. Pescosolido (eds) *Social Networks and Health (Advances in Medical Sociology, Volume 8)*. New York, NY: JAI Press. pp. 223–246.

McLeod, Jane D. and Kathryn J. Lively (2003) Social structure and personality. In J. DeLamater (ed.) *Handbook of Social Psychology*. New York: Kluwer/Plenum. pp. 77–102.

Mechanic, David (1990) The role of sociology in health affairs. *Health Affairs*, 9: 85–97.

Moody, James, Daniel A. McFarland, and Skye Bender-DeMoll (2005) Dynamic network visualization: Methods for meaning with longitudinal network movies. *American Journal of Sociology*, 110: 1206–1241.

Morrissey, Joseph P., Michael O. Calloway, W. Todd Bartko, M. Susan Ridgely, Howard H. Goldman, and Robert I. Paulson (1994) Local mental health authorities and service system change: Evidence from the Robert Wood Johnson Program on Chronic Mental Illness. *The Milbank Quarterly*, 72: 49–80.

O'Reilly, P. 1998 Methodological issues in social support and social network research. *Social Science and Medicine*, 26: 863–873.

Okoro, Catherine A., Tara W. Strine, Lina S. Balluz, John E. Crews, Satvinder Dhingra, Joyce T. Berry, and Ali H. Mokdad (2009) Serious psychological distress among adults with and without disabilities. *International Journal of Public Health*, 54: 52–60.

Orlinsky, D., and K. Howard (1987) A general model of psychotherapy. *Journal of Integrative and Eclectic Psychotherapy*, 6: 6–27.

Ostrom, Elinor (1990) *Governing the Commons: The Evolution of Institutions for Collective Action (Political Economy of Institutions and Decisions)*. Cambridge University Press.

Ostrom, Elinor (2009) A general framework for analyzing sustainability of social-ecological systems. *Science*, 325: 419–422.

Padgett, Deborah K., Ben Henwood, Courtney Abrams, and Robert E. Drake (2008) Social relationships among persons who have experienced serious mental illness, substance abuse, and homelessness: Implications for recovery. *American Journal of Orthopsychiatry*, 78: 333–339.

Pagel, Mark D., William W. Erdly, and Joseph Becker (1987) Social networks: We get by with (and in spite of) a little help from our friends. *Journal of Personality and Social Psychology*, 53: 793–804.

Parsons, Talcott (1951) *The Social System: The Major Exposition of the Author's Conceptual Scheme for the Analysis of the Dynamics of the Social System*. New York, NY: Free Press.

Pearlin, Leonard I., and Carol S. Aneshensel (1986) Coping and social supports: Their functions and applications. In David Mechanic and L.H. Aiken (eds) *Applications of Social Science to Clinical Medicine and Health Policy*. New Brunswick, NJ: Rutgers University Press. pp. 417–437.

Perry, Brea L. (2005) Pre-disease pathways: Integrating biological, psychological, and sociological perspectives on health and illness. In *The Handbook of Medical Sociology*.

Perry, Brea L., and Bernice A. Pescosolido (in press) Functional specificity in discussion networks: Social regulation and the influence of problem-specific networks on health outcomes. In *Social Networks*.

Pescosolido, Bernice A. (1991) Illness careers and network ties: A conceptual model of utilization and compliance. In Gary L. Albrecht and Judith A. Levy (eds) *Advances in Medical Sociology*. CT: JAI Press. pp. 161–184.

Pescosolido, Bernice A. (1992) Beyond rational choice: The social dynamics of how people seek help. *American Journal of Sociology*, 97: 1096–1138.

Pescosolido, Bernice A. (1994) Bringing Durkheim into the 21st century: A social network approach to unresolved issues in the study of suicide. In D. Lester (ed.) *Emile Durkheim: Le Suicide – 100 Years Later*. Philadelphia: The Charles Press. pp. 264–295.

Pescosolido, Bernice A. (2000a) Rethinking models of health and illness behaviour. In M. Kelner, B. Wellman, M. Saks, and B.A. Pescosolido (eds) *Complementary and Alternative Medicine: Challenge and Change*. Harwood Academic Publishers. pp. 175–193.

Pescosolido, Bernice A. (2000b) The role of social networks in the lives of persons with disabilities. In Gary L. Albrecht, Katherine D. Seelman, and Michael Bury (eds) *Handbook of Disability Studies*. Sage Publications. pp. 468–489.

Pescosolido, Bernice A. (2006a) Of pride and prejudice: The role of sociology and social networks in integrating the health sciences. *Journal of Health and Social Behavior*, 47: 189–208.

Pescosolido, Bernice A. (2006b) The sociology of social networks. In Clifton D. Bryant and Dennis L. Peck (eds). *The Handbook of 21st Century Sociology*. Thousand Oaks, CA: Sage Publications. pp. 208–217.

Pescosolido, Bernice A. (2010) Organizing the sociological landscape for the next decades of health and health care research: the Network Episode Model III-R as cartographic subfield guide. In Bernice A. Pescosolido, Jack K. Martin, Jane D. McLeod, and Anne Rogers (eds). *The Handbook of the Sociology of Health, Illness, and Healing*. New York: Springer.

Pescosolido, Bernice A. and Carol A. Boyer (1999) How do people come to use mental health services? Current knowledge and changing perspectives. In Allan V. Horwitz and Teresa L. Scheid (eds) *A Handbook for the Study of Mental Health: Social Contexts, Theories, and Systems*. New York: Cambridge University Press.

Pescosolido, Bernice A. and Carol A. Boyer (2010) Understanding the context and dynamic processes of mental health treatment. In Teresa L. Scheid and Tony N. Brown (eds). *Handbook for the Study of Mental Health: Social Contexts, Theories, and Systems*. Cambridge University Press. pp. 420–438.

Pescosolido, Bernice A., and Sharon Georgianna (1989) Durkheim, religion, and suicide: toward a network theory of suicide. *American Sociological Review*, 54: 33–48.

Pescosolido, Bernice A. and Judith A. Levy (2002) The role of social networks in health, illness, disease and healing: The accepting present, the forgotten past, and the dangerous potential for a complacent future. *Social Networks and Health*, 8: 3–25.

Pescosolido, Bernice A. and Eric R. Wright (2004) The view from two worlds: The convergence of social network reports between mental health clients and their ties. *Social Science and Medicine*, 58: 1795–1806.

Pescosolido, Bernice A., Eric R. Wright, and William P. Sullivan (1995) Communities of care: A theoretical perspective on care management models in mental health. In G. Albrecht (ed.). *Advances in Medical Sociology*. Greenwich, CT: JAI Press. pp. 37–80.

Pescosolido, Bernice A., Carol Brooks-Gardner, and Keri M. Lubell (1998a) How people get into mental health services: Stories of choice, coercion and 'muddling through' from 'first-timers'. *Social Science and Medicine*, 46: 275–286.

Pescosolido, Bernice A., Eric R. Wright, Margarita Alegria, and Mildred Vera (1998b) Social networks and patterns of use among the poor with mental health problems in Puerto Rico. *Medical Care*, 36: 1057–1072.

Pescosolido, Bernice A., Brea L. Perry, J. Scott Long, Jack K. Martin, Jr John I. Nurnberger and Victor Hesselbrock (2008) Under the influence of genetics: how transdisciplinarity leads us to rethink social pathways to illness. *American Journal of Sociology,* 114: S171–S201.

Phongsavan, P., T. Chey, A. Bauman, R. Brooks, and D. Silove (2006) Social capital, socio-economic status and psychological distress among Australian adults. *Social Science and Medicine,* 63: 2546–2561.

Rogers, Anne, Karen Hassell and Gerry Nicolaas (1999) *Demanding Patients? Analysing the Use of Primary Care.* Philadelphia: Open University Press.

Ron, Pnina (2009) Daughters as caregivers of aging parents: The shattering myth. *Journal of Gerontological Social Work,* 52: 135–153.

Rosenfeld, S. and S. Wenzel (1997) social networks and chronic mental illness: a test of four perspectives. *Social Problems,* 44: 200–216.

Segal, S.P. and Jane Holschuh (1995) Reciprocity in support networks of sheltered-care residents. In R.K. Price, B.M. Shea, and H.N. Mookerjee (eds). *Social Psychiatry Across Cultures: Studies from North America, Asia, Europe, and Africa.* New York, NY: Plenum. pp. 73–86.

Shern, D.L., N.Z. Wilson, A.S. Coen, D.C. Patrick, M. Foster, D.A. Bartsch, and J. Demmler (1994) Client outcomes II: Longitudinal client data from the Colorado Treatment Outcome Study. *The Milbank Quarterly,* 72: 123–148.

Shonkoff, Jack P. and Deborah A. Phillips (2000) *From Neurons to Neighborhoods: The Science of Early Childhood Development. Institute of Medicine Committee Report.* Washington DC: National Academy Press.

Simmel, Georg (1955) *Conflict and the Web of Group Affiliations.* New York: Free Press.

Sinokki, M., Hinkka, K. Ahola, K. Koskinen, S. Klaukka, T. Kivimaki, M. Puukka, P. Jouko Lonnqvist, and Virtanen M. (2009) The association between team climate at work and mental health in the Finnish Health, 2000 study. *Occupational and Environmental Medicine,* 66: 523–528.

Song, Lijun and Nan Lin (2009) Social capital and health inequality: Evidence from Taiwan. *Journal of Health and Social Behavior,* 50: 149–163.

Stiffman, Arlene R., Bernice A. Pescosolido, and Leopoldo J. Cabassa (2004) Building a model to understand youth service access: The Gateway Provider Model. *Mental Health Services Research,* 6: 189–198.

Stryker, Sheldon (1980) *Symbolic Interactionism.* Menlo Park, CA: Benjamin/Cummings.

Suitor, Jill J., and Karl Pillemer (2002) Gender, social support, and experiential similarity during chronic stress: The case of family caregivers. In Judith A. Levy and Bernice A. Pescosolido (eds). *Advances in Medical Sociology: Social Networks and Health.* New York, NY: JAI Press. pp. 247–266.

Suitor, J.J., B. Wellman, and D.L. Morgan (1996) It's about time: How, why, and when networks change. *Social Networks,* 19: 1–8.

Thoits, P. (1995) Stress, coping, and social support processes: Where are we? What next? *Journal of Health and Social Behavior.* Extra Issue: 53–79.

Tilly, Charles (1984) *Big Structures, Large Processes, Huge Comparisons.* New York: Russell Sage.

Wasserman, Stanley and Katherine B. Faust (1994) *Social Network Analysis: Methods and Applications.* New York, NY: Cambridge University Press.

Wellman, Barry, Renita Wong, David Tindall, and Nancy Nazer (1996) A decade of network change: Turnover, persistence and stability in personal communities. *Social Networks,* 19: 27–50.

White, Harrison C. (1992) *Identity and Control: A Structured Theory of Social Action.* Princeton, NJ: Princeton University Press.

Willemen, Agnes M., Frits A. Goossens, Hans M. Koot, and Carlo Schuengel (2008) Physiological reactivity to stress and parental support: Comparison of clinical and non-clinical adolescents. *Clinical Psychology and Psychotherapy,* 15: 340–351.

Wong, Daniel Fu Keung, and Grace Leung (2008) The functions of social support in the mental health of male and female migrant workers in China. *Health and Social Work,* 33: 275–285.

Woodward, Amanda Toler, Robert Joseph Taylor, Kai McKeever Bullard, Harold W. Neighbors, Linda M. Chatters, and James S. Jackson (2008) Use of professional and informal support by African Americans and Caribbean blacks with mental disorders. *Psychiatric Services,* 59: 1292–1298.

Wright, Eric R. (1997) The impact of organizational factors on mental health professionals involvement with families. *Psychiatric Services,* 48: 921–927.

Wright, E.R. and B.A. Pescosolido (2002) Sorry, I forgot: The role of recall error in longitudinal personal network studies. *Social Networks and Health,* 8: 113–129.

Index

Figures in **bold**; Tables in *italics*